# Complications of Regional Anesthesia

Second Edition

# Complications of Regional Anesthesia

Second Edition

Brendan T. Finucane, MB, BCh, BAO, FRCA, FRCPC
Professor, Department of Anesthesiology and Pain Medicine, University of Alberta, Edmonton, Alberta, Canada

Editor

Springer

Brendan T. Finucane, MB, BCh, BAO, FRCA, FRCPC
Professor
Department of Anesthesiology and Pain Medicine
University of Alberta
Edmonton, Alberta T6G 2G3
Canada

Library of Congress Control Number: 2006931197

ISBN-10: 0-387-37559-7 eISBN-10: 0-387-68904-3
ISBN-13: 978-0-387-37559-5 eISBN-13: 978-0-387-37559-5

Printed on acid-free paper.



9 8 7 6 5 4 3 2 1

springer.com

*To*
*John Edward Steinhaus*
*Mentor and Friend*

# Foreword

For some readers, the title of this book will immediately raise the question: Why construct a textbook that deals solely with complications? To answer this inquiry, we must refer to the maxim that each of us was taught on the very first day of our medical training: *Primum non nocere*. The discipline of regional anesthesia has seen a major expansion in the last 20 years as a result of better understanding of human anatomy and physiology, and the availability of sophisticated and reliable technology. More and more enthusiastic clinicians apply different regional techniques with great skill and the intention to provide satisfactory anesthesia and analgesia for more than merely the time of surgery. However, such accomplishments may be commended only if associated morbidity is minimized.

Dr. Brendan Finucane is both an accomplished clinician and able teacher who has devoted his career to the advancement of safe regional anesthesia. Who better than him to be charged with the task of assembling a group of fellow illustrious experts to dissect this subject? Regional anesthesia has a very safe record, as is shown in this book. Nevertheless, Dr. Finucane and his colleagues challenge our assurance of these laurels, reminding us that there is no space for complacency because any bad outcome can be disastrous for the patient, family, and medical community. In this book, every aspect of the practice has been scrutinized, with an emphasis on educating the reader to the potential risks associated with frequently performed techniques. I have no doubt that this collection will continue to be the major source not only for the anxious trainee, but also for the experienced and seasoned clinician, who will welcome the wealth of information it provides on every provision of regional anesthesia.

*Francesco Carli, MD, MPhil, FRCA, FRCPC*
Professor of Anesthesia
McGill University
Montreal, Quebec, Canada

# Preface

In 1999, Churchill Livingstone published, what I thought was the first text on *Complications of Regional Anesthesia*. I was subsequently reminded by David C. Moore that Charles C. Thomas published a book with an indentical title in 1955. Dr. Moore generously forgave me for this oversight and provided me with a signed copy of his book which I will always treasure. By the time this edition is complete, eight years will have elapsed since my first edition, and there have been some interesting new developments in regional anesthesia in the intervening period.

What is new about this edition? The contents is expanded by approximately 20% and includes four new chapters along with updating of all the existing ones. The chapter on central neural blockade has been split into two separate chapters, *Complications Associated with Spinal Anesthesia* and *Complications of Epidural Anesthesia* and I have included a new chapter on prevention, *Avoiding Complication of Regional Anesthesia*. The final chapter is entitled *Medicolegal Aspects of Regional Anesthesia* and is quite a provocative treatise on this important topic. Once again I have made an effort to invite individuals from all over the world to be part of the volume, and my success in that goal is in part highlighted by the inclusion of a dedicated chapter, *International Morbidity Studies on Regional Anesthesia*. This section features the perspective of authors from Canada, the United States, Scandinavia, and France.

Reflecting our primary goal as clinicians, the most consistent theme throughout the book is prevention of complications (most of which can be anticipated) and ensuring the highest quality patient care. We, the authors of the chapters, have stressed the importance of proper patient selection, thorough preoperative evaluation, meticulous attention to sterile technique, and careful, deliberate handling of the needle. We emphasized the importance of knowing when to stop. We stressed the importance of patient comfort. The purpose of the exercise of regional anesthesia is defeated if, in the process of performing these techniques, the patient is injured.

In a book of this nature, repetition is difficult to avoid; however, in the process of editing this text I did my best to minimize duplication. Even when there was repetition, the various contributors stressed different aspects of the topics presented. The book is extensively referenced and quite inclusive and up to date. It is my hope that the text will be found extremely useful, and I always welcome the constructive feedback of my colleagues.

*Brendan T. Finucane, MB, BCh, BAO, FRCA, FRCPC*
Edmonton, Alberta, Canada
April 2007

# Acknowledgments

I would like to express my deep gratitude to all of the contributors to this text. I am impressed by the quality of the material presented and their willingness to abide by all of the rules imposed. I would like to thank Beth Campbell for her editorial assistance during earlier phases of this project and Stacy Hague and Barbara Chernow for their assistance during the final phase. I thank Patricia Crossley and Marilyn Blake for assisting me with this effort. I thank my illustrator Steve Wreakes for his timely response to my many requests to reproduce illustrations. Last, but not least, I thank my wife Donna who tolerated my solitude for many months as I toiled to complete this project.

*Brendan T. Finucane, MB, BCh, BAO, FRCA, FRCPC*

# Contents



† Deceased.

# Contributors

*Giuditta Angelini, MD*
Assistant Professor, Department of Anesthesiology, University of Wisconsin Hospital, Madison, WI, USA

*George Arndt, MD*
Professor, Department of Anesthesiology, University of Wisconsin Hospital, Madison, WI, USA

*Yves Auroy, MD*
Professor of Anesthesia, Department of Anesthesia, Hôpital militaire Percy, Clamart, France

*Dan Benhamou, MD*
Professor of Anesthesia, Department of Anesthesia, Hôpital de Bicetre, Le Kremlin-Bicerte, France

*Stephan Blumenthal, MD*
Consultant, Department of Anesthesiology, Orthopedic University Hospital Balgrist, Zurich, Switzerland

*Alain Borgeat, MD*
Professor and Chief of Staff, Department of Anesthesiology, Orthopedic University Hospital Balgrist, Zurich, Switzerland

*Lynn M. Broadman, MD*
Professor Emeritus, West Virginia University, Morgantown, WV, and Clinical Professor of Anesthesiology, Pittsburgh Children's Hospital, Pittsburgh, PA, USA

*David L. Brown, MD*
Edward Rotan Distinguished Professor and Chairman, Department of Anesthesiology and Pain Medicine, M. D. Anderson Cancer Center, Houston, TX, USA

*Andrea Casati, MD*
Associate Professor of Anesthesiology, Department of Anesthesia and Pain Therapy, University of Parma, Parma, Italy

*Dominic A. Cave, MB, BS, FRCPC*
Assistant Clinical Professor, Department of Anesthesiology and Pain Medicine, University of Alberta Hospital, Edmonton, Alberta, Canada

*Vincent W.S. Chan, MD, FRCPC*
Professor, Department of Anesthesia, University of Toronto, Toronto, Ontario, Canada

*Nils Dahlgren, MD, PhD*
Associate Professor, Department of Anesthesia, Landskrona County Hospital, Landskrona, Sweden

*Karen B. Domino, MD, MPh*
Professor, Department of Anesthesiology and Neurological Surgery (adjunct), University of Washington, Seattle, WA, USA

*Guido Fanelli, MD*
Professor of Anesthesiology, Department of Anesthesia and Pain Therapy, University of Parma, Parma, Italy

*F. Michael Ferrante, MD, FABPM*
Director, UCLA Pain and Spine Care and Professor of Clinical Anesthesiology and Medicine, Department of Anesthesiology, David Geffen School of Medicine at University of California–Los Angeles, Santa Monica, CA, USA

*Barry A. Finegan, MB, BCh, FRCPC*
Professor and Chair, Department of Anesthesiology and Pain Medicine, University of Alberta Hospital, Edmonton, Alberta, Canada

*Brendan T. Finucane, MB, BCh, BAO, FRCA, FRCPC*
Professor, Department of Anesthesiology and Pain Medicine, University of Alberta, Edmonton, Alberta, Canada

*Steven J. Fowler, MB, ChB, Dip Obstet, FCARCSI*
Vascular and Neuroanesthesia Fellow, Department of Anesthesia, Auckland City Hospital, University of Auckland, Auckland, New Zealand

*Daniela Ghisi, MD*
Anesthesia Fellow, Department of Anesthesia and Pain Therapy, University of Parma, Parma, Italy

*Admir Hadžić, MD*
Associate Professor of Anesthesia, Department of Anesthesiology, St. Luke's–Roosevelt Hospital Center, Columbia University, New York, NY, USA

*Robert C. (Roy) Hamilton, MB, BCh, FRCPC*
Honorary Clinical Professor, Department of Anesthesiology, University of Calgary, Calgary, Alberta, Canada

*Lloyd Hendrix, MD*
Department of Radiology, Medical College of Wisconsin, Milwaukee, WI, USA

*Nirmala R. Abraham Hidalgo, MD*
Clinical Instructor, Department of Anesthesiology and Assistant Director, UCLA Pain and Spine Care, David Geffen School of Medicine at University of California–Los Angeles, Santa Monica, CA, USA

*Quinn H. Hogan, MD*
Professor, Department of Anesthesiology, Medical College of Wisconsin, Milwaukee, WI, USA

*Ryan A. Holt, MD*
Chief Resident, Department of Anesthesiology, West Virginia University, Morgantown, WV, USA

*Terese T. Horlocker, MD*
Professor of Anesthesiology and Orthopedics, Department of Anesthesiology, Mayo Clinic College of Medicine, Rochester, MN, USA

*Gabriella Iohom, FCARCSI, PhD*
Cork University Hospital and National University of Ireland, Cork, Ireland

*Safwan Jaradeh, MD*
Department of Neurology, Medical College of Wisconsin, Milwaukee, WI, USA

*Andrea Kattula, MB, BS, FANZCA*
Anaesthesia Specialist, Department of Intensive Care and Department of Surgery, The Austin Hospital, Victoria, Australia

*Lorri A. Lee, MD*
Associate Professor, Departments of Anesthesiology and Neurological Surgery (adjunct), University of Washington, Seattle, WA, USA

*John W.R. McIntyre, MD*[†]
Professor Emeritus (deceased), Department of Anesthesiology and Pain Medicine, University of Alberta, Edmonton, Alberta, Canada

*Paul J. O'Connor, MB, FFARCSI*
Consultant Anesthetist, Department of Anesthesia, Letterkenny General Hospital, Letterkenny, County Donegal, Ireland

*Philip W.H. Peng, MBBS, FRCPC*
Assistant Professor, Department of Anesthesia, University of Toronto, Toronto, Ontario, Canada

*Narinder Rawal, MD, PhD*
Professor, Department of Anesthesiology and Intensive Care, University Hospital, Örebro, Sweden

*Per H. Rosenberg, MD, PhD*
Professor of Anesthesiology, Department of Anesthesiology and Intensive Care Medicine, Helsinki University, Helsinki, Finland

*Richard W. Rosenquist, MD*
Professor of Anesthesia, Department of Anesthesia, and Director, Pain Medicine Division, University of Iowa, Iowa City, IA, USA

*David J. Sage, MB, ChB, Dip Obstet, FANZCA*
Clinical Associate, Professor of Anesthesiology, Department of Anesthesia, Auckland City Hospital, University of Auckland, New Zealand

[†] Deceased.

*Albert H. Santora, MD*
Anesthesiologist, Athens, GA, USA

*George Shorten, FFARCSI, FRCA, MD, PhD*
Cork University Hospital and University College Cork, Cork, Ireland

*Kari G. Smedstad, MB, ChB, FRCPC*
Professor Emerita, Department of Anesthesia, McMaster University, Hamilton, Ontario, Canada

*Pekka Tarkkila, MD, PhD*
Associate Professor, Head, Department of Anaesthesia and Intensive Care, Helsinki University Central Hospital, Helsinki, Finland

*Ban C.H. Tsui, MSc, MD, FRCPC*
Assistant Professor, Department of Anesthesiology and Pain Medicine, University of Alberta and Director of Clinical Research, University of Alberta Hospital and Stollery Children's Hospital, Edmonton, Alberta, Canada

*Ciaran Twomey, MB, BCh, BAO (UNI), FCARCSI*
Clinical Fellow, Department of Anesthesiology and Pain Medicine, University of Alberta, University of Alberta Hospital, Edmonton, Alberta, Canada

*William F. Urmey, MD*
Clinical Associate Professor of Anesthesiology, Department of Anesthesiology, Weill Medical College of Cornell University, Hospital for Special Surgery, New York, NY, USA

*Denise J. Wedel, MD*
Professor of Anesthesiology, Department of Anesthesiology, Mayo Clinic College of Medicine, Rochester, MN, USA

# 1 Regional Anesthesia Safety

John W.R. McIntyre[†]

The author of this chapter, Professor John McIntyre (Figure 1-1), is unfortunately no longer with us. He died tragically in a pedestrian accident, very close to the University of Alberta Hospital and to his home, in the spring of 1998.

When I contemplated a second edition of this book, I read his chapter again very carefully and I was just as impressed as I was when I read his first draft. First of all, he is an excellent writer; second, there is great wisdom in his words. He really understood our discipline and even though he did not claim any great expertise in regional anesthesia, he understood the issues better than most people. Even though 8 years or so have gone by since the first edition, Professor McIntyre's contribution is by no means outdated; therefore, I had no hesitation including this chapter in the new edition. Those of us who knew John well miss his humor, enthusiasm and zest for life, and his constant thirst for new information. I took the liberty of making some minor editorial changes to the text with permission from his family. Each time I read his chapter, I learn something new from it.

Professor McIntyre walked the halls of the University of Alberta Hospital for close to 50 years, where he taught 10 generations of residents. He touched the hearts and minds of many people and his influence transcends time.

Respectfully,
Brendan T. Finucane, MB, BCh, BAO, FRCA, FRCPC

Every patient wishes to receive anesthesia care that is safe, in other words, "free from risk, not involving danger or mishap; and guaranteed against failure."[1] The anesthesiologist will present a more realistic view to the patient. The personal view of the hoped-for care will be one in which the clinical outcome is satisfactory and has been achieved without complication (defined as "any additional circumstances making a situation more difficult"[1]) because performance has deviated from the ideal.[2] By this standard, most deviations are trivial or easily corrected by a perfect process, and outcome for the patient and a reasonably stress-free life for the carers are objectives for all anesthesiologists.

The general objective here is to provide information that helps the clinician to minimize complications that may be incurred during the course of regional anesthesia practice. This information is presented under the following headings:

- Complication anticipation
- Equipment
- Behavioral factors and complications

[†] Deceased.

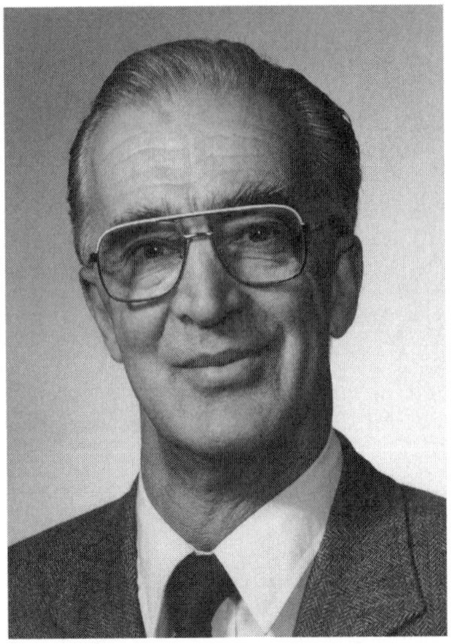

**FIGURE 1-1.** Professor John W.R. McIntyre.

- Complication recognition
- Complications of specific neural blockades
- Complications in the postoperative period
- Complication prevention

## Complication Anticipation: Recognizing Precipitating Factors

### *The Preanesthetic Visit: Patient History*

Some anesthesiologists have a preconceived plan for regional anesthesia before they visit the patient; others gather information before considering what method of anesthesia is appropriate. The following paragraphs about the relationship between regional anesthesia and pathology are intended to aid recognition of potential complications for the patient under consideration and planning of anesthesia to avoid them.

#### The Nervous System

Fundamental issues to be settled during the preoperative visit are how the patient wishes to feel during the procedure and the anesthesiologist's opinion of how well the patient would tolerate the unusual sensations, the posture, and the environment. Whatever decision is made about pharmacologic support, it is absolutely essential that every patient has a clear understanding of reasonable expectations, once a plan has been made, and of the importance of revealing his or her own customary mood-altering medications. This is a convenient occasion to inquire about the patient's and relatives' previous experiences with local, regional, and general anesthesia.

Information should be sought regarding the presence of any degenerative axonal disease involving spinal cord, plexus, or nerve to be blocked and symptoms of thoracic outlet syndrome, spinal cord transection, and lumbar lesions. Strong proponents of regional anesthesia have stated that a wide range of conditions – multiple sclerosis, Guillain-Barré syndrome, residual poliomyelitis, and muscular dystrophy – are unaffected,[3] although difficulty in a patient with Guillain-Barré syndrome has been reported.[4] However, there are reports of permanent neurologic deterioration in patients with unidentified preexisting problems.[5–7] Spinal anesthesia is an effective way of obtunding mass autonomic reflexes in patients with spinal cord transection above T5, but a mass reflex has been described in a patient with an apparently appropriate block.[8] It must be concluded that the uncertainty of outcome when regional anesthesia is used in patients with established neurologic disease demands that the technique be used only when it is clearly advantageous for the patient. It is prudent to seek out symptoms of unrecognized neurologic abnormality when planning which anesthesia technique will be used. Parkinson's disease and epilepsy are not contraindications to regional anesthesia, provided they are habitually well controlled by medications, which should be continued during and after the operative period.

Thus far, the concerns addressed have largely involved the possibility of long-term neuronal damage and uncontrolled muscle activity, but the rapid changes in intracranial pressure during lumbar puncture can be dangerous.[9,10] The lumbar extradural injection of 10 mL of fluid in two patients increased the intracranial pressure from 18.8 to 39.5 mm Hg in the first patient and from 9.3 to 15.6 mm Hg in the second patient.[11] Among patients at risk are those with head injuries, severe eclampsia, and hydrocephalus.

A history of sleep apnea is more a reminder of the need for meticulous monitoring than a contraindication to regional anesthesia. In any case, patients may not recognize their own sleep apnea experiences. They are more likely to know of snoring, daytime hypersomnolence, and restless sleep.

## The Respiratory System

Preoperative pulmonary function tests do not identify definitive values predictive of hypoxia during regional anesthesia, but for practical purposes, if there are spirometric values <50% of predicted, risk is increased.[12] It is certainly so if the values are: FEV < 1.0 L, FVC < 15–20 mL/kg, FEV/FVC < 35%, PEF < 100–200 L/min, and $Pco_2$ > 50 mm Hg. Avoidance of the airway manipulation associated with general anesthesia and preserving coughing ability are advantageous for the patient with asthma or chronic obstructive pulmonary disease. Unfortunately, that can be more than offset by a magnitude of motor blockade that decreases vital capacity, expiratory reserve volume, maximum breathing capacity, and the ability to cough, all of which can result from anesthesia for abdominal surgery. If for some reason the patient is particularly dependent on nasal breathing, as babies are, a block that is complicated by nasal congestion due to Horner's syndrome will cause respiratory difficulty.

Clinical assessment decides the need for acid-base and blood gas measurements. Hypoxia and acidosis enhance the central nervous system and cardiotoxicity of lidocaine.[13–15] In the neonate, these effects are accentuated by poor compensation for metabolic acidosis.

## The Cardiovascular System

Cardiac disease has profound implications for regional anesthesia, as it has for general anesthesia. Among the systems classifying the degree of cardiac risk, Detsky's modification of the Goldman index is useful (Table 1-1).[16]

However, this risk assessment is not patient specific, and there are individual asymptomatic patients with significant coronary artery disease that is unlikely to be detected. Also, chronic and relatively symptom-free chronic valvular dysfunction may lead to sudden and severe circulatory collapse.[17] There are many potential causes of myocardial infarction in patients undergoing extracardiac surgery,[18] as there are for other cardiovascular complications. The role of dipyridamole-thallium scintigraphy and ambulatory (Holter) electrocardiography (ECG) has attracted interest[19,20]; however, physiologic changes that can occur in a patient during the operative period and subsets of patients to whom a specific test applies have yet to be identified with certainty.[17]

When assessing the patient with cardiovascular problems for regional anesthesia and debating the addition, or perhaps sole use, of general anesthesia, the anesthesiologist must make predictions. These are the ability to satisfactorily control preload and afterload, myocardial oxygen supply, and demand and function. If one or more of

Table 1-1. Detsky's Modified Multifactorial Index Arranged According to Point Value

| Variables | Points |
|---|---|
| Class 4 angina* | 20 |
| Suspected critical aortic stenosis | 20 |
| Myocardial infarction within 6 months | 10 |
| Alveolar pulmonary edema within 1 week | 10 |
| Unstable angina within 3 months | 10 |
| Class 3 angina* | 10 |
| Emergency surgery | 10 |
| Myocardial infarction more than 6 months ago | 5 |
| Alveolar pulmonary edema ever | 5 |
| Sinus plus atrial premature beats or rhythm other than sinus on last preoperative electrocardiogram | 5 |
| More than five ventricular premature beats at any time before surgery | 5 |
| Poor general medical status† | 5 |
| Age over 70 years | 5 |

*Sources:* Detsky et al.[16] Copyright 1986, American Medical Association. All rights reserved; Detsky et al.[17] Copyright 1986, Blackwell Publishing. All rights reserved.
*Canadian Cardiovascular Society classification for angina.
†Oxygen tension ($PO_2$) <60 mm Hg; carbon dioxide tension ($Pco_2$) >50 mm Hg; serum potassium <3.0 mEq/L; serum bicarbonate <20 mEq/L; serum urea nitrogen >50 mg/dL; serum creatinine >3 mg/dL; aspartate aminotransferase abnormality; signs of chronic liver disease; and/or patients bedridden from noncardiac causes.

these deviate from optimal limits, will the rate of change that may occur exceed the rate at which the therapeutic management can be developed?

The cardiac dysrhythmias of particular interest are the array of clinical disorders of sinus function (sick sinus syndrome). These are often associated with reduced automaticity of lower pacemakers and conduction disturbances. Local anesthetic drugs that diminish sinoatrial node activity, increase the cardiac refractory period, prolong the intracardiac conduction time, and lengthen the QRS complex, will, in sufficient quantity, aggravate sinus node dysfunction.

It is important to realize that the pharmacokinetics of drugs are influenced by certain cardiac defects. Patients with intracardiac right-to-left shunts are denied protection by the lungs, which normally sequester up to 80% of the intravenous drug. If this is reduced, the likelihood of central nervous system toxicity is increased.[21,22]

## The Gastrointestinal Tract

It is essential that the anesthesiologist obtain reliable information about the food and drink the patient has or will have taken. An elective patient will have received the customary institutional management, which may include one or more of the following: anticholinergic, histamine-receptor blocker (H2), antacid, and benzamide derivative. Based on knowledge up to 1990, the following proposals have been made. First, solid food should *not* be taken on the day of surgery. Second, unrestricted clear fluids should be permitted until 3 hours before scheduled surgery.[23,24]

In a study of the effect of epidural anesthesia on gastric emptying, measured by the absorption of acetaminophen from the upper small intestine, it appeared that block of sympathetic innervation of the stomach (T6–10) did not affect gastric emptying[25]; however, epidural injection of morphine at the T4 level delayed emptying. Nevertheless, with the onset of high spinal anesthesia, antiperistaltic movements and gastric regurgitation may occur and the ability to cough is reduced during a high blockade.

Thus, the value of peripheral neural blockade for a patient with a potentially full stomach cannot be overestimated: subarachnoid and epidural anesthesia do not protect a patient from aspiration. Similarly, paralysis of a recurrent laryngeal nerve, a complication of blockades in the neck region, facilitates aspiration of gastric contents.

In a wide variety of abnormal circumstances, including trauma and near-term pregnancy, it is impossible to predict on the basis of the passage of time what the stomach contains. If the stomach is not empty, there are other vital considerations. In the presence of the blockade, the patient must be able to protect himself from aspiration; alternatively, in the presence of a failed blockade, it must be possible to administer a general anesthetic safely or to abandon the surgical procedure or delivery. Obstetric procedures usually brook no delay, and so it is mandatory that at some time well before the anticipated delivery date, the airway problems of pregnant patients be identified and plans made to cope with any eventuality.

## The Hematologic System

### *Clotting Mechanisms*

A regional anesthesia technique in which a hemorrhage cannot be detected readily and controlled by direct pressure is contraindicated in patients with a coagulation disorder, which might be attributed to diseases such as thrombocytopenia, hemophilia, and leukemia, or to drugs. Drugs having primary anticoagulant effects include unfractionated heparin, low-molecular-weight heparin, coumadin, and aspirin. Other drugs that to some degree influence coagulation are nonsteroidal antiinflammatory medications, urokinase, phenprocoumon, dextran 70, and ticlopidine.

Laboratory measurements determine the presence of a significant coagulation defect. Anticoagulation during heparin therapy is most often monitored by the activated clotting time. This method is not specific for a particular part of the coagulation cascade, and for diagnostic purposes a variety of other tests are used: prothrombin (plasma thromboplastin) time, activated partial thromboplastin time, platelet count, and plasma fibrinogen concentration. Even in combination, however, these fail to provide a complete description of the status of the coagulation system. It is possible that viscoelastic methods are a convenient technique to monitor perioperative bleeding disorders.[26]

Once a detailed history of drug use and laboratory measurements is available, a decision regarding the potential complications of central neural blockade, with or without catheter insertion, may be necessary, as may the influence of an anticoagulated state on postoperative developments.

Clinical experiences with these dilemmas have been comprehensively reviewed,[27,28] the conclusion being that performing epidural or spinal anesthesia in patients treated with drugs that may jeopardize the normal responses of the clotting system to blood vessel damage is a concern. It is clear that major nerve-blocking techniques can be used in some patients who have received or will be receiving anticoagulant drugs. This success is not only dependent on an appreciation of the properties of different anticoagulant managements and a skilled regional anesthesia technique, but also very careful postblockade monitoring. Thus, the advantages of the regional block envisaged must be carefully compared with other anesthesia techniques for the patient and the overall patient care available.

## "Histaminoid" Reactions

*Histaminoid* refers to a reaction whose precise identity – histamine, prostaglandin, leukotremia, or kinin – is unknown. Few patients would recognize that term, and it is wiser to inquire of "allergy or sensitivity experiences." This is particularly valuable information if the patient describes a situation that the anesthesiologist has contemplated repeating.[29] The patient's story should not be discounted by attributing the reported events to epinephrine or a misplaced injection.

The dose or rate of administration does not affect the severity of a histaminoid reaction. Additionally, many studies have shown that reactions occur more often in patients with a history of atopy[30] but that a history of allergy is not predictive of severe clinical anaphylaxis.[31] The patient's history, or lack of it, is important and may guide the anesthesiologist away from certain drugs; however, an unexpected reaction will challenge some anesthesiologists, somewhere, sometime, and that complication will demand immediate recognition and treatment.

### Pseudocholinesterase Dysfunction

If a patient's red cell cholinesterase is deficient or abnormal, drugs metabolized by that enzyme, such as 2-chloroprocaine, will be broken down more slowly, lowering the toxicity threshold.[32,33]

### Methemoglobinemia

Drugs predisposing to methemoglobinemia are aniline dyes, nitrites, nitrates, sulfonamides, and antimalarial medications. It may also be associated with hemoglobinopathies and glucose-6-phosphate dehydrogenase deficiencies. The local anesthetics benzocaine, lidocaine, and prilocaine can contribute to methemoglobinemia.

### Muscle Disease

Inquiries about muscular dystrophy, myasthenia gravis, and malignant hyperthermia are part of the preanesthetic evaluation, regardless of the contemplated anesthetic technique (Chapter 20). These details are significant for regional anesthesia, too, because malignant hyperthermia can still occur. Any drug that releases calcium from the sarcoplasmic reticulum, such as lidocaine, should perhaps be avoided. Although it has been stated that neither amide nor ester-linked local anesthetics are contraindicated in such cases,[34] there seems to be some uncertainty.[35]

If the patient has a muscular dystrophy it is important to know because of associated problems that may be present, such as ECG abnormalities, but regional anesthesia is not contraindicated and may indeed be the technique of choice.

### Diabetes

Diabetic patients usually announce their disease, but some leave the anesthesiologist to find out (Chapter 18). It is important that the anesthesiologist does, because although neural blockade may be the technique of choice in some respects, the peripheral neuropathy and autonomic dysfunction associated with the disease have implications, particularly if they are in the area to be blocked. The preanesthetic symptoms and signs should be carefully documented.

Notably, a central conduction block limits the normal physiologic response to hypoglycemia and a diabetic patient can be unduly sensitive to the normal insulin regimen. This may complicate postoperative care.[36,37]

### Miscellaneous Medications

Neural blockade complications clearly caused by drug interactions are rare, but possibilities can be taken into account during anesthesia planning and in diagnosing any complications detected later.

#### *Aspirin*

Aspirin therapy, because of its antiplatelet activity, may increase the risk of hematoma, which, associated with central blockade, is potentially tragic. The effect of the drug on platelets is irreversible and lasts 7–10 days; thus, some assessment of platelet function should be made in aspirin-treated patients.[38] Presently, measurement of the bleeding time is the only practical test of in vivo platelet function. It may return to normal 72 hours after discontinuation of the drug, but in vitro platelet aggregation tests require much longer. If the bleeding time is 10 minutes or more, the clinician must weigh the relative disadvantages for that patient of other forms of anesthesia and analgesia.

#### *Quinidine and Disopyramide*

Laboratory studies showed that lidocaine metabolites and the metabolites of several antiarrhythmic agents had little effect on lidocaine protein binding. However, bupivacaine, quinidine, and disopyramide caused a significant increase in the lidocaine free fraction. These effects could cause unexpected drug-related complications.[39]

#### *Benzodiazepines*

Diazepam enhances the cardiovascular toxicity associated with bupivacaine and verapamil.[40] Benzodiazepines mask the early signs of systemic toxicity, so that the first evidence of problems may be cardiorespiratory depression.

#### *Verapamil*

Verapamil increases the toxicity of lidocaine and bupivacaine in mice,[41] and cardiovascular collapse in patients has been reported.[42]

#### *Nifedipine*

Nifedipine increases the toxicity of bupivacaine in dogs.[43]

### *The Preanesthetic Visit: Physical Examination*

The routine preoperative examination for anesthesia is described in many textbooks. The following paragraphs address matters that, although interesting at any time, are particularly important for the anesthesiologist contemplating performing a neural blockade. Positive answers to the following questions are not necessarily contraindications to regional anesthesia; indeed, they may support its selection, but they do indicate matters that must be given particular consideration.

Positioning for the Block

- Is the patient so large or heavy that a dangerous strain may be placed on tables, stools, and assistants unless special precautions are taken?

Blood Pressure

- Is the patient hypertensive or hypotensive?

Oxygenation

- Is the patient hypoxic?

Blood Volume

- Is the patient hypovolemic?

Infection

- Is there dystrophic skin or infection at the site of needle entry or infection in the needle track?
- Is there systemic infection in the body?

Previous Surgery

- Are there scars anywhere indicating previous trauma or surgery that the patient has not mentioned?

Abdominal Masses

- Is an abdominal mass present that could impair venous return or respiration?
- Is there a uterus gravid beyond the first trimester that could impair venous return and influence the spread of subarachnoid injections?

Venous Access

- Will venous access for medications or fluids be easily obtained?

The Upper Airway

- In an emergency situation, can the anesthesiologist easily take control of the patient's airway, ventilate the patient, and prevent aspiration?

Technical Difficulty Performing the Proposed Block

- Will arthritis, amputation, or obesity hinder positioning the patient?
- Does obesity obscure bony landmarks?
- Is arthritis likely to hinder neural access?
- Are spinal defects, abnormalities of vertebral fusions, or foreign bodies present to hinder neural access?
- Can the arm be moved into a suitable position?
- Is there a hindrance to positioning a tourniquet?

Lymph Glands

- Are there axillary or femoral lymph glands in the needle path for the proposed block?

Evaluating the Hemodynamic Status of the Limb

- Will a cast or other hindrance prevent monitoring of peripheral blood flow in a limb?

### *Conclusion*

Surprises for an anesthesiologist in the block room are usually stressful, potentially hazardous for the patient, and may delay the operating room schedule. It is cautionary to realize that, in complex processes, be they medical care or industry, dangerous situations result from a sequence of events. Failure to obtain a certain item of information at the preanesthetic visit can be compounded by related events in the surgical or dental suite and the recovery area. The preoperative visit is the opportunity to plan the patient's anesthetic, be it a technique of regional anesthesia, general anesthesia, or a combination. A structured interview and examination is one facet of safe regional anesthesia practice.

## Equipment

The objective for any attempted neural blockade is to produce the anesthesia required, and thus a major complication is block failure. Neural blockade may fail for pharmacologic or pharmacokinetic reasons, because the anesthesiologist lacks mental imagery of the anatomy, manual dexterity, or tactile sensitivity. Well-designed equipment does not make the user skilled, but it can diminish the complication of "failed spinal" and other complications associated with needle placement. The following is a collation of published data criteria believed to influence successful identification of the location for the anesthetic and of the complications associated with these attempts.

## *Spinal Needles*

### Clinical Reports

The size of needles ranging from 18 to 25 gauge do not affect the success rate for subarachnoid tap,[44,45] and Whitacre 25 and 27 gauge, Quincke 25 gauge, and Sprotte have been used satisfactorily.[46–49] Thinner needles (29 and 30 gauge) have a greater tendency to deviate during their passage through ligamentous tissues, and an introducer through which those needles can be passed is essential.[50–52]

Cerebrospinal fluid (CSF) spontaneous flow through a 29-gauge needle appears extremely slowly, if at all, even if the hub is clear plastic instead of metal. Similarly, injection of fluid can be accomplished only slowly, and drug distribution may be affected.[51]

Spinal anesthesia in children can safely be done with 22- or 25-gauge spinal needles or the hollow stylet from a 24-gauge Angiocath.

Headache is primarily a complication of spinal tap in adults. An extensive and critical analysis of clinical reports[53,54] concluded that the smallest-gauge needle with a noncutting tip reduces its likelihood. Thus, choice of needle gauge is a compromise because using a very fine needle is more difficult. It has been suggested that when avoiding headache is paramount, Quincke or Whitacre 27 gauge are the needles of choice.[55] The waiting times for appearance of CSF with the patient in a lateral position using these needles were $10.8 \pm 6.9$ and $10.7 \pm 6.8$ seconds, respectively.

### Laboratory Reports

Laboratory reports address the technical problems about which clinicians speculate and some complications to avoid. The conclusions are summarized next.

#### *Changing the Needle Direction During Insertion*

Deliberate change of direction of a needle is customarily done by almost complete withdrawal and subsequent reentry, and inadvertent deviation during advancement is misleading. A laboratory model[56] demonstrated the occurrence of needle deviation and the influence of needle point design and gauge. It was least with pencil-point spinal needles and greatest with bevelled spinal needles. The needle deviation with bevelled needles was consistent in direction as well as degree, in contrast to pencil-point tip configurations. Thus, rotating a bevelled needle during insertion and redirectioning may hinder future identification of the epidural or subarachnoid space.

#### *Resistance to Penetration of the Dura Mater*

The human dura mater is relatively resistant to penetration by a long, bevelled 21-gauge ($80 \times 0.8$ mm) Quincke-Babcock needle.[57] After entering the epidural space (anatomically believed to vary from 1 to 7 mm in depth), depending on the site of insertion, the needle advanced 7–13 mm within it. This tenting of the dura mater is believed a potential hazard in the thoracic and cervical region because the spinal cord could be impacted.

#### *Detection Time for CSF after Dural Puncture*

Features that determine the effective use of spinal needles include rapid detectability of CSF, and low resistance to injectate. Experiments with a wide variety of needles[58] revealed that all Becton-Dickinson needles had a zero detection time. The Quincke "Spinocan" 26 gauge and Portex pencil-point had the greatest delay, which at an artificial CSF pressure of 20–50 cm $H_2O$ was approximately 8 seconds. The calculated relative resistance to flow through the needles varied from 0.21 (Becton-Dickinson Whitacre 22 gauge) to 2.91 (Quincke, Spinocan 26 gauge).

#### *Rate of CSF Leak Through a Dural Puncture*

The rate of CSF loss through a dural puncture site can be measured in an in vitro model, and experiments demonstrated that, although more force was required to pierce the dura, CSF leakage from pencil-point needles was significantly less than that from Quincke needles of the same external diameter.[59] The authors concluded that the Whitacre 27-gauge needle lacks a clear advantage over the 25-gauge needle, which may be easier to use.

#### *Needle Orifice Shape and Unintended Extra Dural Injection*

A needle whose distal orifice is partially in and partially outside the subarachnoid space may deliver CSF from the hub, but only part of the injectate will be delivered subarachnoidally. The 22-gauge Whitacre needle is preferable to long-orifice needles such as 22-gauge Sprotte, Quincke, and Diamond point.[54,60]

### *Epidural Needles*

A suitable needle has the following characteristics: 1) easy penetration of ligaments, 2) minimally traumatic penetration, 3) minimal difficulty locating the epidural space, and 4) a lumen that facilitates epidural catheter placement. There are three needles that largely incorporate these features.

#### Tuohy Needle

The distal end is curved 20 degrees to direct a catheter into the epidural space. It must be introduced into the epidural space at least to the depth of the orifice. After a catheter has been inserted, it cannot be withdrawn without a serious risk of transection.

#### Crawford Needle

This needle lacks a curved end and so must approach the epidural space obliquely if a catheter is to be inserted. It does not have to penetrate as deeply as the Tuohy needle into the space.

#### Whitacre Needles

Whitacre epidural needles have a blunt tip to reduce the likelihood of dural puncture. The eye of the needle is located laterally, so the distal end must be inserted well into the epidural space.

Needle sizes appropriate to the ages of children are as follows[61]: until 6 to 7 years, 20 gauge; from 7 to 10 years, 19 gauge; over 10 years, 19 or 18 gauge. A 16- or 18-gauge needle is customarily used in adults.

### *Combined Spinal and Epidural Techniques*

The development of combined spinal and epidural (CSE) techniques since their inception in 1937 has been recently reviewed.[62] There are various techniques, and conventional epidural, long spinal needles, catheters, and special devices can be used. The double-segment technique involves the insertion of an epidural needle and a spinal needle one or two segments below. The single-space technique (SST) requires an epidural needle insertion followed by a spinal needle through its lumen once the epidural anesthesia solution has been injected. There are technical complications associated with the combined use of these devices as well as the individual ones, and sets specifically designed for SST have been designed.

### Double-Lumen Needles

In this technique, a Tuohy needle has a parallel tube as a guide for a thinner spinal needle. There are two types – a bent parallel tube and a straight parallel tube. The bent parallel tube consists of a curved 20- to 22-gauge spinal needle of the same length as the Tuohy needle. The straight tube is fixed on the side of a Tuohy needle; the point of the guide is situated 1 cm behind the eye of the Tuohy needle. Spinal needles of normal length can be used. The double-lumen concept allows insertion of the epidural catheter before positioning of the spinal needle.

Another device[50] is a conventional Tuohy needle to which has been added an additional aperture at the end of the longitudinal axis. It is through this that a spinal needle on its way to the subarachnoid space will exit. Favorable clinical reports of CSE techniques have been supplemented by laboratory studies of flow characteristics of long spinal needles and the risk of catheter migration from the epidural space.

#### *Flow Characteristics of Long Spinal Needles*

The 120-mm, 26-gauge Braun Spinocan needle was compared in vitro with the 120-mm, 27-gauge Becton-Dickinson spinal needle. A pressure of 10 cm $H_2O$ caused fluid to drop from the needle after $330 \pm 14.8$ and $129 \pm 20.7$ seconds, respectively. Clinical study findings were 33.5 and 10.85 seconds, respectively. The internal diameter of the 26-gauge needle is 0.23 mm and of the 27-gauge needle, 0.25 mm. The gauge value indicates the outer size, not the lumen.[63]

#### *Catheter Migration*

An epiduroscopic study of cadavers demonstrated that the risk of epidural catheter migration through a dural puncture hole was very small. It was much less likely if the hole had been made by a 25-gauge spinal needle than with a Tuohy needle.[64]

#### *Complications Associated with Spinal and Epidural Catheters*

1. *Insufficient length* to reach from the exit site to the shoulder.
2. *Venous penetration.* The lumen must be sufficient for aspiration. A stylet in the catheter must not project out of the tip.
3. *Dural penetration.* The lumen must be sufficient for aspiration. A stylet in the catheter must not project out of the tip. A closed round-ended catheter with side openings makes penetration less likely.
4. *Kinking.* This is less likely with currently manufactured catheters and with the redesigned version of the Racz catheter.[65]
5. *Knotting.* Interval marking of the catheter is a useful guide to the catheter length within the subarachnoid or epidural space and discourages coiling.
6. *Difficult withdrawal.* A clinical study of forces necessary for lumbar extradural catheter removal (range $1.57 \pm 0.96$ to $3.78 \pm 2.8$ N) and literature review indicated that the original approach to the space was inconsequential. However, the withdrawal force required was greater with the patient sitting than in the lateral position. Thus, the flexed lateral position was recommended for removal.[66,67] This opinion is controversial. It has been recommended that the patient be in the same position used for insertion when it is removed.[68]

#### *Devices for Peripheral Nerve Blockade*

Complications of nerve blockade include intravascular injection, intraneural injection, and failure to locate the nerve to be blocked. Breakage at a weak junction between the hub and stem is unlikely with modern needles, although in some circumstances a security bead can be a useful precaution.

Intravascular needle placement may be impossible to detect by aspiration if the needle lumen is very fine, and a translucent hub is of little help. This has implications for resuscitation arrangements established for minor surgical or dental procedures performed in offices and clinics. Intraneural injection is unlikely, but needles with side-ports provide some protection from that event.

Paresthesias are unusual and unwelcome during the conduct of a central neural blockade, but peripheral nerves are often deliberately located by eliciting paresthesias with the needle, although this depends on the patient and is not absolutely reliable. The causal relationship between paresthesia elicited in this manner and neural damage is controversial, and no statistically significant clinical data indicate that such stimulation produces neuropathy.[69] The animal experiments upon which claims for potential neuropathy are based did not represent clinical practice, although a clinician can never be absolutely certain that the tip of the needle is not actually within a nerve. Indeed, the sterile flexible infusion line between syringe and needle is there to help immobilize the needle when it is in position.

Concerns about mechanically produced paresthesia popularized the introduction of a nerve stimulator to locate the nerve. The needle should ideally be insulated by Teflon coating in order to enhance opportunities to place the needle tip close to the nerve. Paresthesias may occur when the instrument is in use, but its purpose is to elicit visible contraction in a muscle served by the nerve to be blocked.

Ideally, the stimulator should have the following characteristics[70]:

1. Constant current output
2. Clear meter reading to 0.1 mA
3. Variable output
4. Linear output
5. Clearly marked polarity
6. Short pulse width
7. Pulse of 1 Hz
8. Battery indicator
9. High-quality alligator clips
10. High- and low-output settings

Instruments designed for testing neuromuscular transmission do not usually indicate voltage or current at the site of stimulation and so are disadvantageous because they control only voltage, whereas it is current that causes a nerve to depolarize.[71] It is possible to elicit a muscle response when the needle is some distance from the nerve unless the stimulus current is less than 0.5 mA.[72] The concept is attractive and popular with some practitioners, but definitive evidence of its superiority over other methods is lacking and the occurrence of serious complications has been suggested.[69]

Another technique to safely identify the site for injection is visualizing the anatomy by ultrasonography. Not only can this increase the likelihood of successful neural blockade, but it reduces the incidence of pneumothorax associated with the supraclavicular approach to brachial plexus blockade[73] (Chapter 8).

### *Resuscitation Supplies*

Cardiovascular failure, with or without respiratory failure, is a rare complication of regional blockade whether for head, trunk, or limbs. If competent treatment is not *immediately* available, however, the result will be permanent cerebral damage or death.

A standard text[71] states:

> Intravenous access and fluids, a tipping trolley, an oxygen supply, and resuscitation drugs and equipment must be available. The equipment must include an anesthesia machine as

a source of oxygen, a means of lung ventilation, a laryngoscope, oropharyngeal airways, cuffed endotracheal tubes, a stilette, and continuous suction. Thiopentone, diazepam, suxamethonium, ephedrine, and atropine should be immediately available.

Those are the basic requirements of the caregivers trained to provide advanced cardiopulmonary resuscitation and will be present when neural blockade is attempted in the hospital or a large clinic. They are just as necessary in the office where a minor procedure is to be done under neural blockade. Not only must equipment be there, but the persons present should be trained to use it. In light of the magnitude of the potential tragedy, they should be able to communicate with extramural help while continuing their efforts at cardiopulmonary resuscitation.

## Behavioral Factors and Complications

The behavioral factors that lead to complications are of several categories. A lapse of safe habit is the routine failure to check effectively the identity and concentration of fluid to be injected. Another is the lack of a routine method of distinguishing between syringes. An unsafe habit could be the use of an air-filled syringe to identify the epidural space of a child. Other potential causes have been reviewed[74–76] and in general are referred to as *vigilance decrement, vigilance* being a state of maximal and psychological readiness to react to a situation. These can be the cause of temporarily breaking a safe habit or creating an unsafe habit or of missing evidence of a complication. It is an important feature of complication avoidance that anesthesiologists be aware of these behavioral pitfalls and discipline themselves accordingly while establishing safe work scheduling.

### *Effects of Sleep Deprivation*

Sleep deprivation can dramatically impair performance of monitoring tasks, whether the signals are presented in an auditory or visual mode – and particularly if the task is not cognitively exciting. A cumulative sleep debt incurred over days has a detrimental effect; however, there are wide individual differences in responses to acute or chronic sleep loss. Ideally, anesthesiologists should objectively establish their own limitations because an anesthesiologist who has been working most of the night may feel remarkably awake, perhaps euphoric, in the morning, although studies have documented reduced performance, and in the afternoons the situation will have further deteriorated. Napping is not necessarily helpful, particularly if it occurs during a period of REM sleep.

A recommendation[75] supported by evidence from a variety of subjects, including anesthesiologists, for the anesthesiologist who has been working most of the night and is scheduled for a full day's work is this: "Do not work. If work is mandatory do not nap for only 2 hours. If 4 hours is possible, accept it but be prepared for some remaining performance decrement."

### *The Effects of Fatigue*

Hours of continuous cognitively challenging work result in fatigue. The effects of fatigue are accentuated by sleep deprivation and influenced by the position of the activity in the individual's circadian rhythm. Published data support the contention that a fatigued anesthesiologist may be careless and less likely to detect perioperative complications or to respond optimally to evolving clinical situations.[75]

### *The Hazard of Boredom*

A task that is repetitious, uneventful, uninteresting, and undemanding is boring. In such a case, the anesthesiologist has too little work. It is a problem shared by many other real life responsible tasks and results in inappropriate automatic behavior, vigilance decrement, inappropriate interest, and a general feeling of fatigue. Thus, the low-workload situation, similar to the high-workload state, can cause performance decrement, and thus complications, because evidence of their development is overlooked. Anesthesiologists periodically change their location in the operating room[77] or converse with operating room companions, probably in an unconscious effort to maintain vigilance by increasing sensory input. An unsedated patient under regional anesthesia is sometimes a highly entertaining and educational source of information and social commentary, thus keeping the carer close by. During boring cases, the addition of occupations completely unrelated to patient care demand a time-sharing technique that must be learned, and even then their impact on an individual's vigilance for clinically important matters is variable and very difficult to predict. Thus, reading or listening to personal music is controversial behavior in the operating room.

### *The Influences of Physical and Mental Factors*

An anesthesiologist is sometimes anxious in the operating room, but when this is compounded by personal anxieties, planning, decision making, and monitoring may be adversely affected. Substance abuse reduces vigilance and psychomotor performance and there is strong evidence that hangovers from alcohol and marijuana have similar effects. Recent work suggests that pilots should wait at least 14 hours after drinking alcohol before flying, although it is constituent aromatic substances in some beverages that are more likely to cause a problem.

### *Work Environment*

The physical environment for conducting hospital surgery under regional anesthesia is similar to that for general anesthesia in that monitor displays should be discernible from the variety of positions assumed by the anesthesiologist during the course of the procedure.[77]

Recently, verbal communications were found to be responsible for 37% of events that could have resulted in patient deterioration or death in an intensive care unit,[78] supporting other anecdotal reports of communication errors. This confirms the need for an established routine to check the identity and concentration of fluids to be injected in every hospital or clinic location where neural blockades are done or existing blockades reinforced.

Small clinics and professional offices may differ from the hospital environment in one significant respect. In an acute emergency, persons performing cardiopulmonary resuscitation may be unable to communicate with outside help without discontinuing their lifesaving activity, and in some countries or states such behavior is illegal. Protection of patients demands an arrangement that avoids such a situation by ensuring a communication system that can be instantly and conveniently activated.

The "mental environment" in which neural blockade and surgery are performed is as important as the physical environment. It is salutary that anesthesiologists, who are sometimes confronted with injured patients who have suffered because the response to industrial production pressures was to ignore certain defenses against injury, can find themselves faced with the same decision as the industrial worker – and even under similar production pressures. These pressures may be temptations for personal gain or generated by surgeons, dentists, or institutional managers. A recent study concluded that pressure from internal and external sources is a reality for many anesthesiologists and is perceived, in some cases, to have resulted in unsafe actions being performed.[79] The implication is that any effort to increase anesthesia and surgical productivity should be based on methods other than reducing safe practices. Any attempt to achieve it by introducing new technology should be accompanied by a careful analysis and, if necessary, education of the person using it.[80]

## Complication Recognition During Neural Blockade and Surgery

### *Sharing Human and Instrumental Monitoring*

Regional anesthesia conducted expertly on the basis of a careful medical history and examination of the patient is safe, but complications can occur.[81–93] Signs and symptoms, listed by body systems, are matched with the human and instrumental monitoring techniques used for their detection in Table 1-2.

TABLE 1-2. Complication Recognition

| Symptoms and signs to be detected | Detection methods |
|---|---|
| **Nervous System events**<br>• Peroneal numbness and tingling<br>• Dizziness, tinnitus<br>• Hearing impairment<br>• Headache<br>• Reduced vision<br>• Diplopia<br>• Taste in mouth<br>• Dysphagia<br>• Coughing and sneezing<br>• Nausea<br>• Throat numbness<br>• Dysphasia<br>• Pain and paresthesia<br>• Faintness<br>• Restlessness | Patient: Assuming there is no language barrier, the patient may report any of these spontaneously but should be initially instructed to report any unusual sensation.<br>Anesthesiologist: Communication with the patient and observation.<br>Instrument: Instruments do not identify these sensations for the anesthesiologist. |
| Postural pressure or tension on peripheral nerves | Patient: An unreliable source of information<br>Anesthesiologist: Power of observation<br>Instrument: Limited in application. A pulse oximeter at a limb periphery may indirectly indicate a threat to nerve or plexus. |
| Horner's syndrome | Patient: Reports unusual feeling<br>Anesthesiologist: Observation<br>Instrument: – |
| Phrenic nerve paralysis | Patient: Reports unusual feelings<br>Anesthesiologist: Observation<br>Instrument: $Spo_2$ value may diminish |
| Recurrent laryngeal nerve block | Patient: Reports unusual feelings<br>Anesthesiologist: Observation<br>Instrument: – |
| Presence or absence of CSF in hub of needle or dripping from it | Patient: –<br>Anesthesiologist: Observation. After dural puncture, the delay before the first drop of CSF appeared was approximately 11 seconds for a 27-gauge Becton-Dickinson spinal needle, and 33 seconds for a 26-gauge Braun needle.[63]<br>There is considerable variation among commercially available spinal needles.[58] Such details regarding needles used for blocks other than central neural blockade are unavailable.<br>Instrument: – |
| Loss of resistance to injection (epidural space detection) | Patient: –<br>Anesthesiologist: Observation<br>Instrument: Pressure variations in the injection system can be digitized and displayed to show an exponential pressure decline.[94] |

*(Continued)*

Table 1-2. *Continued*

| Symptoms and signs to be detected | Detection methods |
|---|---|
| Blood reaching the hub of a needle and not pulsating | Patient: – <br>Anesthesiologist: Observation. Note, blood will take substantially longer than CSF to pass through a spinal, or other, narrow bore needle. <br>There will be interpatient variability. Thus, a "bloody tap" is evidence that the needle is in a vein or hematoma, but absence of blood is not necessarily definitive evidence that drug will not be injected intravascularly. <br>Instrument: – |
| Cerebral function | Patient: Reports unusual sensation <br>Anesthesiologist: Conversation or intermittent questioning of patient <br>Instrument: – |
| Evidence of planned neural blockade | Patient: Report of unusual sensations <br>Anesthesiologist: Questioning and examining the patient <br>Instrument: Thermography and plethysmography |
| Evidence of unexpected neural blockade | Patient: Report of unusual sensations and/or motor function <br>Anesthesiologist: Observation of blockade area and the patient <br>Instruments: Sphygmomanometer, ECG, pulse meter |
| Vagal stimulation | Patient: Faintness or loss of consciousness <br>Anesthesiologist: Observations <br>Instruments: ECG, pulse oximeter, pulse meter, sphygmomanometer |
| **Respiratory system events** <br>• Respiratory rate changes <br>• Tidal volume change <br>• Apnea <br>• Stertor <br>• Respiratory obstruction <br>• Dyspnea <br>• Bronchospasm | Patient: Dyspnea may be reported but in general patients seem unaware of the significance of respiratory changes, and, if they have been sedated, unaware of them. <br>Anesthesiologist: Observations are valuable but are unlikely to assess function accurately or continuously. <br>Instruments: Pulse oximetry is a late indicator of respiratory dysfunction, relative to end-tidal capnography. <br>The stethoscope in the operating room or PARR is now more of a diagnostic tool to identify such things as atelectasis and pneumothorax than a monitor of respiration but a paratracheal audible respiratory monitor has been described.[95] |
| Erroneous gas delivery to patient | Patient: Comments may be made about odor. <br>Anesthesiologist: Observation of patients behavior. <br>Instrument: An $FIO_2$ monitor with functioning alarms is quicker and more reliable than patient or anesthesiologist. |
| **Cardiovascular system events** | |
| Hypotension <br>Hypertension | Patient: – <br>Anesthesiologist: Sensing error is large <br>Instrument: Automated direct or indirect measurement |

TABLE 1-2. *Continued*

| Symptoms and signs to be detected | Detection methods |
|---|---|
| Bradycardia<br>Tachycardia | Patient: –<br>Anesthesiologist: Accurate observation is possible but may be intermittent.<br>Instruments: A variety are available to provide this information continuously. |
| Cardiac arrhythmia | Patient: The patient may state their heart is beating irregularly.<br>Anesthesiologist: Clinical observation<br>Instrument: Pulse oximeter and precordial stethoscope will indicate irregularity. The ECG provides continuous information upon which a diagnosis can be based. |
| Asystole | Patient: –<br>Anesthesiologist: Suspicion is aroused if at that moment the finger is on a pulse or a precordial stethoscope is in use.<br>Instrument: An ECG is a continuous and definitive indicator.<br>A pulse oximeter can raise a delayed but serious suspicion. |
| Increased or decreased central venous pressure | Patient: Symptoms relative to cardiopulmonary function may be announced.<br>Anesthesiologist: Clinical events indicate a possibility.<br>Instrument: Central venous pressure measurement |
| Cyanosis | Patient: –<br>Anesthesiologist: Visual acuity and environmental circumstances create an undesirable error of assessment.<br>Instruments: Pulse oximetry and blood gas measurements. |
| **Muscle events** | |
| These range from twitching of facial muscles to convulsive movements of major muscle masses | Patient: –<br>Anesthesiologist: Observations<br>Instrument: – |
| **Body temperature events** | |
| Hypothermia | Patient: Patients are aware of cold sometimes but are often poor judges of their real body temperature. There is strong evidence that not only do spinal and epidural anesthesia impair central and peripheral regulatory controls[96–98] but are not perceived by the patient.[99]<br>Anesthesiologist: The observations of the patient may be an unreliable assessment of temperature because shivering is not occurring and, depending on the area felt, the skin may feel warm.<br>Instrument: Thermometry |

The role of the patient is included, as is the anesthesiologist's direct or monitor-assisted sensing. If heavy sedation or a supplementary general anesthetic is used, the clinical situation changes radically. The cost-benefit picture of a specific regional anesthesia plan must be estimated in light of these factors. This is followed by an account of the documented complications for different neural blockades. It would be possible to create monitoring algorithms for individual blocks, but in this author's opinion, such focusing of patient care would be detrimental to the patient's safety because unrelated events might be ignored, threatening though they might be. It is important to realize that, although monitoring devices are invaluable, an astute anesthesiologist will detect signs that are precursors to the resulting events detected by the device. This anticipatory information enables therapy to begin sooner.

## Monitoring Devices

Contemporary recommendations for monitoring of patients under regional anesthesia include the cardiovascular and respiratory systems and body temperature. Whatever the combination of human and instrumental monitoring might be, its purpose is to recognize complications before damage to the patient is inevitable. A vital question is, during what period of patient care should monitoring be in progress? It may not be surprising that reported serious complications threatening patient outcome have occurred any time from the onset of attempted neural blockade until surgery has been in progress for several hours, or even when the patient is in the recovery area.[82] In some instances, a complication has been detected much later. Accordingly, it is prudent to monitor patients carefully from entry into the block room until the effects of the blockade have ended.

When instrumental monitors are used, they should be calibrated correctly and located so that there can be a planned balance of visual attention between patient and instruments, and access by audible alarms. If they are to be used optimally for the early detection of complications, however, the characteristics of these essential pieces of equipment must be appreciated. The following paragraphs concentrate on these limitations but should not undermine their clinical value for caregivers.

### *Pulse Oximetry*[100–106]

Pulse oximeters require a pulse at the site of measurement and provide only a crude indication of peripheral perfusion. Blood flow is barely required. It has been shown that peripheral blood flow can be reduced to only 10% of normal before the pulse oximeter has difficulty estimating a saturation.[107] It does not justify assumptions regarding cardiac output, arterial blood pressure, or cardiac rhythm, which must be assessed by other means. Regarding respiration, a normal saturation measurement when the patient breathes an increased inspired oxygen concentration does not confirm adequacy of ventilation. The hypoxemia that would otherwise accompany the rising carbon dioxide tension is masked.

Most pulse oximeters make measurements and calculations that provide oxygen saturation. The more popular definition of $O_2$ saturation is functional saturation, which is the concentration of oxyhemoglobin divided by the concentration of hemoglobin plus reduced hemoglobin:

$$\text{Functional saturation} = O_2\,\text{Hb}/(\text{RHb} + O_2\,\text{Hb})$$

The met or CO-Hb concentrations used in the algorithms are estimations for the population under consideration; however, the presence of a large percentage of those abnormal hemoglobins can cause overreading of saturation and mask serious hypoxia.

Regional anesthesia can produce profound changes of sympathetic nerve activity in different parts of the body. Evidence has been presented that pulse oximetry during lumbar epidural anesthesia gives falsely low readings when the sensor is placed on a finger.[108]

### *Capnography*[109–112]

Carbon dioxide production, pulmonary circulation, and ventilation are necessary to produce a normal capnogram. Change in the end-tidal carbon dioxide ($ETco_2$) value can have a cardiovascular or respiratory origin, but it is as a monitor of spontaneous breathing that the capnograph has its role in regional anesthesia.

End-tidal capnography sampling in the spontaneously breathing, unintubated patient may be from inside a plastic oxygen mask, a nasal cannula, or a catheter tip in the nasopharynx. The numeric value of the $ETco_2$ and its relationship to the arterial $CO_2$ pressure is influenced by oxygen delivery, ventilation–perfusion ratio, and sampling errors. The value of such monitoring, beyond respiratory rate indication and apnea detection, has been a contentious matter.[113–115] There have been very favorable recent reports of its use in adults and children,[116–120] but certain provisos apply. Small differences in sampling technique affect the accuracy of the values measured, so the technique requires expert evaluation where it is in use. A gas temperature–flow relationship in the nostril has been proposed as a monitor of respiration and refuted.[121,122] Previous attempts to utilize such a relationship were unsuccessful.

### *Cardiac Rate and Rhythm*

A normal ECG can be recorded from a patient who is profoundly hypotensive, hypoxic, or hypercapnic, so although it is valuable as an indicator of heart rate and rhythm, it is a very late indicator of other threatening complications, even if the patient is conscious. Nevertheless, it provides potentially useful diagnostic information not provided by peripheral pulse-activated devices.

This information is more valuable for the diagnosis of arrhythmias than detection of myocardial ischemia, even if a modified V5 lead is used and the right arm electrode of lead I is placed over a position on the intersection of the left anterior axillary line and the fifth intercostal space and the ground electrode is placed on the left shoulder. The principal guides to cardiac ischemic complications are data gathered from monitoring and management of heart rate, mean arterial pressure, hemoglobin concentration, and saturation.

ECG monitoring should be used for major surgery and for patients at cardiac risk, but for routine cases the use of an ECG in preference to a pulse oximeter or capnograph is controversial. Many anesthesiologists favor pulse oximetry or capnography.

### *Systemic Arterial Pressure*

The anesthesiologist predicts an acceptable blood pressure range for the patient and selects the methods of measurement on the basis of the anticipated margin of error. Invasive direct methods have their own sources of error but are more accurate than noninvasive techniques. Although invasive direct methods are possible during regional anesthesia and necessary for major surgery in very poor-risk patients, indirect methods are used for most patients.

### *Manual Indirect Measurement of Blood Pressure*

Methods usually involve the application of a cuff (20% larger than the diameter of the arm), applied snugly to the upper arm. After inflation to above the anticipated systemic pressure, it should be deflated, reducing the pressure at 2–4 mmHg per heartbeat. Detection of the returning pulse by palpation or oximeter provides a crude estimate, as do oscillations of aneroid manometers or mercury columns.

The Korotkoff method of detection requires a sensor under the cuff and over an artery, enabling the Korotkoff sounds to be heard. Although the pressures measured may differ from intraarterial values by only a few millimeters of mercury, systolic, diastolic, and mean arterial pressures may be over- or underestimated by up to 30%.[123] During anesthesia and surgery, the patient's cardiovascular status changes and the magnitude, and even the direction, of error may change.[124] Correlation with direct arterial pressure measurement is poor.[125,126] Additionally, even if the blood pressure remains unchanged, alterations in the vascular tone in the limb, such as may be produced by vasopressor agents, alter Korotkoff sounds. When the patient is very vasoconstricted or hypotensive, Korotkoff sounds are difficult to detect and the palpatory method is reassuring rather than accurate.[127]

### *Automated Oscillometric Measurement*

The inflatable cuff functions as a sensor supplying a pressure transducer within the instrument. The varying oscillations and cuff pressures are analyzed electronically to determine systolic, diastolic, and mean arterial pressures. Comparisons with pressures in the aorta or a peripheral artery have been made,[128–131] and these devices are accurate to ±10mmHg. Another study demonstrated a good correlation only for systolic pressures.[132] Oscillometric diastolic pressures have been found to be higher; however, in a survey of six commercially available devices, errors ranged from –30% to +40% for mean arterial pressures.[124] In general, low pressures were overestimated and high pressures were underestimated. If the patient has cardiac arrhythmia, results may be erroneous.

There is no doubt that automated sphygmomanometers are invaluable, providing blood pressure readings regularly and frequently, particularly when the patient is otherwise inaccessible. However, the anticipated accuracy of measurement does not always meet the anesthesiologist's requirements, and invasive methods are preferable, assuming they are conducted skillfully with the proper equipment. If electronic transducer-amplifier systems are not available, mean arterial pressure may be measured by a calibrated aneroid gauge.[133]

### *Plethysmography*

The finger arterial pressure device (Finapres) consists of a small finger cuff containing an inflatable bladder and an infrared plethysmograph volume transducer that can provide continuous monitoring. It seems that performance is better on a thumb than a finger,[134] and studies have shown the Finapres to be as good as, if not better than, noninvasive oscillometric devices as compared with direct arterial pressure readings.[135] However, lacking precision, the instrument has not been recommended as a substitute for invasive arterial pressure measurement.[135] Since then, it has been shown that even small degrees of cuff misapplication contribute to measurement error as compared with intraarterial cannulation. A comparative study of patients undergoing spinal anesthesia for lower segment cesarean delivery revealed many inconsistencies in some patients, and it was concluded that the Finapres was unsatisfactory for patients in whom sudden hypotension was a threat to outcome.[136] Problems with its use have been reviewed.[137]

### *Thermometrography*

The location of the sensor is important if it is to be used as a predictor of temperature at a site other than its location. The ideal place for a probe is the lower third to fourth of the esophagus, but this site, similar to the nasopharynx, tympanic membrane, and rectum, is uncomfortable for conscious or even mildly sedated patients. The axilla of an adducted area is a useful site for the patient under regional anesthesia, reading approximately 0.5°C less than the oral temperature.

Liquid crystal skin thermometers have been evaluated and are potentially useful as trend indicators during surgery, because they can conveniently be applied to the skin. They are susceptible to drafts, and it is recommended that, before changing exclusively to such a device, it be standardized using a thermocouple method in parallel until adequate experience has been obtained in that working environment.[138]

### *Conclusion*

Conventional practice demands that certain monitoring devices be used routinely; however, funding for them competes in society with all the nonmedical and medical factors that contribute to health in that society. Accordingly, any application for funds and decisions on the dispensation of a global budget must be supported by a valid justification. These are challenging tasks. Outcome studies designed to predict individual risk of complications must be based on very large population.[139,140] They are very expensive and can be confounded to a greater or lesser extent by learning contamination bias during their implementation.[141] Practitioners sometimes develop or improve clinical skills when using a device, and that change affects patient care when the device is not in use. The argument that once learning has occurred with the aid of a monitor the monitor is no longer necessary is invalid, because reinforcement of the learning will be necessary. Additionally, even if convincing studies demonstrating a lack of change in patient outcome were presented, the question of anesthesiologist outcome remains to be addressed. Do these simple monitoring devices render the task less stressful for anesthesiologists and enable them to be more effective members of the hospital personnel and better citizens, once the working day or night is over?

The template proposed for assessing the efficacy of diagnostic imaging[142] has been modified for the assessment of anesthesia technology[140] and has six components: 1) technical efficacy, 2) diagnostic efficacy, 3) diagnostic thinking efficacy and therapeutic efficacy, 4) patient outcome, and 5) societal efficacy. As new devices become commercially available, future studies will be based on the specific problems embraced by regional anesthesia.

Critical features of introducing any new device into the workplace are new educational requirements and the attitudes of the potential users, which will be strongly influenced by the design features, additional work, its perceived value, and health factors.[80]

## Complications of Specific Neural Blockades

The wide variety of symptoms and signs of complications associated with regional blockade have been described as, "Trouble may not come singly but in battalions," so the anesthesiologist must be encouraged to take an overall view of the patient. Nevertheless, initially the emphasis is on the complications of the neural blockade under consideration, because of their role in determining the final anesthesia plan and the matters uppermost in the mind of the anesthesiologist while monitoring that procedure and diagnosing complications during its conduct. Some sources of complications are shared by all patients and will not be described repeatedly for each block (e.g., airway obstruction, drug toxicity, epinephrine side effects, and neural damage).

### *Airway Obstruction*

Traditionally in some institutions, nurses familiar to the patient kept the patient comfortable during major surgery under regional anesthesia. The patient was wide awake, and this was considered an important feature; however, tolerance of the procedure and cooperation must be ensured, not only for the success of the procedure but for satisfaction of all concerned. The choices range from complete consciousness, through a mild state of cortical depression in which the patient is calm and tranquil, to a drug-induced sleep or even general anesthesia supplemented by the regional blockade. The last is usually necessary for infants and children; there are more options for adult patients.

From the anesthesiologist's point of view, some warning signs and symptoms are obtunded in unconscious patients. If the patient is heavily sedated, as opposed to tracheally intubated under general anesthesia, management of respiratory obstruction may be needed. In the awake state, the upper airway muscles help keep that airway patent. In the supine posture, airway patency increases in response to greater airway resistance. During normal sleep, muscle activity is reduced and can be supplemented by drugs such as alcohol, benzodiazepines, and barbiturates.[143–145] Thus, respiratory obstruction is a potential problem throughout the procedure that must be immediately recognized and successfully managed. The hazard is compounded in patients who normally experience episodes of sleep apnea, from the influence of deafferentation and central effects of the local anesthetic agent, including respiratory depression.

### *Local Anesthetic Focal Complications*

In a conscious, unsedated patient, the first symptoms or signs of focal complications are drowsiness or light-headedness. As toxic activity increases, the characteristic sequence is circumoral and lingual numbness, tinnitus, visual disturbances, dysarthria, and restlessness. Muscular twitching, often facial, progresses to convulsions, coma, and respiratory and circulatory depression. The quantity of drug reaching activity sites and time after injection are influenced not only by distribution, elimination, and drug characteristics, but by the site of injection. Sometimes all the vital systems are depressed simultaneously. This dangerous situation is compounded by inability of the patient to report symptoms. In the case of pregnant patients at term, neonatal depression can occur and hypotonia has a prominent role.[146–148] Bradycardia, heart block, and ventricular tachycardia have been reported.[149,150]

### *Epinephrine Complications*

Epinephrine complications in regional anesthesia are related to vasoconstriction at the site of the injected fluid. As such, they are more likely to be evidenced in the postoperative period. However, if absorbed into the general circulation at the time of neural blockade, temporary hypertension is associated with tachycardia or reflex bradycardia. Cardiac arrhythmias, including ventricular fibrillation, occur when the quantity entering the general circulation is sufficient.

### *Complications of Neural Blockade*

The complications of neural blockade are directly related to the anatomy of the route of the needle and the body into which fluid or air has been introduced. Thus, the anesthesiologist with a good mental image of the relevant anatomy can predict events that may occur, particularly if the preoperative visit has been informative. Those events comprise a mix of the symptoms and signs outlined as complications to be recognized during neural blockade, surgery, and recovery. Risks depend not only on the skill and care of the anesthesiologist, but also on the drugs, equipment, the environment, and unanticipated scenarios. Their early detection and management depend on the competence of all those with care responsibilities and their performance. In view of this multifactorial situation, it is virtually impossible to know the chances of a specific complication for a specific patient, although low reported incidences can be an encouraging guide. Table 1-3 lists the complications that have been associated with various neural blockades and can be correlated with previous sections about detection methods. Complications associated with narcotics are described elsewhere in this volume. The complications identified have been gathered largely from references 61, 71, 72, and 81 to 93.

### *Miscellaneous Neural Blockade Complications*

Neural blockades are created at a wide variety of sites in the upper and lower limbs, the lumbar and sacral nerves, the scalp, and nerves supplying the mandible and maxilla. These complications are similar in character, and on occasion their development is sudden and severe.

TABLE 1-3. Complications of Neural Blockade*

| Orbital regional blockade | |
|---|---|
| **Local effect by needle, catheter, or injected volume** | **Conductor blockade effects** |
| • Venous penetration causing retrobulbar hematoma<br>• Arterial penetration causing a retrobulbar hematoma and local ischemia<br>• Vascular occlusion of the central retinal artery<br>• Optic nerve penetration<br>• Penetration of the globe<br>• Penetration of the optic stem<br>• Oculocardiac reflex | • Brain stem anesthesia associated with optic nerve sheath penetration resulting in<br>• Increasing or decreasing cardiovascular vital signs, pulmonary edema, cardiac arrest, shivering, convulsions, hyperreflexia, hemiplegia, paraplegia, quadriplegia, contralateral amaurosis, contralateral oculomotor paralysis, facial palsy, deafness, vertigo, aphasia, loss of neck muscle power, loss of consciousness, vagolysis, respiratory depression, apnea (Chapter 6). |
| **Cervical plexus blockade complications** | |
| **Local effect by needle, catheter, or injected volume** | **Conductor blockade effects** |
| • Entry to epidural space<br>• Entry to subarachnoid space<br>• Intravenous penetration<br>• Intraarterial penetration<br>• Penetration of esophagus (associated with the anterior approach to the ganglion)<br>• Pneumothorax (especially on the patient's right side)<br>• Nasal congestion | • High spinal anesthesia with cardiovascular and respiratory failure<br>• Aphasia and hemiparesis<br>• Blindness |
| **Supraclavicular brachial plexus blockade complications** | |
| **Local effect by needle, catheter, or injected volume** | **Conductor blockade effects** |
| • Vascular penetration of subclavian and axillary arteries or veins, the vertebral artery, and external jugular vein. Ischemic arm problems may develop, particularly in children<br>• Penetration of apical pleura, causing a pneumothorax<br>• Epidural space entry<br>• Subarachnoid space entry<br>• Nerve trauma<br>• Vasovagal episodes in patients in the sitting position | • Stellate ganglion block producing Horner's syndrome<br>• Phrenic nerve block which in children impairs respiration<br>• Recurrent laryngeal in block causing hoarseness and possibility of aspiration<br>• Epidural anesthesia with cardiovascular and respiratory depression<br>• Spinal anesthesia with cardiovascular and respiratory depression |
| **Infraclavicular brachial plexus blockade complications** | |
| **Local effect by needle, catheter, or injected volume** | **Conductor blockade effects** |
| • Axillary artery puncture, sometimes with a brief vascular insufficiency<br>• Venous penetration causing a hematoma<br>• Apical pleura penetration and ensuing pneumothorax is possible but unusual. | |

(*Continued*)

TABLE 1-3. *Continued*

| Epidural blockade complications | |
|---|---|
| **Local effect by needle, catheter, or injected volume** | **Conductor blockade effects** |
| • Epidural vessel penetration<br>• Epidural hematoma<br>• Dural puncture<br>• Back pain<br>• Neural trauma<br>• Air embolism (especially in children) if an air-filled syringe has been used to locate the epidural space<br><br>If a catheter has been inserted:<br>• Subdural space catheterization<br>• Intravascular catheterization<br>• Infection<br>• Headache associated with supplementary injections | • Hypotension<br>• Respiratory depression failure<br>• Bradycardia<br>• Total spinal anesthesia<br>• Horner's syndrome<br>• Trigeminal nerve paralysis |
| **Caudal epidural blockade complications** | |
| **Local effect by needle, catheter, or injected volume** | **Conductor blockade effects** |
| • Subcutaneous injection<br>• Penetration of dura mater<br>• Penetration into epidural vein<br>• Hematoma<br>• Intraosseous penetration<br>• Pelvic visceral penetration<br>• Infection, particularly if a caudal–epidural catheter is in situ | • Accidental spinal anesthesia with cardiovascular and respiratory involvement<br>• Urinary retention |
| **Subarachnoid block complications** | |
| **Local effect by needle, catheter, or injected volume** | **Conductor blockade effects** |
| • Epidural vessel penetration<br>• Epidural hematoma<br>• Neural trauma<br>• Headache | • Total spinal anesthesia<br>• Hypotension<br>• Respiratory depression/failure<br>• Dyspnea<br>• Bradycardia/asystole |
| **Intercostal nerve blockade complications** | |
| **Local effect by needle, catheter, or injected volume** | **Conductor blockade effects** |
| • Pneumothorax<br>• Penetration of intercostal vessels<br>• Penetration of pleural space<br>• Entry to paravertebral space<br>• Entry to epidural space<br>• Entry to subarachnoid space | • Hemodynamic depression<br>• Respiratory depression/failure<br>• Depressed cough reflex<br>• Blockade of spinal nerves |

TABLE 1-3. *Continued*

| Intravenous regional anesthesia (IVRA, Bier's block) complications (Chapter 12) | |
|---|---|
| Local effect by needle, catheter, or tourniquet | Conductor blockade effects |
| • Tourniquet discomfort<br>• Tourniquet leak<br>• Tourniquet release less than 20 minutes after local anesthetic injection<br>• Vomiting followed by aspiration of recent food or drink<br>• Neural damage caused by prolonged tourniquet time, or the cuff too close to the elbow joint<br>• Necrosis caused by ischemia created in an already injured limb | |
| **Thoracic paravertebral anesthesia** | |
| Local effect by needle catheter | Conductor blockade effects |
| • Paravertebral vessel puncture<br>• Pneumothorax<br>• Intrapleural catheter placement or migration<br>• Headache<br>• Sepsis<br>• Intercostal nerve trauma and pain | • Hypotension<br>• Respiratory paralysis<br>• Epidural analgesia<br>• Horner's syndrome (possibly bilateral)<br>• Phrenic nerve paralysis (possibly bilateral) |

*For an explanation of central effects, see the section Local Anesthetic Focal Complications.

- Vascular penetration and hematoma
- Vascular penetration followed by the local anesthetic focal complications (LAFC) that may culminate in cardiac and respiratory arrest
- Neural trauma
- Local vasoactive effects of epinephrine resulting in gangrene
- Cardiac arrhythmias produced by epinephrine
- Bradycardia

## Complications in the Postoperative Period

Patients who have been neurally blocked or received centrally administered narcotics require meticulous surveillance if complications are to be detected while therapy has an excellent chance of being effective. Specific training of personnel is necessary for these tasks.

### *Admitting the Patient – History and Physical Examination*

The activities of caregivers in recovery rooms and intensive care units have much in common, and there is anecdotal as well as research evidence in intensive care units that a significant complication is failure of communication between physicians and nurses.[78] This complication can occur in recovery rooms as well. The nurse accepting responsibility for a patient from the operating room is entitled to a report of the baseline data about vital systems and other information that relates to the neurally blocked patient. Presented verbally with a completed written protocol, recovery room complications may be a continuation of intra-operating room or in-transit events on new developments. They manifest themselves in several categories.

**Cardiovascular System**

- Blood pressure, pulse rate, and cardiac rhythm: when vasopressor drugs were administered, and whether their waning effect will unmask residual sympathetic blockade or hypovolemia
- Details of any evidence of circulatory overload during surgical irrigation of the bladder
- Fluid balance
- Perfusion of peripheral vascular beds

**Respiratory System**

- Respiratory rate, tidal volume, and apparent oxygenation
- Administration of respiratory depressant drugs epidurally or by any other route, and any antidote administration
- Airway management in the operating room

**Central Nervous System**

- Sedative or analgesic drugs
- The likelihood that the patient will arouse before sensory and motor block have disappeared and then will become agitated
- State of consciousness and responses to sensory stimuli
- Analgesia preparations for recovery room sojourn
- Antinausea preparations administered

**Peripheral Nervous System**

- The existing neural blockade and when it is expected to have disappeared
- The nerves in an anesthetized area that need protection (e.g., ulnar or lateral peroneal nerves)
- An epidural or subarachnoid catheter in situ

**Bladder Distention**

- Presence of a urinary catheter, its drainage, and the state of the bladder

**Perioperative Anticoagulant Therapy**

- The drugs administered and anticipated effects on prothrombin time or other measurements of coagulation

**Endocrine Pathology**

- Diabetes and its management in the operating room
- Steroid medications given in the operating room or elsewhere

**Body Temperature**

- Evidence of hypo- or hyperthermia

**Muscle Activity**

- Restlessness
- Shivering
- Muscle twitching

### *Monitoring the Patient*

The demand for recognition of complications in the recovery room is similar in most respects to recognition in the operating room and as described in a previous section. It is a judicious combination of human and instrumental sensing, the former being the fundamental component of recovery room care. Analysis of recovery room complications in adults and children[151] reveals that they were identifiable largely by clinical observation rather than instrumental monitoring. Nevertheless, certain instruments are invaluable for recovery room care because they provide for patients at risk; they provide more precise information and supply the caregiver with continuous vital information. Instruments invaluable for recovery room care are an ECG, pulse meter, pulse oximeter, automated sphygmomanometer, thermometer, and stethoscope.

Complications monitoring includes evaluation of respiration, hemodynamics, level of consciousness, adequacy of analgesia, degree of motor blockade, and other side effects on admission to the postanesthesia recovery room. There are certain complications for which early detection, followed by early diagnosis and treatment, reduces the chance of a permanent neurologic deficit. They are those associated with central neural blockade, and presenting symptoms include backache[152,153] pain in thighs, calves, or buttocks,[153] headache, muscle twitching, and increase in neural blockade or its failure to regress. The detection of these complications can be made difficult by postoperative sedation[154] and analgesia and the normal variation in block duration. Although these complications, indicative of a wide variety of pathology, are chronologically related to the neural blockade, they may be attributable to concomitant pathology,[155] and headache accompanying epidural supplementation can be attributable to an increase in intracranial pressure during labor,[156] trauma, or another intracranial lesion.

### *Discharging the Patient*

Ambulatory patients are discharged home with a companion when the effects of the neural blockade have worn off and complications such as nausea, pain, and dizziness have been treated. Exceptions are patients who have had dental and very minor surgical procedures, for whom the residual effects of sedation determine fitness for discharge from the office or clinic, rather than the disappearance of neural blockade effects. Subsequent complications are detected by a follow-up call, visit 24 hours later, or an emergency communication from patient or relative.

The situation for hospitalized patients who have often received a central neural blockade is somewhat different. When the neural blockade has worn off, any pain and nausea have been treated, and pharmacologic, neurologic, cardiovascular, and respiratory complications resolved, the patient is transferred to a ward or intensive care unit. It is there that the delayed, but potentially permanent, complications occur 2 or 3 days later, whose outcome is determined by the time between detection and therapeutic intervention. The presenting symptoms and signs associated with different complications often include pain and evidence of increasing (rather than decreasing) neural blockade that may end in permanent disability. These complications are discussed elsewhere in this volume. It suffices to say that it is likely to be helpful if patient and caregivers are aware of the need to keep in touch regarding symptoms of these rare complications.

## Complication Prevention

Complication reduction, and ultimate abolition, depends on consistent application of current knowledge and skills to patient care plus further development of expertise. In 1940, the leading article of the first issue of the *Journal of the American Society of Anesthesiologists* (today *Anesthesiology*) concluded with this statement: "The important decision is what man shall give the anesthetic [in contrast to the drug or technique]."[157] The implications for training and practice remain.

The baseline competence reached at the inception of independent anesthetic practice is established by certifying authorities but the significant variation among certificants[158] probably represents other training programs. This is partly attributable to limited clinical experience[159,160] and, particularly relevant for regional anesthesia, a possibly doubtful correlation between knowledge and skills.[161] Thus, any further move toward complication prevention must, among other things, include better regional anesthesia training. This is occurring on several counts. Virtual reality techniques that register in a three-dimensional manner on a computer screen can radically change the pattern of training.[160] Mental imagery of anatomy is an integral part of the anatomic reasoning while performing neural blockade. Three-dimensional computer-based methods of presenting anatomic relations have great potential for overcoming existing limitations of conventional teaching.[162] Last, more critical evaluation techniques can assess training methods and establish levels of competence reached in manual skills.[163,164] However, improvement in the training of future anesthesiologists does little to reduce complications perpetuated by recently training and established anesthesiologists.

Contrasting characteristics of two competing perspectives of safe practice are presented in Table 1-4.[165]

Anesthesiologists' attitudes consistent with the same characteristics of normal accident theory have been documented.[166] These reflect certain problems facing persons who wish to implement factors supporting a high reliability theory, for example the five hazardous thinking patterns: antiauthority, impulsivity, invulnerability, macho, and resignation.

Ever since anesthesia has been practiced, a variety of case reports and collations of mortality and morbidity have been published under the auspices of individuals, groups, or institutions. Nevertheless, controversy and democracy have remained pre-eminent, and resistance "on principle" to external imposition of medical practice was firmly entrenched until the last decade, when such independence was seriously challenged and many anesthesiologists perceived certain changes to be in their own interests as well as those of patients.

The Department of Anesthesia of Harvard Medical School, Boston, in 1986 published specific, detailed, mandatory standards for minimal patient monitoring during anesthesia.[167] These were to be implemented in its nine component teaching hospital

Table 1-4. Competing Perspectives on Safety

High reliability theory
- Complications can be prevented through good organization and management.
- Safety is the priority of the organization.
- Duplicating tasks and devices increases safety.
- Continuous quality improvement with simulations creates and maintains safety.
- Trial and error learning from complications can be effective.

Normal accidents theory
- Complications are inevitable in any complex system.
- Safety is only a competing objective, "We cannot necessarily do that here."
- Duplication encourages risks and reduces safety.
- Discipline and socialization are incompatible with democratic values.
- Organizations cannot train for the unimagined. "Intuition is better than algorithms."
- Learning efforts from critical incidents and complications are crippled by faulty reporting and denial of responsibility.

*Source:* Modified from Sagan.[165] Copyright 1993, Princeton University Press, 1995 paperback edition. Reprinted by permission of Princeton University Press.

departments and published for the interest of other practitioners, organizations, and institutions. The motivation was anesthetic complications that incurred substantial financial settlements, and that were thought to have been preventable and strongly influenced by a report of critical incidents. Included in those standards were these references to regional anesthesia:

- An attending or resident anesthesiologist or nurse anesthesiologist shall be present in the operating room at all times during its conduct.
- The arterial blood pressure and heart rate shall be measured at least every 5 minutes, where not clinically impractical.
- The ECG shall be continuously displayed from the institution of anesthesia until preparing to leave the anesthetizing location, unless clinically impractical.

The effect of these standards on complications of regional anesthesia have not been published, but there has been a favorable association between the adoption of the standards and diminishing cost of malpractice insurance.

The Canadian Anesthesiologists' Society (CAS) has promoted its guidelines to the practice of anesthesia[168] for more than a decade. A standard is a definite level of excellence or adequacy demanded by an organization. Clinical practice guidelines (CPGs) are systematically developed statements to inform practitioners about appropriate care in specific clinical circumstances. Implicit in this is planned avoidance of complications. The word *guidelines*, as opposed to *standards*, was used advisedly, because although mandatory requirements could be reasonable for a hospital or group of institutions, it was deemed inappropriate to address all Canadian anesthesiologists in such a manner. The Canadian guidelines promulgated for regional anesthesia in 1996 are as follows.

### *Patient Monitoring*

The only indispensable monitor is the presence, at all times, of an appropriately trained and experienced physician. Mechanical and electronic monitors are, at best, aids to vigilance. Such devices help the anesthesiologist to ensure the integrity of the vital organs, and in particular the adequacy of tissue perfusion and oxygenation. The healthcare facility is responsible for the provision and maintenance of monitoring equipment that meets current published equipment standards.

The chief of anesthesiology is responsible for advising the healthcare facility on the procurement of monitoring equipment and for establishing policies for monitoring to help ensure patient safety.

The anesthesiologist is responsible for monitoring patients receiving care and *must ensure* that appropriate monitoring equipment is available and working property. *A preanesthetic checklist (such as found in Table 1-5 or equivalent) must be completed before initiation of anesthesia.* Monitoring guidelines for standard patient care apply to all patients receiving regional anesthesia or intravenous sedation.

Monitoring equipment may be classified either as *required* for each anesthetized patient (that is, the device is attached, or dedicated exclusively, to each patient) or *immediately available* (the device is available for the anesthetized patient without inappropriate delay).

### *Required Equipment*

- Pulse oximeter
- Apparatus to measure blood pressure
- Stethoscope, precordial, esophageal, or paratracheal
- ECG monitor
- Capnograph for an intubated patient
- Apparatus to measure temperature
- Appropriate lighting to visualize the exposed portion of the patient

Table 1-5. Preanesthetic Checklist

A. Gas pipelines
   Secure connections between terminal units (outlets) and anesthetic machine.
B. Anesthetic machine
1. Turn on machine master switch and all other necessary electrical equipment.
   Line oxygen (40–60psi) (275–415 $KP_a$)
   Line nitrous oxide (40–60psi) (275–415 $KP_a$)
   Adequate reserve cylinder oxygen pressure
   Adequate reserve cylinder nitrous oxide content
   Check for leaks and turn off cylinders
   Flow meter function of oxygen and nitrous oxide over the working range
2. Vaporizer filled
   Filling ports pin-indexed and closed
   Ensure "on/off" function and turn off
3. Functioning oxygen bypass (flush)
4. Functioning oxygen fail-safe device
5. Oxygen analyzer calibrated and turned on functioning mixer (where available)
   Attempt to create a hypoxic $O_2/N_2O$ mixture and/or verify correct changes in flow alarm
6. Functioning common fresh gas outlet
7. Ventilator function verified
8. Backup ventilation equipment available and functioning

If an anesthesiologist uses the same machine in successive cases, departmental policy may permit performing an abbreviated checklist between cases.

C. Breathing circuit
1. Correct assembly of circuit to be used
2. Patient circuit connected to common fresh gas outlet
3. Oxygen flow meter turned on
4. Check for exit of fresh gas at face mask pressurize. Check for leaks and integrity at circuit (e.g., Pethick test for coaxial)
5. Functioning high-pressure relief valve
6. Unidirectional valves and soda lime
7. Functioning adjustable pressure relief valve

D. Vacuum system
   Suction adequate
E. Scavenging system
   Correctly connected to patient circuit and functioning
F. Routine equipment
1. Airway
   Functioning laryngoscope (backup available)
   Appropriate tracheal tubes: patency of lumen and integrity of cuff
   Appropriate oropharyngeal airways
   Stylet
   Magill forceps
2. IV supplies
3. Blood pressure cuff of appropriate size
4. Stethoscope
5. ECG monitor
6. Pulse oximeter
7. Capnograph
8. Temperature monitor
9. Functioning low- and high-pressure alarm

G. Drugs
1. Adequate supply of frequently used drugs and IV solutions
2. Appropriate doses of drugs in labeled syringes

H. Location of special equipment in each anesthetizing location
1. Defibrillators
2. Emergency drugs
3. Difficult intubation kit

### *Immediately Available Equipment*

- Peripheral nerve stimulator
- Respirometer (tidal volume)

It is recognized that brief interruptions of continuous monitoring may be unavoidable. Furthermore, there are certain circumstances when a monitor may fail; thus, continuous vigilance by the anesthesiologist is essential.

The use of agent-specific anesthetic gas monitors is encouraged.

### *Epidural Anesthesia During Childbirth*

Experience since publication of the guidelines in the September 1986 issue of the CAS newsletter has shown that the incidence of major complications associated with continuous low-dose epidural infusion for obstetric analgesia is extremely low. Consequently, it is not necessary for an anesthesiologist to remain physically present or immediately available during maintenance of continuous infusion epidural analgesia. Instead, the following requirements suffice: 1) an appropriate protocol for the management of these epidurals is in place; 2) an anesthesiologist can be contacted for the purpose of advice and direction.

In contrast to continuous infusion epidural analgesia, bolus injection of local anesthetic into the epidural space can be associated with immediate life-threatening complications. In recognition of this, the CAS recommends the following:

- When a bolus dose of local anesthetic is injected into the epidural space, an anesthesiologist must be available to intervene appropriately should complications arise.
- The intent of the phrase *available to intervene appropriately* is that individual departments of anesthesiology shall make their own determinations of *availability* and *appropriateness*. This determination must be made after each individual department of anesthesiology has considered the possible risks of bolus injection of local anesthetic and the methods of dealing with any emergency situation that might arise from the performance of the procedure in their facility.

### *Practice of Anesthesia Outside a Hospital*

The basic principles, training requirements, techniques, equipment, and drugs used for the practice of anesthesia are noted in other sections of the guidelines. The following guidelines are for certain aspects peculiar to anesthetic practice outside a hospital.

#### Patient Selection

Patients should be classified by physical status in a manner similar to that in use by the American Society of Anesthesiologists (ASA). Usually, only patients in the ASA classifications I and II should be considered for an anesthetic outside a hospital. Patients in classification III may be accepted under certain circumstances.

#### Preoperative Considerations

The patient must have had a recent and recorded history, physical examination, and appropriate laboratory investigations. This may be performed by another physician or anesthesiologist. The duration of fasting before anesthesia should conform to the previously stated guidelines. The patient should be given an information sheet with pre- and postanesthetic instructions.

#### Conduct of Anesthesia

The anesthetic and recovery facilities shall conform to hospital standards published by the Canadian Standards Association, as defined in other sections. The standards of care and monitoring shall be the same in all anesthetizing locations. The Canadian guidelines are comprehensive and include the organization of hospital anesthesia services, the responsibilities of the chief of anesthesiology, and anesthetic equipment and anesthetizing locations.

Intuitively, CPGs are useful for collaboration with lay persons in a managerial capacity and with physicians, and they have been generated for a variety of reasons,[169] including quality assurance and the assistance of practitioners in their decision making. However, a cause-and-effect relationship between guidelines and anesthesia complications has been neither demonstrated nor sought.[170] Indeed, formal evaluation of CPGs in Canada is rare, and there is concern that CPGs, lacking policies to ensure compliance, will be ineffective. It is expected that guidelines unsupported by peer review and prominent personalities will be ignored; nevertheless, whether referred to as *audit, quality assurance, or continuous quality improvement* or CPG, developments continue. It is noteworthy that it was insistence of the government of the United Kingdom that motivated the Confidential Enquiry into Perioperative Deaths there, and pressures elsewhere for establishing actual standards of practice come from governments, insurers, and the general public. In a definitive analysis of guidelines,[170] the need for a clear target if they are to be effective improvers of patient care is emphasized and that they must be oriented to practitioners, managers, and planners as well as other stakeholders. Achieving consensus is itself a difficult task, but guidelines for this process have been promulgated.[171]

## Conclusion

Safety – avoidance of complications – in regional anesthesia is dependent on the cooperative efforts of anesthesiologists, other care providers, and persons with management responsibilities. The deficiencies at any moment in time may be inadequacies in the state of the art or defects in what is a very complex system. It may be that differences between general and regional anesthesia detected in comparative studies are affected by factors in the patient care systems other than differences intrinsic to the techniques.

In 1858, the redoubtable John Snow published rules for chloroform administration. These were not rules in the regulatory sense but advice or recommendations from a respected figure. What would have been his views about competing perspectives on safety will remain unknown; however, his efforts for the greater good of patients can be emulated by taking advantage of superior opportunities to promote safe regional anesthesia practice, not only by improving training, practice, and research but by international dissemination of information.

## References


1. The Oxford English Dictionary. New York: Oxford University Press; 1971.
2. Allnutt MF. Human factors in accidents. Br J Anaesth 1987;59:856–864.
3. Crawford JS, James FM, Nolte H, et al. Regional anaesthesia for patients with chronic neurological disease and similar conditions. Anaesthesia 1981;36:821–822.
4. Perel A, Reches A, Davidson JT. Anaesthesia in the Guillain-Barre syndrome. A case report and recommendations. Anaesthesia 1977;32:257–260.
5. Chaudhari LS, Kop BR, Dhruva AJ. Paraplegia and epidural analgesia. Anaesthesia 1978;33:722–725.
6. Hirlekar G. Paraplegia after epidural analgesia associated with an extradural spinal tumour. Anaesthesia 1980;35:363–364.
7. Ballin NC. Paraplegia following epidural blockade. Anaesthesia 1981;36:952–953.
8. Lambert DH, Deane RS, Mazuzan JE. Anesthesia and the control of blood pressure in patients with spinal cord injury. Anesth Analg 1982;61:344–348.
9. Duffy GP. Lumbar puncture in the presence of raised intracranial pressure. Br Med J 1969;1:407.
10. Richards PG, Towv-Aghanste F. Dangers of lumbar puncture. Br Med J 1986;292: 605–606.
11. Hilt H, Gramm HJ, Link J. Changes in intracranial pressure associated with extradural anaesthesia. Br J Anaesth 1986;58:676–680.
12. Brown LK. Surgical considerations: effects of surgery on lung function, preoperative evaluation. In: Miller A, ed. Pulmonary Function Tests: A Guide for the Student and House Officer. Orlando, FL: Grune and Stratton; 1987.
13. Englesson S, Matousek M. Central nervous system effects of local anaesthetic agents. Br J Anaesth 1975;47:241–246.
14. Rosen M, Thigpen JW, Shnider SM, et al. Bupivacaine-induced cardiotoxicity in hypoxic and acidotic sheep. Anesth Analg 1985;64:1089–1096.

15. Freysz M, Timour Q, Bertrix L, et al. Bupivacaine hastens the ischemia-induced decrease of the electrical ventricular fibrillation threshold. Anesth Analg 1995;80:657–663.
16. Detsky AS, Abrams HB, Forbath N, et al. Cardiac assessment for patients undergoing non-cardiac surgery, a multifactorial clinical risk index. Arch Int Med 1986;146:2131–2134.
17. Detsky AS, Abrams HB, McLaughlin TR, et al. Predicting cardiac complications in patients undergoing non-cardiac surgery. J Gen Intern Med 1986;1:211.
18. Mangano DT. Perioperative cardiac morbidity. Anesthesiology 1990;72:153–184.
19. Mangano DT. Preoperative risk assessment: many studies, few solutions. Anesthesiology 1995;83:897–901.
20. Fleisher LA, Rosenbaum SH, Nelson AH, et al. Preoperative dipyridamole thallium imaging and ambulatory electrocardiographic monitoring as a predictor of perioperative cardiac events and long-term outcome. Anesthesiology 1995;83:906–917.
21. Lofstrom B. Tissue distribution of local anaesthetics with special reference to the lung. Int Anesthesiol Clin 1978;16:53.
22. Jorfeldt L, Lewis DH, Lofstrom B, et al. Lung uptake of lidocaine in healthy volunteers. Acta Anaesthesiol Scand 1979;23:567–574.
23. Splinter WM, Stewart JA, Muir JG. Large volumes of apple juice preoperatively did not affect gastric pH and volume in children. Can J Anaesth 1990;37:36–39.
24. Goresky GV, Maltby JR. Fasting guidelines for elective surgical patients. Can J Anaesth 1990;37:493–495.
25. Thoren T, Wattwil M. Effects on gastric emptying of thoracic epidural anesthesia with morphine or bupivacaine. Anesth Analg 1988;67:687–694.
26. Hett DA, Walker D, Pilkington SN, et al. Sonoclot analysis. Br J Anaesth 1995;75:771–776.
27. Wildsmith JAW, McClure JH. Anticoagulant drugs and central nerve blockade. Anaesthesia 1991;46:613–614.
28. Vandermeulen EP, Van Aken H, Vermylen J. Anticoagulants and spinal epidural anesthesia. Anesth Analg 1994;79:1165–1177.
29. McKinnon RP, Wildsmith JAW. Histaminoid reactions in anaesthesia. Br J Anaesth 1995;74:217–228.
30. Dundee JW, Fee JPH, McDonald JR, Clarke RS. Frequency of atopy and allergy in an anaesthetic patient population. Br J Anaesth 1978;50:793–798.
31. Fisher MM, Outhred A, Bowey CJ. Can clinical anaphylaxis to anaesthetic drugs be predicted from allergic history? Br J Anaesth 51987;9:690–692.
32. Kuhnert BR, Philipson EH, Pimental R, et al. A prolonged chloroprocaine epidural block in a postpartum patient with abnormal pseudo-cholinesterase. Anesthesiology 1982;56:477–478.
33. Smith AR, Hur D, Resano F. Grand mal seizures after 2 chloroprocaine epidural anaesthesia in a patient with plasma cholinesterase. Anesth Analg 1987;66:677–678.
34. Paasuke RT, Brownell AKW. Amide local anaesthetics and malignant hyperthermia. Can Anaesth Soc J 1986;33:126.
35. Moore DC. Ester or amide local anesthetics in malignant hyperthermia – who knows? Anesthesiology 1986;64:294–296.
36. Romano E, Gullo A. Hypoglycemic coma following epidural analgesia. Anaesthesia 1980;35:1084–1086.
37. Traynor C, Paterson JL, Ward D, et al. Effects of extradural analgesia and vagal blockade on the metabolic and endocrine responses to upper abdominal surgery. Br J Anaesth 1982;54:319–323.
38. MacDonald R. Aspirin and extradural blocks. Br J Anaesth 1991;66:1–3.
39. McNamara PJ, Slaughter RL, Pieper JA. Factors influencing serum protein binding of lidocaine in humans. Anesth Analg 1981;60:395–400.
40. Yong CL, Kunka RL, Bates TR. Factors affecting the plasma binding of verapamil and norverapamil in man. Res Commun Chem Pathol Pharmacol 1980;30:329.
41. Rosenblatt RM, Weaver JM, Wang Y, et al. Verapamil potentiates the toxicity of local anesthetics. Anesth Analg 1984;63:269.
42. Collier C. Verapamil and epidural bupivacaine. Anaesth Intensive Care 1985;13:101.
43. Howie MB, Candler E, Mortimer W, et al. Does nifedipine enhance the cardiovascular toxicity of bupivacaine? Anesthesiology 1985;64:A225.

44. Manchikanti L, Hadley C, Markwell SJ, et al. A retrospective analysis of failed spinal anesthetic attempts in a community hospital. Anesth Analg 1987;66:363–366.
45. Munhall RJ, Sukhani R, Winnie AP. Incidence and etiology of failed spinal anesthetics in a university hospital. A prospective study. Anesth Analg 1988;67:843–848.
46. Parker RK, DeLeo BC, White PF. Spinal anesthesia: 25 GA Quincke vs 25 GA or 27 GA Whitacre needles. Anesthesiology 1992;77:A485.
47. Campbell DC, Douglas MJ, Pavy TJG, et al. Comparison of the 25-gauge Whitacre with the 24-gauge Sprotte spinal needle for elective caesarean section: cost implications. Can J Anaesth 1993;40:1131–1135.
48. Kang SB, Romeyn RL, Shenton DW, et al. Spinal anesthesia with 27-gauge needles for outpatient knee arthroscopy in patients 12 to 18 years old. Anesthesiology 1991;75: A1103.
49. Kang SB, Goodnough DE, Lee YK, et al. Spinal anesthesia with 27-gauge needles for ambulatory surgery patients. Anesthesiology 1990;73:A2.
50. Lifschitz R, Jedeikin R. Spinal anaesthesia. A new combination system. Anaesthesia 1992;47:503–505.
51. Lesser P, Bembridge M, Lyons G, Macdonald R. An evaluation of a 30-gauge needle for spinal anaesthesia for caesarean section. Anaesthesia 1990;45:767–768.
52. Dahl JB, Schultz P, Anker-Moller E, et al. Spinal anaesthesia in young patients using a 29-gauge needle: technical considerations and an evaluation of postoperative complaints compared with general anaesthesia. Br J Anaesth 1990;64:178–182.
53. Halpern S, Preston R. Postdural puncture headache and spinal needle design. Metaanalyses. Anesthesiology 1994;81:1376–1383.
54. Fritz T, Matthew A. How to establish accurate estimates of the effectiveness of three spinal needles in decreasing postdural puncture headache (PDPH) and other complications. A meta analysis. Reg Anesth 1994;19:4.
55. Lynch J, Kaspar SM, Strick K, et al. The use of Quincke and Whitacre 27 gauge needles in orthopedic patients: incidence of failed spinal anaesthesia and postdural puncture headache. Anesth Analg 1994;79:124–128.
56. Kopacz DJ, Allen HW. Comparison of needle deviation during regional anesthetic techniques in a laboratory model. Anesth Analg 1995;81:630–633.
57. Zarzur E, Goncalves J. The resistance of the human dura to needle penetration. Reg Anesth 1992;17:216.
58. Carson DF, Serpell MG. Clinical characteristics of commonly used spinal needles. Anaesthesia 1995;50:523–525.
59. Westbrook JL, Uncles DR, Sitzmann BT, et al. Comparison of the force required for dural puncture with different spinal needles and subsequent leakage of cerebrospinal fluid. Anesth Analg 1994;79:769–772.
60. Sayeed YG, Sosis M, Braverman B, et al. An in vitro investigation of the relationship between spinal needle design and failed spinal anesthesia. Reg Anesth 1993;18:85.
61. Epidural anesthesia. In: Dalens BJ, ed. Pediatric Regional Anesthesia. Boca Raton, FL: CRC Press; 1990:386.
62. Felsby S, Juelsgaard P. Combined spinal and epidural anesthesia. Anesth Analg 1995; 80:821–826.
63. Patel M, Samsoon G, Swami A, et al. Flow characteristics of long spinal needles. Anaesthesia 1994;49:223–225.
64. Holmstrom B, Rawal N, Axelsson K, et al. Risk of catheter migration during combined spinal epidural block: percutaneous epiduroscopy study. Anesth Analg 1995;80:747–753.
65. Racz GB, Sabonghy M, Gintavtas J, et al. Intractable pain therapy using a new epidural catheter. JAMA 1982;248:579–581.
66. Frankhouser PL. Hazard of a new epidural catheter. Anesthesiology 1983;58:593.
67. Boey SK, Carrie LES. Withdrawal forces during removal of lumbar extradural catheters. Br J Anaesth 1994;73:833–835.
68. Morris GN. Removal of lumbar extradural catheters. Br J Anaesth 1995;74:722.
69. Moore DC, Mulroy MF, Thompson GE. Peripheral nerve damage and regional anaesthesia. Br J Anaesth 1994;73:435–436.
70. Ford DJ, Pither CE, Raj PP. Electrical characteristics of nerve stimulators: implications for nerve localization. Reg Anesth 1984;9:42.

71. Wildsmith JAW, Armitage EN, eds. Principles and Practice of Regional Anaesthesia. 2nd ed. New York: Churchill Livingstone; 1993:58.
72. Prithvi Raj P, ed. Clinical Practice of Regional Anesthesia. New York: Churchill Livingstone; 1991:167.
73. Kapral S, Krafft P, Eibenberger K, et al. Ultrasound-guided supraclavicular approach for regional anesthesia of the brachial plexus. Anesth Analg 1994;78:507–513.
74. Cooper JB, Gaba DM. A strategy for preventing accidents. Int Anesthesiol Clin 1989; 27:148–152.
75. Weinger MB, Englund CE. Ergonomic and human factors affecting anesthetic vigilance and monitoring performance in the operating room environment. Anesthesiology 1990; 73:995–1021.
76. Gaba DM. Human error in anesthetic mishaps. Int Anesthesiol Clin 1989;27:137–147.
77. McIntyre JWR. Implication of anaesthesiologists varying location during surgery. Int J Clin Monit Comput 1995;12:33.
78. Donchin Y, Gopher D, Olin M, et al. A look into the nature and causes of human errors in the intensive care unit. Crit Care Med 1995;23:294.
79. Gaba DM, Howard S, Jump B. Production pressure in the work environment: California anesthesiologists' attitudes and experiences. Anesthesiology 1994;81:488–500.
80. McIntyre JWR. Anaesthesia monitoring: the human factors component of technology transfer. Int J Clin Monit Comput 1993;10:23.
81. Gribomont BG. Sudden complications in regional anesthesia. Acta Anaesth Belg 1988;39(suppl 2):165.
82. McIntyre JWR. Monitoring regional anaesthesia. Int J Clin Monit Comput 1990;7:241.
83. Finucane BT. Regional anaesthesia: complications and techniques. Can J Anaesth 1991; 38:R3–10.
84. Douglas MJ. Potential complications of spinal and epidural anaesthesia for obstetrics. Semin Perinatol 1991;15:368–374.
85. Crosby ES, Reid D, Elliott RD. Obstetrical anaesthesia and analgesia in chronic spinal cord-injured women. Can J Anaesth 1992;39(5PE-1):487–494.
86. Harris AP, Michitsch RV. Anesthesia and analgesia for labor. Curr Opin Obstet Gynecol 1992;4:813.
87. Fox MAL, Webb RK, Singleton R, et al. Problems with regional anaesthesia: an analysis of 2000 incident reports. Anaesth Intensive Care 1993;21:646–649.
88. Peyton PJ. Complications of continuous spinal anaesthesia. Anaesth Intensive Care 1992;20:417–438.
89. Wong DHW. Regional anaesthesia for intraocular surgery. Can J Anaesth 1993;40:635.
90. Rubin AP. Complications of local anaesthesia for ophthalmic surgery. Br J Anaesth 1995;75:93–96.
91. Beers RA, Thomas S, Martin RJ, et al. Severe lumbar back pain following epidural injection of local anesthetic for epidural anesthesia. Reg Anesth 1995;20:69.
92. Liu S, Carpenter RL, Neal JM. Epidural anaesthesia, analgesia: their role in postoperative outcome. Anesthesiology 1995;82:1474–1506.
93. Goldman LJ. Complications in regional anaesthesia. Paediatr Anaesth 1995;5:3.
94. Rodiera J, Calabuig L, Aliaga W, et al. Mathematical analysis of epidural space location. Int J Clin Monit Comput 1995;12:213.
95. Eldor J, Alder D, Mahler Y, et al. Para-tracheal audible respiratory monitor (PTARM). Can J Anaesth 1987;34:329.
96. Giesbrecht GG. Human thermo regulatory inhibition by regional anesthesia. Anesthesiology 1994;81:277–281.
97. Ozaki M, Kurz A, Sessler DI, et al. Thermoregulatory thresholds during epidural and spinal anesthesia. Anesthesiology 1994;81:282–288.
98. Joris J, Ozaki M, Sessler DI, et al. Epidural anesthesia impairs both central and peripheral thermoregulatory control during general anesthesia. Anesthesiology 1994; 80:268–277.
99. Vasilieff N, Rosencher N, Sessler DI. Shivering thresholds during spinal anesthesia is reduced in elderly patients. Anesthesiology 1995;83:1162–1166.
100. Ralston AC, Webb RK, Runciman WB. Potential errors in pulse oximetry. I. Pulse oximeter evaluation. Anaesthesia 1991;46:202–206.
101. Webb RK, Ralston AC, Runciman WB. Potential errors in pulse oximetry. II. Effects of change in saturation and signal quality. Anaesthesia 1991;46:207–212.

102. Ralston AC, Webb RK, Runciman WB. Potential errors in pulse oximetry. III. Effects of interference, dyes, dyshaemoglobins and other pigments. Anaesthesia 1991;46:291–295.
103. Clayton DG, Webb RK, Ralston AC, et al. A comparison of the performance of 20 pulse oximeters under conditions of poor perfusion. Anaesthesia 1991;46:3–10.
104. Clayton DG, Webb RK, Ralston AC, et al. Pulse oximeter probes. A comparison between finger, nose, ear and forehead probes under conditions of poor perfusion. Anaesthesia 1991;46:260–265.
105. Runciman RB, Webb RK, Barker L. The pulse oximeter: applications and limitations – an analysis of 2000 incident reports. Anaesth Intensive Care 1993;21:543–550.
106. Hutton P, Clutton-Brock T. The benefits and pitfalls of pulse oximetry. Br Med J 1993; 307:457.
107. Tremper KK. Interpretation of non-invasive oxygen and carbon dioxide data. Can J Anaesth 1990;37:SIxxvii–SIxxxii.
108. Peduto VA, Tani R, Pani S. Pulse oximetry during lumbar epidural anaesthesia: reliability of values measured at the hand and foot. Anesth Analg 1994;78:921–924.
109. Stock MC. Noninvasive carbon dioxide monitoring. Crit Care Clin 1988;4:511.
110. Paulus DA. Capnography. Int Anesthesiol Clin 1989;27:167–175.
111. Williamson JA, Webb RK, Cockings J, et al. The capnograph: applications and limitations – an analysis of 2000 incident reports. Anaesth Intensive Care 1993;21: 551–557.
112. Campbell FA, McLeod ME, Bissonette B, et al. End-tidal carbon dioxide measurement in infants and children during and after general anaesthesia. Can J Anaesth 1994; 41:107–110.
113. Urmey WF. Accuracy of expired carbon dioxide partial pressure sampled from a nasal cannula. Anesthesiology 1988;68:961.
114. Goldman JM. Accuracy of expired carbon dioxide partial pressure sampled from a nasal cannula. Anesthesiology 1988;68:961.
115. Dunphy JA. Accuracy of expired carbon dioxide sampled from a nasal cannula. Anesthesiology 1988;67:960–961.
116. Barton CW, Wang ESJ. Correlation of end-tidal $CO_2$ measurements to arterial $Pa{CO_2}$ in nonintubated patients. Ann Emerg Med 1994;23:560–563.
117. Tobias JD, Flanagan JFK, Vuheeler TJ, et al. Noninvasive monitoring of end tidal $CO_2$ via nasal cannulas in spontaneously breathing children during the perioperative period. Crit Care Med 1994;22:1805.
118. Flanagan JFK, Garrett JS, McDuffee A, et al. Noninvasive monitoring of end tidal carbon dioxide tension via nasal cannulas in spontaneously breathing children with profound hypocarbia. Crit Care Med 1995;23:1140–1142.
119. Abramo TJ, Cowman MR, Scott SM, et al. Comparison of pediatric end-tidal $CO_2$ measured with nasal/oral cannula circuit and capillary $P{CO_2}$. Am J Emerg Med 1995; 13:30.
120. Oberg B, Waldau T, Larsen VH. The effect of nasal oxygen flow and catheter position on the accuracy of end-tidal carbon dioxide measurements by a pharyngeal catheter in unintubated, spontaneously breathing subjects. Anaesthesia 1995;50:695–698.
121. Amin HM, Cigado M, Fordyce WE, et al. Noninvasive monitoring of respiratory volume. Anaesthesia 1993;48:608–610.
122. Drummond GB. Breath monitoring device. Anaesthesia 1994;49:352–353.
123. Van Bergen FH. Comparison of indirect and direct methods of measuring arterial blood pressure. Circulation 1954;10:481.
124. Rutten AJ, Ilsley AH, Skowronski GA, et al. A comparative study of the measurement of mean arterial blood pressure using automatic oscillations, arterial cannulation, and palpation. Anaesth Intensive Care 1986;14:58–65.
125. Bruner JM, Krenis LJ, Kunsman JM, et al. Comparison of direct and indirect methods of measuring arterial blood pressure. Part I. Med Instrum 1981;15:11–21.
126. Bruner JM, Krenis IJ, Kunsman JM, et al. Comparison of direct and indirect methods of measuring arterial blood pressure. Part II. Med Instrum 1981;15:97.
127. Cohn JN. Blood pressure measurement in shock. Mechanisms of inaccuracy in ausculatory and palpatory methods. JAMA 1967;199:118–122.
128. Ramsey M III. Noninvasive automatic determination of mean arterial pressure. Med Biol Eng 1979;17:11.

129. Yelderman M, Ream AK. Indirect measurement of mean blood pressure in anesthetised patients. Anesthesiology 1979;50:253–256.
130. Hutton P, Dye J, Prys-Roberts C. An assessment of the Dynamap 845. Anaesthesia 1984;39:261.
131. Borow KM, Newburger JW. Noninvasive estimation of central aortic pressure using the oscillometric method for analysing systemic arterial pulsatile flow. Am Heart J 1982;103:879.
132. Hystrom E, Reid KH, Bennett R, et al. A comparison of two automated indirect blood pressure meters: with recordings from a radial artery catheter in anaesthetised surgical patients. Anesthesiology 1985;62:526–530.
133. Runciman WB, Ludbrook GL. Monitoring. In: Nimmo WS, Rowbotham DJ, Smith G, eds. Anaesthesia. 2nd ed. Cambridge, MA: Blackwell Science; 1994:711.
134. Kurki T, Smith NT, Head N, et al. Noninvasive continuous blood pressure measurement from the finger: optimal measurement conditions and factors affecting reliability. J Clin Monit 1987;3:6.
135. Jones RDM, Kornberg JP, Roulson CJ, et al. The Finapres 2300e finger cuff. The influence of cuff application on the accuracy of blood pressure measurement. Anaesthesia 1994;48:611.
136. Wilkes MP, Bennett A, Hall P, et al. Comparison of invasive and non-invasive measurement of continuous arterial pressure using the Finapres in patients undergoing spinal anaesthesia for lower segment caesarean section. Br J Anaesth 1994;73:738–743.
137. Lake CL, ed. Clinical Monitoring for Anesthesia and Critical Care. 2nd ed. Philadelphia, PA: WB Saunders; 1994:106.
138. Mackenzie R, Asbury AJ. Clinical evaluation of liquid crystal skin thermometers. Br J Anaesth 1994;72:246–249.
139. Myles PS, Williams NJ, Powell J. Predicting outcome in anaesthesia: understanding statistical methods. Anaesth Intensive Care 1994;22:447.
140. Byrick RJ, Cohen MM. Technology assessment of anaesthesia monitors: problems and future directions. Can J Anaesth 1995;42:224.
141. Roizen MF, Toledano A. Technology assessment and the “learning contamination” bias. Anesth Analg 1994;79:410–412.
142. Fryback DG, Thornbury DR. The efficacy of diagnostic imaging. Med Decis Making 1991;11:88–94.
143. Drummond GB. Influence of thiopentone on upper airway muscles. Br J Anaesth 1989; 63:12–21.
144. Montravers P, Diureuil B, Desmonts JM. Effects of IV midazolam on upper airway resistance. Br J Anaesth 1992;68:27–31.
145. Nishino T, Kochi T. Effects of sedation produced by thiopentone on responses to nasal occlusion in female adults. Br J Anaesth 1993;71:388–392.
146. Abboud TK, Khoo SS, Miller F, et al. Maternal, fetal, and neonatal responses after epidural anesthesia with bupivacaine, 2-chloroprocaine or lidocaine. Anesth Analg 1982;61:638–644.
147. Kuhnert BR, Harrison MJ, Lin PL, et al. Effects of maternal epidural anesthesia on neonatal behaviour. Anesth Analg 1984;63:301–308.
148. Wiener PC, Hogg MI, Rosen M. Neonatal respiration, feeding and neurobehavioural state – effect of intrapartum bupivacaine, pethidine and pethidine reversed by naloxone. Anaesthesia 1979;34:996–1004.
149. Van Dorsten JJP, Miller FC. Fetal heart rate change after accidental intrauterine lidocaine. Obstet Gynecol 1981;57:257–260.
150. Garner L, Stirt JA, Finholt DA. Heart block after intravenous lidocaine in an infant. Can J Anaesth 1985;32:425.
151. Wood CE, Goresky GV, Klassen KA, et al. Complications of continuous epidural infusions for postoperative analgesia in children. Can J Anaesth 1994;41:613.
152. Bougher RJ, Ramage D. Spinal subdural haematoma following combined spinal epidural anaesthesia. Anaesth Intensive Care 1995;23:111.
153. Tarkkila P, Huhtala J, Tuominen M. Transient radicular irritation after spinal anaesthesia with hyperbaric 5% lignocaine. Br J Anaesth 1995;74:328–329.
154. Horlocker TT, Cabanela ME, Wedel DJ. Does postoperative epidural analgesia increase the risk of peroneal nerve palsy after total knee arthroplasty? Anesth Analg 1994; 79:495–500.

155. Mills GH, Howell SJL, Richmond MN. Spinal cord compression immediately following but unrelated to, epidural analgesia. Anaesthesia 1994;49:954.
156. Murthy BV, Fogarty DJ, Fitzpatrick K, Brady MM. Headache during epidural top-ups in labour—a sign of reduced intracranial compliance. Anaesth Intensive Care 1995;23: 744–746.
157. Haggard HW. The place of the anesthetist in American medicine. Anesthesiology 1940;1:1.
158. Slogoff S, Hughes FP, Hug CC, et al. A demonstration of validity for certification by the American Board of Anesthesiology. Acad Med 1994;69:740–746.
159. Duncan PG, Cohen MM, Yip R. Clinical experiences associated with anesthesia training. Ann RCPSC 1993;26:363.
160. Burt DER. Virtual reality in anaesthesia. Br J Anaesth 1995;75:472–480.
161. Sivarajan M, Miller E, Hardy C, et al. Objective evaluation of clinical performance and correlation with knowledge. Anesth Analg 1984;63:603–607.
162. Rosse C. The potential of computerized representations of anatomy in the training of health care providers. Acad Med 1995;70:499.
163. Kestin IG. A statistical approach to measuring the competence of anaesthetic trainees at practical procedures. Br J Anaesth 1995;75:805–809.
164. Ellis FR. Measurement of competence. Br J Anaesth 1995;75:673–674.
165. Sagan SD. The Limits of Safety. Princeton, NJ: Princeton University Press; 1993:46.
166. Rudge BA. Decision-making in anaesthesia. Anaesth Intensive Care 1995;23:597.
167. Eichhorn JH, Cooper JB, Cullen DJ, et al. Standards for patient monitoring during anesthesia at Harvard Medical School. JAMA 1986;256:1017.
168. Guidelines to the practice of anaesthesia as recommended by the Canadian Anesthesiologists Society. Can J Anaesth 1996;43(3 suppl 2).
169. Battista RN, Hodge MJ. Clinical practice guidelines: between science and art. Can Med Assoc J 1993;148:385.
170. Carter AO, Battista RN, Hodge MJ, et al. Report on activities and attitudes of organizations active in the clinical practice guidelines field. Can Med Assoc J 1995;153:901.
171. Lomas J. Words without action? The production, dissemination, and impact of consensus recommendations. Annu Rev Public Health 1991;12:41–65.

# 2 Outcome Studies Comparing Regional and General Anesthesia

Gabriella Iohom and George Shorten

## Outcome Measures

Substantial increase in healthcare costs has contributed to the development of outcomes research in the United States. Outcomes research evaluates the effectiveness of healthcare interventions in many aspects of patient care (clinical outcomes, functional health status, patient satisfaction, health-related quality of life) and reflects national trends in determining appropriateness, value, and quality of health care.[1] Outcomes research in regional anesthesia has traditionally focused on clinically oriented outcomes, such as overall mortality and major morbidity (cardiovascular, pulmonary, coagulation, cognitive, gastrointestinal, immune, stress response).[2] This chapter examines the currently available evidence comparing regional and general anesthesia in terms of clinically oriented outcomes.

Although postoperative pain per se is neither a traditional outcome measure nor an independent predictor of duration of hospital stay, inadequate control of postoperative pain is an important cause of readmission after ambulatory surgery.[3] Because pain is often the predominant symptom of the postoperative period, it can be considered an important outcome of surgery. Patients relate improved pain control to improved postoperative outcome.[4] Therefore, the role of regional anesthesia and analgesia as part of multimodal analgesic regimens is also considered.

## Challenges of Data Interpretation

Although the worth of data from prospective randomized, controlled studies (RCTs) and metaanalyses is well established, there are inherent difficulties complicating their interpretation.

Prospective RCTs are the "gold standard" in evaluating the effect of an intervention on patient outcomes. Significant drawbacks include the cost, time, and need for large sample sizes when evaluating rare outcomes.[5] For example, a sample size of 24,000 patients would be needed to determine if regional anesthesia would decrease the overall mortality after a specific procedure by 50% (power 80%) when compared with that from general anesthesia.[6] Although multicenter trials are possible, protocol deviation and institutional differences may affect the results.[7] Other disadvantages include ethical concerns and less external validity ("generalizability" of the findings of a study).[5] In addition, RCTs comparing regional with general anesthesia are necessarily unblinded (with very few exceptions), allowing for the introduction of bias.[2] Other methodologic issues with studies examining outcome after regional anesthesia include the use of surrogate end points, inappropriate selection of postoperative analgesic regimens, and inadequate assessment of pain.[2]

Metaanalysis using strict criteria for the inclusion of studies and appropriate statistical methods is a valuable means of drawing meaningful conclusions from studies with similar objectives. One of its disadvantages is that conclusions are based on data derived from studies that may vary widely in design, subject population (sample), and selected outcomes.[8] Small differences in one of several factors may affect whether a trial meets the inclusion criteria, and thus potentially alter the conclusions of the metaanalysis.[9] Metaanalyses may also contain publication biases (inclusion of older outdated studies, exclusion of non-English language trials, and the initial failure to publish negative results).[10] These factors tend to increase the likelihood of demonstrating an effect of treatment.

Patient management has changed considerably over the last two decades, making some alleged benefits of regional anesthesia less impressive. For instance, low-molecular-weight heparins, used routinely for thromboprophylaxis in patients undergoing hip and knee surgery, have considerably decreased the incidence of deep venous thrombosis.[11] This tends to make the earlier described benefits of epidural analgesia less relevant in current practice. Similarly, a number of RCTs support the perioperative use of β-blockers to reduce the morbidity and mortality associated with noncardiac surgery in patients at risk for cardiac complications.[12] In addition, laboratory tests or radiologic investigations used to diagnose certain complications have changed (plasma concentration of troponin Ic for the diagnosis of postoperative myocardial infarction (PMI) or computed tomography for identifying pulmonary atelectasis), making the results of some earlier studies unreliable.[4]

In view of the above, the analysis and conclusions of metaanalyses must be interpreted carefully.

Reliable and valid conclusions about therapies in controversial areas of clinical practice require not only that systematic reviews or metaanalyses indicate the likely sizes of effects of such therapies, but also that the findings be independently confirmed in at least one, and preferably more, high-quality RCT.[13] Ideally, findings of metaanalyses should be confirmed by large RCTs to examine the effects of regional anesthesia on outcome. There are many specific reasons to explain why conclusions from metaanalyses may not correlate with those from subsequent large-scale RCTs.[9] These include problems inherent in the study design and problems in execution.[14]

## Neuraxial Blockade

Blockade of afferent neural stimuli from the surgical area by local infiltration, peripheral nerve blocks, or neuraxial (spinal and epidural) blockade decreases the endocrine-metabolic response after major surgery. These effects are further enhanced if the blockade is maintained postoperatively.[15]

Hypothesis: That epidural anesthesia and analgesia is preferable in high-risk patients undergoing major surgery, because it can attenuate the neurohumoral stress response to surgery,[16] improve cardiorespiratory function postoperatively, and decrease the incidence and/or severity of complications.

Several small RCTs support this hypothesis,[17–19] but none had sufficient power to convincingly establish a benefit in postoperative outcome.

### *Reviews (Metaanalyses and Systematic Reviews)*

In a metaanalysis of data from 141 RCTs available before January 1, 1997 including 9559 patients (Table 2-1), Rodgers et al.[20] showed that the use of epidural or spinal

TABLE 2-1. Metaanalyses

| Author | Year | Setting | Intervention (groups) | Outcome | Result |
|---|---|---|---|---|---|
| Rodgers et al.[20] | 2000 | All types of surgery | Neuraxial blockade ± GA versus GA | Overall 30-day mortality | Neuraxial blockade superior (OR, 0.70; 95% CI, 0.54–0.90 |
| | | | | DVT | Neuraxial superior (OR decreased by 44%) |
| | | | | Pulmonary embolism | Neuraxial superior (OR decreases by 55%) |
| | | | | Transfusion requirements | Neuraxial superior (OR decreased by 50%) |
| | | | | Pneumonia | Neuraxial superior (OR decreased by 39%) |
| | | | | Respiratory depression | Neuraxial superior (OR decreased by 59%) |
| Urwin et al.[21] | 2000 | Hip fracture surgery | Neuraxial blockade versus GA | 30-day mortality | Neuraxial superior (OR, 0.66; 95% CI, 0.47–0.96) |
| | | | | DVT | Neuraxial superior (OR, 0.41; 95% CI, 0.23–0.72) |
| Parker et al.[22] | 2004 | Hip fracture surgery | Neuraxial blockade versus GA | 30-day mortality | Neuraxial superior (RR, 0.69; 95% CI, 0.71–1.21) |
| | | | | Postoperative confusion | Neuraxial superior (RR, 0.50; 95% CI, 0.26–0.95) |
| Liu et al.[23] | 2004 | Coronary artery bypass surgery | Central neuraxial blockade (thoracic epidural, intrathecal) + GA versus GA | Dysrhythmias | Thoracic epidural superior (OR, 0.52) |
| | | | | Pulmonary complications | Thoracic epidural superior (OR, 0.41) |
| | | | | Time to tracheal extubation | Thoracic epidural superior |
| | | | | Pain VAS scores at rest and with activity | Thoracic epidural superior |
| Ballantyne et al.[24] | 1998 | Abdominal and thoracic surgery | Postoperative epidural opioids and local anesthetics versus systemic opioids | Atelectasis | Epidural opioids superior (RR, 0.54; 95% CI, 0.33–0.85) |
| | | | | Pulmonary infections | Epidural local anesthetics superior (RR, 0.36; 95% CI, 0.21–0.65) |
| | | | | Overall pulmonary complications | Epidural local anesthetics superior (RR, 0.58; 95% CI, 0.42–0.80) |
| Beattie et al.[25] | 2001 | Abdominal, aortic, peripheral vascular surgery | Postoperative epidural analgesia >24 hours | Postoperative analgesia | Epidural superior |
| | | | | Postoperative MI | TEA superior (rate difference, –5.3%; 95% CI, –9.9%, –0.7%) |
| Block[26] | 2003 | All types of surgery | Postoperative epidural analgesia versus systemic opioids | Postoperative analgesia | Epidural superior on each postoperative day |

GA, general anesthesia; DVT, deep vein thrombosis; MI, myocardial infarction; VAS, visual analog scale.

block (with or without general anesthesia) resulted in a 30% reduction ($P = .006$) in the overall 30-day mortality after surgery [odds ratio (OR), 0.70; 95% confidence interval (CI), 0.54–0.90]. Furthermore, neuraxial blockade reduced the odds of deep vein thrombosis by 44%, pulmonary embolism by 55%, transfusion requirements by 50%, pneumonia by 39%, and respiratory depression by 59% (all $P < .001$). There were also reductions in the incidence of perioperative myocardial infarction and renal failure. Although the authors acknowledge the limited power to assess subgroup effects, they conclude that the proportional reductions in mortality did not differ by surgical group, type of neuraxial blockade (spinal or epidural), or in those trials in which neuraxial blockade was combined with general anesthesia compared with trials in which neuraxial blockade was used alone.[20] Thus, it seemed that the benefits were principally attributable to the use of neuraxial blockade, and the technique by which this was achieved was less relevant.

This metaanalysis has been criticized on the following grounds: the management of postoperative patients had changed over the preceding 20 years (i.e., thromboprophylaxis after hip and knee surgery), making some alleged benefits of regional anesthesia less impressive; regional anesthesia only improved mortality in patients undergoing orthopedic surgery and had no effect in patients undergoing general, urologic, and vascular surgery (because more than half the trials with at least 10 deaths per trial involved patients with hip fracture, thus enhancing the contribution of the findings of these trials to the overall result); although thoracic epidural and spinal analgesia significantly improved mortality, lumbar epidural analgesia was ineffective.[27]

Another metaanalysis of randomized trials regarding the effects of general versus regional anesthesia on outcome after hip fracture surgery was published in 2000.[21] Fifteen trials comprising a total of 2162 patients with hip fractures were included. A lesser 30-day mortality was reported in the regional anesthesia group (6.4% versus 9.4%; OR, 0.66; 95% CI, 0.47–0.96), but this advantage did not extend to 3 months or beyond. In addition, neuraxial blockade was associated with a decrease in deep vein thrombosis (30.2% versus 46.9% in the regional and general anesthesia group, respectively; OR, 0.41; 95% CI, 0.23–0.72). These results were mostly derived from trials that had used routine venography. No such difference was identified for incidence of pulmonary embolism (OR, 0.84; 95% CI, 0.33–2.13), need for transfusion (OR, 1.02; 95% CI, 0.58–1.80), or incidence of pneumonia (OR, 0.92; 95% CI, 0.53–1.59). However, the incidence of fatal pulmonary embolism was less in patients who had undergone regional anesthesia. Although these latter results represent a subgroup analysis, they support the contention that regional anesthesia may have a protective effect against major thromboembolism. It is recognized that routine use of thromboembolism prophylaxis (mentioned in only three studies) might negate such a benefit.

This metaanalysis was recently updated to include newly available data.[22] Twenty-two trials comprising a total of 2567 predominantly female and elderly patients were included. Although all trials had methodologic flaws and many did not reflect current anesthetic practice, pooled results from eight trials showed regional anesthesia to be associated with a lesser 30-day mortality (6.9% versus 10.0%). However, this was of borderline statistical significance (relative risk, 0.69; 95% CI, 0.71–1.21). In fact, removal of data from an early study (McLaren 1978) with an unusually high mortality rate in the general anesthesia group (28%) resulted in a statistically nonsignificant difference in mortality at 1 month (relative risk, 0.79; 95% CI, 0.56–1.12). The decrease in the incidence of deep venous thrombosis (30% versus 47% in the regional versus general anesthesia group; relative risk, 0.64; 95% CI, 0.48–0.86) was considered insecure because of possible selection bias in the subgroup in whom this outcome was measured.[22] Interestingly, but not unexpectedly, regional anesthesia was associated with a lesser risk of postoperative confusion (9.4% versus 19.2%; relative risk, 0.50; 95% CI, 0.26–0.95). The authors concluded that overall, there was insufficient evidence available from trials comparing regional versus general anesthesia to rule out clinically important differences.[22]

A recent systematic review of data from 24 published trials including a number of patients ranging from 30 to 9598 addressed the effect of intraoperative neuraxial anesthesia versus general anesthesia on postoperative cognitive dysfunction (POCD) and delirium.[28] The authors concluded that, in the presence of methodologic and study-design issues related to the unelucidated pathophysiology of POCD, the use of intraoperative neuraxial anesthesia does not seem to decrease the incidence of POCD when compared with general anesthesia.[28]

In 2004, a metaanalysis of 15 trials (comprising 1178 patients) examined the effects of perioperative central neuraxial blockade on outcome after coronary artery bypass surgery.[23] Outcomes were compared in patients randomized to general anesthesia versus general anesthesia – thoracic epidural analgesia (TEA) or general anesthesia – intrathecal analgesia. TEA did not affect incidences of mortality or myocardial infarction. TEA significantly reduced the risk of dysrhythmias (OR, 0.52), pulmonary complications (OR, 0.41), time to tracheal extubation by 4.5 hours, and visual analog pain scores at rest and with activity (by 7.8 and 11.6mm, respectively). It had no significant effect on incidences of mortality, myocardial infarction, dysrhythmias, nausea/vomiting, or time to tracheal extubation. It decreased systemic morphine consumption by 11mg and visual analog scale pain scores by 16mm.

The authors concluded that, although no differences in the rates of mortality or myocardial infarction were observed, central neuraxial analgesia for coronary artery bypass grafting was associated with shorter intervals to tracheal extubation, fewer pulmonary complications and cardiac dysrhythmias, and less pain postoperatively.[23]

A comprehensive, cumulative metaanalysis published in 1998 focused on comparative effects of postoperative analgesic therapies on pulmonary outcome.[24] Compared with systemic opioids, epidural opioids decreased the incidence of atelectasis [risk ratio (RR), 0.53; 95% CI, 0.33–0.85] and had a weak tendency to decrease the incidence of pulmonary infections and pulmonary complications overall. Epidural local anesthetics increased $Pao_2$ by 4.6mm Hg (95% CI, 0.06–9.08) and decreased the incidence of pulmonary infections (RR, 0.36; 95% CI, 0.21–0.65) and pulmonary complications overall (RR, 0.58; 95% CI, 0.42–0.80) compared with systemic opioids. There were no clinically or statistically significant differences in the surrogate measures of pulmonary function such as forced expiratory volume in 1 second, functional vital capacity, or peak expiratory flow rate. The authors concluded that clinical measures of pulmonary outcome (incidence of atelectasis, infection, and other complications) were significantly improved by epidural opioid and epidural local anesthetic treatments in the postoperative period.[24]

In 2001, a metaanalysis of 11 RCTs (comprising a total of 1173 patients) examined the effect of postoperative epidural analgesia continued for more than 24 hours on the incidence of PMI.[25] Postoperative epidural analgesia resulted in superior analgesia for the first 24 hours after surgery and was associated with a lesser incidence of PMI (rate difference, −3.8%; 95% CI, −7.4%, −0.2%; $P$ = .049). The incidences of in-hospital death (3.3%) were similar in the epidural and nonepidural groups. Of note, the proportion of patients taking β-blockers was identical in the two groups. The incidence of PMI in patients who received epidural analgesia via the thoracic route was less than in those who received systemic analgesia (rate difference, −5.3%; 95% CI, −9.9%, −0.7%; $P$ = .04). The authors concluded that, in high-risk cardiac patients, postoperative epidural analgesia is indicated.[25]

In 2003, a metaanalysis of 100 RCTs examined the efficacy of postoperative epidural analgesia in adults.[26] Weighted mean pain scores, weighted mean differences in pain score, and weighted incidences of complications were determined using a fixed-effect model. Epidural analgesia provided better overall postoperative analgesia compared with parenteral opioids ($P < .001$). Epidural analgesia was better than that achieved using parenteral opioids on each postoperative day ($P < .001$). In conclusion, epidural analgesia, regardless of analgesic agent, location of catheter placement, and type and time of pain assessment, provided superior postoperative analgesia compared with parenteral opioids.[26]

### *Recent, Large RCTs*

A multicenter, randomized, controlled, unblinded study conducted in 15 United States Veterans Affairs hospitals set out to determine the effects of intraoperative epidural anesthesia and postoperative epidural analgesia on outcome after major abdominal surgery (Table 2-2).[29] This study compared (1) general anesthesia intraoperatively plus parenteral opioids postoperatively with (2) epidural bupivacaine analgesia and light general anesthesia intraoperatively plus epidural morphine postoperatively in 1021 patients undergoing four types of surgery: intraabdominal aortic, gastric, biliary, or colonic surgery. The primary outcome was the combined end point of 30-day all-cause mortality, myocardial infarction, congestive heart failure, ventricular tachyarrhythmia, complete atrioventricular block, severe hypotension, cardiac arrest, pulmonary embolism, respiratory failure, stroke, and renal failure. The secondary outcomes were angina, respiratory depression, pneumonia, sepsis, gastrointestinal bleeding, epidural hematoma, and reoperation. Postoperative pain at

TABLE 2-2. Recent RCTs

| Author | Year | Setting | Intervention | Outcome | Result |
|---|---|---|---|---|---|
| Park et al.[29] | 2001 | Major abdominal surgery | Epidural LA analgesia + GA intraoperatively + epidural morphine postoperatively versus GA + parenteral opioids postoperatively | VAS pain score<br>30-day mortality<br>Duration of tracheal intubation and ICU stay | Epidural superior ($P \leq .03$ on the first, third, and seventh postoperative day<br>Epidural superior in abdominal aortic surgical patients (22% versus 37%, $P < .01$)<br>Epidural superior |
| Norris et al.[30] | 2001 | Abdominal aortic surgery | Thoracic epidural anesthesia + light GA or GA followed by epidural PCA postoperatively or morphine PCA (four treatment groups) | Time to extubation | Epidural PCA superior ($P = .002$) |
| Rigg and the MASTER group[31] | 2002 | High-risk patients undergoing major abdominal surgery or esophagectomy | Intraoperative epidural anesthesia with GA and postoperative epidural analgesia for 72 hours | Respiratory failure<br>VAS pain scores | Epidural superior (23% versus 30%, $P = .02$)<br>Epidural superior |
| Foss et al.[32] | 2005 | Hip fracture surgery | Continuous postoperative epidural analgesia with local anesthetics + opioids | Dynamic analgesia | Epidural superior |

VAS, visual analog scale; LA, local anesthetic; GA, general anesthesia.

rest, physical mobilization, and durations of intensive care unit (ICU) and hospital stay were also evaluated.

The two groups were similar in terms of the frequencies of primary or secondary outcomes, the average postoperative physical performance scores, and durations of ICU or hospital stays. Visual analog pain scores were lesser in the epidural group ($P \leq .03$) on the first, third, and seventh postoperative day. For abdominal aortic surgical patients, the incidence of primary end points was less in the epidural group (22% versus 37%, $P < .01$). This difference stemmed from differences in the incidence of new myocardial infarction, stroke, and respiratory failure. In the epidural group, the duration of tracheal intubation was 13 hours shorter, which translated into a 3.5 hours shorter ICU stay. The authors concluded that the effect of anesthetic and postoperative analgesic techniques on perioperative outcome varies with the type of operation performed. Overall, epidural analgesia provides better postoperative pain relief. In addition, epidural anesthesia and analgesia improves the overall outcome and shortens the intubation time and intensive care stay in patients undergoing abdominal aortic operations.[29] Critics of this study have argued that in addition to being underpowered (to demonstrate a reduction in major morbidity and mortality up to 30 days postoperatively), the intervention may not have been adequate.[33] This study used intraoperative lumbar or thoracic epidural local anesthetic without opioids for abdominal surgery followed by postoperative analgesia with epidural opioids alone. As we have pointed out, two metaanalyses demonstrated that only thoracic, and not lumbar, epidural analgesia decreases the incidence of mortality[20] or perioperative myocardial infarction.[25] In addition, it seems that an epidural local anesthetic is essential to improve pulmonary, cardiac, and gastrointestinal outcome. Epidurally administered local anesthetics, but not opioids, produce their beneficial effects in pulmonary outcome by promoting the postoperative recovery of diaphragmatic contractility.[14]

A prospective, double-blind, randomized clinical trial was designed to compare four combinations of intraoperative anesthesia and postoperative analgesia with respect to postoperative outcomes in patients undergoing surgery of the abdominal aorta.[30] One hundred sixty-eight patients were randomly assigned to receive either thoracic epidural anesthesia plus a light general anesthesia or general anesthesia alone intraoperatively combined with either intravenous or epidural patient-controlled analgesia (PCA) postoperatively (four treatment groups). PCA was continued for at least 72 hours. Duration of hospital stay and direct medical costs for patients surviving to discharge were similar among the four treatment groups. Postoperative outcomes were similar among the four treatment groups with respect to death, myocardial infarction, myocardial ischemia, reoperation, pneumonia, and renal failure. The only difference observed was a shorter time to extubation ($P = .002$) in the epidural PCA group. Times to ICU discharge, ward admission, first bowel sounds, first flatus, tolerance of clear liquid intake, tolerance of regular diet, and independent ambulation were similar among the four treatment groups. Postoperative pain scores were also similar among the treatment groups.

This study concluded that in patients undergoing surgery of the abdominal aorta, thoracic epidural anesthesia combined with a light general anesthesia and followed by either intravenous or epidural PCA offers no major advantage over general anesthesia alone followed by either intravenous or epidural PCA.[30]

An important limitation of this trial is that generalization of the conclusion, beyond the very select patient population studied and the very specific anesthetic and analgesic regimens used, may not be possible. When used for postoperative pain control after aortic aneurysm repair, epidural techniques may yield outcome benefits provided that (1) adequate concentrations are used, and (2) the infusion rates are adjusted swiftly, with boli where needed, to respond to individual patient and changing antinociceptive needs.[34] Other authors caution against the "overstated" conclusions of Norris et al. and the more general interpretation that epidural anesthesia – analgesia is not beneficial.[35] The lack of a rigorous recovery protocol, use of opioids in all patients, and selection of an insensitive primary outcome measure (duration of hospital stay) may have contributed to the negative findings of this study.

The Multicentre Australian Study of Epidural Anaesthesia (the MASTER Anaesthesia Trial) was designed to have adequate power to test the proposed beneficial effect of epidural techniques,[17] while allowing for a smaller difference observed as a result of improvements in perioperative management that have occurred since 1987.[31] The RCT by Yeager et al.[17] conducted in the mid-1980s, comparing general anesthesia with or without perioperative epidural anesthesia and analgesia in high-risk patients undergoing major surgery, was stopped for ethical reasons after 53 patients had been studied, because of the impressive improvement in mortality and morbidity observed in patients who received epidurals. The MASTER trial targeted the highest-risk patients (with one or more of the following comorbidities: morbid obesity, diabetes mellitus, chronic renal failure, respiratory insufficiency, cardiac failure, acute myocardial infarction, exertional angina, myocardial ischemia, severe hepatocellular disease, age >75 years plus at least two criteria) undergoing major abdominal operations or esophagectomy. The authors argued that this combination of high-risk patients and high-risk procedures defines an area of practice in which major perioperative complications are concentrated and consequently maximizes the power of a study of given size.[36] Nine hundred fifteen patients were randomly allocated to receive either intraoperative epidural anesthesia (site selected to provide optimum block) with general anesthesia and postoperative epidural analgesia for 72 hours or control (general anesthesia and postoperative systemic opioids for analgesia). The primary end points were death at 30 days or major postsurgical morbidity.

There was no difference in the 30-day mortality rate between groups, and only one of eight categories of morbid end points in individual systems (respiratory failure; 23% versus 30%, $P = .02$) occurred less frequently in patients managed with epidural techniques. However, postoperative epidural analgesia was associated with lesser pain scores during the first three postoperative days, despite most participants in the control group receiving multimodal analgesia.

The authors concluded that most major postoperative complications in high-risk patients undergoing major abdominal surgery are not decreased by the use of combined epidural and general anesthesia combined with postoperative epidural analgesia.[31] However, they advocate the use of combined general and epidural anesthesia intraoperatively with continuing postoperative epidural analgesia in high-risk patients undergoing major intraabdominal surgery, based on improvement in analgesia, and the decrease in incidence of respiratory failure.

A subsequent subgroup analysis of the data from the MASTER trial, published in 2003, identified no difference in outcome between epidural and control groups in patients at increased risk of respiratory or cardiac complications or undergoing aortic surgery, nor in a subgroup with failed epidural block.[37] There was a small reduction in the duration of postoperative ventilation in the epidural group compared with controls ($P = .048$). No differences were found in duration of intensive care or hospital stay. Perioperative epidural analgesia did not influence the incidence of serious morbidity or mortality after major abdominal surgery.[37]

It seems that this study lacked adequate sample size and power to demonstrate a difference in overall mortality or cardiac morbidity between epidural and systemic treatments. Mortality at 30 days was low in both groups (epidural 5.1% versus control 4.3%). It is conceivable that the true benefit associated with the use of epidural techniques is 3.6%, as observed in this study (57.1% of patients in the epidural group and 60.7% in the control group had at least one morbidity end point or died, $P = .29$). A trial of 6000 patients at high risk would be required to give an 80% chance of declaring statistically significant an absolute difference of 3.6% in the rate of death or major complications.[36] Similarly, to demonstrate a 30% reduction in the incidence of myocardial infarction, as suggested by Rodgers et al.,[20] a study with a 5% type I error rate and 80% power would require at least 9500 patients. Nearly 50% of patients in the epidural group were not fully compliant with the study protocol and thoracic epidural – previously shown to decrease the incidence of mortality and perioperative myocardial infarction – was not mandatory.[33]

More recently, a randomized, double-blind, placebo-controlled trial looked at the effect of postoperative epidural analgesia on rehabilitation and pain after hip fracture surgery.[32] Sixty elderly patients were randomly allocated to receive either 4 days of continuous postoperative epidural infusion of 4mL/hour bupivacaine 0.125% plus 50μg/mL morphine or placebo. Both groups received balanced analgesia and intravenous nurse-controlled analgesia with morphine. Patients followed a multimodal rehabilitation program. Postoperative epidural analgesia provided superior dynamic analgesia without motor dysfunction compared with placebo. However, under the conditions of this study, superior analgesia did not translate into enhanced rehabilitation.[32]

## *Alternatives to RCT*

In 2000, O'Hara et al.[38] published a retrospective cohort study of 9425 consecutive patients with hip fracture, aged >60 years, who underwent surgical repair at one of 20 study hospitals between 1983 and 1993. They demonstrated that older and more ill patients were more likely to receive regional anesthesia. The 30-day mortality rate in the general anesthesia group was 4.4% compared with 5.4% in the regional anesthesia group (unadjusted OR, 0.80; 95% CI, 0.66–0.97). After controlling for differences in patient characteristics, the authors found no association between type of anesthesia and mortality or morbidity. Their findings suggest that unadjusted differences in outcome between regional and general anesthesia are mainly a result of comorbidities, and not of a protective effect of one anesthetic technique.[38]

In 2003, Wu et al.[39] offered an extensive database analysis (study of effectiveness) as an alternative to an RCT (study of efficacy) in which large numbers would be needed to examine the effect of postoperative epidural analgesia on morbidity and mortality after total hip replacement surgery. From a 5% nationally random sample of Medicare claims from 1994 to 1999, 23,136 patients who underwent total hip arthroplasty were identified (of whom 2591 had and 20,545 had not received postoperative epidural analgesia). The unadjusted 7- and 30-day mortality rates were less for patients who had received epidural analgesia (1.9/1000 versus 3.9/1000, $P = .04$ at 7 days and 5.8/1000 versus 9.9/1000, $P = .01$ at 30 days). However, multivariate regression analysis revealed no difference between groups with regard to mortality or major morbidity with the exception of an increase in deep venous thrombosis in patients who received epidural analgesia. Although this is one of the largest data sets to date to examine this issue, the results should be interpreted with caution because of limitations in using such databases. The authors warn that insertion of a postoperative epidural catheter per se does not confer improved patient outcome; benefit may only occur with appropriate utilization of the epidural catheter.[39]

In summary, it seems that results from recent metaanalyses are not substantiated by subsequent large RCTs. Metaanalyses suggested advantages of (1) intraoperative neuraxial blocks such as lower 30-day mortality and less deep venous thrombosis in orthopedic patients,[20,21] less transfusion requirement, and fewer incidences of pulmonary embolism, pneumonia, respiratory depression, myocardial infarction, and renal failure,[20] fewer dysrhythmia, pulmonary complications, and better analgesia associated with the use of thoracic epidural anesthesia,[23] and (2) postoperative neuraxial blockade is associated with fewer pulmonary complications (atelectasis and infection),[24] fewer PMIs[25] (in the case of TEA), and overall better pain scores.[25,26]

Of these, RCTs support the contention that perioperative epidural techniques are associated with fewer incidences of respiratory failure in high-risk patients undergoing major abdominal surgery,[31] with a decrease in the incidence of 30-day mortality, respiratory failure, PMI, and stroke in patients undergoing abdominal aortic surgery,[29] and superior analgesia.[29,31,32]

## Peripheral Nerve Blocks

Despite superior analgesia and possible physiologic benefits provided by peripheral nerve blocks, there is no large-scale RCT that has examined the efficacy of these techniques in decreasing perioperative mortality or morbidity in surgical patients. However, a number of individual studies have independently shown that better pain management through peripheral regional blocks may improve the functional result of surgery and shorten the duration of rehabilitation, resulting in economic benefit.

Capdevila et al.[40] tested the hypothesis that postoperative analgesic techniques influence surgical outcome and the duration of convalescence after major knee surgery. They demonstrated that regional analgesic techniques (continuous femoral block or continuous epidural infusion) improved rehabilitation after major knee surgery by effectively controlling pain during continuous passive motion in the postoperative period.[40]

Similarly, Chelly et al.[41] examined the effects of continuous femoral infusion of local anesthetic on recovery after total knee arthroplasty. Ninety-two patients were randomly assigned to receive general anesthesia (1) alone followed by PCA with morphine, (2) plus 3-in-1 and sciatic blocks followed by continuous femoral infusions of local anesthetic, or (3) plus epidural analgesia with local anesthetic followed by a continuous epidural infusion of local anesthetic and opioid. Blocks decreased postoperative morphine requirements by 74% and 35% compared with PCA and epidurals ($P < .05$) and provided superior recovery. The use of blocks was associated with a reduction of postoperative bleeding and allowed better performance on continuous passive motion, which translated into a 2-day decrease in the duration of hospitalization. Also, it was associated with a 90% decrease in the total incidence of postoperative serious complications (including hypoxia and mental changes, hypotension, deep venous thrombosis, myocardial infarction, cerebrovascular accident, atelectasis, upper gastrointestinal bleed).[41]

## Current Opinion

Given the difficulty of proving efficacy relating to rare adverse outcomes and of evaluating the role of one factor among many in the perioperative period, our inability to document a “global” superiority of regional techniques should not detract from their clinical use. Nor should they impede further clinical research to establish the relationship between these techniques and important health outcomes.

Future studies evaluating the potential benefits of regional anesthesia and analgesia techniques should use a multimodal approach with aggressive postoperative rehabilitation. In addition, such studies should focus on patient-meaningful and resource outcomes, rather than the occurrence of rare events (or those of intermediate rarity) with an unknown relationship to meaningful health outcomes. Progress in the evolution of multimodal postoperative rehabilitation may eventually establish regional anesthesia and analgesia techniques as critical to the process.[42] There is increasing evidence to suggest that postoperative ileus is decreased by continuous epidural analgesia with local anesthetics. Preliminary data from studies using aggressive multimodal rehabilitation including continuous epidural analgesia after major abdominal and thoracic operations suggest that the positive impact on pain and paralytic ileus will facilitate early recovery (i.e., early mobilization and nutrition).[43]

The aim of analgesic regimens is not only to reduce pain intensity but also to decrease the incidences of adverse effects of analgesic agents and to improve patient comfort. Moreover, adequate pain control is a prerequisite for the use of rehabilitation programs to accelerate recovery from surgery.[4]

The concept of multimodal pain management or balanced analgesia is to provide sufficient pain relief through additive and synergistic effects, using different analgesics, with a concomitant reduction of adverse effects attributed to the lesser doses of individual drugs. Peripheral nerve blocks are the cornerstone of balanced analgesic regimens in combination with nonopioid analgesics (acetaminophen, nonsteroidal antiinflammatory drugs, $\alpha_2$-agonists, N-methyl D-aspartate antagonists, etc). They facilitate the use of opioids only when required (breakthrough pain and block resolution), thus decreasing the incidence of their systemic adverse effects. Continuous regional anesthesia is likely to enhance the quality of postoperative analgesia and patient satisfaction.[44] Harrop-Griffiths and Picard[45] ask, "If continuous regional anesthesia can, with the right equipment in trained hands, provide perfect or excellent analgesia after painful limb surgery, can we afford not to use it?" The information supporting the use of these regional techniques has become so extensive that the United States Veterans' Health Administration and the Department of Defense have made recommendations for procedure-specific analgesic regimens emphasizing regional analgesia.[46]

The clinical implications of adequately controlled postoperative pain are manifold. After orthopedic surgery, better analgesic control can improve the functional result of surgery and shorten the duration of rehabilitation, leading to a substantial economic benefit.[40] After abdominal surgery, patients who receive epidural analgesia have a more rapid recovery of bowel motility, allowing prompt oral intake; they mobilize more rapidly and are ready for hospital discharge earlier.[47]

Uncontrolled postoperative pain has been identified as a risk factor in the development of chronic postsurgical pain syndrome.[48] Chronic postsurgical pain has been defined as that which develops after a surgical procedure, is of at least 2 months' duration, for which other causes have been excluded (e.g., malignancy or chronic infection), and for which the possibility of pain continuing from a preexisting condition has been explored and exclusion attempted.[49] Chronic postsurgical pain has been reported after thoracotomy, mastectomy, hernia repair, and limb amputation, with all surgical procedures having the potential of developing this debilitating condition.[48,49] Compared with pain-free patients, those with significant acute postoperative pain are more likely to develop chronic postsurgical pain.[50] Furthermore, the severity of acute pain (more importantly, movement-evoked pain) correlates with the incidence of chronic pain.[51] This suggests that adequate pain relief, particularly movement-evoked pain relief, may reduce the risk of persistent postoperative pain.

Regional anesthesia techniques such as epidural analgesia and continuous peripheral nerve blockade have been shown to provide superior dynamic pain relief. Senturk et al.[52] compared the effects of TEA with bupivacaine and morphine (either initiated preoperatively or postoperatively) and those of intravenous (IV)-PCA with morphine. Compared with patients receiving IV-PCA, patients who received preoperative TEA had a lesser incidence of pain at 6 months (78% versus 45%). Similarly, Obata et al.[53] in a prospective, randomized, single-blind study demonstrated a significant effect of combined intra- and postoperative epidural analgesia when compared with postoperative epidural analgesia alone for posterolateral thoracotomy (decreasing the incidence of pain at 6 months from 67% to 33%).

Thus, in the absence of convincing generalizable evidence that regional anesthesia and analgesia decreases mortality and morbidity, an increasing body of evidence supports the excellent pain relief it provides after surgery, which alone is sufficient to justify its use, especially in view of the long-term benefits of adequate intra- and postoperative pain control on rehabilitation and prevention of chronic postsurgical pain. This is best achieved with a multimodal approach, of which regional anesthesia is an essential component.

## References

1. Orkin FK. Application of outcomes research to clinical decision making in cardiovascular medicine. In: Tuman K, ed. Outcome Measurements. Baltimore: Williams & Wilkins; 1999:39–66.
2. Wu CL, Fleisher LA. Outcomes research in regional anesthesia and analgesia. Anesth Analg 2000;91:1232–1242.
3. Gold BS, Kitz DS, Lecky JH, Neuhaus JM. Unanticipated admission to the hospital following ambulatory surgery. JAMA 1989;262:3008–3010.
4. Bonnet F, Marret E. Influence of anaesthetic and analgesic techniques on outcome after surgery. Br J Anaesth 2005;95(1):52–58.
5. Hearst N, Grady D, Barron HV, Kerlikowske K. Research using existing data: secondary data analysis, ancillary studies, and systematic reviews. In: Hulley SB, Cummings SR, eds. Designing Clinical Research. An Epidemiologic Approach. Philadelphia: Lippincott Williams & Wilkins; 2001:195–215.
6. Bode RH Jr, Lewis KP, Zarich SW, et al. Cardiac outcome after peripheral vascular surgery: comparison of general and regional anesthesia. Anesthesiology 1996;84:3–13.
7. Fisher DM. How do we obtain outcome data: randomized clinical trials versus observational databases. In: Tuman K, ed. Outcome Measurements. Baltimore: Williams & Wilkins; 1999:23–37.
8. Capelleri JC, Ioannidis JPA, deFerranti SD, et al. Large trials versus meta-analyses of smaller trials: how do their results compare? JAMA 1996;276:1332–1338.
9. LeLorier J, Gregoire G, Benhaddad A, et al. Discrepancies between meta-analyses and subsequent large randomised controlled trials. N Engl J Med 1997;337:536–542.
10. Gregoire G, Derderian F, Le Lorier J. Selecting the language of the publications included in a meta-analysis: is there a Tower of Babel bias? J Clin Epidemiol 1995;48:159–163.
11. Anderson FA, Hish J, White K, Fitzgerald RH, for the hip and knee registry investigators. Temporal trend in prevention of venous thromboembolism following primary total hip replacement or knee arthroplasty 1996–2001. Chest 2003;124:349S–356S.
12. Auerbach AD, Goldman L. Beta-blockers and reduction of cardiac events in non-cardiac surgery. JAMA 2002;287:1435–1444.
13. Collins R, Gray R, Godwin J, Peto R. Avoidance of large biases and large random errors in the assessment of moderate treatment effects: the need for systematic overviews. Stat Med 1987;6:245–254.
14. de Leon-Casasola OA. When it comes to outcome, we need to define what a perioperative epidural technique is. Anesth Analg 2003;96:315–318.
15. Kehlet H, Dahl JB. Anaesthesia, surgery, and challenges in postoperative recovery. Lancet 2003;362:1921–1928.
16. Liu S, Carpenter RL, Neal JM. Epidural anesthesia and analgesia. Their role in postoperative outcome. Anesthesiology 1995;82:1474–1506.
17. Yeager MP, Glass DD, Neff RK, Brinck-Johnsen T. Epidural anesthesia and analgesia in high risk surgical patients. Anesthesiology 1987;66:729–736.
18. Tuman KJ, McCarthy RJ, March RJ, et al. Effects of epidural anesthesia and analgesia on coagulation and outcome after major vascular surgery. Anesth Analg 1991;73:696–704.
19. Christopherson R, Beattie C, Frank SM, et al. Perioperative morbidity in patients randomized to epidural or general anesthesia for lower extremity vascular surgery. Anesthesiology 1993;79:422–434.
20. Rodgers A, Walker N, Schug S, et al. Reduction of post-operative mortality and morbidity with epidural or spinal anaesthesia: results from overview of randomised trials. BMJ 2000;321:1493–1497.
21. Urwin SC, Parker MJ, Griffiths R. General versus regional anaesthesia for hip fracture surgery: a meta-analysis of randomized trials. Br J Anaesth 2000;84:450–455.
22. Parker MJ, Handoll HHG, Griffiths R. Anesthesia for hip fracture surgery in adults. Cochrane Database Syst Rev 2004;(4):CD000521.

23. Liu SS, Block B, Wu CL. Effects of perioperative central neuraxial analgesia on outcome after coronary artery bypass surgery: a meta-analysis. Anesthesiology 2004;101:153–161.
24. Ballantyne JC, Carr DB, deFerranti S, et al. The comparative effects of postoperative analgesic therapies on pulmonary outcome: cumulative meta-analyses of randomized, controlled trials. Anesth Analg 1998;86:598–612.
25. Beattie WS, Badner NH, Choi P. Epidural analgesia reduces postoperative myocardial infarction: a meta-analysis. Anesth Analg 2001;93:853–858.
26. Block BM, Liu SS, Rowlingson AJ, et al. Efficacy of postoperative epidural analgesia: a meta-analysis. JAMA 2003;290:2455–2463.
27. Hall GM. Regional anesthesia versus general anesthesia: is there an impact on outcome after major surgery? IARS 2005 Review Course Lectures, Supplement to Anesthesia & Analgesia.
28. Wu CL, Hsu W, Richman JM, Raja SN. Postoperative cognitive function as an outcome of regional anesthesia and analgesia. Reg Anesth Pain Med 2004;29:257–268.
29. Park WY, Thompson JS, Lee KK. Effect of epidural anesthesia and analgesia on perioperative outcome: a randomized, controlled Veteran Affairs cooperative study. Ann Surg 2001;234:560–571.
30. Norris EJ, Beattie C, Perler BA, et al. Double-masked randomized trial comparing alternate combinations of intraoperative anesthesia and postoperative analgesia in abdominal aortic surgery. Anesthesiology 2001;95:1054–1067.
31. Rigg JRA, Jamrozik K, Myles PS. Epidural anaesthesia and analgesia and outcome of major surgery: a randomised trial. Lancet 2002;359:1276–1282.
32. Foss NB, Kristensen MT, Kristensen BB, Jensen PS, Kehlet H. Effect of postoperative epidural analgesia on rehabilitation and pain after hip fracture surgery: a randomized, double-blind, placebo-controlled trial. Anesthesiology 2005;102:1197–1204.
33. Ganapathy S, McCartney CJL, Beattie WS, Chan VWS. Best evidence in anesthetic practice. Can J Anaesth 2003;50:143–146.
34. Andreae M. Underdosing the epidural invalidates a good clinical trial. Anesthesiology 2002;97:1026–1027.
35. Karanikolas M, Kalauokalani D, Swarm R. Epidural anesthesia and analgesia: is there really no benefit? Anesthesiology 2002;97:1027.
36. Rigg JRA, Jamrozik K, Clarke M. How can we demonstrate that new developments in anesthesia are of real clinical importance? Anesthesiology 1997;86:1008–1010.
37. Peyton PJ, Myles PS, Silbert BS, et al. Perioperative epidural analgesia and outcome after major abdominal surgery in high-risk patients. Anesth Analg 2003;96:548–554.
38. O'Hara DA, Duff A, Berlin JA, et al. The effect of anesthetic technique on postoperative outcomes in hip fracture repair. Anesthesiology 2000;92:947–957.
39. Wu CL, Anderson GF, Herbert R, Lietman SA, Fleisher LA. Effect of postoperative epidural analgesia on morbidity and mortality after total hip replacement surgery in Medicare patients. Reg Anesth Pain Med 2003;28:271–278.
40. Capdevila X, Barthelet Y, Biboulet P, et al. Effects of perioperative analgesic technique on the surgical outcome and duration of rehabilitation after major knee surgery. Anesthesiology 1999;91:8–15.
41. Chelly JE, Greger J, Gebhard R, et al. Continuous femoral blocks improve recovery and outcome of patients undergoing total knee arthroplasty. J Arthroplasty 2001;16:436–445.
42. Basse L, Hjort Jakobsen D, Billesbolle P, Werner M, Kehlet H. A clinical pathway to accelerate recovery after colonic resection. Ann Surg 2000;232:51–57.
43. Holte K, Kehlet H. Epidural anaesthesia and analgesia – effects on surgical stress responses and implications for postoperative nutrition. Clin Nutr 2002;21:199–206.
44. Grant SA, Nielsen KC, Greengrass RA, Steele SM, Klein SM. Continuous peripheral nerve block for ambulatory surgery. Reg Anesth Pain Med 2001;26:209–214.
45. Harrop-Griffiths W, Picard J. Continuous regional analgesia: can we afford not to use it? Anaesthesia 2001;56:299–301.
46. Rosenquist RW, Rosenberg J. Postoperative pain guidelines. Reg Anesth Pain Med 2003;28:279–288.
47. Carli F, Mayo N, Kluben K, et al. Epidural analgesia enhances functional exercise capacity and health-related quality of life after colonic surgery: results of a randomized trial. Anesthesiology 2002;97:540–549.
48. Perkins FM, Kehlet H. Chronic pain as an outcome of surgery. A review of predictive factors. Anesthesiology 2000;93:1123–1133.

49. Macrae WA. Chronic pain after surgery. Br J Anaesth 2001;87:88–98.
50. Callesen B, Kehlet H. Prospective study of chronic pain after hernia repair. Br J Surg 1999;86:1528–1531.
51. Katz J, Jackson M, Kavanagh BP, Sandler AN. Acute pain after thoracic surgery predicts long-term post-thoracotomy pain. Clin J Pain 1996;12:50–55.
52. Senturk M, Ozcan PE, Talu GK, et al. The effects of three different analgesia techniques on long-term postthoracotomy pain. Anesth Analg 2002;94:11–15.
53. Obata H, Saito S, Fujita N, et al. Epidural block with mepivacaine before surgery reduces long-term post-thoracotomy pain. Can J Anaesth 1999;46:1127–1132.

# 3 Avoiding Complications in Regional Anesthesia

Richard W. Rosenquist

There is widespread conviction among anesthesiologists that regional anesthesia offers significant advantages over general anesthesia in certain settings. At the same time, there is a fear of complications related to the performance of regional anesthetic techniques that is held with almost equal intensity. Complications related to regional anesthesia have been described by many authors, although our understanding of the numerous factors leading to these complications is limited. Auroy et al.[1] described the risk of complications related to regional blocks as lower than 5 in 10,000 patients in their series, which included spinal, epidural, and peripheral nerve blocks. In the case of spinal or epidural hematoma, the relative risk has been described as 1:220,000 and 1:150,000, respectively, a rate that approaches the risk of routine general anesthesia.[2] However, the risk of neurologic complications after central neuraxial block can be markedly elevated (1:1,800) in patients with risk factors such as female sex, osteoporosis, or concurrent use of anticoagulants.[3] Despite the relatively infrequent occurrence of complications related to regional anesthesia, the fear of complications exceeds their actual occurrence. This may be attributable in part to widespread misperceptions regarding the role of regional anesthesia in producing neurologic injury on the part of patients, surgeons, anesthesiologists, and other healthcare providers. The absence of a clear understanding often leads to blame being assigned to the regional anesthetic without careful assessment and diagnosis of the neurologic deficit to determine its etiology. These misconceptions have also led to "chart wars," in which written statements assigning blame before establishment of a clear diagnosis are placed in the medical record. These statements often obscure the truth and serve as a barrier to effective communication between physicians caring for patients with neurologic deficits after surgery. They may also serve as fodder for the malpractice attorney and make it difficult to defend a physician practicing within the "standard of care," regardless of their specialty. Although it is impossible to prevent all neurologic injuries related to regional anesthesia, it may be possible to reduce their occurrence by avoiding well-defined risk factors and using meticulous technique at all times.

## Scope of the Problem

Lee et al.[4] described the "Injuries Associated with Regional Anesthesia in the 1980's and 1990's" based on a closed claims analysis of 134 cases. Axillary blocks made up 44% of claims, intravenous regional block 21%, interscalene blocks 19%, and supraclavicular blocks 7%. The damaging event was related to the block in 51% of peripheral block claims. Death or brain damage was present in 11%. The damaging event in high-severity claims was variable and included block technique (n = 3), wrong drug or dose (n = 3), allergic reactions (n = 2), inadequate ventilation (n = 2), high block (n = 1), difficult intubation (n = 1), no event (n = 1), and unknown (n = 1). Permanent nerve damage was present in 29% of peripheral block claims and temporary injury in 58% of claims.

### *Bleeding*

The potential risk of bleeding complications resulting from the performance of regional anesthesia is readily apparent given the almost universal association of nerve plexuses with vascular bundles including an artery and a vein. Complications related to bleeding include minor issues such as oozing or bruising at the site of needle insertion. In addition, the potential for significant blood loss is present as well. Small amounts of oozing or minor bruising at the needle insertion site are common and should not be considered complications, but rather an expected part of the procedure. There is also a risk for significant hematoma formation or blood loss. This may be related to vascular puncture or injury related to needle insertion. The degree of concern for this complication is directly related to size of the needle, the number of times the vascular structure or tissues are punctured, the ability to compress the vessel, and any underlying coagulation abnormalities. Major bleeding complications related to the performance of regional anesthesia have been reported and include persistent Horner's syndrome, peripheral nerve injury, hematoma formation, and blood loss requiring transfusion. The potential for significant blood loss is increased by the presence of inherent anticoagulation abnormalities or medically administered anticoagulants. Ekatodramis et al.[5] reported two cases of prolonged Horner's syndrome caused by hematoma formation after continuous interscalene block.[5] Several authors have reported peripheral nerve or brachial plexus injuries related to hematoma formation during axillary brachial plexus block.[6–9] A case report by Nielsen[10] describes bleeding after a series of intercostal nerve blocks performed for analgesia after cholecystectomy in a patient receiving heparin. After the fourth set of blocks, the patient's hematocrit decreased from 33–40 to 20 and eventually to 15. Transfusion of eight units of packed red blood cells was required to maintain a hematocrit above 30. The small hematoma present after the third set of blocks expanded to cover a 30 × 65 cm area. The patient had no long-term sequelae, but had pain in the right flank and hip for 4 weeks in the area of the hematoma. In the case of lumbar plexus blocks, numerous case reports of psoas hematoma with and without neurologic complications and with and without anticoagulants have been reported.[11–14] In addition, renal subcapsular hematoma in association with lumbar plexus block has been reported.[15] Although there is sparse literature to support this, some authorities have suggested that the *ASRA Consensus Guidelines for the Performance of Neuraxial Anesthesia in the Presence of Anticoagulants* be applied to the performance of peripheral nerve blocks as well.[2] In the case of deep nerve blocks in noncompressible sites such as cervical, thoracic, and lumbar paravertebral, there may be merit to this approach. However, some degree of latitude may be appropriate in those situations in which a block is performed in an area that is readily compressible such as the femoral or axillary region. However, this cannot be recommended as entirely safe, because case reports of neurologic injury related to hematoma formation in association with axillary block have been published. It is vitally important that preblock history determine if there is a history of coagulation abnormality or if medications or oral dietary supplements are being taken that can affect coagulation.

### *Infection*

The potential for infection associated with the performance of regional anesthesia is an obligatory part of every regional anesthesia discussion (see Chapter 19). The usual maxims to avoid performing blocks in patients with sepsis, placing needles through an obvious skin infection, or avoiding the performance of blocks in infected extremities have been conventional wisdom. The occurrence of infection related to the performance of single-shot peripheral nerve blocks is rare, which may reflect the relatively low infectious risk of sterile needle insertion and/or the antimicrobial effects of local anesthetics.[16] There is a greater risk associated with the performance of continuous peripheral nerve block techniques. When indwelling catheters are present, it is common for these catheters to become colonized.[17,18] However, if left in for short periods of time, progression to frank infection or sepsis is uncommon. The most common organisms encountered are staphylococcus species although enterococcus, other gram-positive cocci, gram-negative bacillus, and others are found as well.[16] The risk of infection can best be reduced by using meticulous technique including careful cleansing of the skin before needle insertion, using agents such as Betadine or chlorhexidine, using sterile needles, and using sterile gloves if palpation of the site or contact with the needle is anticipated. In the case of indwelling catheters, the routine use of a hat, mask, and sterile gloves is warranted. The use of a sterile gown may not be required in all cases, but if contact with the catheter during insertion is likely, this extra precaution is recommended. Attempts to demonstrate a difference in infection rate between catheters inserted with and without the use of a sterile gown during epidural catheter insertion have not been successful in demonstrating any significant change in outcome.[18] There is no evidence to support the routine use of preblock antibiotics for single-shot blocks and little to support the use of preinsertion antibiotics in the case of continuous nerve blocks, although they do reduce the incidence of colonization. Colonization seems to be increased by frequent dressing changes. Efforts should be made to dress catheters well initially and minimize the total number of dressing changes or breaks in the integrity of infusions.[18]

### *Allergic Reaction*

Allergic reactions to local anesthetics are uncommon and avoiding this complication is something that should be accomplished by taking a thorough drug and allergy history. A history of prior allergic reaction to local anesthetics or a history of allergic reaction to paraaminobenzoic acid–containing compounds should be recorded. In this setting, ester local anesthetics should be avoided. It is also possible that allergic reactions may be attributable to preservatives such as methylparaben or metabisulfite in the local anesthetic solution.[19–21]

### *Drug Toxicity*

There are several types of toxicity associated with the use of local anesthetics for peripheral nerve blocks. These include central nervous system (CNS) toxicity related either to the total dose administered or the site of injection, cardiac toxicity, neurotoxicity, and myotoxicity.

The risk of CNS toxicity related to injection of local anesthetic may be reduced by careful aspiration of the needle before injection of local anesthetic, injection of a test dose of local anesthetic containing epinephrine and looking for mild signs of CNS toxicity or effects of intravenous epinephrine, injection of small volumes of local anesthetic followed by frequent aspiration and allowing sufficient time for drug to circulate before administering additional local anesthetic. In the case of blocks such as interscalene in which the carotid or vertebral arteries may be encountered, seizure activity may be produced by a large injection or as little as 0.5–1 mL of local anesthetic.[22,23] This is significantly different from CNS toxicity, that results from administering doses of local anesthetic too large for an individual's body size, age, weight, or general state of health.[24–28] Information about the patient's age, weight, general state of health, number of blocks to be performed, and site of local anesthetic administration should be taken into consideration when choosing a total dose of local anesthetic.

It is well established that local anesthetics have neurotoxic effects. These effects have been much more prominent and well studied within the subarachnoid space in association with spinal anesthesia where both concentration and dose seem to have a role in the observed changes.[29–31] There is little direct evidence to correlate the use of local anesthetic for peripheral nerve block with significant direct neurotoxicity.[32] However, the combination of local anesthetic with or without adjuvants and peripheral nerve injury or intraneural injection may be related to worsened outcome.

Myotoxicity is a well-known side effect of local anesthetics.[33] It has been used with theoretic advantage in the treatment of myofascial trigger points, but complications related to the myotoxicity resulting from local anesthetic used in the performance of peripheral nerve block have been rare.[34,35] The performance of single-shot peripheral nerve blocks has not been associated with significant myotoxicity. However, significant complications related to the performance of continuous regional anesthesia with resultant long-term muscular injury have been reported. Marginal block performance and the need for multiple large boluses of local anesthetics should be carefully evaluated to avoid repeated intramuscular injections. The potential for drug toxicity related to other drugs inserted via indwelling peripheral nerve catheters exists and may lead to catastrophic consequences. However, there are no reports in the peer-reviewed medical literature regarding this complication.

### *Equipment*

Regional anesthesia techniques have been enhanced by the use of various types of equipment. This includes the nerve stimulators, ultrasound imaging devices, and pressure manometers. Nerve stimulators have been used to facilitate the location of peripheral nerve bundles transcutaneously, which aids in selecting the correct needle insertion site.[36] They have had more widespread use as a means of providing visual cues to needle location and have become commonplace in this setting. Once a needle has been advanced toward a peripheral nerve, the presence of motor or sensory pulsations may be used as an indicator of needle-tip location. It has been assumed that there is a direct correlation between the current required to elicit a motor response and the distance of the needle tip away from the nerve structure. It is widely accepted that performance of peripheral nerve blocks with currents of 0.5 mA or less is more likely to result in a favorable outcome than nerve blocks performed with higher currents. There are many under the false assumption that the presence of a motor response at a reasonable current not only indicates proximity, but also indicates the absence of needle insertion to the nerve with a resultant increase in safety. Although a motor response at an extremely low current may indicate intraneural needle placement, this is not always true. The converse is also not true. Studies comparing the response of patient-reported paresthesias to nerve stimulation and nerve stimulation to ultrasound have demonstrated that reliance on current alone is insufficient to prevent nerve injury.[37,38] Perlas et al.[39] have demonstrated that paresthesias may be perceived by patients in the absence of a motor response even at currents as high as 1.5 mA. Although nerve stimulators are excellent tools, their use alone does not confer an automatic safety advantage with respect to the avoidance of nerve injury. However, if motor stimulation is present at an extremely low current, it is prudent to withdraw the needle until the twitch disappears and then increase the current to see if the twitch may be reestablished. Avoiding injection in the patient with a motor response at an extremely low current may help to avoid complications, although this cannot be guaranteed.

Recent years have seen an explosion in the use of imaging techniques for the performance of regional anesthesia. The largest growth in this area has been in the use of ultrasound. These devices allow the imaging of bones, soft tissue structures, nerves, vascular bundles, and the needle approaching the nerve. In addition, they demonstrate the flow of local anesthetic either around the nerve in the desired manner or away from the nerve, allowing time to reposition the needle to facilitate greater success in the block. They may also demonstrate intraneural injection.[40] These techniques have the significant advantage of allowing direct visualization of the important structures and may provide greater safety in years to come. At present, the size, expense, and overall lack of experience in the larger community of regional anesthesiologists has limited application of these techniques. However, the explosion of courses and the rapidly advancing ultrasound technology and reduced costs of new devices will help to increase their acceptance and use.

It is also a widely held belief that there is a certain "feel" to the syringe during the injection of local anesthetic associated with a normal injection. If this normal feel is not apparent and the injection requires markedly increased pressures, it may be because the needle tip is either against or within the nerve. Early work has been reported outlining the use of pressure manometers to evaluate injection pressure during the performance of nerve injections in animal models.[41] The authors contend that high injection pressures at the onset of injection may indicate intraneural needle placement and lead to severe fascicular injury and persistent neurologic deficits. This is strictly experimental at the present time and its future applicability in the clinical setting is yet to be determined.

### *Operator Factors*

Although the patient is the one who experiences the complication, there should be no doubt that the practitioner handling the needle has an intimate and critical role in the development of complications. Although many attempts have been made to simplify the performance of regional anesthesia with the use of various surface landmarks, mnemonics, peripheral nerve stimulators, and imaging devices, the simple fact remains that regional anesthetic techniques are more readily performed by those who have a solid understanding of the anatomy. This includes knowledge of anatomy that goes beyond the simple surface landmarks drawn to facilitate needle insertion and extends to the three-dimensional anatomy of the nerves, muscles, and blood vessels below the surface of the skin. This anatomic knowledge should incorporate not only the standard understanding of various nerves and their plexuses, but should also include a simple understanding of various anatomic variations that may be present. These variations may lead to either altered nerve location or motor and sensory responses, which although different from the standard, are nonetheless valid. A sound knowledge of anatomy also helps to prevent errors related to excessive needle insertion depth. This error is frequently observed during the early stages of learning regional anesthesia and results from the desire on the part of that person performing the technique to encounter the targeted nerve, believing that if only they will go deeper they will sooner or later encounter what they are looking for. This is a dangerous way of thinking and has produced many devastating complications. Interscalene blocks have been a far too frequent example of this complication. In this block, the nerve plexus is typically 1–1.5 cm below the surface of the skin. Evidence of needles inserted too far with this particular technique have been reported in the literature in the form of spinal cord injuries.[42] Other examples include pneumothorax during thoracic paravertebral block and kidney hematoma and peritoneal catheter insertion during lumbar paravertebral blocks.[15,43,44] The accomplished regional anesthesia practitioner must also learn to listen to the patient. Patient reports of unusual paresthesias or pain during needle insertion or injection should be noted and evaluated. They may be reporting the pain that occurs with direct nerve contact, needle insertion into the nerve, or intraneural injection. The ability to use the patient as a source of information for the practitioner has created great controversy, especially surrounding the performance of regional anesthetics on patients who are awake, heavily sedated, or asleep. In most cases, performance of regional anesthetic techniques should not be excessively painful, and reassurance and a gentle hand should allow the procedure to be performed on the awake or mildly sedated patient without difficulty.[45,46] In the case of young children, the mentally unstable, or the patient with an unstable fracture who is unable to tolerate positioning or nerve stimulation, the use of heavy sedation or general anesthesia may be necessary and should be discussed at the time that consent is obtained. Finally, the practitioner should carefully evaluate the indications for selecting a given block for a given patient. If there are significant contraindications to the performance of a block such as preexisting neurologic deficit, changing neurologic deficit, or inability to conduct appropriate postoperative neurologic evaluation, choice of another technique may be appropriate. Performance of regional anesthetics on the wrong limb has been an ongoing problem. This requires care on the part of all involved to reconfirm correct limb selection. Attempts to reduce the incidence of error have stimulated the use of preanesthetic site verification and the "time-out" process.[47]

Finally, the importance of appropriate education and training in regional anesthesia techniques cannot be overemphasized. This should occur during residency training and at continuing medical education courses on an ongoing basis, in order to stay current with contemporary techniques.

### *Patient Factors*

There are numerous patient factors that may contribute to complications associated with the performance of regional anesthesia. Preexisting disease such as diabetes may change neuroconductivity and result in the need for higher nerve stimulator currents to produce the desired effect.[48] The underlying nerve dysfunction in these patients may also predispose them to additional neurologic injury. This is not an absolute contraindication to doing blocks in these patients, but rather should be taken into consideration during the performance and the discussion of risks related to the procedure preoperatively. The same is true of other causes of peripheral neuropathy. Patient factors such as morbid obesity in which landmark identification may be challenging must be taken into consideration.[49] In some patients, this may prevent successful performance of the block. Other patient factors, such as trauma resulting in anatomic abnormality or the potential for complications such as compartment syndrome, may prevent the performance of blocks, and in this setting, altered anesthetic and postoperative analgesic techniques may be more appropriate.

## Conclusion

Numerous factors contribute to the development of complications related to the performance of peripheral nerve blocks. A thorough knowledge of anatomy, indications and contraindications for block performance, meticulous attention to preparation and performance of regional anesthetic techniques, careful selection of local anesthetic drug and dose, and use of available technical devices to facilitate performance of regional anesthesia will help to minimize long-term complications related to these techniques.

## References

1. Auroy Y, Benhamou D, Bargues L, et al. Major complications of regional anesthesia in France: The SOS Regional Anesthesia Hotline Service. Anesthesiology 2002;97:1274–1280.
2. Horlocker TT, Wedel DJ, Benzon H, et al. Regional anesthesia in the anticoagulated patient: defining the risks (the second ASRA Consensus Conference on Neuraxial Anesthesia and Anticoagulation). Reg Anesth Pain Med 2003;28:172–197.
3. Moen V, Dahlgren N, Irestedt L. Severe neurological complications after central neuraxial blockades in Sweden 1990–1999. Anesthesiology 2004;101:950–959.

4. Lee LA, Posner KL, Domino KB, et al. Injuries associated with regional anesthesia in the 1980s and 1990s: a closed claims analysis. Anesthesiology 2004;1001:143–152.
5. Ekatodramis G, Macaire P, Borgeat A. Prolonged Horner syndrome due to neck hematoma after continuous interscalene block. Anesthesiology 2001;95:801–803.
6. Bergman BD, Hebl JR, Kent J, Horlocker TT. Neurologic complications of 405 consecutive continuous axillary catheters. Anesth Analg 2003;96:247–252.
7. Tsao BE, Wilbourn AJ. Infraclavicular brachial plexus injury following axillary regional block. Muscle Nerve 2004;30:44–48.
8. Cockings E. Axillary block complicated by hematoma and radial nerve injury. Reg Anesth Pain Med 2000;25:103.
9. Ben-David B, Stahl S. Axillary block complicated by hematoma and radial nerve injury. Reg Anesth Pain Med 1999;24:264–266.
10. Nielsen CH. Bleeding after intercostals nerve block in a patient anticoagulated with heparin. Anesthesiology 1989;71:162–164.
11. Hsu DT. Delayed retroperitoneal haematoma after failed lumbar plexus block. Br J Anaesth 2005;94:395.
12. Aveline C, Bonnet F. Delayed retroperitoneal haematoma after failed lumbar plexus block. Br J Anaesth 2004;93:589–591.
13. Weller RS, Gerancher JC, Crews JC, Wade KL. Extensive retroperitoneal hematoma without neurologic deficit in two patients who underwent lumbar plexus block and were later anticoagulated. Anesthesiology 2003;98:581–585.
14. Klein SM, D'Ercole F, Greengrass RA, et al. Enoxaparin associated with psoas hematoma and lumbar plexopathy after lumbar plexus block. Anesthesiology 1997;87:1576–1579.
15. Aida S, Takahashi H, Shimoji K. Renal subcapsular hematoma after lumbar plexus block. Anesthesiology 1996;84:452–455.
16. Aydin ON, Eyigor M, Aydin N. Antimicrobial activity of ropivacaine and other local anaesthetics. Eur J Anaesthesiol 2001;18:687–694.
17. Capdevilla X, Pirat P, Bringuier S, et al. Continuous peripheral nerve blocks in hospital wards after orthopedic surgery: a multicenter prospective analysis of the quality of postoperative analgesia and complications in 1,416 patients. Anesthesiology 2005;103: 1035–1045.
18. Morin AM, Kerwat KM, Klotz M, et al. Risk factors for bacterial catheter colonization in regional anaesthesia. BMC Anesthesiol 2005;5:1–9.
19. Jacobsen RB, Borch JE, Bindslev-Jensen C. Hypersensitivity to local anaesthetics. Allergy 2005;60:262–264.
20. Riemersma WA, Schuttelaar ML, Coenraads PJ. Type IV hypersensitivity to sodium metabisulfite in local anaesthetic. Contact Dermatitis 2004;51:148.
21. Finucane BT. Allergies to local anesthetics – the real truth. Can J Anaesth 2003;50: 869–874.
22. Korman B, Riley RH. Convulsions induced by ropivacaine during interscalene brachial plexus block. Anesth Analg 1997;85:1128–1129.
23. Crews JC, Rothman TE. Seizure after levobupivacaine for interscalene brachial plexus block. Anesth Analg 2003;96:1188–1190.
24. Finucane BT. Ropivacaine cardiac toxicity – not as troublesome as bupivacaine. Can J Anaesth 2005;52:449–453.
25. Petitjeans F, Mion G, Puidupin M, et al. Tachycardia and convulsions induced by accidental intravascular ropivacaine injection during sciatic block. Acta Anaesthesiol Scand 2002; 46:616–617.
26. Mullanu Ch, Gaillat F, Scemama F, et al. Acute toxicity of local anesthetic ropivacaine and mepivacaine during a combined lumbar plexus and sciatic block for hip surgery. Acta Anaesthesiol Belg 2002;53:221–223.
27. Cox B, Durieux ME, Marcus MA. Toxicity of local anaesthetics. Best Pract Res Clin Anaesthesiol 2003;17:111–136.
28. Tsui BC, Wagner A, Finucane B. Regional anaesthesia in the elderly: a clinical guide. Drugs Aging 2004;21:895–910.
29. Sakura S, Kirihara Y, Mugurama T, et al. The comparative neurotoxicity of intrathecal lidocaine and bupivacaine in rats. Anesth Analg 2005;101:541–547.
30. Radwan IAM, Saito S, Goto F. The neurotoxicity of local anesthetics on growing neurons: a comparative study of lidocaine, bupivacaine, mepivacaine, and ropivacaine. Anesth Analg 2002;94:319–324.

31. Kasaba T, Onizuka S, Takasaki M. Procaine and mepivacaine have less toxicity in vitro than clinically used local anesthetic. Anesth Analg 2003;97:85–90.
32. Kroin JS, Penn RD, Levy FE, Kerns JM. Effect of repetitive lidocaine infusion on peripheral nerve. Exp Neurol 1986;94:166–173.
33. Zink W, Graf BM. Local anesthetic myotoxicity. Reg Anesth Pain Med 2004;29: 333–340.
34. Zink W, Bohl JRE, Hacke N, et al. The long term myotoxic effects of bupivacaine and ropivacaine after continuous peripheral nerve blocks. Anesth Analg 2005;101:548–554.
35. Hogan Q, Dotson R, Erickson S, et al. Local anesthetic myotoxicity: a case and review. Anesthesiology 1994;80:942–947.
36. Urmey WF, Grossi P. Percutaneous electrode guidance: a noninvasive technique for prelocation of peripheral nerves to facilitate peripheral plexus or nerve block. Reg Anesth Pain Med 2002;27:261–267.
37. Choyce A, Chen V, Middleton W, et al. What is the relationship between paresthesia and nerve stimulation for axillary brachial plexus block? Reg Aneseth Pain Med 2001; 26:100–104.
38. Bollini CA, Urmey WF, Vascello L, Cacheiro F. Relationship between evoked motor response and sensory paresthesia in interscalene brachial plexus block. Reg Anesth Pain Med 2003;2:384–388.
39. Perlas A, Chan VWS, Simons M. Brachial plexus examination and localization using ultrasound and electrical stimulation. Anesthesiology 2003;99:429–435.
40. Chan VWS. Ultrasound evidence of intraneural injection. Anesth Analg 2005;101:610–611.
41. Hadzic A, Dilberovic F, Shah S, et al. Combination of intraneural injection and high injection pressure lead to fascicular injury and neurologic deficits in dogs. Reg Anesth Pain Med 2004;29:417–423.
42. Benumof JL. Permanent loss of cervical spinal cord function associated with interscalene block performed under general anesthesia. Anesthesiology 2000;93:1541–1544.
43. Lonnqvist PA, MacKenzie J, Soni AK, Conacher ID. Paravertebral blockade: failure rate and complications. Anaesthesia 1995;50:813–815.
44. Capdevila X, Coimbra C, Choquet O. Approaches to the lumbar plexus: success, risks, and outcome. Reg Anesth Pain Med 2005;30:150–162.
45. Borgeat A, Ekatodramis G, Gaertner E. Performing an interscalene block during general anesthesia must be the exception. Anesthesiology 2001;85:1302–1303.
46. Choquet O, Jochum D, Estebe JP, et al. Motor response following paresthesia during interscalene block: methodological problems may lead to inappropriate conclusions. Anesthesiology 2003;98:587–588.
47. Edmonds CR, Liguori GA, Stanton MA. Two cases of a wrong-site peripheral nerve block and a process to prevent this complication. Reg Anesth Pain Med 2005;30:99–103.
48. Sites BD, Gallagher J, Sparks M. Ultrasound-guided popliteal block demonstrates an atypical motor response to nerve stimulation in 2 patients with diabetes mellitus. Reg Anesth Pain Med 2003;28:479–482.
49. Nielsen DC, Guller U, Steele SM, et al. Influence of obesity on surgical regional anesthesia in the ambulatory setting: an analysis of 9,038 blocks. Anesthesiology 2005;102:181–187.

# 4 Local Anesthetic Toxicity

David L. Brown

Effective regional block is not possible without the use of local anesthetics. Even though local anesthetics have been used for more than 115 years, details about balancing risks of their toxic effects with the benefits of their therapeutic effects remain poorly focused for many clinicians. In this chapter, the most frequent toxic effect of local anesthetics – local anesthetic systemic toxicity – will be covered, as will the less-frequent clinical situations of allergy to local anesthetics and myelotoxicity.

## History of Local Anesthetic Systemic Toxicity

Local anesthetic toxicity was recognized even before cocaine was introduced as a surgical anesthetic in humans. In 1868, the first report of cocaine-induced seizures in animals was cited by Moreno y Maiz.[1] At the same time, Maiz also reported cutaneous anesthesia and asked whether cocaine might be used as a local anesthetic.[2] Almost 20 years passed before Koller introduced regional anesthesia to the world by applying cocaine to the eye.[3] Shortly after the introduction of cocaine as a topical anesthetic, physicians across the world began injecting cocaine near peripheral nerves, as well as into the spinal and epidural spaces.[1] Within 10 years of the introduction of regional anesthesia, reviews of "cocaine poisoning" appeared in the literature. Mattison[4] cited more than 125 cases of toxic reactions to cocaine, including seven deaths, with the initial report.

Despite this cocaine toxicity, the use of cocaine for peripheral nerve block was a real advantage during the later half of the 19th century, when general anesthetic techniques were still in their infancy. Nevertheless, although knowledge about the pharmacodynamics of cocaine accumulated, individuals paid a price in terms of toxicity and time. Rapid absorption limited the safe quantity of cocaine to 30mg and the useful duration of anesthesia to 10–15 minutes.[3] Reclus suggested that during infiltration anesthesia with cocaine, a weak solution be used to avoid toxic reactions and fatalities. It seems that Reclus clearly understood that the basic cause of accidental deaths during cocaine anesthesia was from the use of unnecessarily high concentrations and, thus, high total doses.[5] It was this toxicity of cocaine, coupled with its tremendous advantages for surgery, which led to a search for less-toxic substitutes. In 1904, such a substitute – procaine (Novocain) – was introduced by Einhorn.[6]

The introduction of a safer local anesthetic did not stop interest in local anesthetic toxicity. In 1919, Eggleston and Hatcher[7] published a comprehensive summary of the prevention and treatment of local anesthetic reactions. At this early time, they were able to identify most issues of importance in the prevention and treatment of local anesthetic systemic toxicity. They found that animals were a suitable experimental model, that different local anesthetics were additive in their toxicity, that the combination of artificial respiration and stimulation of the heart by intravenous epinephrine allowed twice the average fatal dose of local anesthetics to be administered to cats, and that the addition of epinephrine to subcutaneous injection of local anesthetics significantly reduced local anesthetic systemic toxicity. In 1925, Tatum, Atkinson, and Collins matured the concepts of Eggleston and Hatcher by identifying that artificial respiration alone was insufficient to increase the minimal fatal dose of cocaine in the rabbit, whereas the prophylactic administration of barbiturates to the dog produced a condition in which the tolerance to a toxic dose increased fourfold.[8] Likewise, they identified that seizures related to local anesthetic systemic toxicity are completely, practically, and instantaneously controlled by barbiturate injection and that the likelihood of recovery from such a reaction to cocaine in the dog is roughly inversely proportional to the duration the seizures were permitted to continue.

In addition to the insights about local anesthetic systemic toxicity provided by these early researchers, Vandam[9] identified two other major contributions to the understanding and treatment of local anesthetic reactions. He believed that Tanaka and Yamasaki's[10] report on the selective blocking of cortical inhibitory synapses by lidocaine (a surrogate for other local anesthetics) with the excitatory synapses being more resistant to the drug was a major contribution. He outlined a second major contribution by Englesson, who in 1974 reported the observance of seizure activity in the amygdala on cortical electroencephalography (EEG) after the intravenous infusion of several different local anesthetics in the cat. These two contributions helped mature physicians' understanding of the anatomic and neurophysiologic locus of local anesthetic-induced seizures and led to more complete knowledge of the basic science of a local anesthetic reaction.

## Basic Science

As the researchers detailed, local anesthetic systemic toxic responses are related to blood levels of the local anesthetic and, more specifically, to the levels found in the central nervous system (CNS). There is an initial generalized excitatory phase of a local anesthetic systemic toxic reaction related to increasing levels of local anesthetic in the blood of the CNS, which again is a result of a blocking of inhibitory pathways in the amygdala. This inhibition allows facilitatory (excitatory) neurons to function unopposed.[11] As levels of local anesthetic in the blood and brain increase further, both inhibitory and facilatory pathways are inhibited, eventually resulting in CNS depression. Can this brief and simplified view of neurophysiologic anatomy and reaction to local anesthetic systemic toxicity be expanded to deepen our understanding?

The amygdala is indeed central to understanding a local anesthetic-induced seizure and is part of the limbic system. It is located anterior to and partly superior to the tips of the inferior horn of the lateral ventricle[12] (Figure 4-1). The amygdala itself can be divided into basilateral and corticomedial nuclear groups, of which the former is highly developed in humans. Afferent pathways to the amygdala include dual olfactory sensory pathways, and efferent paths projecting to the hypothalamus, the thalamus, and the reticular formation.[13] The function of the amygdala is complex. In humans, ablation of lesions in the amygdala results in a decrease in aggressive behavior[14,15] and electrical stimulation of the amygdala in animals reveals changes in both visceral and autonomic function. With electrical stimulation, animals often turn their head and eyes to the contralateral side and demonstrate chewing, licking, and swallowing movements, as well as reactions of attention, rage, and fear.[16] Amygdala stimulation in humans results in confusional states and amnesia.[17]

Although most information suggests that the amygdala is the main and initial neurophysiologic focus for local anesthetic-induced seizures, some investigators have

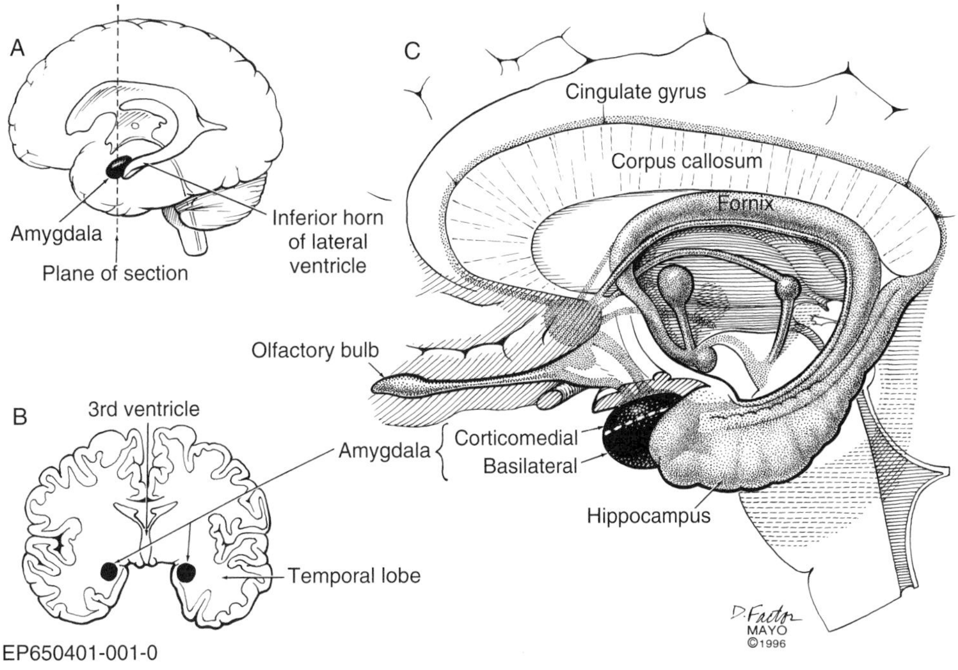


**FIGURE 4-1.** Anatomy of the amygdala and neuronal pathways connecting it to other CNS structures. The neuronal pathways to and from the amygdala are stippled in the illustration. **(A)** Parasagittal image of amygdala, lateral ventricle, and brain. **(B)** Cross-sectional image through the amygdala in the temporal lobe. **(C)** Expanded parasagittal image of structures immediately adjacent to the amygdala, including the corticomedial and basilateral areas of the amygdala. (Brown DL. Complications of Regional Anesthesia. New York: Churchill Livingstone; 1999:94–104. By permission of Mayo Foundation for Medical Education and Research. All rights reserved.)

demonstrated that the hippocampus is a secondary focus.[13] Despite this secondary focus, the amygdala seems necessary for local anesthetic-induced seizures to develop, because they fail to occur during typical cocaine-induced local anesthetic systemic toxic reactions in rats when the amygdala has been ablated.[18] With the amygdala as the initial limbic structure activated through local anesthetic systemic toxic reactions, the seizure activity both electrically and behaviorally mimics temporal lobe epilepsy, with subsequent progression to generalized seizures.[19–21] It seems that cerebral blood flow more than compensates for the increased oxygen demands in the cortex during lidocaine-induced seizures.[22] Furthermore, animal behavior data show that if local anesthetic-induced seizures are brief, no permanent neurologic or behavioral sequelae are produced.[23] With these brief basic science observations as a background, what can we learn from clinical episodes of systemic toxicity to local anesthetics?

## Clinical Science

During clinical care, the systemic toxic responses to local anesthetic drugs are the result of either an unintentional intravascular injection of the drug or administration of excessive amounts of the local anesthetic to a given patient. Clinically, it seems that most local anesthetic-induced seizures are a result of unintentional injection into the vascular system rather than uptake from excessive doses administered during regional block.[24] Part of the reason that most local anesthetic-induced seizures result from unintentional vascular injection rather than absorptive uptake is that the lung uptake of local anesthetic seems to exceed 90% of the drug. The lung seems to have a very important function as a buffer to unintentional vascular injection.[25] Nevertheless, this buffering action in the lung is saturable. Again, for emphasis, both central nervous excitation and cardiovascular manifestations of systemic toxic responses are attributable to blood levels of local anesthetic.

Before the classic local anesthetic-induced seizure develops, patients may experience various symptoms and signs leading up to the seizure (Figure 4-2). Some of the early symptoms include light-headedness and dizziness, both frequently associated with difficulty in focusing the eyes and the development of tinnitus. As blood levels increase, shivering, muscle twitching, and tremors are displayed. Often the tremors involve facial musculature and distal parts of the extremities, similar to the effects of amygdala stimulation in animals.[13] As blood and brain levels of anesthetic further increase, then the generalized tonic clonic convulsions occur.[26] Many clinicians suggest that numbness of the tongue, or circumoral numbness, may be one of the first symptoms of a systemic toxic reaction, and Scott[27] suggested that this is not a CNS effect but rather a result of drug leaving the vascular space and affecting the sensory nerve endings in the extravascular space.

In addition to these typical signs and symptoms developing during local anesthetic systemic toxic reactions, many clinical variables affect their development. For example, CNS depressant drugs often modify the clinical presentation of a systemic toxic reaction. In general, CNS depressant drugs minimize the signs and symptoms of CNS excitation, thus contributing to an appearance that CNS and cardiovascular toxicity occur nearer the same plasma concentration of local anesthetic.[28,29] Some have even suggested that sedative drugs used before a regional block mask the "early warning" that CNS excitation provides.[30] Nevertheless, most clinicians continue to appropriately provide anxiolysis and analgesia before administration of regional blocks.

Furthermore, the local anesthetic systemic toxic reactions are influenced by a patient's acid-base status. Generally, the convulsive threshold of local anesthetics is inversely proportional to the patient's $Paco_2$.[26] If there is an increase in $Paco_2$ or a decrease in pH, the convulsive threshold is decreased or the incidence of a systemic toxic reaction is increased. Presumably, effects of hypercapnia on cerebral blood flow explain this effect. Increasing $Paco_2$ increases cerebral blood flow, which may lead to increased uptake of local anesthetic by the brain. Additionally, plasma protein binding is decreased in the presence of acidosis or hypercapnia (or both), which results in an increased free drug level.[31]

Despite the basic science evidence, attempts to correlate EEG changes with the subjective and objective signs of CNS activity after administration of local anesthetic have been difficult. There does not seem to be a good correlation between changes in EEG activity and the subjective symptoms of CNS excitation in clinical situations.[32]

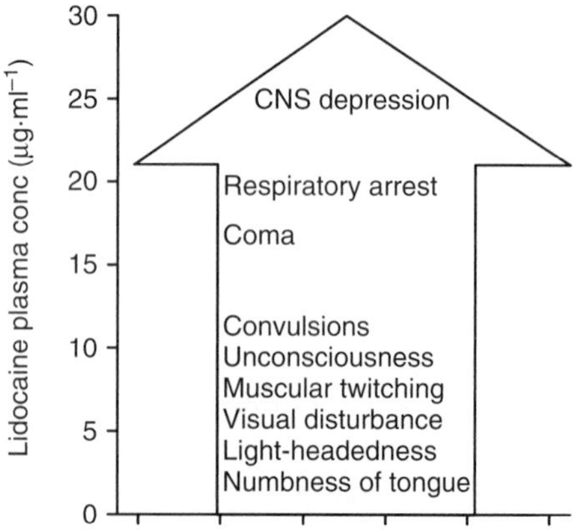


**FIGURE 4-2.** Local anesthetic systemic toxic symptoms are represented on a scale corresponding to the typical plasma lidocaine concentration producing respective symptoms.

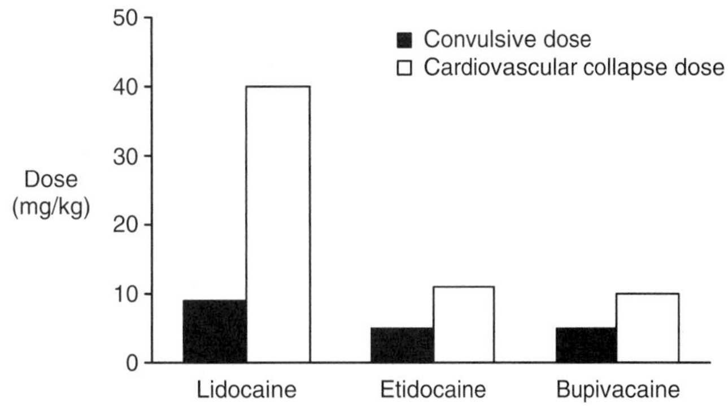


**FIGURE 4-3.** Relationship among doses of lidocaine, etidocaine, and bupivacaine that cause toxic responses in the CNS and doses that produce cardiovascular collapse. (Covino.[26] Reproduced with permission from the publisher.)

As outlined, the cardiovascular system is typically more resistant to the effects of local anesthetic drugs than the CNS; that is, the CNS toxic responses occur at lower blood levels than the cardiovascular system toxic responses. This general dictum is modified by the individual drug used. Each local anesthetic has an individual "circulatory collapse/CNS excitation ratio." For example, potent, long-acting local anesthetics such as bupivacaine and etidocaine have a lower circulatory collapse/CNS excitation ratio than other, less-potent aminoamides[33] (Figure 4-3).

Local anesthetic toxicity in the cardiovascular system results from drug effects on both vascular smooth muscle and cardiac muscle. The local anesthetics have dual effects on the heart, affecting both electrical and mechanical activities. Early during a systemic toxic reaction, sympathetic discharge may predominate and hypertension and tachycardia may be associated with an excitatory phase of CNS toxic response. As blood levels of local anesthetic increase, this initial phase may be followed by myocardial depression, moderate hypertension, and decreased cardiac output. Finally, as the severity of toxicity progresses, there is peripheral vasodilatation, profound hypotension, myocardial conduction abnormalities, sinus bradycardia, ventricular arrhythmias, and ultimately cardiovascular collapse. In general, basic science studies suggest that doses of local anesthetic agents that cause significant cardiovascular effects are approximately three times higher than the doses that will have distinct effects on the CNS.[32]

When the clinical science of the cardiac effects of local anesthetic systemic toxic reactions are examined, it is clear that the cardiac effects of local anesthetics are related to inhibition of sodium channels in the cardiac membranes, similar to the sought-after effect of local anesthetics on sodium channels in nerve membranes. There are also local anesthetic effects on potassium and calcium channels,[34] although understanding the effects of the drugs on the sodium channels allows the mechanism of systemic toxicity and its treatments to be easily conceptualized.

This sodium channel inhibition in the myocardium results in a decreased maximal rate of depolarization ($V_{max}$) of Purkinje fibers and ventricular muscle as well as decreased action potential duration and effective refractory period.[35–37] At high blood levels, local anesthetics prolong conduction time, and at even higher levels, these drugs depress spontaneous pacemaker activity.[25] In addition to these electrophysiologic effects, local anesthetics exhibit a negative inotropic action on the myocardium. As outlined, the more potent local anesthetics typically have a greater arrhythmogenic potential and cardiovascular depressive potential than do drugs such as lidocaine and mepivacaine. Albright[38] highlighted these cardiovascular systemic toxic effects with the potent local anesthetics in his 1979 editorial. Since that time, there has been extensive basic science and clinical investigation of the cardiovascular effects of potent, long-acting local anesthetics.

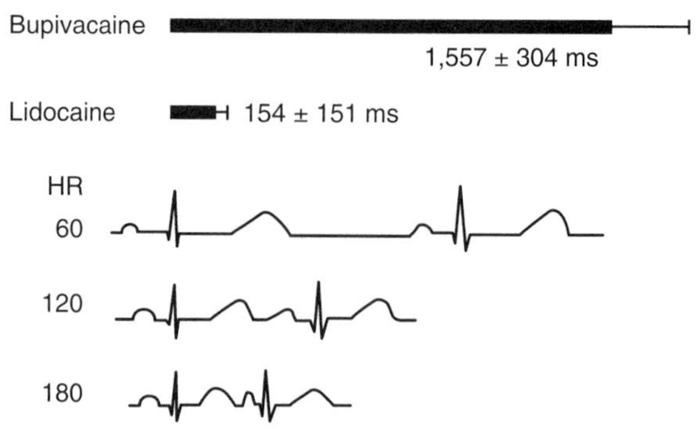


**FIGURE 4-4.** Comparison of time course of recovery after sodium channel block with lidocaine and bupivacaine. The dark "time bars" (lidocaine and bupivacaine) indicate the amount of time necessary for recovery of sodium channel availability in guinea pig papillary muscle. The simulated electrocardiographic traces [heart rate (HR): 60, 120, and 180 bpm] indicate that after bupivacaine block there is not an opportunity for sodium channel recovery even at slow heart rates, whereas with lidocaine the sodium channel has an opportunity to recover even at heart rates of 180 bpm. (Modified after data from Arlock P. Actions of three local anaesthetics: lidocaine, bupivacaine and ropivacaine on guinea pig papillary muscle sodium channels ($V_{max}$). Pharmacol Toxicol 1988;63:96–104. Reproduced with permission from Blackwell Publishing.)

A logical question is why the potent agents, with bupivacaine as the primary example, should cause more profound clinical effects. It was Clarkson and Hondeghem[37] who performed electrophysiologic studies on guinea pig ventricular muscle with bupivacaine and lidocaine and showed that block development and recovery are different with two drugs. In their study, lidocaine rapidly blocked inactivated and open sodium channels during the action potential, whereas bupivacaine block developed more slowly at low concentrations but rapidly at higher concentrations; additionally, recovery from the bupivacaine block was significantly slower than that from lidocaine. These authors developed a concept that lidocaine blocks sodium channels in a "fast-in fast-out fashion" and bupivacaine should be considered to block sodium channels in either a "slow-in slow-out manner" at low concentrations or in a "fast-in slow-out manner" at higher concentrations. Figure 4-4 demonstrates that at typical heart rates after lidocaine sodium channel blockade, the lidocaine has time to leave the sodium channel before the next QRS complex, whereas with bupivacaine the "slow-out" sodium channel effect prevents sodium channel release of the bupivacaine before the next QRS cycle.

The peripheral vascular effects of local anesthetics have been demonstrated to have a biphasic action on the smooth muscle of the peripheral blood vessels.[39] Typically, at low concentrations local anesthetics may cause increased tone in vascular beds, whereas at higher concentrations they produce a decrease in vascular tone. At extremely high blood levels, there is profound peripheral dilatation because of a direct relaxing effect on vascular smooth muscle in almost all beds. It should be remembered that cardiovascular collapse is also a result of the profound negative inotropic action of the local anesthetics at these extremely high blood levels.

## Recommended Doses of Local Anesthetic

In an effort to minimize local anesthetic systemic toxic reactions, many anesthesiologists look to recommended maximal doses as an absolute ceiling for local anesthetic administration. As Scott[40] suggested, acceptance of a maximal recommended dose of any particular drug may be a welcome "piece of information" for anesthesiologists; nevertheless, those recommendations are illogical and without scientific foundation. Presumably, the purpose of stating a maximal recommended dose for local anesthetics is to prevent the administration of an excessive amount, which then might result in systemic toxicity. For example, recommendations for "maximal doses" can be found in several anesthesia texts.[41,42] These maximal recommended doses have been developed for the clinical situation in which "too much drug" is injected. In reality, and as outlined, the cause of most episodes of local anesthetic systemic toxicity is unintentional intravascular injection of local anesthetic.[24] In that clinical situation, maximal recommended doses are irrelevant (Chapter 8). Another clinical factor that makes maximal recommended doses problematic is that the site of injection alters the rate of absorption, and thus the eventual local anesthetic blood levels.[43,44] Figure 4-5 demonstrates that the uptake is most rapid after interpleural or intercostal block and least rapid after spinal injection.

One other factor that affects peak blood levels is the addition of vasoconstrictors (usually epinephrine) to the local anesthetic solution. Epinephrine in a 1:100,000 to 1:200,000 concentration causes an approximately 50% decrease in peak plasma concentration of lidocaine after subcutaneous infiltration, but only a 20%–30% decrease after intercostal, epidural, or brachial plexus block.[45–48] Additionally, epinephrine decreases the peak blood level of bupivacaine significantly less than that of lidocaine, thus further confounding real understanding of establishing maximal doses of local anesthetics.[49–51] Pälve and colleagues[52] further highlighted the difficulties with maximal recommended doses during a study of adult patients undergoing brachial plexus block with 1.5% lidocaine plus epinephrine. After a dose of 900 mg of lidocaine plus epinephrine, the 17 patients (all more than 50 kg in weight) had a peak mean lidocaine value of 2.9 μg/mL, and the highest individual plasma concentration of lidocaine was 5.6 μg/mL. This highest individual level resulted from a patient receiving approximately 18 mg/kg. The investigators suggested that maximal doses of local anesthetics need to be individualized but leave "individualization" of dose undefined.

Another clinical example of the difficulties in establishing maximal doses is that shown by Samdal and colleagues,[53] who administered dilute (0.1%) lidocaine with epinephrine (1:1,000,000) in patients undergoing suction-assisted lipectomy of the abdomen, flanks, and lower extremities. In the 12 patients, the total dose of 1260–2880 mg of lidocaine (corresponding to 10.5–34.4 mg/kg) was administered with an

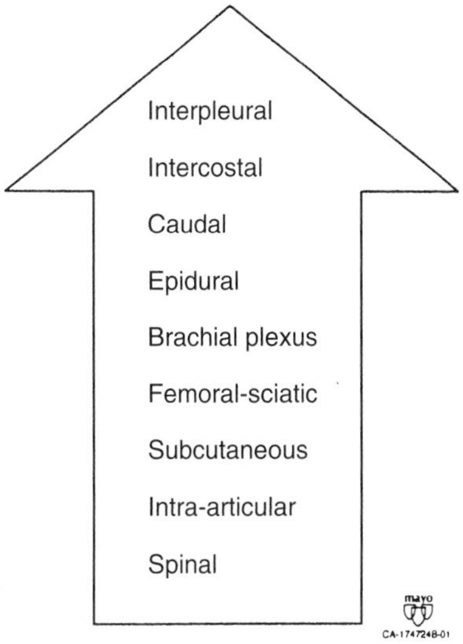


**FIGURE 4-5.** Ranking of the peak blood levels of local anesthetics after a wide variety of regional blocks. (Modified after Carpenter RL, Mackey DC. Local anesthetics. In: Barash PG, Cullen BF, Stoelting RK, eds. Clinical Anesthesia. Philadelphia: JB Lippincott; 1989:371–403; de Jong RH. Local Anesthetics. St. Louis: Mosby; 1994:152; and Covino BG, Vassallo HG. Local Anesthetic: Mechanism of Action and Clinical Use. New York: Grune and Stratton; 1976:97.)

injection speed of 60–78 mL per minute. In these patients, the peak concentration of lidocaine varied from 0.9 to 3.6 μg/mL and occurred between 6 and 12 hours postoperatively. These investigators also suggested that the maximal recommended dose needs to be individualized, but they went on to suggest that in addition to individualizing maximal recommended dose, the period of postprocedure observation should also be individualized. In their clinical setting, they suggested at least 18 hours of observation be applied to patients undergoing the large-volume subcutaneous injections of lidocaine.

## Treatment of Local Anesthetic Systemic Toxicity

Similar to most clinical recommendations, Feldman[1] suggested that the best treatment for local anesthetic toxicity is prevention. Because most local anesthetic systemic toxic reactions result from unintentional intravascular injection, efforts should be made to minimize that potential. This can be accomplished by both aspiration via the needle after the needle has been positioned for the regional block, and inclusion of "intravascular markers" such as epinephrine in the local anesthetic solution. When epinephrine-containing solution is injected, the heart rate increases; if dosing of the regional block is incremental, the total dose administered may be minimized before recognition of unintentional intravascular injection. This is the rationale behind the epidural test dose advocated by Moore and Batra.[54]

Brown and colleagues[24] showed that of 26 patients experiencing local anesthetic-induced systemic toxicity during regional block, all developed seizures without cardiovascular collapse. These data are supported by similar findings in a French survey of major complications with regional anesthesia, when none of the 24 patients experiencing local anesthetic systemic toxicity developed cardiovascular toxicity.[55] Fourteen of these French patients received bupivacaine, whereas 16 of Brown's patients did. These data highlight that most anesthesiologists focus on managing the CNS toxic responses (seizure) during the treatment of a systemic toxic reaction. Many anesthesiologists reflexively reach for sedatives or hypnotics at the onset of seizure activity, and it is known that barbiturates as well as benzodiazepines will effectively treat many of the local anesthetic-induced seizures.[56–60] Doses of these sedatives and hypnotics are important because their associated myocardial depression seems to be additive to that of the local anesthetic-induced myocardial depression (personal communication with Dan Moore, 1989). Moore and Bridenbaugh[61] suggested more than 30 years ago that the key to successful treatment of local anesthetic-induced CNS toxicity is provision of oxygen and the use of succinylcholine if it is needed to allow adequate oxygenation. Critics of this approach suggest that the succinylcholine simply masks local anesthetic-induced seizures, whereas Moore and colleagues emphasized that one of the reasons for using succinylcholine is to minimize the rapid development of acidosis that occurs from the motor seizures accompanying the local anesthetic-induced CNS excitation.[62,63] It is not mandatory to intubate a patient's trachea if an adequate airway can be maintained during the local anesthetic-induced seizure. Rather similar to maximal recommended doses of local anesthetics, this decision needs to be individualized.

If cardiovascular depression is present during a local anesthetic systemic toxic reaction, the first step is to concentrate on correcting the physiologic derangements that may potentiate the cardiac toxicity of local anesthetics (particularly bupivacaine), including hypoxemia, acidosis, and hyperkalemia.[64] There is little information regarding the best treatment of cardiovascular toxicity in humans, although investigators have highlighted some interesting new concepts. One of the new concepts is partitioning the lipid-soluble long-acting local anesthetics into a lipid-soluble medium. Weinberg and colleagues[65] have introduced the concept that bolus injection of intralipid may be a clinically effective method in patients unresponsive to basic resuscitative maneuvers. A more novel approach is to incorporate the lipid-soluble medium on the interior of a nanoparticle, and use injection of the nanoparticles to "sponge up" the long-acting local anesthetics on the interior of the nanoparticles, thus effectively reducing the systemic blood levels.[66] Others have explored insulin and glucose infusions in animal models, and this may hold promise.[67]

There are data from animals to suggest that large doses of epinephrine may be necessary to support heart rate and blood pressure, and there is more recent evidence that vasopressin (40 units(u) intravenous, once) may be used in place of, or in addition to, epinephrine.[68] Furthermore, atropine may be useful to treat bradycardia, direct current cardioversion often is successful, ventricular arrhythmias are probably better treated with amiodarone than with lidocaine, and cardiopulmonary bypass may be a useful adjunct to resuscitation.[3,68–73] Amiodarone, an inotropic agent, increases intracellular cyclic AMP and calcium via the inhibition of phosphodiesterase fraction 3. Again, the most effective treatment for cardiovascular toxic reactions associated with local anesthetic toxicity is prevention.

## Other Local Anesthetic Toxicity

### *Allergic Reactions*

Allergic reactions to local anesthetics are rare.[74] Nevertheless, clinical reactions associated with local anesthetics seem to be common, and often they are difficult for non-anesthesiologists to differentiate from true allergic reactions.[75–77] This clinical confusion seems to explain why many patients are labeled "allergic" to local anesthetics even when signs and symptoms are more consistent with an adverse reaction.

The amino-ester local anesthetics such as procaine, chloroprocaine, and tetracaine are all derivatives of paraaminobenzoic acid (PABA). PABA is known to be an allergen and is, in fact, a byproduct of the hydrolysis of the amino-ester local anesthetics. Allergic reactions to amino-ester compounds are much more common than those to amino-amide compounds. Confounding this further, some commercial preparations of amino-amide agents use methylparaben as a preservative. Methylparaben is also chemically related to PABA and has been identified as a true allergen.[75] When an amino-amide is linked to an allergic reaction, the allergy is likely attributable to the preservative rather than to the amino-amide local anesthetic. If PABA-like compounds are linked to allergic reactions, why are they added to local anesthetics?

One of the primary reasons for the use of the paraben-esters is the excellent bacteriostatic and fungistatic properties associated with the compounds. These compounds are widely used in multidose local anesthetic preparations, other drugs, cosmetics, and foods. Thus, a large percentage of the population has been exposed to the parabens, whether or not they have ever received local anesthetic compounds.[78]

It has been suggested that provocative skin testing is safe and effective in differentiating patients with adverse and true allergic reactions to local anesthetics.[76,79] The proponents of testing suggest that if the local anesthetic skin test and progressive challenge is negative, it is safe to use a local anesthetic. It should be emphasized that this concept of skin testing with local anesthetics is not universally shared, and some question the reliability of the skin testing.[76,80]

### *Myotoxicity*

Local anesthetic injection into muscle may cause focal necrosis, and usually this focal necrosis is followed by rapid regeneration within a few weeks.[81] When the longer-acting drug bupivacaine is injected into muscle, muscle repair is slower. It should be emphasized that the myotoxicity is limited to muscle and does not involve nerves[82] (Chapter 6). Bupivacaine seems to create myotoxicity by suppressing muscle protein synthesis through the inhibition of amino acylation of RNA.[83] The recognition experimentally that bupivacaine can be linked to myotoxicity needs to be correlated with the widespread use of bupivacaine in mixtures for muscle trigger-point injections.[84] One may speculate that some of the effects of trigger-point injection are produced through a beneficial myotoxicity mechanism. It should be remembered that in typical clinical situations, bupivacaine, lidocaine, procaine, and tetracaine seem to produce only isolated, localized myotoxicity, which does not spread to neural structures.[85]

## References


1. Feldman HS. Toxicity of local anesthetic agents. In: Rice SA, Fish KJ, eds. Anesthetic Toxicity. New York: Raven Press; 1994:107–133.
2. Holmstedt B, Fredga A. Sundry episodes in the history of coca and cocaine. J Ethnopharmacol 1981;3:113–147.
3. Fink BR. History of neural blockade. In: Cousins MJ, Bridenbaugh PO, eds. Neural Blockade in Clinical Anesthesia and Management of Pain. Philadelphia: JB Lippincott; 1988: 3–15.
4. Mattison JB. Cocaine poisoning. Med Surg Rep 1891;60:645–650.
5. Reclus P. Analgésie locale par la cocaïne. Rev Chir 1889;9:913.
6. Braun H. Ueber einige neuerörtliche Anesthetica (Stovain, Alypin, Novocain). Dtsch Klin Wochenschr 1905;31:1667.
7. Eggleston C, Hatcher RA. A further contribution to the pharmacology of the local anesthetics. J Pharmacol Exp Ther 1919;13:433.
8. Tatum AL, Atkinson AJ, Collins KH. Acute cocaine poisoning, its prophylaxis and treatment in laboratory animals. J Pharmacol Exp Ther 1925;26:325–335.
9. Englesson S. The influence of acid-base changes on central nervous system toxicity of local anaesthetic agents. Acta Anaesthesiol Scand 1974;18:79–87.
10. Tanaka K, Yamasaki M. Blocking of cortical inhibitory synapses by intravenous lidocaine. Nature 1966;209:207–208.
11. Wagman IH, DeJong RH, Prince DA. Effects of lidocaine on the central nervous system. Anesthesiology 1967;28:155–172.
12. Truex RC, Carpenter MB. The basal ganglia and rhinencephalon, olfactory and limbic system pathways. In: Human Neuroanatomy. 6th ed. Baltimore: Williams & Wilkins; 1971: 498–542.
13. Garfield JM, Gugino L. Central effects of local anesthetic agents. In: Strichartz G, ed. Local Anesthetics. Vol 81. New York: Springer-Verlag; 1987:253–284.
14. Green JD, Duisberg REH, McGrath WB. Focal epilepsy of psychomotor type. A preliminary report of observations on effects of surgical therapy. J Neurosurg 1951;8:157–172.
15. Pool JL. Neurophysiological symposium: visceral brain in man. J Neurosurg 1954;11: 45–63.
16. MacLean PD, Delgado JMR. Electrical and chemical stimulation of fronto-temporal portion of limbic system in the waking animal. Electroencephalogr Clin Neurophysiol 1952;5:91–100.
17. Feindel W, Penfield W. Localization of discharge in temporal lobe automatism. AMA Arch Neurol Psychiatry 1954;72:605–630.
18. Eidelberg E, Lesse H, Gaulta FP. An experimental model of temporal lobe epilepsy. Studies of the convulsant properties of cocaine. In: Glaser GH, ed. EEG and Behavior. New York: Basic Books; 1963:Chapter 10.
19. DeJong RH. Central nervous system effects. In: DeJong RH, ed. Local Anesthetics. 2nd ed. Springfield, IL: Charles C. Thomas; 1977:84–114.
20. Stein PA, Michenfelder JD. Neurotoxicity of anesthetics. Anesthesiology 1979;50:437–453.
21. Moore DC. Administer oxygen first in the treatment of local anesthetic-induced convulsions. Anesthesiology 1980;53:346–347.
22. Maekawa T, Oshibuchi T, Takao, Takeshita H, Imamura A. Cerebral energy state and glycolytic metabolism during lidocaine infusion in the rat. Anesthesiology 1981;54:278–283.

23. DeJong RH, Heavner JE. Diazepam prevents local anesthetic seizures. Anesthesiology 1971;34:523–531.
24. Brown DL, Ransom DM, Hall JA, Leicht CH, Schroeder DR, Offord KP. Regional anesthesia and local anesthetic-induced systemic toxicity: seizure frequency and accompanying cardiovascular changes. Anesth Analg 1995;81:321–328.
25. Löfström JB. Physiologic disposition of local anesthetics. Reg Anesth 1982:33–38.
26. Covino BG. Pharmacology of local anesthetic agents. In: Rogers MC, Tinker JH, Covino BG, et al., eds. Principles and Practice of Anesthesiology. St. Louis: Mosby Year Book; 1993:1235–1257.
27. Scott DB. Toxic effects of local anaesthetic agents on the central nervous system. Br J Anaesth 1986;58:732–735.
28. Gerard JL, Edouard A, Berdeaux A, Duranteau J, Ahmad R. Interaction of intravenous diazepam and dupivacaine in conscious dogs. Reg Anesth 1989;14:298–303.
29. Bernards CM, Carpenter RL, Rupp SM, et al. Effect of midazolam and diazepam premedication on central nervous system and cardiovascular toxicity of bupivacaine in pigs. Anesthesiology 1989;70:318–323.
30. Ausinsch B, Malagodi MH, Munson ES. Diazepam in the prophylaxis of lignocaine seizures. Br J Anaesth 1976;48:309.
31. Englesson S. The influence of acid-base changes on central nervous system toxicity of local anaesthetic agents. I. An experimental study in cats. Acta Anaesthesiol Scand 1974;18: 79–87.
32. Covino BG. Toxicity and systemic effects of local anesthetic agents. In: Brown DL, ed. Local Anesthesia. Vol 81. New York: Springer-Verlag; 1987:187–212.
33. Concepcion M. Acute complications and side effects of regional anesthesia. In: Regional Anesthesia and Analgesia. Philadelphia: WB Saunders; 1996:Chapter 23.
34. Heavner JE. Cardiac toxicity of local anesthetics in the intact isolated heart model: a review. Reg Anesth Pain Med 2002;27:545–555.
35. Lynch C III. Depression of myocardial contractility in vitro by bupivacaine, etidocaine, and lidocaine. Anesth Analg 1986;65:551–559.
36. Moller RA, Covino BG. Cardiac electrophysiologic effects of lidocaine and bupivacaine. Anesth Analg 1988;67:107–114.
37. Clarkson CW, Hondeghem LM. Mechanism for bupivacaine depression of cardiac conduction: fast block of sodium channels during the action potential with slow recovery from block during diastole. Anesthesiology 1985;62:396–405.
38. Albright GA. Cardiac arrest following regional anesthesia with etidocaine or bupivacaine [editorial]. Anesthesiology 1979;51:285–287.
39. Blair MR. Cardiovascular pharmacology of local anaesthetics. Br J Anaesth 1975;47: 247–252.
40. Scott DB. "Maximal recommended doses" of local anaesthetic drugs. Br J Anaesth 1989; 63(4):373–374.
41. Strichartz GR, Berde CB. Local anesthetics. In: Miller RD, ed. Anesthesia. 4th ed. New York: Churchill Livingstone; 1994:489–521.
42. DiFazio CA, Woods AM. Drugs commonly used for nerve blocking: pharmacology of local anesthetics. In: Prithi R, ed. Practical Management of Pain. 2nd ed. St. Louis: Mosby Year Book; 1992:685–700.
43. Braid DP, Scott DB. The systemic absorption of local analgesic drugs. Br J Anaesth 1965; 37:394–404.
44. Rosenberg PH, Veering BT, Urmey WF. Maximum recommended doses of local anesthetics: a multifactorial concept. Reg Anesth Pain Med 2004;29:564–575.
45. Braid DP, Scott DB. The effect of adrenaline on the systemic absorption of local anaesthetic drugs. Acta Anaesthesiol Scand 1996;(suppl 23):334–346.
46. Raj RP, Rosenblatt R, Miller J, Katx RL, Corden E. Dynamics of local anesthetic compounds in regional anesthesia. Anesth Analg 1977;56:110–117.
47. Mather LE, Tucker GT, Murphy TM, Stanton-Hicks M, Bonica JJ. Effect of adding adrenaline to etidocaine and lignocaine in extradural anaesthesia. II. Pharmacokinetics. Br J Anaesth 1976;48:989–994.
48. Wildsmith JAW, Tucker GT, Cooper S, Scott DB, Covino BG. Plasma concentrations of local anaesthetics after interscalene brachial plexus block. Br J Anaesth 1977;49:461–466.

49. Wilkinson GR, Lund PC. Bupivacaine levels in plasma and cerebrospinal fluid following peridural administration. Anesthesiology 1970;33:482–486.
50. Appleyard TN, Witt A, Atkinson RE, Nicholas ADG. Bupivacaine carbonate and bupivacaine hydrochloride: a comparison of blood concentrations during epidural blockade for vaginal surgery. Br J Anaesth 1974;46:503–533.
51. Abdel-Salam AR, Vonwiller JB, Scott DB. Evaluation of etidocaine in extradural block. Br J Anaesth 1975;47:1081–1086.
52. Pälve H, Kirvelä O, Olin H, Syvälahti E, Kanto J. Maximum recommended doses of lignocaine are not toxic. Br J Anaesth 1995;74:704–705.
53. Samdal F, Amland PF, Bugge JF. Plasma lidocaine levels during suction-assisted lipectomy using large doses of dilute lidocaine with epinephrine. Plast Reconstr Surg 1994;93(6): 1217–1223.
54. Moore DC, Batra MS. The components of an effective test dose prior to epidural block. Anesthesiology 1981;55(6):693–696.
55. Auroy Y, Benhamou D, Bargue L, et al. Major complications in regional anesthesia in France: the SOS regional anesthesia hotline service. Anesthesiology 2002;97:1274–1280.
56. Liu P, Feldman HS, Covino BM, Giasi R, Covino BG. Acute cardiovascular toxicity of intravenous amide local anesthetics in anesthetized ventilated dogs. Anesth Analg 1982; 61:317–322.
57. Feldman HS, Arthur GR, Covino BG. Comparative systemic toxicity of convulsant and supraconvulsant doses of intravenous ropivacaine, bupivacaine, and lidocaine in the conscious dog. Anesth Analg 1989;69:794–801.
58. Feldman HS, Arthur GR, Pitkanen M, Hurley R, Doucette AM, Covino BG. Treatment of acute systemic toxicity after the rapid intravenous injection of ropivacaine and bupivacaine in the conscious dog. Anesth Analg 1991;73:373–384.
59. Covino BG. Toxicity and systemic effects of local anesthetic agents. In: Strichartz G, ed. Local Anesthesia. New York: Springer-Verlag; 1987:187–209.
60. Davis NL, deJong RH. Successful resuscitation following massive bupivacaine overdose. Anesth Analg 1982;61:62–64.
61. Moore DC, Bridenbaugh LD. Oxygen: the antidote for systemic toxic reactions from local anesthetic drugs. JAMA 1960;174:842–847.
62. Moore DC, Crawford RD, Scurlock JE. Severe hypoxia and acidosis following local anesthetic-induced convulsions. Anesthesiology 1980;53(3):259–260.
63. Moore DC, Thompson GE, Crawford RD. Long-acting local anesthetic drugs and convulsions with hypoxia and acidosis. Anesthesiology 1982;56(3):230–232.
64. Reis S, Nath S. Cardiotoxicity of local anaesthetic agents. Br J Anaesth 1986;58: 736–746.
65. Weinberg G, Ripper R, Feinstein DL, Hoffman W. Lipid emulsion infusion rescues dogs from bupivacaine-induced cardiac toxicity. Reg Anesth Pain Med 2003;28:198–202.
66. Varshney M, Morey TE, Shah DO, et al. Pluronic microemulsions as nanoreservoirs for extraction of bupivacaine from normal saline. J Am Chem Soc 2004;126:5108–5112.
67. Kim JT, Jung CW, Lee KH. The effect of insulin on the resuscitation of bupivacaine-induced severe cardiovascular toxicity in dogs. Anesth Analg 2004;99:728–733.
68. Weinberg GL. Current concepts in resuscitation of patients with local anesthetic toxicity. Reg Anesth Pain Med 2002;27:568–575.
69. Bennett A. The physiological action of coca. Br Med J 1874;1:510.
70. Freud S. Über Coca. Zentralbl Ges Ther 1884;2:289–314.
71. Bull CS. The hydrochlorate of cocaine as a local anaesthetic in ophthalmic surgery. NY Med J 1884;40:643–644.
72. Hall RJ. Hydrochlorate of cocaine. NY Med J 1884;40:609–611.
73. Corning JL. Spinal anaesthesia and local medication of the cord. NY Med J 1885;42: 483–485.
74. Adriani J. Reactions to local anesthetics. JAMA 1966;196:119.
75. Aldrete JA, Johnson DA. Evaluation of intracutaneous testing for investigation of allergy to local anesthetic agents. Anesth Analg 1970;49:173.
76. Incaudo G, Schatz M, Patterson R, et al. Administration of local anesthetics to patients with a history of prior adverse reaction. J Allergy Clin Immunol 1978;61:339.
77. Brown DT, Beamish D, Wildsmith JAW. Allergic reaction to an amide local anaesthetic. Br J Anaesth 1981;53:435.

78. Nagel JE, Fuscaldo JT, Fireman P. Paraben allergy. JAMA 1977;237:1594.
79. DeShazo RD, Nelson HS. An approach to the patient with a history of local anaesthetic hypersensitivity: experience with 90 patients. J Allergy Clin Immunol 1979;63:387.
80. Fisher MM. Intradermal testing in the diagnosis of acute anaphylaxis during anaesthesia – results of five years' experience. Anaesth Intensive Care 1979;7:58.
81. Benoit PW, Belt WD. Some effects of local anesthetic agents on skeletal muscle. Exp Neurol 1972;34:264–278.
82. Hall-Craggs ECB. Rapid degeneration and regeneration of a whole skeletal muscle following treatment with bupivacaine (Marcaine). Exp Neurol 1974;43:349–358.
83. Johnson ME, Jones GH. Effects of Marcaine, a myotoxic drug, on macromolecular synthesis in muscle. Biochem Pharmacol 1978;27:1753–1757.
84. Zink W, Graf BM. Local anesthetic myotoxicity. Reg Anesth Pain Med 2004;29: 333–340.
85. Foster AH, Carlson BM. Myotoxicity of local anesthetics and regeneration of the damaged muscle fibers. Anesth Analg 1980;59:727–736.

# 5 Mechanisms of Neurologic Complications with Peripheral Nerve Blocks

Alain Borgeat, Stephan Blumenthal, and Admir Hadžić

Although there are relatively few published reports of anesthesia-related nerve injury associated with the use of peripheral nerve blocks (PNBs), it is likely that the commonly cited incidence (0.4%) of severe injury is underestimated because of underreporting.[1–3] The less frequent clinical application of lower-extremity nerve blocks may be the main reason that there are even fewer reports of anesthesia-related nerve injury associated with lower-extremity PNBs as compared with upper-extremity PNBs. Although neurologic complications after PNBs can be related to a variety of factors related to the block (e.g., needle trauma, intraneuronal injection, neuronal ischemia, and toxicity of local anesthetics), a search for other common causes should also include surgical factors (e.g., positioning, stretching, retractor injury, ischemia, and hematoma formation). In some instances, the neurologic injury may be a result of a combination of these factors.

In this chapter, we will discuss mechanisms and consequences of acute neurologic injury related to the nerve block procedures. Specific nerve injuries associated with upper and lower nerve block techniques, neuraxial anesthesia, and local anesthetic toxicity will be discussed elsewhere in the text.

## Functional Histology of the Peripheral Nerves

To understand the mechanisms of peripheral nerve injury, one must be familiar with the functional histology of the peripheral nerve. Peripheral nerves are complex structures consisting of fascicles held together by the *epineurium* – an enveloping, external connective sheath (Figure 5-1). Each fascicle contains many nerve fibers and capillary blood vessels embedded in a loose connective tissue, *the endoneurium*.[4] The *perineurium* is a multilayered epithelial sheath that surrounds individual fascicles and consists of several layers of perineural cells. Therefore, in essence, a fascicle is a group of nerve fibers surrounded by *perineurium*. Of note, fascicles can be organized in one of three common arrangements: *monofascicular* (single, large fascicle); *oligofascicular* (few fascicles of various sizes); and *polyfascicular* (many fascicles of various sizes).[5]

Nerve fibers can be myelinated or unmyelinated; sensory and motor nerves contain both in a ratio of 4:1, respectively. Unmyelinated fibers are composed of several

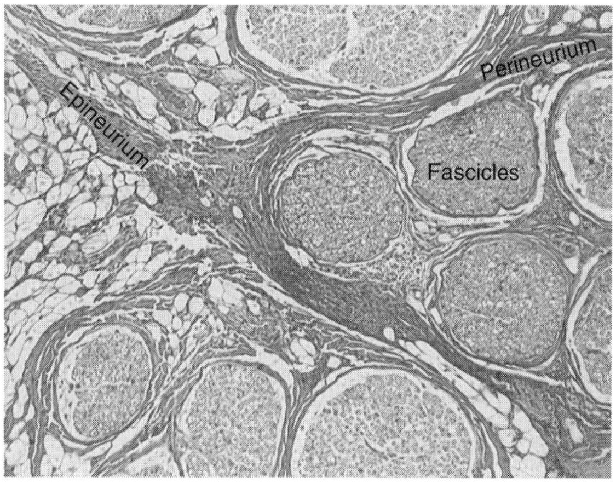


**FIGURE 5-1.** Histology of the peripheral nerve. A peripheral nerve is a complex structure consisting of fascicles held together by the epineurium. Fascicles contain many nerve fibers and capillary blood vessels embedded in a loose connective tissue, the endoneurium. The perineurium is a multilayered epithelial sheath that surrounds individual fascicles.

axons, wrapped by a single Schwann cell. The axons of myelinated nerve fibers are enveloped individually by a single Schwann cell. A thin layer of collagen fibers, the *endoneurium*, surrounds the individually myelinated or groups of unmyelinated fibers.

Nerve fibers depend on a specific endoneurial environment for their function. Peripheral nerves are richly supplied by an extensive vascular network in which the endoneurial capillaries have endothelial "tight junctions," a peripheral analogy to the "blood-brain barrier." The neurovascular bed is regulated by the sympathetic nervous system, and its blood flow can be as high as 30–40 mL/100 g/minute. In addition to conducting nerve impulses, nerve fibers also maintain axonal transport of various functionally important substances, such as proteins, and precursors for receptors and transmitters. This process is highly dependent on oxidative metabolism. Any of these structures and functions can be deranged during a traumatic nerve injury, with the possible result of temporary or permanent impairment or loss of neural function.

## Mechanisms of Peripheral Nerve Injury

The etiology of peripheral nerve injury related to the use of PNBs falls into one of four categories (Table 5-1). *Laceration* results when the nerve is cut partially or completely, such as by a scalpel or a large-gauge cutting needle. *Stretch injuries* to the nerves may result when nerves or plexuses are stretched in a nonphysiologic or exaggerated physiologic position, such as during shoulder manipulation under an interscalene block. *Pressure*, as a mechanism of nerve injury, is relatively common. A typical example of this mechanism is chronic compression of the nerves by neighboring structures, such as fibrous bands, scar tissue, or abnormal muscles, where they pass through fibro-osseous spaces if the space is too small, such as the carpal tunnel. Such chronic compression syndromes are called *entrapment neuropathies*. Examples of pressure injuries applicable to PNBs include external pressure over a period of hours (e.g., a "Saturday night palsy" resulting from pressure of a chair back on the radial nerve of an intoxicated person). The pressure may be repeated and have a cumulative effect (e.g., an ulnar neuropathy resulting from habitually leaning on the elbow). Such a scenario is conceivable, for instance, with a patient who positions the anesthetized arm (e.g., long-acting or continuous brachial plexus block) in a nonphysiologic position for a few hours. Another example of pressure-related nerve injury is prolonged use

TABLE 5-1. Mechanism of Peripheral Nerve Injury Related to PNBs

| |
|---|
| Mechanical-acute |
| Laceration |
| Stretch |
| Intraneural injection |
| Vascular |
| Acute ischemia |
| Hemorrhage |
| Pressure |
| Extraneural |
| Intraneural |
| Compartment syndrome |
| Chemical |
| Injection of neurotoxic solutions |

of a high-pressure tourniquet. Finally, an intraneural injection may lead to sustained high intraneural pressure, which exceeds capillary occlusion pressure, leading to nerve ischemia.[6] *Vascular nerve damage* after nerve blocks can occur when there is acute occlusion of the arteries from which the vasa nervora are derived or from a hemorrhage within a nerve sheath. With *injection injuries*, the nerve may be directly impaled and the drug injected directly into the nerve, or the drug may be injected into adjacent tissues, causing an acute inflammatory reaction or chronic fibrosis, both indirectly involving the nerve. *Chemical nerve injury* is the result of tissue toxicity of injected solutions (e.g., local anesthetic toxicity or neurolysis after alcohol or phenol injections).

## Clinical Classification of Acute Nerve Injuries

Classification of acute nerve injuries is useful in considering the physical and functional state of damaged nerves. In his classification, Seddon[7] introduced the terms *neurapraxia*, *axonotmesis*, and *neurotmesis*; Sunderland[8] subsequently proposed a five-grade classification system.

*Neurapraxia* refers to nerve dysfunction lasting several hours to 6 months after a blunt injury to the nerve. In neuropraxia, the nerve axons and connective tissue structures remain intact. The nerve dysfunction probably results from several factors, of which *focal demyelination* is the most important abnormality. Intraneural hemorrhage, changes in the vasa nervora, disruption of the blood-nerve barrier and axon membranes, and electrolyte disturbances all may add to the impairment of nerve function. Because the nerve dysfunction is rarely complete, clinical deficits are partial and recovery usually occurs within a few weeks, although some neurapraxic lesions (with minimal or no axonal degeneration) may take several months to recover.

*Axonotmesis* consists of *physical interruption of the axons* but within intact Schwann cell tubes and intact connective tissue structures of the nerve (i.e., the endoneurium, perineurium, and epineurium). Sunderland subdivided this group, depending on which of the three structures were involved (Table 5-2). With axonotmesis, the nerve sheath remains intact, enabling regenerating nerve fibers to find their way into the distal segment. Consequently, efficient axonal regeneration can eventually take place.

*Neurotmesis* refers to a *complete interruption of the entire nerve* including the axons and all connective tissue structures (epineurium included). Clinically, there is total nerve dysfunction. With both axonotmesis and neurotmesis, axonal disruption leads to Wallerian degeneration, from which recovery occurs through the slow process of axonal regeneration. However, with neurotmesis, the two nerve ends may be

TABLE 5-2. Classification of Nerve Injuries

| Seddon | Sunderland | Structural and functional processes |
|---|---|---|
| Neurapraxia | 1 | Myelin damage, conduction slowing, and blocking |
| Axonotmesis | 2 | Loss of axonal continuity, endoneurium intact, no conduction |
| | 3 | Loss of axonal and endoneurial continuity, perineurium intact, no conduction |
| | 4 | Loss of axonal, endoneurial, and perineurial continuity; epineurium intact; no conduction |
| Neurotmesis | 5 | Entire nerve trunk separated; no conduction |

*Source:* Based on data from Seddon,[7] Sunderland,[8] and Lundborg.[9]

completely separated, and the regenerating axons may not be able to find the distal stump. For these reasons, effective recovery does not occur unless the severed ends are sutured or joined by a nerve graft. With closed injuries, the only way to distinguish clearly between axonotmesis and neurotmesis is surgical exploration and intraoperative inspection of the nerve.

It should be noted that most acute nerve injuries are mixed lesions.[7] Different fascicles and nerve fibers typically sustain different degrees of injury, which may make it difficult to assess the type of injury and predict outcome even by electrophysiologic means. Recovery from a mixed lesion is characteristically biphasic; it is relatively rapid for fibers with neurapraxic damage, but much slower for axons that have been totally interrupted and have undergone Wallerian degeneration.

## Mechanical Nerve Injury

### *Intraneural Injection*

As opposed to a relatively clean injury caused by a needle, intraneural injection has the potential to create structural damage to the fascicle(s) that is more extensive and less likely to heal (Figure 5-2). Indeed, the devastating sequelae of sensory and motor loss after injection of various agents into peripheral nerves has been well documented.[10]

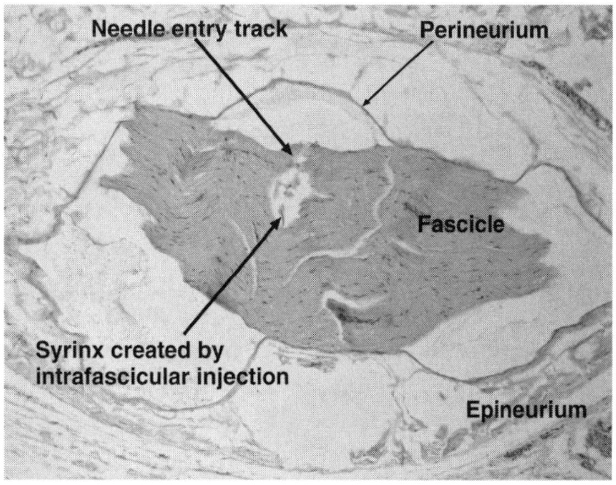


**FIGURE 5-2.** Mechanical nerve injury after an intraneural injection in a sciatic nerve of a rat. Shown are bulging of the perineurium, needle insertion track, and a syrinx created by intrafascicular injection. (Reproduced with permission from Deschner S, Borgeat A, Hadzic A. Neurologic complications of peripheral nerve blocks. In Hadzic A, ed. Regional Anesthesia and Acute Pain Management, 2007;967–997. McGraw-Hill, New York).

Nearly, all experimental studies on this subject have demonstrated that the site of injection is critical in determining the degree and nature of injury. More specifically, to induce neurologic injury, the injectate must be injected intrafascicularly; extrafascicular injections of the same substance typically do not cause nerve injury.[11] Thus, the main factor leading to a severe peripheral nerve damage associated with injection techniques is injection of local anesthetic into a fascicle or group of faciles bound together. This causes mechanical destruction of the fascicular architecture and sets into motion a cascade of pathophysiologic changes including inflammation, cellular infiltration, axonal degeneration, and others, all possibly leading to nerve scarring.

Histologic features after intraneural injection are rather nonspecific and range from simple mechanical disruption and delamination to fragmentation of the myelin sheath and marked cellular infiltration. A vast array of cellular changes occur after peripheral nerve trauma, and these have been documented using a variety of animal models.[11] The extent of actual neurologic damage occurring after an intrafascicular injection can range from neuropraxia with minimal structural damage to neurotmesis with severe axonal and myelin degeneration, depending on the needle–nerve relationship, agent injected, and dose of the drug used.[12–15] In general, subperineural changes tend to be more prominent, compared with the central area of the fascicle.[16] Additionally, injury to primary sensory neurons, which is not detectable histologically, causes a shift in membrane channel expression, sensitivity to algogenic substances, neuropeptide production, and intracellular signal transduction, both at the injury site and in the cell body in the dorsal root ganglion. All of this leads to increased excitability and the occurrence of acute or chronic pain, often experienced by patients with neurologic injury. It should be noted that intraneural injection and its resultant mechanical injury are merely the inciting mechanisms; a host of additional changes occur involving inflammatory reactions such as chemical neuritis and intraneural hemorrhage, all of which eventually may lead to nerve scarring and chronic neuropathic pain (Figure 5-3).

## *Prevention of Intraneural Injection*

### Pain on Injection

Little is known about how to avoid an intraneuronal injection. Pain with injection has long been thought of as the cardinal sign of intraneuronal injection; consequently, it is frequently suggested that blocks be avoided in heavily premedicated or anesthetized patients. However, case reports suggest that pain may not be reliable as a sole warning sign of impending nerve injury, and it may be present in only a minority of cases.[17–20] For instance, Fanelli and colleagues[3] have reported unintended paresthesia in 14% of patients in their study; however, univariate analysis of potential risk factors for

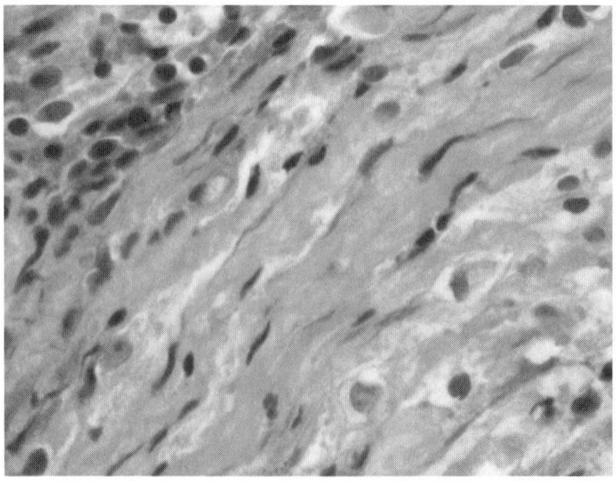

**FIGURE 5-3.** Inflammatory changes in a nerve fascicle after an intraneural injection.

postoperative neurologic dysfunction failed to demonstrate paresthesia as a risk factor. In addition, the sensory nature of the pain-paresthesia can be difficult to interpret in clinical practice.[21] A certain degree of discomfort on injection ("pressure paresthesia") is considered normal and affirmative of impending successful blockade because it indicates that injection of local anesthetic has been made in the vicinity of the targeted nerve.[21] In clinical practice, however, it can be difficult to discern when pain-paresthesia on injection is "normal" and when it is the ominous sign of an intraneural injection.[22] Moreover, it is unclear how pain or paresthesia on injection, even when present, can be used clinically to prevent development of neurologic injury. For instance, in a prospective study on neurologic complications of regional anesthesia by Auroy and colleagues,[2] neurologic injuries occured even when the participating anesthesiologists did not continue to inject local anesthetic when pain on injection was reported by the patients.

### Intensity of the Stimulating Current

In current clinical practice, development of nerve localization and injection monitoring techniques to reliably prevent intraneural injection remain inconclusive.[18] Nerve stimulators are very useful for nerve localization; however, the needle–nerve relationship cannot be adequately, precisely, and reliably ascertained as early literature suggested.[23] Response to nerve stimulation with a frequently used current intensity (1 mA) may be absent even when the needle makes physical contact with or is inserted into a nerve.[24,25] Occurrence of nerve injuries despite using nerve stimulation to localize the nerve further suggests that nerve stimulators can, at best, provide only a rough approximation of the needle–nerve relationship.[1] The current interest in ultrasound-assisted nerve localization holds promise for facilitating nerve localization and administration of nerve blocks; however, the image resolution of this technology is insufficient to visualize nerve fascicles and prevent intrafascicular injection.

The optimal current intensity resulting in accurate localization of a nerve has been a topic of controversy for many years.[23,26–29] For instance, stimulation at currents higher than 0.5 mA may result in block failure because the needle tip is distant from the nerve, whereas stimulation at currents lower than 0.2 mA theoretically may pose a risk of intraneuronal injection (http://www.nysora.com, January 1, 2003). Some authors suggest that a motor response with a current intensity between 1.0 and 0.5 mA is sufficient for accurate placement of the block needle,[23] whereas others advise using a current of much lower intensity (0.5–0.1 mA).[26,28] Others simply suggest stimulating with currents less than 0.75 mA,[29,30] or progressively reducing the current to as low a level as possible while still maintaining a motor response.[27] Methods in most recently published reports have suggested obtaining nerve stimulation with currents of 0.2–0.5 mA (100 ms) before injecting local anesthetics, believing that motor response with current intensities lower than 0.2 mA may be associated with intraneural needle placement. However logical these beliefs might sound, there are no published reports substantiating these concerns.

### Resistance to Injection

Assessing resistance to injection is a common practice, similar to loss of resistance to injection of air or saline using a "syringe feel" during administration of epidural, paravertebral, or lumbar plexus blocks. Similarly, assessing tissue resistance and injection compliance is another means of estimating the anatomic location of the needle tip during the practice of PNBs. For this, many clinicians use a syringe feel to estimate what may be an abnormal resistance to nerve block injection and thus reduce the risk of intraneural injection.[6,28,31] However, this practice has significant inherent limitations.[32] For instance, the resistance to injection is greater with smaller needles that are used for nerve blocks, introducing a confusion factor as to what is "normal" or "abnormal" resistance. Second, as opposed to "loss of resistance" in an epidural injection, there is no baseline pressure information or a change in tissue compliance during nerve block injection. In a study by Claudio and colleagues,[32] all anesthesiologists detected a change in pressure of as little as 0.5 psi during a simulated nerve block injection. However, when gauging the absolute pressure, they substantially varied (by as much as 40 psi) in their perception of what constituted an appropriate resistance to injection. Finally, until recently, no information has been available on what constitutes "normal" and "abnormal" injection pressure during nerve block performance. For these reasons, subjective estimation of resistance to injection is at least as inaccurate as perhaps estimating blood pressure by palpating the radial artery pulse. Objective means of assessing resistance to injection should be far superior in standardizing injection force and pressure.

To explain the mechanisms responsible for development of neuraxial anesthesia after an interscalene block,[33,34] Selander and Sjostrand[35] injected solutions of local anesthetic into rabbit sciatic nerves and traced the spread of the anesthetic along the nerve sheath. They postulated that an intraneural injection results in significant spread of local anesthetic *within the nerve sheath*. In their model, these investigators incidentally noticed that intraneural injections often resulted in higher pressures (up to 9 psi) than those required for perineural injections (<4 psi). Injection into a nerve fascicle resulted in rupture of the *perineurium* and histologic evidence of disruption of the fascicular anatomy. This study, however, used a small-animal model, microinjections (10–200 μL), miniature needles, clinically irrelevant injection rates (100–300 μL/min), and did not include neurologic evaluation after intraneural injections. It is perhaps for these reasons that their foretelling results on the association of injection pressure with intrafascicular injection did not gain the deserved acceptance in clinical practice.

More recent studies, however, have used clinically more-applicable injection speeds and volumes of local anesthetic in a canine model of nerve injury.[36] The results of these studies unequivocally suggested that high-injection pressures (>20 psi) may indicate intrafascicular injection and carry a risk of neurologic injury (Figure 5-4).[37] Specifically, intraneural injections resulting in pressures >20 psi have been associated with clinically detectable neurologic deficits as well as histologic evidence of injury to nerve fascicles (Figure 5-5).

Current evidence suggests that neurologic injury does not always develop after an intraneural injection.[38] In fact, injection after an intraneural needle placement is more likely to result in deposition of the local anesthetic between and not into the fascicles.[36] Intraneural, but *extrafascicular* (interfascicular) injection probably occurs more fre-

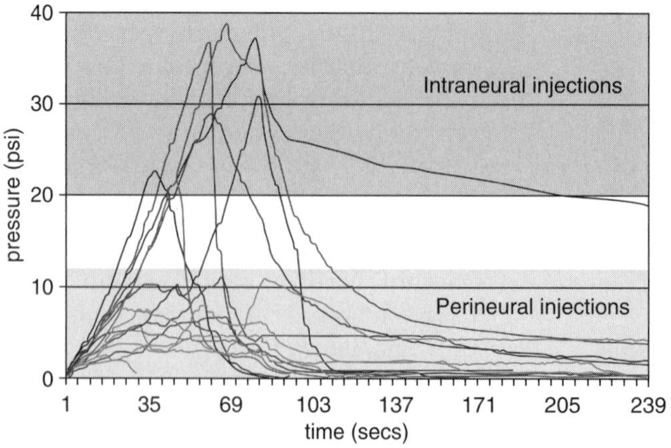


**FIGURE 5-4.** Injection pressure tracings during sciatic nerve blockade in a canine model. Perineural injections result in low pressures, whereas intraneural, intrafascicular injections are associated with significantly higher injection pressures.

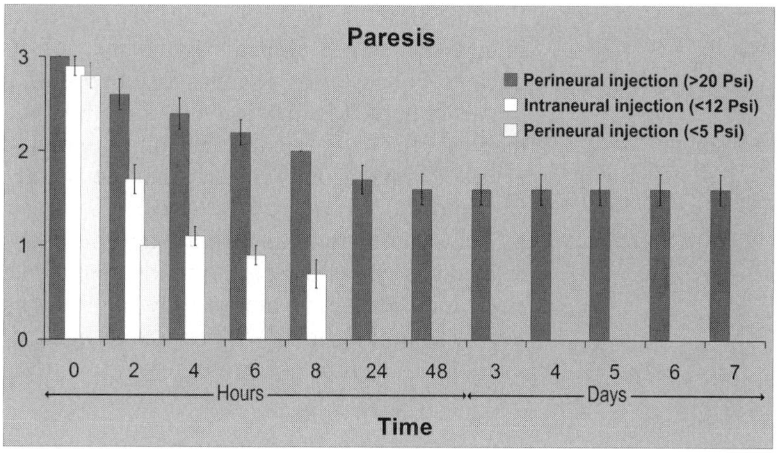


**FIGURE 5-5.** Duration of sciatic nerve blockade in the canine model of sciatic block. Perineural injections with 2% lidocaine result in motor block lasting up to 3 hours; intraneural but extrafascicular injections result in denser and longer blockade (up to 8 hours) but no permanent injury; intraneural intrafascicular injections (pressures >20 psi) result in blockade lasting >7 days and neurologic injury. (Reprinted with permission from Acta Anaesthesiol Scand. November 1, 2006 [Epub ahead of print]).

quently than thought in clinical practice.[38] Such an injection results in a block of unusually fast onset and long duration rather than in a neurologic injury. This is because an intraneural but extrafascicular injection leads to intimate exposure of nerve fascicles to high concentrations and doses of local anesthetics. However, permanent neurologic injury does not develop because the local anesthetic is deposited *outside* the fascicles and the blocks slowly resolve after the injection, without evidence of histologic derangement.

### *Needle Design and Direct Needle Trauma*

Needle tip design and risk of neurologic injury have been matters of considerable debate for more than 3 decades. Nearly 30 years ago, Selander and colleagues[39] suggested that the risk of perforating a nerve fascicle was significantly lower when a short-bevel (e.g., 45°) needle was used as opposed to a long-bevel (12°–15°) needle. The results of their work are largely responsible for the prevalent trend of using short-bevel needles (i.e., angles 30°–45°) for the majority of major peripheral nerve conduction blocks. However, the work by Rice and McMahon[40] suggests that short-beveled needles, when placed intraneurally, tend to cause more mechanical damage than the long-beveled needles. In their experiment in a rat model, after deliberately penetrating the largest fascicle of the sciatic nerve with 12°- to 27°-beveled needles, the degree of neural trauma on histologic examination was greater with short-beveled needles. Their work suggests that sharp needles produce cleaner, more-likely-to-heal cuts, whereas blunt needles produced noncongruent cuts and more extensive damage. In addition, the cuts produced by the sharper needles were more likely to recover faster and more completely than were the irregular, more traumatic injuries caused by the blunter, short-beveled needles. Although the data on needle design and nerve injury have not been clinically substantiated, the theoretical advantage of short-beveled needles in reducing the risk of nerve penetration has influenced both practitioners and needle manufacturers. Consequently, whenever practical, most clinicians today prefer to use short-beveled needles for major conduction blocks of the peripheral nerves and plexuses. Sharp beveled, small-gauge needles, however, continue to be used routinely for many nerve block procedures, such as axillary transarterial brachial plexus block, wrist and ankle blocks, cutaneous nerve block, and others.

Regardless of the considerations related to the needle design and risk of nerve injury, the actual clinical significance of isolated, direct needle trauma remains unclear. For instance, it is possible that both paresthesia and nerve stimulation techniques of nerve localization may often lead to unrecognized intraneural needle placement, yet the risk of neurologic injury remains relatively low. Similarly, during femoral arterial cannulation, it is likely that the needle is often inserted into the femoral nerve, yet reported injuries to the nerve are rare, and when they occur, they are usually attributed to hematoma formation rather than needle injury. It is possible that needle-related trauma without accompanying intraneural injection results in injury of a relatively minor nature, which readily heals and may go clinically undetected. In contrast, needle trauma coupled with injections of local anesthetics into the nerve fascicle carry a risk of much more severe injury.[37]

### *Toxicity of Injected Solution*

Nerves can be injured by direct contact with a needle, injection of a drug into or around the nerve, pressure from a hematoma, or scarring around the nerve.[41–44] Experimental studies have shown that the degree of nerve damage after an injection depends on the exact site of the injection and the type and quantity of the drug used.[45] The most severe damage is produced by intrafascicular injections, although extrafascicular (subepineurial) injections of some particularly noxious drugs can also produce nerve damage.[14,46] Benzylpenicillin, diazepam, and paraldehyde are the most damaging, but certain other antibiotics, analgesics, sedatives, and antiemetic medications are also capable of damaging peripheral nerves when injected experimentally or accidentally.[45]

Local anesthetics produce a variety of cytotoxic effects in cell cultures, including inhibition of cell growth, motility, and survival, as well as morphologic changes. The extent of these effects is proportionate to the length of time the cells are exposed to the local anesthetic solutions and occur in concentrations normally used in clinical practice. Within normal ranges, the cytotoxic changes are greater as concentrations increase. In the clinical setting, the exact site of local anesthetic deposition has a critical role in determining the pathogenic potential.[47] After applying local anesthetics outside a fascicle, the regulatory function of the perineural and endothelial blood-nerve barrier is only minimally compromised. High concentrations of extrafascicular anesthetics may produce axonal injury independent of edema formation and increased endoneural fluid pressure.[48] As with the effects of local anesthetics in cell cultures, the duration of exposure and concentration of local anesthetic determine the degree and incidence of local-anesthetic–induced residual paralysis. Neurotoxicity of local anesthetics will be discussed in greater detail elsewhere in this textbook.

### *Neuronal Ischemia*

Lack of blood flow to the primary afferent neuron results in metabolic stress. The earliest response of the peripheral sensory neuron to ischemia is depolarization and generation of spontaneous activity, symptomatically perceived as paresthesias. This is followed by blockade of slow-conducting myelinated fibers and eventually all neurons, possibly through accumulation of excess intracellular calcium, which accounts for the loss of sensation with initiation of limb ischemia. Nerve function returns within 6 hours if ischemic times are less than 2 hours. Ischemic periods of up to 6 hours may not produce permanent structural changes in nerves. However, detailed pathologic examination after ischemia initially shows minimal changes, but with 3 hours or more of reperfusion, edema and fiber degeneration develops that lasts for 1–2 weeks, followed by a phase of regeneration lasting 6 weeks. In addition to neuronal damage, oxidative injury associated with ischemia and reperfusion also affects the Schwann cells, initiating apoptosis.

The perineurium is a tough and resistant tissue layer. An injection into this compartment or a fascicle can also result in a prolonged increase in endoneurial pressure, exceeding the capillary perfusion pressure. This pressure, in turn, can lead to endoneural ischemia.[35] The addition of vasoconstricting agents theoretically can enhance ischemia because of the resultant vasoconstriction and reduction in blood flow. The addition of epinephrine has been shown, in vitro, to decrease the blood supply to intact nerves in the rabbit. However, in patients undergoing lower-extremity surgery, addition of epinephrine to the local anesthetic solution used in combined femoral and sciatic nerve blocks has not been shown to be a risk factor for developing postblock nerve dysfunction.[3]

### *Tourniquet Neuropathy*

Tourniquet-induced neuropathy is well documented in the orthopedic literature and ranges from mild neuropraxia to permanent neurologic injury. The incidence of tourniquet paralysis has been reported to be 1 in 8000 operations. A prospective study of lower-extremity nerve blockade suggests that higher tourniquet inflation pressures (>400 mm Hg) were associated with an increased risk of transient nerve injury.[3] Current recommendations for appropriate use of the tourniquet include: the maintenance of a pressure of no more than 150 mm Hg greater than the systolic blood pressure and deflation of the tourniquet every 90–120 minutes.[49] Even with these recommendations, post-tourniquet-application neuropraxia may occur, particularly in the setting of preexisting neuropathy.

### *Compressive Hematoma*

Few data exist regarding the safety of PNB in patients treated with anticoagulants. Compressive hematoma formation leading to neuropathy has been associated with needle misadventures when performing lower extremity PNB, particularly with concomitant treatment with anticoagulants. However, as opposed to spinal or epidural hematoma, peripheral neuropathy from this etiology typically resolves completely.[50,51] Regardless, these reports emphasize the important differences in the risk–benefit ratio of PNBs compared with neuraxial blocks in patients receiving anticoagulant therapy.

## Conclusion

The published data suggest that neurologic complications of PNBs are relatively rare. However, the severity of consequences and lack of prevention strategies continue to present a source of concern for both clinicians and patients. The main inciting mechanism of neurologic injury with PNBs seems to be an intrafascicular or intraneural injection. However, it is fortunate that peripheral nerves possess an inherent natural protection. Intraneural injections do not always result in intrafascicular needle placement and, therefore, do not necessarily lead to nerve injury. It is often suggested that the use of short-beveled needles and avoidance of excessive sedation and general anesthesia to decrease the risk of nerve injury. However, these frequently voiced recommendations have recently been challenged. In addition, avoidance of adequate premedication may have a significant negative impact by decreasing the patient's acceptance and satisfaction with PNBs. The relatively low incidence rate of complications with PNBs, coupled with the lack of objective documentation and means to more precisely monitor administration of nerve blocks, make retrospective analyses of cases of nerve injury largely speculative with regard to the actual mechanism of nerve injury in clinical practice.

Few publications have had a greater impact on the clinical practice of anesthesiology than the American Society of Anesthesiologists (ASA) practice guidelines.[52]

These practice guidelines have been designed to enhance and promote the safety of anesthetic practice and have made the practice of general anesthesia much safer. Such guidelines are much needed but currently do not exist with regard to the practice of PNBs. This is likely because administration of PNBs has been traditionally based on individual preferences, clinical impressions, and other subjective methods. Future efforts should be directed toward developing more objective and exacting nerve localization and injection monitoring techniques to more reliably detect and prevent intraneural intrafascicular injection. The results of these efforts will inevitably be of crucial importance to the future of PNBs and their role in practice of modern anesthesiology.

## References

1. Auroy Y, Benhamou D, Bargues L. Major complications of regional anesthesia in France: the SOS regional anesthesia hotline service. Anesthesiology 2002;97:1274–1280.
2. Auroy Y, Narchi P, Messiah A, et al. Serious complications related to regional anesthesia: results of a prospective study in France. Anesthesiology 1997;87:479–486.
3. Fanelli G, Casati A, Garancini P, et al. Nerve stimulator and multiple injection technique for upper and lower limb blockade: failure rate, patient acceptance, and neurologic complications. Study Group on Regional Atesthesia. Anesth Analg 1999;88:847–852.
4. Sunderland S. Nerve and Nerve Injury. Edinburgh: Churchill Livingstone; 1978:31–32.
5. Millesi H, Terzis JK. Nomenclature in peripheral nerve surgery. Clin Plast Surg 1984;11:3–8.
6. Selander D. Peripheral nerve injury after regional anesthesia. In: Finucane B, ed. Complications of Regional Anesthesia. New York: Churchill Livingstone; 1999:105–115.
7. Seddon HJ. Three types of nerve injury. Brain 1943;66:236–288.
8. Sunderland S. A classification of peripheral nerve injuries producing loss of function. Brain 1951;74:491–516.
9. Lundborg G. Nerve Injury and Repair. New York: Churchill Livingstone; 1988.
10. Hudson AR, Kline D, Gentili F. Management of peripheral nerve problems. In: Omer G, Spinner M, eds. Peripheral Nerve Injection Injury. Philadelphia: WB Saunders; 1980: 639–653.
11. Mackinnon SE, Dellon AL. Classification of nerve injuries as the basis of treatment. In: Mackinnon SE, Dellon AL, eds. Surgery of the Peripheral Nerve. New York: Thieme Medical Publishers; 1988:35–63.
12. Gentili F, Hudson A, Kline D, et al. Early changes following injection injury of peripheral nerves. Can J Surg 1980;23:177–182.
13. Mackinnon SE, Hudson AR, Gentili F, et al. Peripheral nerve injury with steroid agents. Plast Reconstr Surg 1982;69:482–489.
14. Mackinnon SE, Hudson AR, Llamas F, et al. Peripheral nerve injury by chymopapain injection. J Neurosurg 1984;61:1–8.
15. Strasberg JE, Atchabahian A, Strasberg SR, et al. Peripheral nerve injection injury with antiemetic agents. J Neurotrauma 1999;16:99–107.
16. Hadzic A, Dilberovic F, Shah S, et al. Combination of intraneural injection and high injection pressure leads to fascicular injury and neurologic deficits in dogs. Reg Anesth Pain Med 2004;29:417–423.
17. Bhananker SM, Domino KB. What actions can be used to prevent peripheral nerve injury. In: Fleisher LA, ed. Evidence-based Practice of Anesthesiology. New York: Elsevier; 2004: 228–235.
18. Fremling MA, Mackinnon SE. Injection injury to the median nerve. Ann Plast Surg 1996;37:561–567.
19. Lim E, Pereira R. Brachial plexus injury following brachial plexus block. Anesthesia 1984; 39:691–694.
20. Gillespie JH, Menk EJ, Middaugh RE. Reflex sympathetic dystrophy. A complication of interscalene block. Anesth Analg 1987;66:1316–1317.
21. Winnie AP. Interscalene brachial plexus block. Anesth Analg 1970;49:455–466.
22. Barutell C, Vidal F, Raich M, et al. A neurological complication following interscalene brachial plexus block. Anaesthesia 1980;35:365–367.

23. Raj PP, De Andrés J, Grossi P, et al. Aids to localization of peripheral nerves. In: Raj P, ed. Textbook of Regional Anesthesia. New York: Churchill Livingstone; 2002:251–284.
24. Urmey WF, Stanton J. Inability to consistently elicit a motor response following sensory paresthesia during interscalene block administration. Anesthesiology 2002;96:552–554.
25. Choyce A, Chan VW, Middleton WJ, et al. What is the relationship between paresthesia and nerve stimulation for axillary brachial plexus block? Reg Anesth Pain Med 2001; 26:100–104.
26. Brown DL. Local anesthetics and regional anesthesia equipment. In: Brown DL, ed. Atlas of Regional Anesthesia. Philadelphia: WB Saunders; 1992:3–11.
27. Chelly J. Nerve stimulator. In: Chelly J, ed. Peripheral Nerve Blocks. A Color Atlas. Philadelphia: Lippincott Williams & Wilkins; 1999:7–10.
28. Jankovic D, Wells C. Brachial plexus. In: Jankovic D, Wells C, eds. Regional Nerve Blocks. Berlin: Blackwell Publishers; 2001:58–86.
29. Jankowski CJ, Hebl JR, Stuart MJ, et al. A comparison of psoas compartment block and spinal and general anesthesia for outpatient knee arthroscopy. Anesth Analg 2003; 97:1003–1009.
30. Tonidandel WT, Mayfield JB. Successful interscalene block with a nerve stimulator may also result after a pectoralis major motor response. Reg Anesth Pain Med 2002;27:491–493.
31. Weaver MA, Tandatnick CA, Hahn MB. Peripheral nerve blockade. In: Raj P, ed. Regional Anesthesia. New York: Churchill Livingstone; 2002:857–870.
32. Claudio RE, Hadzic A, Shih H, et al. Injection pressures by anesthesiologists during simulated peripheral nerve block. Reg Anesth Pain Med 2004;29:201–205.
33. Passannante AN. Spinal anesthesia and permanent neurologic deficit after interscalene block. Anesth Analg 1996;82:873–874.
34. Dutton RP, Eckhardt WF 3rd, Sunder N. Total spinal anesthesia after interscalene blockade of the brachial plexus. Anesthesiology 1994;80:939–941.
35. Selander D, Sjostrand J. Longitudinal spread of intraneurally injected local anesthetics. An experimental study of the initial neural distribution following intraneural injections. Acta Anaesthesiol Scand 1978;22:622–634.
36. Hadzic A. Combination of intraneural injection and high-injection pressure leads to fascicular injury and neurologic deficit in dogs. Reg Anesth Pain Med 2005;30:309–310.
37. Hadzic A, Dilberovic F, Shah S, et al. Combination of intraneural injection and high injection pressure leads to severe fascicular injury and neurologic deficits in dogs. Reg Anesth Pain Med 2004;29:417–423.
38. Sala-Blanch X, Pomes J, Matute P, et al. Intraneural injection during anterior approach for sciatic nerve block. Anesthesiology 2004;101:1027–1030.
39. Selander D, Dhuner K, Lundborg G. Peripheral nerve injury due to injection needles used for regional anesthesia. Acta Anaesthesiol Scand 1977;21:182–189.
40. Rice ASC, McMahon SB. Peripheral nerve injury caused by injection needles used in regional anaesthesia: influence of bevel configuration, studied in a rat model. Br J Anaesth 1992;9:433–438.
41. Sunderland S. The sciatic nerve and its tibial and common peroneal divisions: anatomical and physiological features. In: Sunderland S, ed. Nerves and Nerve Injuries. Edinburgh: Churchill Livingstone; 1978:925–991.
42. Rousseau JJ, Reznik M, LeJeune GN, et al. Sciatic nerve entrapment by pentazocine-induced muscle fibrosis: a case report. Arch Neurol Psychiatry 1979;36:723–724.
43. Obach J, Aragones JM, Ruano D. The infrapiriformis foramen syndrome resulting from intragluteal injection. J Neurol Sci 1983;58:135–142.
44. Napiontek M, Ruszkowski K. Paralytic drop foot and gluteal fibrosis after intramuscular injections. J Bone Joint Surg Br 1993;75:83–85.
45. Gentili F, Hudson AR, Hunter D. Clinical and experimental aspects of injection injuries of peripheral nerves. Can J Neurol Sci 1980;7:143–151.
46. Mackinnon SE, Hudson AR, Gentili F, et al. Peripheral nerve injury with steroid agents. Plast Reconstr Surg 1982;69:482–489.
47. Selander D. Neurotoxicity of local anesthetics: animal data. Reg Anesth 1993;18:461–468.
48. Kaneko S, Matsumoto M, Tsuruta S, et al. The nerve root entry zone is highly vulnerable to intrathecal tetracaine in rabbits. Anesth Analg 2005;101:107–114.
49. Sharrock NE, Savarese JJ. Anesthesia for orthopedic surgery. In: Miller R, ed. Anesthesia. New York: Churchill Livingstone; 2000:2118–2139.

50. Klein SM, D'Ercole F, Greengrass RA, et al. Enoxaparin associated with psoas hematoma and lumbar plexopathy after lumbar plexus block. Anesthesiology 1997;87:1576–1579.
51. Weller RS, Gerancher JC, Crews JC, et al. Extensive retroperitoneal hematoma without neurologic deficit in two patients who underwent lumbar plexus block and were later anticoagulated. Anesthesiology 2003;98:581–585.
52. American Society of Anesthesiologists. Policy statement on practice parameters. In: ASA Standards, Guidelines and Statements. American Society of Anesthesiologists Publication; October 3, 1999.

# 6 Complications of Ophthalmic Regional Anesthesia

Robert C. (Roy) Hamilton

Administering anesthesia blocks for ophthalmic surgery was, in the past, the exclusive domain of the ophthalmologist; however, more and more anesthesiologists are now performing these blocks worldwide. Anesthesiologists now routinely perform many ophthalmic blocks at eye clinics or surgery centers and most of them have expertise that is equal or superior to that of the average ophthalmologist. When anesthesiologists perform ophthalmic blocks, it is advisable to communicate with the ophthalmologist about the relevant anatomy of the eye in question.

## Training of the Ophthalmic Regional Anesthesiologist

Sound knowledge of orbital anatomy, ophthalmic physiology, and the pharmacology of anesthesia and ophthalmic drugs are prerequisites before embarking on orbital regional anesthesia techniques; such information should then be augmented by training in techniques obtained in clinical settings from practitioners with wide experience and knowledge in the field.[1] Neophytes go through an obligatory "learning curve," the gradient of which can be greatly reduced by exposure to expert instruction and supervision.[2] Cadaver dissection is an excellent means of gaining the necessary anatomic knowledge of the orbit.[3]

## Optimal Management of Patients Undergoing Ophthalmic Regional Anesthesia

The advantages of regional anesthesia easily surpass those of general anesthesia, in terms of safety, efficacy, and patient comfort. All patients require a thorough preoperative assessment, including history and physical examination with open communication with the patients about risks and potential complications of the procedure. Each patient is expected to provide a list of all current medications to ensure that essential therapy is continued through the perioperative period and to minimize the risk of drug interactions. Laboratory and radiologic investigations are ordered only when indicated and appropriate to the management of the case.[4] The majority of patients presenting for ophthalmic surgery are elderly and many of them have hypertension, coronary artery disease, chronic obstructive pulmonary disease, diabetes, and obesity, which present additional challenges to the operating team. Every effort must be made to have patients in the best possible medical condition before surgery. Most ophthalmic surgery is elective, therefore there is ample opportunity to optimize patients' medical conditions in advance.

The monitoring requirements for ophthalmic anesthesia/surgery, in the awake patient, are no different than those required for procedures being performed under general anesthesia.[5] The elderly require less sedation at the time of surgery than do young patients, and take the discomforts of life "in their stride." If sedation is required, it must be prescribed judiciously and in small increments so that the patient will be comfortable yet remain alert, calm, and cooperative. The advantages of regional anesthesia can be quickly negated with excessive use of sedation.[6] A recent multicenter study confirmed that intravenous anesthetic agents administered to reduce pain and anxiety are associated with an increased incidence of side effects and adverse medical events.[7] Incomplete regional anesthesia is best managed with block supplementation until complete; to operate in the presence of obvious block failure is to subject the patient to an unpleasant and stressful experience. It is hazardous and inappropriate to use intravenous sedation to cover up for gross block inadequacy.

In cataract surgery, a precise axial length measurement of the eye is usually available because it is required for intraocular lens diopter power calculation. It is of the utmost importance to know the axial length of the eye in advance of needle placement to reduce the risk of globe perforation in those patients with longer-than-average axial lengths.

## Complications of Ophthalmic Regional Anesthesia

### *Hemorrhage*

Retrobulbar hemorrhages vary in severity. Some are of venous origin and spread slowly. Signs of severe arterial hemorrhage are a rapid and taut orbital swelling, marked proptosis with immobility of the globe, and massive blood staining of the lids and conjunctiva.[8] Serious impairment of the vascular supply to the globe may result.[9] More usually, however, an excellent surgical outcome can be achieved.[10,11] Bleeding can be minimized and confined by rapid application of digital pressure over a gauze pad applied to the closed lids, and by constant vigilance and keen observation of the patient immediately after needle withdrawal. The incidence of serious retrobulbar bleeding is reported to be in the range of 1%–3% in one article[12] and as 0.44% in a series of 12,500 cases.[13] Gentle and smooth needle insertion without pivotal or slicing movement is less likely to cause bleeding.[12,13] A strong argument can be made in favor of using small-gauge, disposable needles as opposed to larger-gauge needles,[14–16] on the grounds that if a vessel is perforated, the amount of bleeding that occurs is reduced and less precipitous because of a smaller tear in the vessel. Furthermore, patients tolerate smaller-gauge needles and usually do not experience pain or require sedation during needle placement.

Blood vessels are smaller in the anterior orbital region than in the posterior region. In the interest of avoiding hemorrhage, sites that are relatively avascular are preferred for needle placement. The inferior temporal quadrant and directly nasally in the compartment that is on the nasal side of the medial rectus muscle[17] are recommended. The superior nasal quadrant of the orbit should be avoided because the end vessels of the ophthalmic arterial system are located there, as is the complex trochlear mechanism of the superior oblique muscle. Because orbital blood vessels are largest in the posterior orbit, deep needle placement must be avoided if at all possible (see next section).

### *Brainstem Anesthesia*

The most likely situation that may warrant cardiopulmonary resuscitation in ophthalmic regional anesthesia is brainstem anesthesia, which is a form of central nervous system (CNS) toxicity.[18] Brainstem anesthesia is not caused by increasing levels of local anesthetics in the systemic circulation (including CNS) but by direct spread of local anesthetic to the brain from the orbit, along submeningeal pathways (Figure 6-1). The usual doses of local anesthetics used for eye surgery do not result in plasma levels of local anesthetic that result in systemic toxicity.

Brainstem anesthesia is reported to occur in 1 in 350–500 intraconal local anesthesia injections.[18] Typically, the patient first describes symptoms within 2 minutes of the orbital injection. Frequently, the zenith is reached at 10–20 minutes and resolves over 2–3 hours. Because this is a potential complication on each occasion that orbital blocks are performed, patients should not be draped for surgery until 15 minutes have elapsed after completion of the block, otherwise identification and corrective treatment may be dangerously delayed. Ophthalmic regional anesthesia should not be performed in any location unless all the necessary monitoring and resuscitation equipment is immediately available.[8,15,19–22] The clinical picture of brainstem anesthesia is protean in manifestation,[23] producing signs that vary from mild confusion through marked shivering or convulsant behavior,[24] bilateral brainstem nerve palsies (including motor nerve blocking to the contralateral orbit with amaurosis),[25,26] dysarthria,[27] or hemi-, para-, or quadriplegia, with or without loss of consciousness, to apnea with marked cardiovascular instability.[18,28–30] Treatment of these differing manifestations of central spread includes reassurance, ventilatory support with oxygen, intravenous fluid therapy, and pharmacologic circulatory support with vagolytics, vasopressors, vasodilators, or adrenergic blocking agents as appropriate and as dictated by close monitoring of the vital signs.

Much is known about prevention of this syndrome. Unsöld and coworkers[31] in 1981 revealed the danger of the elevated, adducted globe, as advocated by Atkinson[32] during inferior temporal needle placement. This position places the optic nerve closer to the advancing needle. They demonstrated, using computed tomography studies in the fresh cadaver, that with the globe in primary gaze, the optic nerve is less vulnerable. Avoidance of deep penetration of the orbit in any technique is advisable both to prevent this and other serious block complications. Katsev et al.[33] advised that maximum penetration from the orbital rim should not exceed 31 mm. Modern

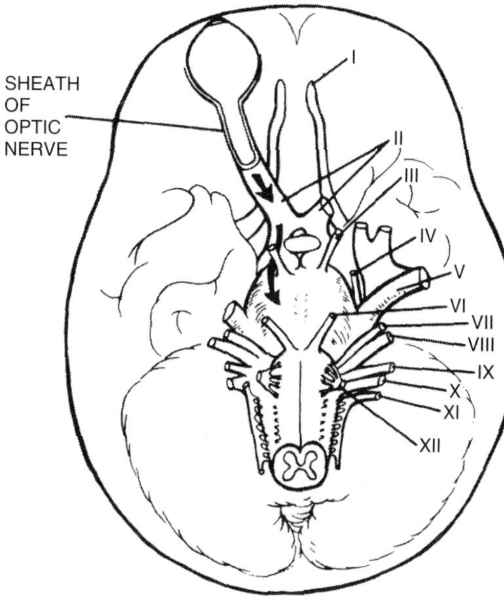


**FIGURE 6-1.** Illustration of the base of the brain and the pathway for spread of local anesthetics inadvertently injected into the subarachnoid space surrounding the optic nerve. Note that this pathway includes the cranial nerves, pons, and midbrain. (Reprinted from Javitt et al.[21] Copyright 1987, with permission from the American Academy of Ophthalmology.)

techniques avoid deep orbital placement and instead promote accurate injection at limited orbital depth and recommend increasing the volume of injectate in order to achieve critical blocking concentration at the apex.

## *Globe Penetration and Perforation*

The ability to detect subtle changes in tissue densities during needle advancement is a vital part of safe regional anesthesia; it is an acquired skill that requires experience and ongoing practice.[34] Needle advancement within the confines of the orbit is essentially a blind procedure and has the potential for serious complications. In view of the many eye block procedures performed annually, the incidence of globe perforation is low; however, even rare complications become significant.[33] The Atkinson "up and in" globe positioning[30] has been discredited. During inferior temporal needle insertion with the globe elevated and adducted, the optic nerve is brought closer to the needle tip and the macular area is more exposed to damage.[19,29,31,34] Optic nerve sheath penetration, optic nerve trauma, and ocular penetration or perforation by the needle may result. The posterior pole of the globe is endangered, particularly in the ovoid globes of myopic patients.[14] In patients with gross myopia (axial length greater than 29 mm), there is a higher incidence of staphyloma usually located inferior to the posterior pole of the globe; single medial canthal blockade[17] is safer in these patients rather than inferior temporal placement.[35] Many serious complications are avoided by having patients direct their eyes in primary gaze position during needle placement and subsequent injection. In the literature, there was a considerable lobby for the use of dull needles to reduce the incidence of bleeding and of ocular penetration.[36–38] The superiority of blunt- over sharp-tipped needles in reducing these complications has not been demonstrated in a controlled trial.[39] Tactile discrimination is progressively reduced with increasing needle size; the increased resistance caused by a blunt needle is not appreciated because of the necessarily greater preload.[14] To avoid scleral penetration (entrance wound only) or perforation (entrance and exit wounds), the importance of block technique and needle type are stressed. "The equator of the globe, with the eye in the primary position, is the greatest diameter in the coronal plane. Any needle entering the orbital region anteriorly must be directed in such a manner as to avoid encountering the sclera. Only by accurately judging the position of the equator can a needle be inserted in safety."[1] Penetration or perforation of the eye using larger dull needles causes more serious damage than when fine disposable needles are used.[40] The use of blunt-tipped needles does not protect against penetration and perforation.[40,41] Blunt-tipped needles are painful for the patient and require sedation during insertion, whereas fine disposable needles cause much less discomfort and sedatives are usually not required during insertion. The use of blunt-tipped, wider-gauge needles should be abandoned.[42]

Although there are proponents of both intraconal and periconal techniques, safe anesthesia can be accomplished using either method; likewise, serious complications can arise with either technique if performed incorrectly. A faster onset of anesthesia is achieved when blocking within the muscle cone.[15,43] Approximately 10% of peribulbar blocks are considered failures because they do not provide adequate ocular analgesia.[44] Chemosis is more common with periconal blocks.[45] Although it is possible to achieve effective blocks with small-volume injection at the apex of the orbit,[46] the risks are too great. Needles should never be advanced beyond 31 mm as measured from the orbit rim[33] nor should a needle advancing from an inferior temporal entry be allowed to cross the midsagittal plane of the eye (Figure 6-2).[14] All needles used for intraconal and periconal insertion should be orientated tangentially to the globe with the bevel opening faced toward the globe.[15,47] If a tangentially aligned needle contacts the sclera, globe penetration is less likely to occur than a needle approaching at a greater angle. All needles in the orbit are potentially hazardous in the wrong hands; careful supervision and training in technique have great relevance in the avoid-

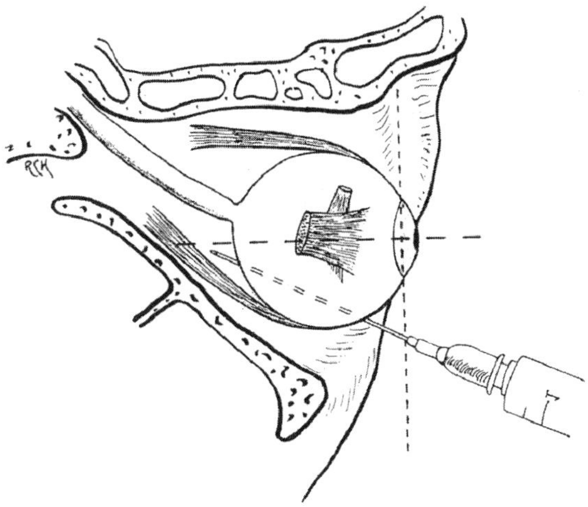


**FIGURE 6-2.** Globe in primary gaze. Fine dashed line indicates the plane of the iris; coarse dashed line indicates the midsagittal plane of the eye and the visual axis through the center of the pupil. The optic nerve lies on the nasal side of the midsagittal plane of the eye. Note how the temporal orbit rim is set back from the rest of the orbit rim at or about the globe equator, making for easy needle access to the retrobulbar compartment. A 31-mm needle is advanced beyond the equator of the globe, and then directed toward an imaginary point behind the macula, being careful not to cross the midsagittal plane of the eye. In a globe with normal axial length as illustrated here, when the needle/hub junction has reached the plane of the iris, the tip of the needle lies 5–7 mm beyond the hind surface of the globe. (From Gimbel Educational Services, with permission.)

ance of serious complications.[1] Techniques requiring multiple needle placements are associated with an increased incidence of complications when compared with a single or reduced number of injections.

The author, with an experience of more than 33,000 retrobulbar (intracone) blocks, routinely uses and recommends a percutaneous approach from a more lateral inferior temporal entry point than frequently practiced[48] after preliminary local anesthesia of the skin (Figure 6-3).[49] By using a percutaneous entry, patients with narrow palpebral fissures, and those with excessive blinking strength, present no problem.

Ocular penetration or perforation is more likely in patients with elongated myopic eyes. Patients presenting for retinal detachment or refractive surgery (such as laser in situ keratomileusis) have a higher propensity of longer globes than patients having cataract surgery. In myopic patients, the incidence may be as high as 1 in 140.[50] This complication has been reported with both the intraconal and the periconal methods. Nonakinetic anesthesia methods have been developed (see below), partly to avoid the serious complications associated with needle blocks. The diagnosis of penetration may be suspected in the presence of hypotony, poor red reflex, vitreous hemorrhage, and "poking through sensation"[51]; however, more than 50% of iatrogenic needle penetrations of the globe go unrecognized at the time of their occurrence.[52] The patient may report marked pain at the time of the penetration,[53] particularly if the anesthetic is inadvertently injected intraocularly. Funduscopy confirms the diagnosis, if the media are sufficiently clear. Cases involving retinal tears only, with minimal blood-staining of the vitreous, can be managed with laser photocoagulation, cryotherapy, or on occasion observation only. When so much blood is present that the fundus is not visible early vitrectomy may be indicated. Without surgical intervention, vitreous hemorrhage after penetrating injury frequently leads to proliferative vitreoretinopathy with resultant detachment of the retina. Once retinal detachment is diagnosed, whether associated with clear or cloudy media, prompt surgical treatment is indicated. The appropriate management of scleral penetration and perforation is complex and often

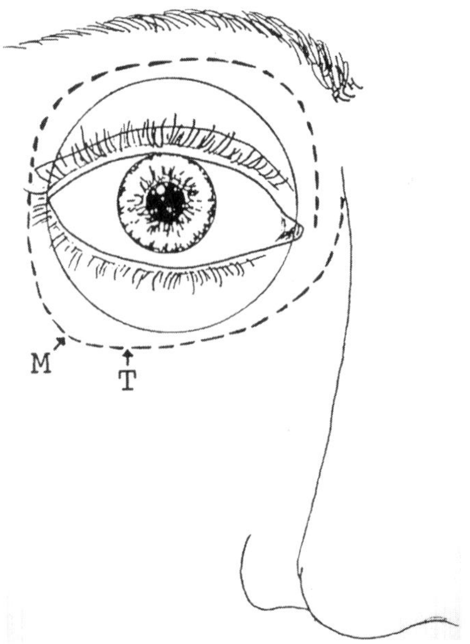


**FIGURE 6-3.** The outline of the globe is superimposed on a template of the orbit rim. The traditional inferior block injection site ("T") is just inside the orbit rim at the junction of the medial two-thirds and lateral third of the inferior orbital rim. The author's modified injection site ("M") is just inside the orbit rim at the junction of the inferior and lateral orbital rims. Injection at the modified site is best done percutaneously, the entry point on the skin being 4–5 mm inferior to the lateral canthus. (From Gimbel Educational Services, with permission.)

drawn out over some weeks involving difficult judgment calls on the part of the ophthalmologist.[54]

Ocular explosion associated with orbital blockade has been described.[55,56] This is a devastating complication with catastrophic visual outcome. It typically occurs in deeply sedated patients, after unrecognized ocular penetration, associated with the use of excessive force of local anesthetic injection. To date, eight cases have been described in the literature. There is a strong argument here to avoid deep sedation. Patients who are fully alert experience severe pain in these circumstances. The precautions described above, if followed, should greatly reduce the likelihood of this complication.

### *Myotoxicity*

Prolonged extraocular muscle malfunction may follow regional anesthesia of the orbit.[15,57,58] Diplopia and ptosis are common for 24–48 hours postoperatively when long-acting local anesthetics have been used in large volume. However, when this persists for days or weeks, or fails to recover, it may be evidence of toxic change within muscle. In those patients in whom muscle recovery is delayed more than 6 weeks, 25% turn out to be permanent. It is indeed a complication of the greatest magnitude for a patient to have an excellent optical result and end up with devastating diplopia because the eyes are misaligned. Studies of the myotoxicity of local anesthetics have been published.[59–61] Higher concentrations of local anesthetic agents are more likely to result in myotoxicity.[61] A common cause of prolonged muscle malfunction, whatever concentration has been used, is intramuscular injection.[59,61–63] The etiologies of these muscle malfunctions, however, include not only local anesthetic myotoxicity,[59–61] but also surgical trauma, inappropriately placed antibiotic injection,[64] and ischemic contracture of the Volkmann's type after trauma or hemorrhage.[65] Increasing age is associated with poor recovery from anesthesia-induced muscle damage.[66] It is imperative to have a good three-dimensional knowledge of the anatomy of the orbit and its contents to accurately place injections. Of particular note are the number of articles indicating damage to the inferior rectus muscle,[58,62–65] likely caused by inadequate elevation of the needle tip from the orbit floor during attempted intracone placement (Figure 6-4). By meticulous attention to detailed placement of anesthetic needles and with precise knowledge of the anatomy of the six extraocular muscles, the incidence of muscle damage/malfunction can be eliminated. Aiming the retrobulbar needle "midway between the inferior and lateral rectus muscles" to gain clear entry into the intraconal space, avoiding trauma to the inferior rectus muscle is stressed.[65] Extraocular muscles are more easily avoided by using a fully inferior temporal orbital entry point for the retrobulbar injection (Figure 6-3).[48] This more lateral entry point for the retrobulbar block allows for easy and safe access to the intraconal space, because the temporal orbit rim is set back from the rest of the orbit rim. Inferior oblique muscle injury and trauma to its motor nerve by regional anesthesia injection have been reported.[66] Less frequently affected are the superior oblique,[67] the medial rectus,[17] and the lateral rectus muscles.[68] A persistent strabismus may be caused by contracture of an antagonist muscle reacting to an initial temporary paresis of its agonist muscle.[69] For additional information on this topic, please refer to Chapter 5.

## *Globe Ischemia*

The risk imposed on the blood supply of the globe from retrobulbar hemorrhage has been discussed above.

In intraocular surgery, it is considered advantageous if the intraocular pressure is low and pressure fluctuations are kept to a minimum.[70] In a previous era, it was considered particularly important to maintain a "soft eye" in the avoidance of complications, particularly suprachoroidal hemorrhage.[71] Phacoemulsification techniques, which require a smaller surgical incision, are associated with smaller swings in intraocular pressure than the older intracapsular or extracapsular methods. After completion of regional anesthetic blocks, mechanical orbital decompression devices[72–75] are frequently used to promote ocular hypotony and a reduction in vitreous volume,[76] especially when larger volumes of orbital injectate have been used (as in periconal blocks). Because blood flow to the retina, choroid, and optic nerve depend on the balance between the intraocular pressure and the mean local arterial blood pressure,

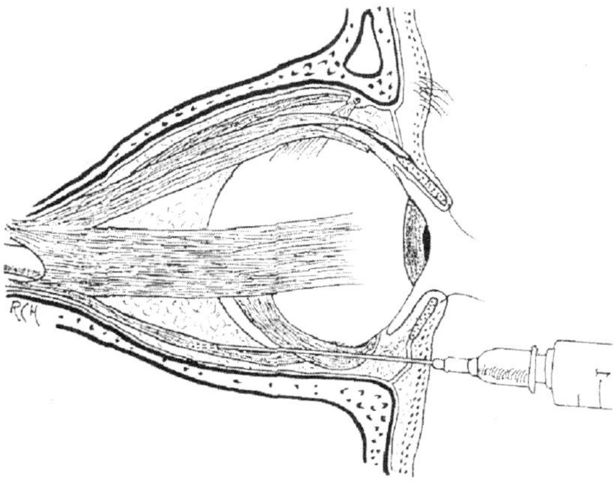

**FIGURE 6-4.** A straight 31-mm needle being advanced from the inferotemporal quadrant in an attempt to enter the intraconal space has failed to adequately clear the orbit floor. The needle tip has entered the belly of the inferior rectus muscle. Hemorrhage into the muscle with subsequent fibrosis, or intramuscular injection of local anesthetic with subsequent myotoxicity, may result in prolonged or permanent imbalance between the superior and inferior rectus muscles and vertical diplopia. (From Gimbel Educational Services, with permission.)

it is possible for these devices to induce global ischemia.[77,78] In the presence of significant local arterial disease, orbital hemorrhage, or in patients with glaucoma, vascular occlusion may result.[79] It may be prudent to omit epinephrine from the anesthesia injectate in these cases.[14,43]

### *Optic Nerve Damage*

Injection at the orbital apex, as was advocated in the distant past,[46] has the potential of frank optic nerve injury (Figure 6-5). The needle length introduced beyond the orbital rim for both intraconal and periconal injections should not exceed 31 mm to assuredly avoid damage to the optic nerve in all patients.[33] In the execution of orbital blocks, it is possible for the needle tip to enter the optic nerve sheath and produce not only brainstem anesthesia, as described above, but also tamponade of the retinal vessels within the nerve and/or the small vessels supplying the nerve itself either by the volume of drug injected or by initiating intrasheath hemorrhage.[12,16,80–82] Even without trauma to the optic nerve, the increased orbital pressure of retrobulbar hemorrhage may tamponade its small nutrient vessels, explaining those cases of profound visual loss in which the findings of retinal vascular occlusion were not seen and late optic atrophy developed.[8,79] Preexisting small vessel disease such as is seen in diabetes mellitus may increase the likelihood of this complication.

### *Other Nerve Injury*

It is possible for autonomic,[83,84] sensory, or motor nerves[61] in the orbit to be traumatized by a needle. The motor nerve to the inferior oblique muscle may be damaged by a needle entering insufficiently lateral (Figure 6-6) with resultant diplopia.[66]

### *Therapeutic Misadventures (Including Systemic Toxicity)*

Orbital injections of depot steroid medications and antibiotics are frequently used at the time of ophthalmic surgery for their antiinflammatory and antiinfective properties. The anesthesiologist may be asked to administer such agents and should be aware of the risks involved. Their inadvertent injection into the vitreous has serious implications.[85–91] In delivering steroids and antibiotics in a planned extraocular location, it is important to aspirate before injection to check for inadvertent intravascular needle-tip placement. There are many reports of retinal, ciliary, and choroidal arterial embolism of these medications, often with irreversible vision deterioration.[92–94] Intraocular antibiotics are used to treat established endophthalmitis and are being increasingly used prophylactically in its prevention. The preparation of the special concentration

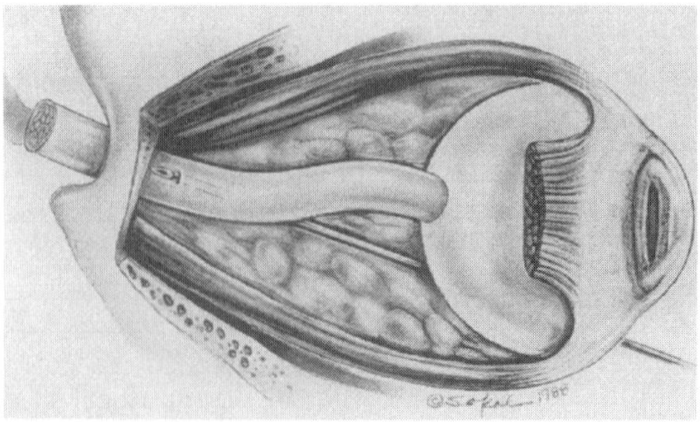

**FIGURE 6-5.** Injections into the deep orbit may perforate the optic nerve or injure other important structures, including vessels, tightly packed at the apex. (Reprinted from Katsev et al.[33] Copyright 1989, with permission from the American Academy of Ophthalmology.)

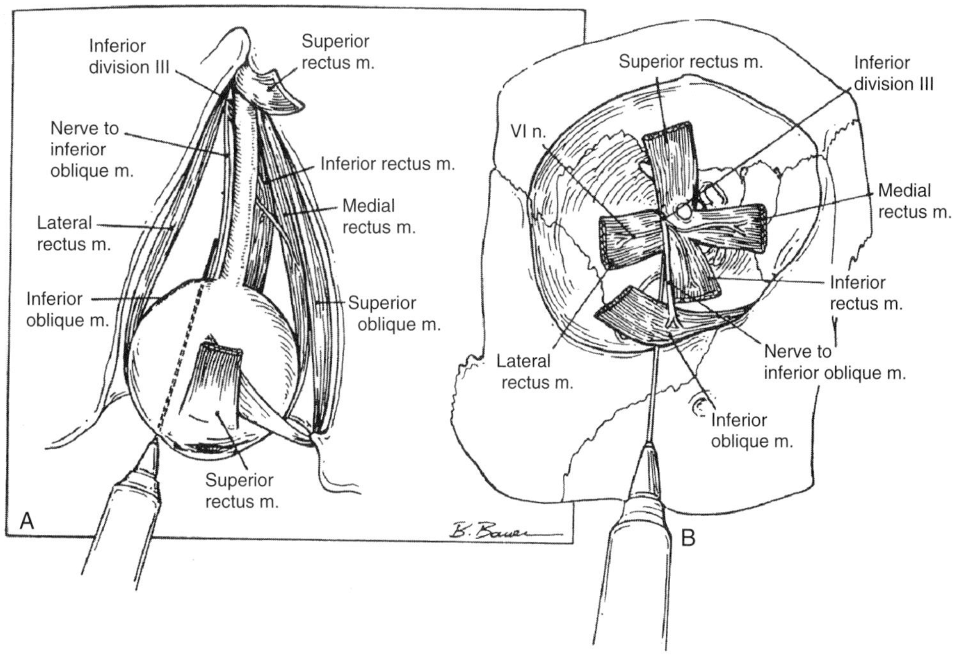


**FIGURE 6-6.** Right orbit. **(A)** View from above. **(B)** View from in front with the globe removed. Observe the proximity of the needle path to the inferior oblique muscle belly, its motor nerve, and the lateral border of the inferior rectus muscle. One or more of these three structures can be damaged by a traditionally placed retrobulbar needle. (Reprinted from Hunter et al.[66] Copyright 1995, with permission from the American Academy of Ophthalmology.)

required must be done correctly and is probably best delegated to a pharmacist so as to avoid devastating and irreversible retinotoxic iatrogenic damage.[95]

The incidence of systemic toxicity with local anesthetics is related to total dose given, vascularity of site of injection, drug used, speed of injection, and whether epinephrine has been used as an additive to delay systemic release. The amount of local anesthesia agent required to be effective in ophthalmic anesthesia is relatively small in comparison with regional anesthesia requirements for most other types of surgery, so systemic toxicity is unlikely. Unintentional intravenous injection of the total mass of local anesthetic required for an eye block if given rapidly may result in systemic toxicity with the usual target organs being those with the more excitable membranes, namely, the CNS and myocardium. Aspirating before injection and injecting slowly reduces the likelihood of this complication. Inadvertent intraarterial injection of local anesthetics with retrograde flow to the cerebral circulation may result in an acute grand mal seizure.[96,97]

### *Seventh Nerve Block Complications*

An isolated facial nerve block is rarely necessary in modern ophthalmic practice. Complications associated with blocking of the main trunk of the facial nerve at the base of the skull have been reported.[98,99] In these cases, patients experienced difficulty swallowing and respiratory obstruction related to unilateral vagus, glossopharyngeal, and spinal accessory nerve blockade. For facial blockade at this site, it is prudent to inject no deeper than 12 mm and to avoid hyaluronidase in the injectate.[99,100] Bilateral facial nerve block is not recommended.[101]

### *Allergy*

True allergy to local anesthetics is extremely rare.[102] Allergic reactions are almost exclusively confined to the ester-linked drugs. The breakdown product of the esters, paraaminobenzoic acid, is thought to trigger an allergic reaction in certain individuals. Reaction with preservatives, such as methylparabens, in multidose vials is possible; hence, it may be better to use preservative-free vials where a history of the problem exists.[103] A myasthenia-like response to various agents including local anesthetics has been reported[104] and also two well-documented cases of true allergy to amide drugs have been reported.[105,106]

## Alternative Methods of Ophthalmic Anesthesia

Ongoing reports of the rare but serious complications of intraconal anesthesia stimulated editorials and reintroduced the concept of alternative nonakinetic methods of regional anesthesia for ophthalmic surgery.[107,108] These fall into three groups: subconjunctival (perilimbal)[107,109–112]; injection of local anesthetic by needle or cannula within Tenon's capsule[113–116]; and solely topical corneoconjunctival anesthesia.[117–119] With these methods, the surgeon encounters a varying degree of muscle action affecting the globe and lids, and sensitivity of intraocular contents (particularly the iris and ciliary muscle with solely topical anesthesia).[109] A systematic search of the literature concluded that retrobulbar block provided better pain control than topical anesthesia.[120]

## Anticoagulants and Antiplatelet Therapy

It has been common practice in surgery, including ophthalmic, to reduce or discontinue anticoagulant therapy for some days before an operation. Whereas this action may be appropriate for more major ophthalmic surgical procedures, such as scleral buckling, its advisability for the cataract surgery patient has been questioned.[121,122] Discontinuation of anticoagulant medication may result in thrombotic complications such as cerebral vascular accident, pulmonary embolism, and death.[123] In two reports, the minor hemorrhagic complications associated with continuance of anticoagulants had no long-term effects on visual acuity.[124,125] This implies that the risk of stopping anticoagulants for this type of surgery is probably greater than any risk imposed by their continuance. A recent publication reviews the current literature.[126] Patients receiving antiplatelet therapy may also continue their drugs through cataract surgery if medical reasons dictate.[127]

## References


1. Hawkesworth NR. Peribulbar anaesthesia [letter]. Br J Ophthalmol 1992;76:254.
2. Kopacz DJ, Neal JM, Pollock MD. The regional anesthesia "learning curve." What is the minimum number of epidural and spinal blocks to reach consistency? Reg Anesth 1996;21:182–190.
3. Wong DHW. Regional anaesthesia for intraocular surgery [review]. Can J Anaesth 1993;40:635–657.
4. Schein OD, Katz J, Bass E, et al. The value of routine preoperative medical testing before cataract surgery: a randomized trial. N Engl J Med 2000;342:168–175.
5. Rubin AP. Anaesthesia for cataract surgery – time for change? [editorial] Anaesthesia 1990;45:717–718.
6. Smith DC, Crul JF. Oxygen desaturation following sedation for regional analgesia. Br J Anaesth 1989;62:206–209.
7. Katz J, Feldman MA, Bass EB, et al. Adverse intraoperative medical events and their association with anesthesia management strategies in cataract surgery. Ophthalmology 2001;108(10):1721–1726.
8. Feibel RM. Current concepts in retrobulbar anesthesia. Surv Ophthalmol 1985;30: 102–110.

9. Puustjarvi T, Purhonen S. Permanent blindness following retrobulbar hemorrhage after peribulbar anesthesia for cataract surgery. Ophthalmic Surg 1992;23:450–452.
10. Ahmed S, Grayson MC. Retrobulbar haemorrhage: when should we operate? Eye 1994;8:336–338.
11. Cionni RJ, Osher RH. Retrobulbar hemorrhage. Ophthalmology 1991;98:1153–1155.
12. Morgan CM, Schatz H, Vine AK, et al. Ocular complications associated with retrobulbar injections. Ophthalmology 1988;95:660–665.
13. Edge KR, Nicoll JMV. Retrobulbar hemorrhage after 12,500 retrobulbar blocks. Anesth Analg 1993;76:1019–1022.
14. Grizzard WS. Ophthalmic anesthesia. In: Reinecke RD, ed. Ophthalmology Annual. New York: Raven Press; 1989:265–294.
15. Hamilton RC, Gimbel HV, Strunin L. Regional anaesthesia for 12,000 cataract extraction and intraocular lens implantation procedures. Can J Anaesth 1988;35:615–623.
16. Pautler SE, Grizzard WS, Thompson LN, Wing GL. Blindness from retrobulbar injection into the optic nerve. Ophthalmic Surg 1986;17:334–337.
17. Hustead RF, Hamilton RC, Loken RG. Periocular local anesthesia: medial orbital as an alternative to superior nasal injection. J Cataract Refract Surg 1994;20:197–201.
18. Hamilton RC. Brain-stem anesthesia as a complication of regional anesthesia for ophthalmic surgery. Can J Ophthalmol 1992;27:323–325.
19. Fletcher SJ, O'Sullivan G. Grand mal seizure after retrobulbar block. Anaesthesia 1990;45:696.
20. Hamilton RC. Brain stem anesthesia following retrobulbar blockade. Anesthesiology 1985;63:688–690.
21. Javitt JC, Addiego R, Friedberg HL, et al. Brain stem anesthesia after retrobulbar block. Ophthalmology 1987;94:718–724.
22. Morgan GE. Retrobulbar apnea syndrome: a case for the routine presence of an anesthesiologist [letter]. Reg Anesth 1990;15:106–107.
23. Jackson K, Vote D. Multiple cranial nerve palsies complicating retrobulbar eye block. Anaesth Intensive Care 1998;26:662–664.
24. Lee DS, Kwon NJ. Shivering following retrobulbar block. Can J Anaesth 1988; 35:294–296.
25. Friedberg HL, Kline OR. Contralateral amaurosis after retrobulbar injection. Am J Ophthalmol 1986;101:688–690.
26. Antoszyk AN, Buckley EG. Contralateral decreased visual acuity and extraocular muscle palsies following retrobulbar anesthesia. Ophthalmology 1986;93:462–465.
27. Rosen WJ. Brainstem anesthesia presenting as dysarthria. J Cataract Refract Surg 1999;25:1170–1171.
28. Ahn JC, Stanley JA. Subarachnoid injection as a complication of retrobulbar anesthesia. Am J Ophthalmol 1987;103:225–230.
29. Nicoll JM, Acharya PA, Ahlen K, et al. Central nervous system complications after 6000 retrobulbar blocks. Anesth Analg 1987;66:1298–1302.
30. Ruusuvaara P, Setala K, Tarkkanen A. Respiratory arrest after retrobulbar block. Acta Ophthalmol (Copenh) 1988;66:223–225.
31. Unsöld R, Stanley JA, DeGroot J. The CT-topography of retrobulbar anesthesia. Albrecht Von Graefes Arch Klin Exp Ophthalmol 1981;217:125–136.
32. Atkinson WS. Retrobulbar injection of anesthetic within the muscular cone (cone injection). Arch Ophthalmol 1936;16:494–503.
33. Katsev DA, Drews RC, Rose BT. An anatomic study of retrobulbar needle path length. Ophthalmology 1989;96:1221–1224.
34. Brown DL, Wedel DJ. Introduction to regional anesthesia. In: Miller RD, ed. Anesthesia. 3rd ed. New York: Churchill Livingstone; 1990:1369–1375.
33. Vivian AJ, Canning CR. Scleral perforation with retrobulbar needles. Eur J Implant Ref Surg 1993;5:39–41.
34. Liu C, Youl B, Moseley I. Magnetic resonance imaging of the optic nerve in extremes of gaze. Implications for the positioning of the globe for retrobulbar anaesthesia. Br J Ophthalmol 1992;76:728–733.
35. Vohra SB, Good PA. Altered globe dimensions of axial myopia as risk factors for penetrating ocular injury during peribulbar anaesthesia. Br J Ophthalmol 2000;85: 242–245.
36. Callahan A. Ultrasharp disposable needles [letter]. Am J Ophthalmol 1966;62:173.

37. Davis DB, Mandel MR. Posterior peribulbar anesthesia: an alternative to retrobulbar anesthesia. J Cataract Refract Surg 1986;12:182–184.
38. Kimble JA, Morris RE, Witherspoon CD, Feist RM. Globe perforation from peribulbar injection. Arch Ophthalmol 1987;105:749.
39. Dhaliwal R, Demediuk OM. A comparison of peribulbar and retrobulbar anesthesia for vitreoretinal surgical procedures [comment]. Arch Ophthalmol 1996;114:502.
40. Grizzard WS, Kirk NM, Pavan PR, Antworth MV, Hammer ME, Roseman RL. Perforating ocular injuries caused by anesthesia personnel. Ophthalmology 1991;98:1011–1016.
41. Hay A, Flynn HW, Hoffman JI, Rivera AH. Needle penetration of the globe during retrobulbar and peribulbar injections. Ophthalmology 1991;98:1017–1024.
42. Gardner S, Ryall D. Local anaesthesia within the orbit. Curr Anaesth Crit Care 2000; 11:299–305.
43. Loots JH, Koorts AS, Venter JA. Peribulbar anesthesia. A prospective statistical analysis of the efficacy and predictability of bupivacaine and a lignocaine/bupivacaine mixture. J Cataract Refract Surg 1993;19:72–76.
44. McGoldrick KE. Anesthesia for Ophthalmic and Otolaryngologic Surgery. Philadelphia: Saunders; 1992:272–290.
45. Weiss JL, Deichman CB. A comparison of retrobulbar and periocular anesthesia for cataract surgery. Arch Ophthalmol 1989;107:96–98.
46. Gifford H. Motor block of extraocular muscles by deep orbital injection. Arch Ophthalmol 1949;41:5–19.
47. Gills JP, Loyd TL. A technique of retrobulbar block with paralysis of orbicularis oculi. J Am Intraocul Implant Soc 1983;9:339–340.
48. Hamilton RC. Retrobulbar block revisited and revised. J Cataract Refract Surg 1996; 22:1147–1150.
49. Hamilton RC. Retrobulbar anesthesia. Operative techniques in cataract and refractive surgery. 2000;3:116–121.
50. Duker JS, Belmont JB, Benson WE, et al. Inadvertent globe perforation during retrobulbar and peribulbar anesthesia. Ophthalmology 1991;98:519–526.
51. Gentili ME, Brassier J. Is peribulbar block safer than retrobulbar? [letter] Reg Anesth 1992;17:309.
52. Ginsburg RN, Duker JS. Globe perforation associated with retrobulbar and peribulbar anesthesia. Semin Ophthalmol 1993;8:87–95.
53. Seelenfreund MH, Freilich DB. Retinal injuries associated with cataract surgery. Am J Ophthalmol 1980;89:654–658.
54. Rinkoff JS, Doft BH, Lobes LA. Management of ocular penetration from injection of local anesthesia preceding cataract surgery. Arch Ophthalmol 1991;109:1421–1425.
55. Magnante DO, Bullock JD, Green WR. Ocular explosion after peribulbar anesthesia: case report and experimental study. Ophthalmology 1997;104:608–615.
56. Bullock JD, Warwar RE, Green WR. Ocular explosions from periocular anesthetic injections. A clinical, histopathologic, experimental, and biophysical study. Ophthalmology 1999;106:2341–2353.
57. Carlson BM, Emerick S, Komorowski TE, Rainin EA, Shepard BM. Extraocular muscle regeneration in primates. Ophthalmology 1992;99:582–589.
58. Rao VA, Kawatra VK. Ocular myotoxic effects of local anesthetics. Can J Ophthalmol 1988;23:171–173.
59. Foster AH, Carlson BM. Myotoxicity of local anesthetics and regeneration of the damaged muscle fibers. Anesth Analg 1980;59:727–736.
60. Rainin EA, Carlson BM. Postoperative diplopia and ptosis: a clinical hypothesis on the myotoxicity of local anesthetics. Arch Ophthalmol 1985;103:1337–1339.
61. Yagiela JA, Benoit PW, Buoncristiani RD, Peters MP, Fort NF. Comparison of myotoxic effects of lidocaine with epinephrine in rats and humans. Anesth Analg 1981;60: 471–480.
62. O'Brien CS. Local anesthesia. Arch Ophthalmol 1934;12:240–253.
63. Ong-Tone L, Pearce WG. Inferior rectus muscle restriction after retrobulbar anesthesia for cataract extraction. Can J Ophthalmol 1989;24:162–165.
64. Kushner BJ. Ocular muscle fibrosis following cataract extraction. Arch Ophthalmol 1988;106:18–19.
65. Hamed LM. Strabismus presenting after cataract surgery. Ophthalmology 1991;98: 247–252.

66. Hunter DG, Lam GC, Guyton DL. Inferior oblique muscle injury from local anesthesia for cataract surgery. Ophthalmology 1995;102:501–509.
67. Erie JC. Acquired Brown's syndrome after peribulbar anesthesia. Am J Ophthalmol 1990;109:349–350.
68. Barrere M. Cut risk of strabismus. Ophthalmol Times 1995;March 27–April 2:12.
69. Grimmett MR, Lambert SR. Superior rectus muscle overaction after cataract extraction. Am J Ophthalmol 1992;114:72–80.
70. Mackool RJ. Intraocular pressure fluctuations [letter]. J Cataract Refract Surg 1993; 19:563–564.
71. Atkinson WS. Observations on anesthesia for ocular surgery. Trans Am Acad Ophthalmol Otolaryngol 1956;60:376–380.
72. Buys NS. Mercury balloon reducer for vitreous and orbital volume control. In: Emery J, ed. Current Concepts in Cataract Surgery. St. Louis: CV Mosby; 1980:258.
73. Davidson B, Kratz R, Mazzocco T. An evaluation of the Honan intraocular pressure reducer. J Am Intraocul Implant Soc 1979;5:237–238.
74. Drews RC. The Nerf ball for preoperative reduction of intraocular pressure. Ophthalmic Surg 1982;13:761.
75. Gills JP. Constant mild compression of the eye to produce hypotension. J Am Intraocul Implant Soc 1979;5:52–53.
76. Palay DA, Stulting RD. The effect of external ocular compression on intraocular pressure following retrobulbar anesthesia. Ophthalmic Surg 1990;21:503–507.
77. Jay WM, Aziz MZ, Green K. Effect of Honan intraocular pressure reducer on ocular and optic nerve blood flow in phakic rabbit eyes. Acta Ophthalmol 1986;64:52–57.
78. Loken RG, Coupland SG, Deschênes MC. The electroretinogram during orbital compression following intraorbital (regional) block for cataract surgery. Can J Anaesth 1994;41:802–806.
79. Carl JR. Optic neuropathy following cataract extraction. Semin Ophthalmol 1993;8: 144–148.
80. Brod RD. Transient central retinal occlusion and contralateral amaurosis after retrobulbar anesthetic injection. Ophthalmic Surg 1989;20:643–646.
81. Giuffrè G, Vadala M, Manfrè L. Retrobulbar anesthesia complicated by combined central retinal vein and artery occlusion and massive vitreoretinal fibrosis. Retina 1995;15: 439–441.
82. Sullivan KL, Brown GC, Forman AR, Sergott RC, Flanagan JC. Retrobulbar anesthesia and retinal vascular obstruction. Ophthalmology 1983;90:373–377.
83. Lam S, Beck RW, Hall D, Creighton JB. Atonic pupil after cataract surgery. Ophthalmology 1989;96:589–590.
84. Saiz A, Angulo S, Fernandez M. Atonic pupil: an unusual complication of cataract surgery. Ophthalmic Surg 1991;22:20–22.
85. Brown GC, Eagle RC, Shakin EP, Gruber M, Arbizion VV. Retinal toxicity of intravitreal gentamicin. Arch Ophthalmol 1990;108:1740–1744.
86. Campochiaro PA, Conway BP. Aminoglycoside toxicity – a survey of retinal specialists: implications for ocular use. Arch Ophthalmol 1991;109:946–950.
87. Jain VK, Mames RN, McGorray S, Giles CL. Inadvertent penetrating injury to the globe with periocular corticosteroid injection. Ophthalmic Surg 1991;22:508–511.
88. Nianiaris NA, Mandelcorn M, Baker G. Retinal and choroidal embolization following soft-tissue maxillary injection of corticosteroids. Can J Ophthalmol 1995;30:321–323.
89. Pendergast SD, Eliott D, Machemer R. Retinal toxic effects following inadvertent intraocular injection of Celestone Soluspan [letter]. Arch Ophthalmol 1995;113:1230–1231.
90. Schlaegal TF, Wilson FM. Accidental intraocular injection of depot corticosteroids. Trans Am Acad Ophthalmol Otolaryngol 1974;78:847–855.
91. Verma LK, Goyal M, Tewari HK. Inadvertent intraocular injection of depot corticosteroids. Ophthalmic Surg Laser 1996;27:73–74.
92. Ellis PP. Occlusion of the central retinal artery after retrobulbar corticosteroid injection. Am J Ophthalmol 1978;85:352–356.
93. McLean EB. Inadvertent injection of corticosteroid into the choroidal vasculature. Am J Ophthalmol 1975;80:835–837.
94. Shorr N, Seiff SR. Central retinal artery occlusion associated with periocular corticosteroid injection for juvenile hemangioma. Ophthalmic Surg 1986;17:229–231.

95. McDonald HR, Schatz H, Johnson RN. Aminoglycoside toxicity. Semin Ophthalmol 1993;8:136–143.
96. Aldrete JA, Romo-Salas F, Arora S, Wilson R, Rutherford R. Reverse arterial blood flow as a pathway for central nervous system toxic responses following injection of local anesthetics. Anesth Analg 1978;57:428–433.
97. Meyers EF, Ramirez RC, Boniuk I. Grand mal seizures after retrobulbar block. Arch Ophthalmol 1978;96:847.
98. Koenig SB, Snyder RW, Kay J. Respiratory distress after a Nadbath block. Ophthalmology 1988;95:1285–1287.
99. Lindquist TD, Kopietz LA, Spigelman AV, Nichols BD, Lindstrom RL. Complications of Nadbath facial nerve block and review of the literature. Ophthalmic Surg 1988; 19:271–273.
100. Nadbath RP, Rehman I. Facial nerve block. Am J Ophthalmol 1963;55:143–146.
101. Rabinowitz L, Livingston M, Schneider H, Hall A. Respiratory obstruction following the Nadbath facial nerve block [letter]. Arch Ophthalmol 1986;104:1115.
102. Philip BK, Covino BG. Local and regional anesthesia. In: Wetchler BV, ed. Anesthesia for Ambulatory Surgery. 2nd ed. Philadelphia: JB Lippincott; 1991:357.
103. Incaudo G, Schatz M, Patterson R, Rosenberg M, Yamamoto F, Hamburger RN. Administration of local anesthetics to patients with a history of prior adverse reaction. J Allergy Clin Immunol 1978;61:339–345.
104. Meyer D, Hamilton RC, Gimbel HV. Myasthenia gravis-like syndrome induced by topical ophthalmic preparations. A case report. J Clin Neuroophthalmol 1992;12: 210–212.
105. Brown DT, Beamish D, Wildsmith JAW. Allergic reaction to an amide local anaesthetic. Br J Anaesth 1981;53:435–437.
106. McLeskey CH. Allergic reaction to an amide local anaesthetic [letter]. Br J Anaesth 1981;53:1105–1106.
107. Smith RJH. Cataract extraction without retrobulbar anaesthetic injection. Br J Ophthalmol 1990;74:205–207.
108. Lichter PR. Avoiding complications from local anesthesia [editorial]. Ophthalmology 1988;95:565–566.
109. Redmond RM, Dallas NL. Extracapsular cataract extraction without retrobulbar anaesthesia. Br J Ophthalmol 1990;74:203–204.
110. Hatt M. Cataract extraction with intraocular lens implantation under subconjunctival local anaesthesia. Klin Monatsbl Augenheilkd 1990;196:307–309.
111. Furuta M, Toriumi T, Kashiwagi K, Satoh S. Limbal anesthesia for cataract surgery. Ophthalmic Surg 1990;21:22–26.
112. Petersen WC, Yanoff M. Subconjunctival anesthesia: an alternative to retrobulbar and peribulbar techniques. Ophthalmic Surg 1991;22:199–201.
113. Swan KC. New drugs and techniques for ocular anesthesia. Trans Am Acad Ophthalmol Otolaryngol 1956;60:368–375.
114. Tsuneoka H, Ohki K, Taniuchi O, Kitahara K. Tenon's capsule anaesthesia for cataract surgery with IOL implantation. Eur J Implant Refract Surg 1993;5:29–34.
115. Stevens JD. A new local anaesthesia technique for cataract extraction by one quadrant sub-Tenon's infiltration. Br J Ophthalmol 1992;76:670–674.
116. Greenbaum S. Parabulbar anesthesia [letter]. Am J Ophthalmol 1992;114:776.
117. Dillman DM. Topical anesthesia for phacoemulsification. Ophthalmol Clin North Am 1995;8:419–427.
118. Novak KD, Koch DD. Topical anesthesia for phacoemulsification: initial 20-case series with one month follow-up. J Cataract Refract Surg 1995;21:672–675.
119. Kershner RM. Topical anesthesia for small incision self-sealing cataract surgery: a prospective evaluation of the first 100 patients. J Cataract Refract Surg 1993;19: 290–292.
120. Friedman DS, Bass EB, Lubomski LH, et al. Synthesis of the literature on the effectiveness of regional anesthesia for cataract surgery. Ophthalmology 2001;108: 519–529.
121. Hall DL, Steen WH, Drummond JW, Byrd WA. Anticoagulants and cataract surgery. Ophthalmic Surg 1988;19:221–222.
122. McMahan LB. Anticoagulants and cataract surgery. J Cataract Refract Surg 1988;14: 569–571.

123. Stone LS, Kline OR Jr, Sklar C. Intraocular lenses and anticoagulation and antiplatelet therapy. J Am Intraocul Implant Soc 1985;11:165–168.
124. Gainey SP, Robertson DM, Fay W, Ilstrup D. Ocular surgery on patients receiving long-term warfarin therapy. Am J Ophthalmol 1989;108:142–146.
125. Robinson GA, Nylander A. Warfarin and cataract extraction. Br J Ophthalmol 1989; 3:702–703.
126. Konstantatos A. Anticoagulation and cataract surgery: a review of the current literature. Anaesth Intensive Care 2001;29:11–18.
127. Shuler JD, Paschal JF, Holland GN. Antiplatelet therapy and cataract surgery. J Cataract Refract Surg 1992;18:567–571.

# 7 Complications of Paravertebral, Intercostal Nerve Blocks and Interpleural Analgesia

Nirmala R. Abraham Hidalgo and F. Michael Ferrante

Paravertebral, intercostal nerve blocks and interpleural analgesia are used to provide intermittent, temporary, or continuous anesthesia or analgesia in the thoracic and abdominal regions. These regional techniques may be appropriate alternatives to the standard methods of providing analgesia (i.e., epidural analgesia, intravenous opioids) for selected groups of patients. These analgesic techniques have been used to treat pain related to thoracotomy,[1,2] rib fractures,[3–5] trauma,[6] and chronic pain.[7] In recent years, utilization of these techniques has been extended to include breast surgery,[8,9] shoulder surgery,[10,11] laparoscopic cholecystectomy,[12] and inguinal hernia repair.[13] Paravertebral blocks have recently been described as an effective means of providing analgesia after hepatectomy.[14]

The advantage of these techniques over thoracic epidural analgesia is related to the unilateral nature of these blocks and a less extensive sympathetic block, and therefore an attendant decrease in overall physiologic trespass (e.g., lack of hypotension).[15,16] When compared to intravenous opioid analgesia, these regional analgesic techniques provide excellent pain relief without interfering with respiratory drive.[4,17,18]

When appropriately used and performed, there is substantive evidence that paravertebral and intercostal nerve blocks and interpleural analgesia provide excellent pain relief. In deciding which block will be appropriate for a particular case, it is important to consider the type of anesthesia and/or analgesia one hopes to obtain. There are many different approaches to these techniques and there are numerous potential complications.

We will first describe the pertinent thoracic anatomy. We will then describe how to perform the technique and discuss the potential complications. It is important to note that in recent years, paravertebral blocks have experienced a renaissance, whereas interpleural analgesia has fallen out of favor. Thus, the review of interpleural analgesia will be largely for the sake of completeness.

## Thoracic Anatomy

Thoracic anatomy relevant to these analgesic techniques is portrayed in Figures 7-1 and 7-2.

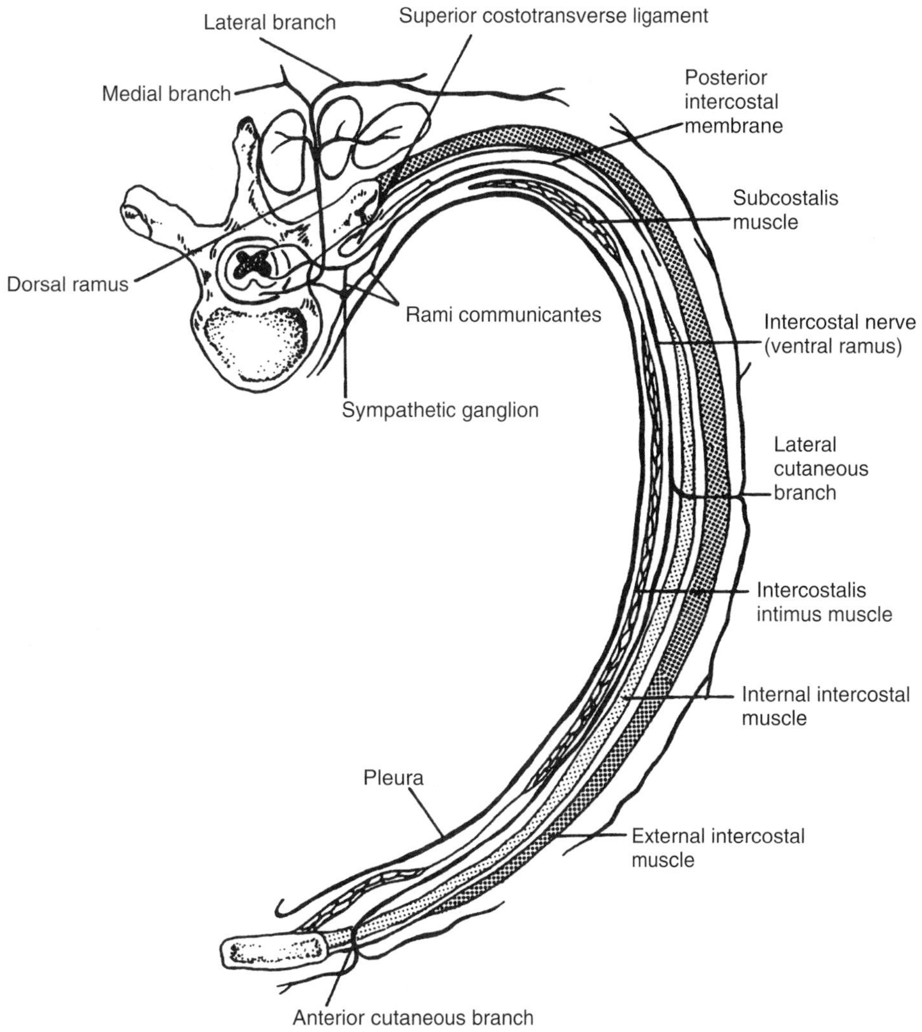


**FIGURE 7-1.** A transverse section through a typical thoracic dermatome at the level of the intervertebral foramen. (Reprinted from Ferrante FM, VadeBoncouer TR. Postoperative Pain Management. New York: Churchill Livingstone; 1993, with permission from Elsevier.)

## *Paravertebral Anatomy*

The paravertebral space (Figure 7-3) is the shape of a four-sided pyramid with its apex facing posteriorly into the neural foramen and its base bordered anteriorly by the parietal pleura. The thoracic paravertebral space is defined by the following four borders: 1) the bone and articular capsules of the rib and transverse process above, 2) the rib below, 3) medially by the vertebral body, and 4) laterally by the intercostal space and the costotransverse ligament. The costotransverse ligament runs from the transverse process to the superior aspect of the inferior rib. The paravertebral space contains the spinal nerve root and its continuation, the intercostal nerve. The intercostal nerve branches into dorsal and ventral rami in the paravertebral space. Gray and white rami communicantes course through the space to and from the respective sympathetic ganglion at that level, which is also contained within the paravertebral space. Other contents include areolar tissue, fat, and blood vessels. It is important to keep in mind that the paravertebral space is contiguous with the epidural and intercostal spaces as it lies between these two other spaces. Any substance injected into the paravertebral space may potentially spread cephalad and caudad to adjacent paravertebral spaces as well as medially and laterally to the epidural and intercostal

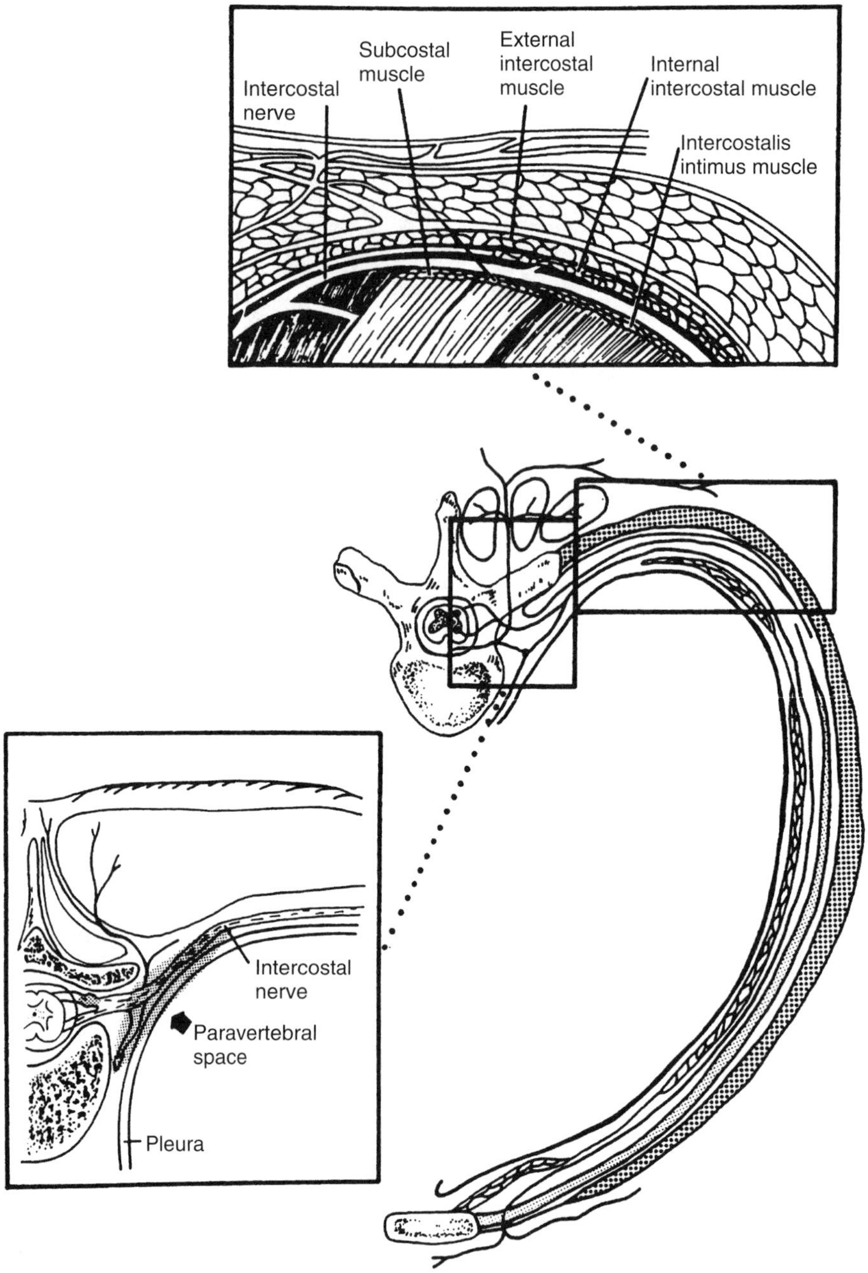


**FIGURE 7-2.** Paravertebral nerve blocks and interpleural nerve blocks act in the area of the lower box. Intercostal nerve blocks are applied to the anatomy depicted in the upper box. (Reprinted from Ferrante FM, VadeBoncouer TR. Postoperative Pain Management. New York: Churchill Livingstone; 1993, with permission from Elsevier.)

spaces, respectively.[19] Rarely, an injection into the paravertebral space will spread to the contralateral space, and this has been demonstrated radiologically.[19–21]

In general, topographic spread is variable and difficult to predict.[22,23] Naja et al.[24] performed a series of paravertebral blocks using nerve-stimulator guidance to determine the effect of varying injection points on spread of solution. Their findings indicated that injection in the more ventral aspect of the thoracic paravertebral space resulted in a multisegmental longitudinal spreading pattern. Injecting at the dorsal aspect of the space showed a cloud-like spread with limited distribution to adjacent segments (Figure 7-4).

**FIGURE 7-3.** The paravertebral space is defined by four borders: 1) medial, vertebral body; 2) lateral, intercostal space and the costotransverse ligament; 3) superior, bone and articular capsules of the rib and transverse process above; and 4) inferior, the rib below. In three dimensions, the space is a four-sided pyramid with its base at the pleura and apex at the intervertebral foramen. (Reprinted from Ferrante FM, VadeBoncouer TR. Postoperative Pain Management. New York: Churchill Livingstone; 1993, with permission from Elsevier.)

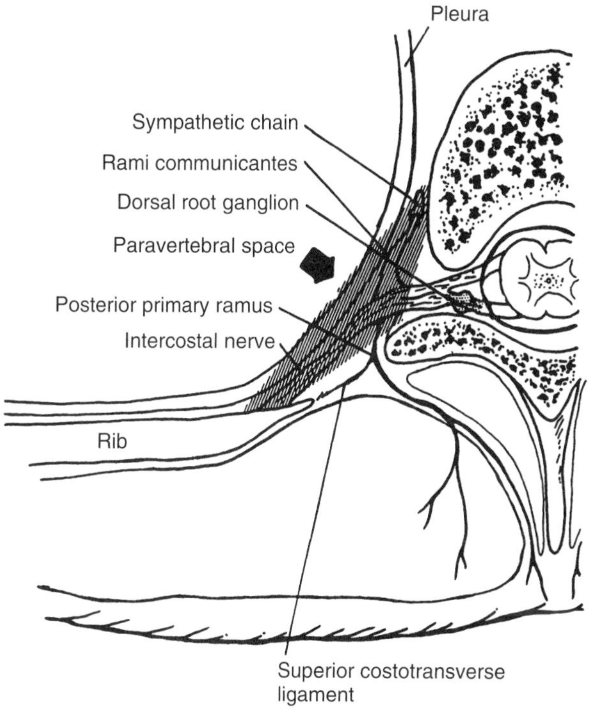


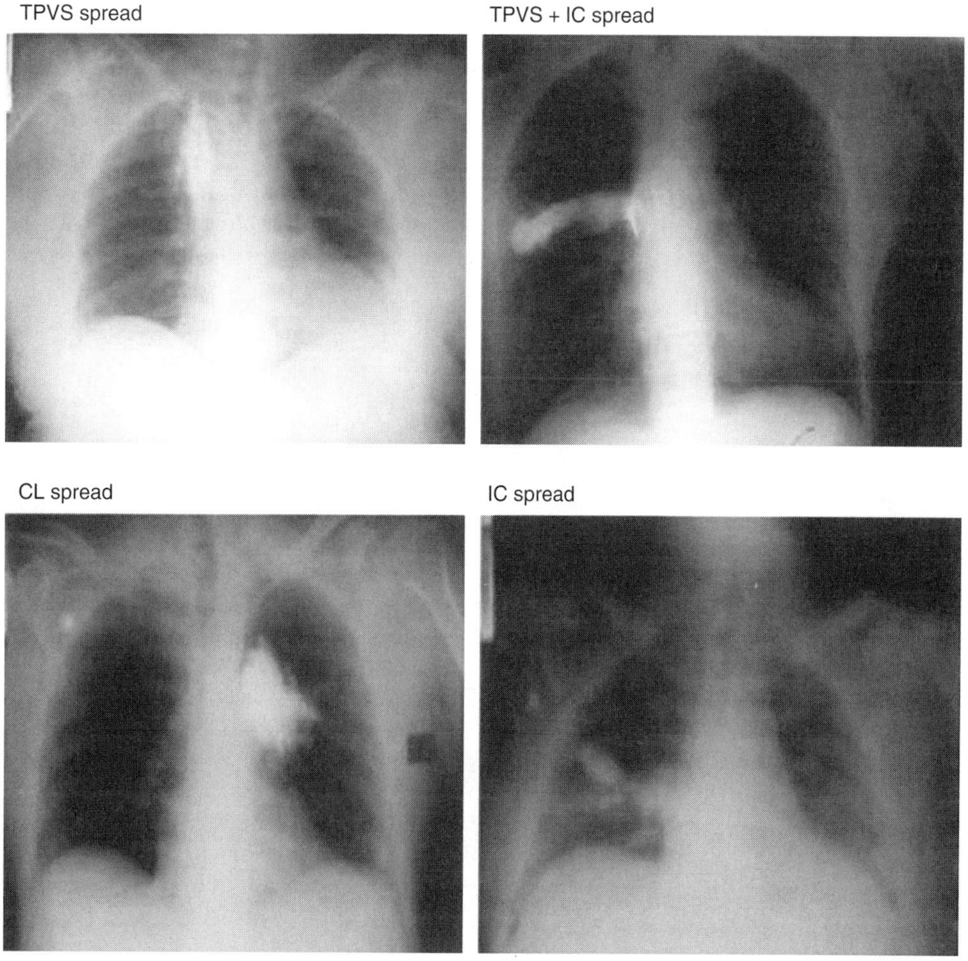


**FIGURE 7-4.** Images of four patterns of spread: TPVS, thoracic paravertebral space; TPVS + IC, thoracic paravertebral space and intercostal; CL, cloud-like; IC, intercostal. (From Naja et al.[24] Reprinted with permission from Blackwell Publishing.)

The similarity in the anatomic distribution and density of block produced by continuous paravertebral block and continuous epidural infusion would seem to indicate that some cases of unilateral "epidural" block may be attributable to inadvertent continuous paravertebral blockade. This phenomenon has been confirmed radiologically.[25]

### *Intercostal Anatomy*

The anatomy of the intercostal nerves and spaces is depicted in Figures 7-1 and 7-5. Intercostal nerves are derived from the spinal roots of the respective thoracic segments. They are composed of dorsal horn sensory afferent fibers, ventral horn motor efferent fibers, and postganglionic sympathetic nerves that join the nerve via the paravertebral gray rami communicantes. Thus, each intercostal nerve has autonomic and somatic sensory and motor functions. Soon after the sympathetic contribution occurs within the paravertebral space, the intercostal nerve divides into ventral and dorsal rami. The dorsal ramus provides sensory innervation to the posteromedial structures of the back (synovium, periosteum, fascia, muscles, and skin) and motor innervation to the erector spinae muscles. The ventral ramus travels between the ribs. It is protected within the subcostal groove by the rib and two layers of intercostal muscle.

Each intercostal nerve (ventral ramus) is associated with a vein and artery. The intercostal vein is derived from the confluence of venules along the thoracic cage and empties into the azygous vein on the right and the hemiazygous vein on the left. The most cephalad intercostal veins join and empty into the respective brachiocephalic veins bilaterally. The intercostal arteries are derived directly from the aorta.

The neurovascular structures are always superficial to the parietal pleura and thin aponeurotic-areolar tissue called the intercostalis intimus muscle. The aponeurotic-areolar tissue has muscle fibers embedded within its substance, and despite its name, its classification as a true muscle is a matter of debate among anatomists. There is various cutaneous branching of the ventral rami. In general, there are anterior and lateral branches, which divide and innervate skin and intercostal muscles of an individual segment along with variable collateral innervation of the adjacent segments. Because of this collateral innervation, it is necessary to block a level above and below

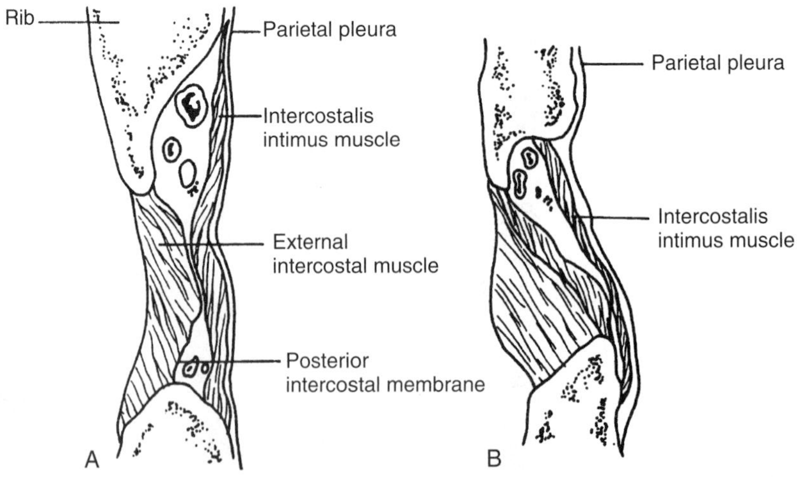


**FIGURE 7-5.** Anatomic cross-section through the intercostal space at **(A)** the angle of the rib and **(B)** laterally at the posterior axillary line. (Reprinted from Ferrante FM, VadeBoncouer TR. Postoperative Pain Management. New York: Churchill Livingstone; 1993, with permission from Elsevier.)

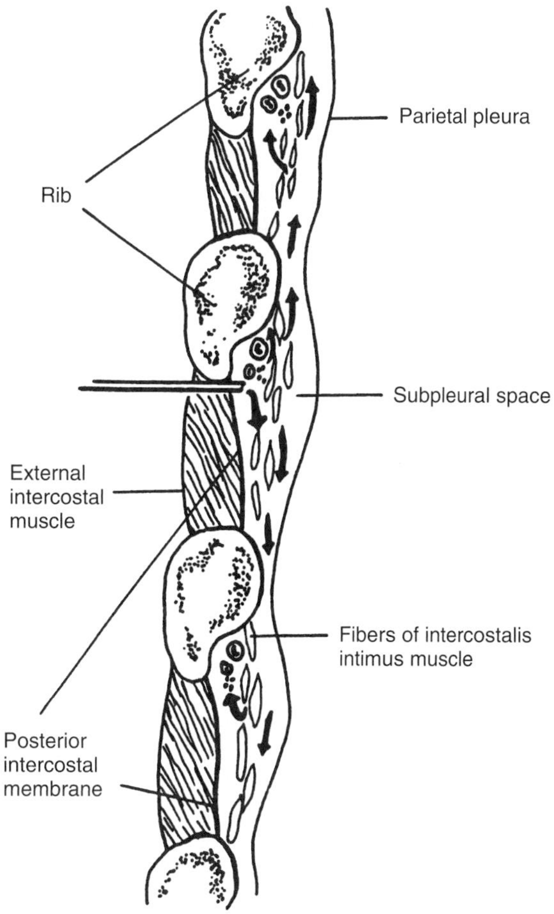


**FIGURE 7-6.** The aponeurosis or the intercostalis intimus does not impede spread of injectate to adjacent intercostal spaces when the needle or catheter is placed in the correct tissue plane. (Reprinted from Ferrante FM, VadeBoncouer TR. Postoperative Pain Management. New York: Churchill Livingstone; 1993, with permission from Elsevier.)

the desired level. Because there is minimal adhesion of the aponeurosis to the parietal pleura, and the intercostalis intimus muscle is a rather flimsy structure, cephalad and caudad spread of injected solution to the adjacent intercostal spaces is not impeded (Figure 7-6). It is important to keep in mind that the intercostal and paravertebral spaces are contiguous at all levels. Spread of local anesthetic to the paravertebral space produces unilateral segmental sympathetic blockade.

### *Pleural Anatomy*

The lungs are sheathed in a glossy membrane called the visceral pleura. This membrane develops embryonically from the lung tissue. This closely attached serous membrane is continuous with the membrane that lines the chest wall, mediastinum, and diaphragm, where it is called the parietal pleura. The cupola of the lung is adjacent to a portion of cervical parietal pleura. The potential space between the visceral and parietal pleura, the pleural cavity, is only evident when filled with air (pneumothorax), pus (empyema), or fluid (hydro- or hemothorax). The costal and diaphragmatic parietal pleurae meet and descend in a groove with no lung tissue between them, caudad and anterior to T6 and posterior to T10. This is the costophrenic sulcus, which opens to accommodate vital capacity lung expansion.

## Neural Blockade

### *Paravertebral Nerve Block Techniques*

Patient comfort during performance of a paravertebral block is improved by good technique, the use of small-gauge needles, and the avoidance of paresthesias while performing the block.[26] Generous infiltration of local anesthetic also makes the procedure more tolerable. Sedation before the procedure is strongly recommended and adds greatly to patient comfort.

#### Classic Technique – Lateral Approach

The classic technique for paravertebral blockade involves insertion of a needle 4.0cm lateral to the midline, level to the caudad aspect of the spinous process one level above the level to be blocked (Figure 7-7). The caudad angle of the thoracic spinous process brings the inferior tip of the spinous process to the superior aspect of the spinous process at the level below.[27] The needle is advanced perpendicular to the skin in all planes until it contacts the transverse process. The depth of the needle is noted. A sterile hemostat can be clamped to the needle to mark the depth of the needle at the skin. The needle is then "walked off" the transverse process in a cephalad direction and advanced 1cm, placing the tip of the needle in the paravertebral space. Modification of this technique by advancing the needle medially to contact the vertebral body affords relative confidence that an intraneural or subarachnoid injection will not occur. (See detailed description below.) Because the epidural space is contiguous with the paravertebral space via the intervertebral neural foramen, epidural spread is always possible if enough volume is injected.

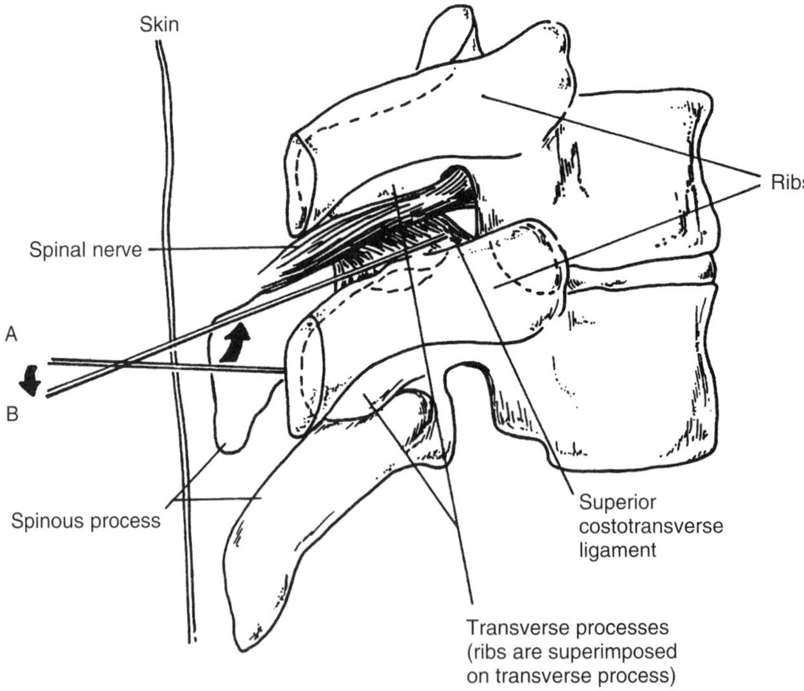


**FIGURE 7-7.** The needle is inserted at the level of the caudad tip of the spinous process one segment above the level to be blocked. This brings the needle to the transverse plane of the transverse process immediately below. **(A)** The needle is advanced to contact the transverse process. **(B)** The needle is then "walked off" the transverse process in a cephalad direction, to pass through the costotransverse ligament. (Reprinted from Ferrante FM, VadeBoncouer TR. Postoperative Pain Management. New York: Churchill Livingstone; 1993, with permission from Elsevier.)

### Medial Approach

To avoid intrathecal injection, Shaw[28] recommends a medial approach. The needle insertion point is approximately 1 cm from midline. The needle is advanced until the lamina is contacted and then directed laterally off the bone. With this technique, the tip of the needle is directed away from the neuraxis, but intraneural injection and epidural extravasation is still possible. Tenicela and Pollan[16] modified and strongly advocate performance of the medial approach in the following manner: after a skin wheal is placed, generous infiltration of local anesthetic into the paraspinal muscles is performed 3–4 cm lateral to the midline in the thoracic region and 2–3 cm lateral to midline in the lumbar region. A 22-gauge, 9-cm spinal needle is inserted and advanced at a 45-degree angle to the transverse plane in a medial direction until the lamina is contacted. The approximate depth required to make contact with the lamina is 5–6 cm in males and somewhat less in females. Gentle aspiration is performed to confirm negative return of blood or cerebrospinal fluid (CSF). At this point, a small amount of local anesthetic is injected at the periosteum. A sterile hemostat is clamped to the shaft of the needle about 1–1.5 cm from the skin, marking the depth of the lamina. The needle is then withdrawn and guided laterally off the lamina and advanced until the hemostat is flush with the skin. After negative aspiration for blood, CSF, and air, a test dose of 3 mL is given. The remaining dose can be given if there was no adverse response to the test dose. If bone is contacted at increasingly superficial levels, the needle has contacted the transverse process and is too cephalad. It must be reinserted approximately 1 cm caudad. These authors claim good to excellent results in 97% of 380 performances of paravertebral block. The complications encountered are discussed below.

### Continuous Technique

Further modification of the injection technique allows placement of a catheter for continuous infusion. Eason and Wyatt[29] proposed that this technique achieves the closest possible approximation of the needle tip with the common intercostal nerve (i.e., before division into dorsal and ventral rami). By using an epidural needle, a catheter can be advanced for repeated bolus dosing or continuous infusion. Beginning 3 cm lateral to midline, a needle is passed perpendicular to the skin in all planes. The needle is advanced until it contacts bone, which may be rib or transverse process. From this point, the needle is walked cephalad off the bone. This technique was proposed to be safer than using the caudad direction for performance of the block (Figure 7-8). Loss of resistance with an air-filled syringe is used to identify entrance of the needle tip into the paravertebral space. When the needle is in the costotransverse ligament, there is significant resistance to attempted injection of air. Once the needle tip passes into the loose areolar tissue of the paravertebral space, the air can be injected. If a catheter is advanced, it should have a single orifice at the tip to ensure that aspiration will give accurate information about the location of the tip. An insertion depth of 1 cm is suggested.

The authors report that manipulation of the epidural needle may be necessary to actually insert the catheter into the paravertebral space. An easily advancing catheter may indicate interpleural localization.[21] Injection of 15 mL of 0.375% bupivacaine reliably blocks four dermatomes.

### Complications of Paravertebral Blockade

The most important factors for safe performance of paravertebral neural blockade are a solid knowledge of pertinent anatomy, meticulous attention to injection technique, and anticipation of all possible physiologic changes associated with the block. The clinician must have a comprehensive understanding of the potential complications. Early recognition facilitates rapid treatment, thus minimizing more serious

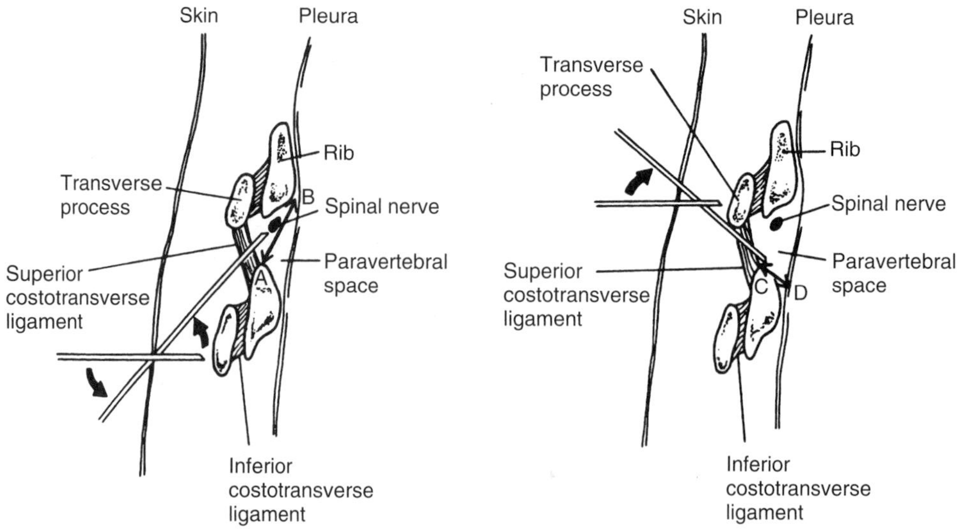


**FIGURE 7-8.** The distance from the superior costotransverse ligament to the pleura is longer with the cranial approach (line **A-B**) than it is with a caudad approach (line **C-D**). The risk of pneumothorax may therefore be decreased with a superior approach. (Reprinted from Ferrante FM, VadeBoncouer TR. Postoperative Pain Management. New York: Churchill Livingstone; 1993, with permission from Elsevier.)

sequelae. Utilization of a nerve-stimulator guided technique is associated with a higher success rate and fewer complications than standard techniques.[30] It is strongly suggested that an intravenous line be in place before performing the block.

It is imperative that low-osmolarity contrast agents be used when performing these blocks, because spread of high-osmolarity solutions into the subarachnoid space can lead to significant neurologic harm. The proximity of the paravertebral space to the central nervous system creates the obvious potential for needle entrance into either the epidural or subarachnoid space. Iodinated contrast has been injected into the epidural space with and without spread into the paravertebral space. In performing 45 paravertebral blocks, Purcell-Jones et al.[19] showed contrast confined to the paravertebral space in only 18% of procedures. There was epidural extravasation in 70% and exclusive epidural spread in 31% of cases.

In addition to epidural[13] and subdural[31] injection, unrecognized subarachnoid puncture can occur. Headaches not associated with obvious dural puncture occurred in 3 of 24 cases in one series of paravertebral blocks. Aspiration was negative for CSF before injection.[32] Negative aspiration for CSF is not an absolute guarantee of proper needle placement, especially with small-gauge needles or long, small-bore catheters. The headaches resolved with conservative management within 5–14 days postoperatively. The medial approach proposed by Shaw[28] and modified by Tenicela and Pollan[16] has shown excellent results with low complication rates. Of the 384 blocks performed by Tenicela and Pollan, there was one incident of pneumothorax (0.26%), one recognized dural puncture, two intrathecal injections of the test dose, 18 incidents of hypotension (4.6%), five bilateral blockades (1.3%), and 27 incidents of fair to poor block (7.0%). Poor results were attributed to centralized pain disorders. There were no incidents of serious or permanent sequelae.

Intravenous, intraarterial, and intraneural injection can occur using any approach to the paravertebral space.[30] In addition, infection, hematoma formation, or damage to the neural fascicle may occur from dry needling. The type of needle can also affect the incidence of sequelae. Short-beveled needles have been shown to cause less nerve damage than long-beveled needles.[33]

Aspiration will not reveal the presence of an intrafascicular needle tip. Injectate can dissect back through an epineural injection to the contiguous pia mater.[34] This mode of access to the subarachnoid space has been clearly demonstrated in experimental models.[35] These investigations were driven by the occurrence of severe sequelae (death,[36] paraplegia,[37] transverse myelitis[38]) from injection of a long-acting formulation of procaine. The diffuse tissue necrosis was attributed to the carrier solution.[39] For this reason, the use of fluoroscopy and injection of low-osmolarity iodinated contrast to confirm proper needle placement are recommended when performing paravertebral blockade.

When using a continuous technique, there is always a risk of shearing the catheter if it is withdrawn back through the needle. Predictably, there will almost always be some pain at the site of needle insertion. Infection and hematoma are also possible risks. Monoplatythela (unilateral flat nipple) may occur with a successful block.[40]

Other potential complications involve interpleural or intrapulmonary injections. If the tip of the needle is in the interpleural space, aspiration should reveal air. Injection of a small volume of radiocontrast under live fluoroscopy can quickly and easily detect an interpleural or intrapulmonary injection.

Prolonged anesthesia and motor block after inguinal hernia repair under general anesthesia with paravertebral blockade was observed in a patient with multiple sclerosis.[41] Abnormal uptake of local anesthetics into the spinal cord secondary to the presence of demyelination was proposed as the mechanism.

Contraindications to paravertebral block are infection at the site, patient refusal, and allergy to any of the solutions to be injected.

### *Intercostal Nerve Block Techniques*

Intercostal neural blockade can be achieved intermittently, continuously, or permanently in one or several segments, depending on the technique used. Careful attention to technique decreases the rate of complication. Percutaneous injection of 2–5 mL of local anesthetic in at least three adjacent levels will ensure anesthesia/analgesia in the distribution of the middle intercostal nerve because of collateral innervation. Although relief is temporary, this technique is very effective in alleviating somatic pain in the chest wall and abdominal wall. Prolonged blockade requires either multiple reinsertions with the attendant risk of pneumothorax, placement of a catheter for bolus dosing or continuous infusion,[42] injection with a neurolytic agent,[43] or cryoablation.[44]

Another important risk to keep in mind is local anesthetic toxicity. Blood levels of local anesthetic after intercostal blockade and interpleural analgesia are significantly greater than after any other frequently performed regional anesthetic techniques. Tucker et al.[45] performed epidural, caudal, intercostal, brachial plexus, and sciatic/femoral nerve blocks with a single injection of mepivacaine 500 mg (1% and 2% solutions) with and without epinephrine. When measuring arterial plasma levels, the highest levels were found after intercostal nerve blocks without epinephrine (5–10 µg/mL). When epinephrine was added to the solution (1:200,000 concentration), the plasma level decreased to 2–5 µg/mL. Epinephrine should be uniformly added to local anesthetic for performance of intercostal nerve block to minimize the potential for systemic toxicity.

#### **Posterior Approach**

Traditionally, intercostal nerve blocks are performed with a posterior approach at the angle of the rib, 6–8 cm lateral to the respective spinous process.[46] This target point allows direct palpation of the rib in most patients. It also allows blockade of the lateral intercostal cutaneous branch, which usually originates distal to the angle of the rib, ensuring good medial as well as lateral analgesia. The immediately adjacent intercostal nerves must also be blocked, because there is collateral innervation from the levels above and below. Neurolytic injections and cryoablative procedures must also be performed in a similar manner.

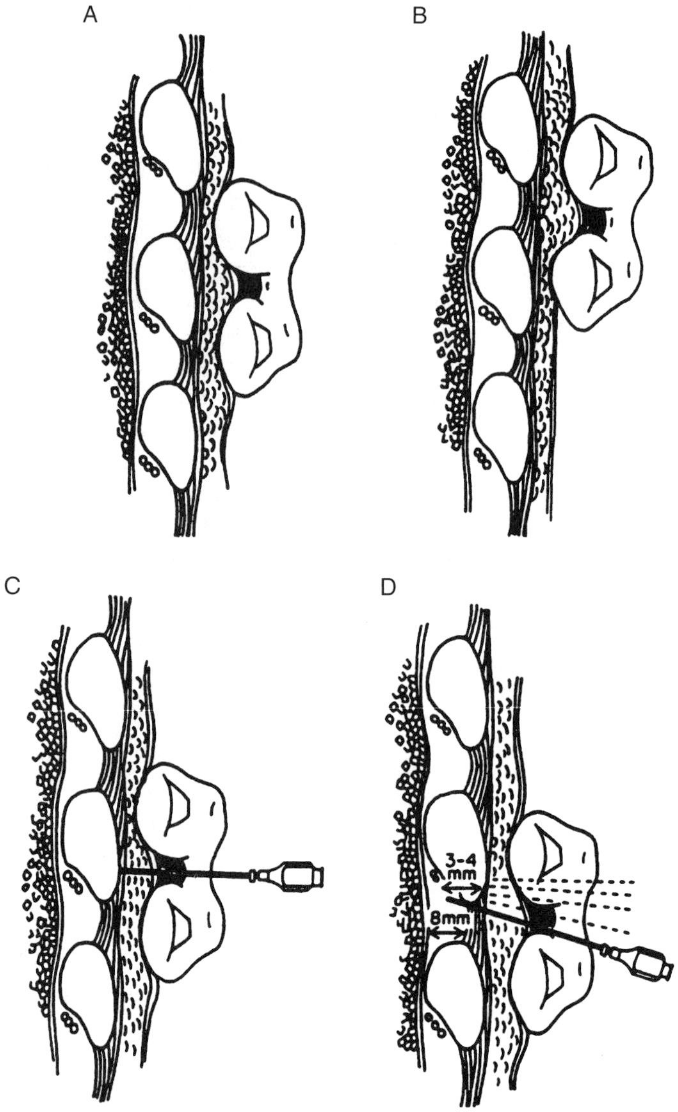


**FIGURE 7-9.** Technique for intercostal nerve block. **(A,B)** The skin is retracted cephalad by two fingers straddling a rib. **(C)** A 25-gauge needle is advanced toward the inferior aspect of the rib until bone is contacted. **(D)** The cephalad traction on the skin is released, the needle is "walked off" the inferior border of the rib and advanced 3–5 mm beyond the rib to pass through the external and internal intercostal muscles. (Reprinted from Ferrante FM, VadeBoncouer TR. Postoperative Pain Management. New York: Churchill Livingstone; 1993, with permission from Elsevier.)

Figure 7-9 shows a technique for safely performing an intercostal nerve block. The skin above one intercostal space is retracted in a cephalad direction by the index and middle fingers of the nondominant hand. The rib corresponding to the nerve to be blocked is now between the fingers. A short-beveled, 25-gauge needle is advanced toward the inferior margin of the rib until bone is gently contacted. The fingers then release the skin to its original position. The needle is carefully walked off the inferior margin of the rib and advanced 3–5 mm, passing the external and internal intercostal muscles and placing the tip in the intercostal space. The width of the posterior intercostal space at the angle of the rib is approximately 8 mm.[46] Aspiration must be negative for blood and air. A volume of 2–5 mL of local anesthetic with 1:200,000 epinephrine is then slowly injected. This exact procedure is then repeated at the level above and below the targeted intercostal nerve. If multiple dermatomes need to be blocked, one level above and one below the targeted levels must also be blocked.

For pain associated with video-assisted thoracoscopy procedures, the utilization of intercostal nerve blockade with 0.375% bupivacaine resulted in a significant decrease in the postoperative use of intravenous morphine.[2] This technique may be particularly useful for outpatient video-assisted thoracoscopy procedures.

### Lateral Approach

A variation of this technique is entry at the posterior or midaxillary lines. These approaches may be adequate for blocking the anterior chest or abdominal wall, but will often miss the lateral cutaneous branch, thus providing less than satisfactory blockade of the back and flank regions (Figure 7-4).

In patients undergoing thoracotomy, the surgeon may perform the blocks under direct visualization just before closure. However, these blocks are often placed at a site more medial than what would be chosen for a percutaneous approach. Thus, there seems to be a higher incidence of complications because of the proximity to the spinal nerve roots.

### Continuous Technique

Nunn and Slavin[46] described the ability of a single intercostal injection of India ink to spread subpleurally to multiple intercostal spaces. The minimally adherent parietal pleura and the thin intercostalis intimus muscle did not hinder the multidirectional spread of the injectate (Figure 7-5).

Based on morphometric measurements of the intercostal space, Nunn and Slavin placed the needle tip 3mm past the inferior margin of the rib, leaving approximately 5mm to the pleura. In a study by O'Kelly and Garry,[47] a continuous catheter was placed through a 19-gauge epidural needle with the tip directed medially. After first injecting 10mL of solution through the needle, the catheter was advanced 2cm and then secured to the skin. Appropriate spread of local anesthetic was confirmed by radiographic imaging.

Satisfactory analgesia has been documented using continuous infusion.[48] Seventy-five patients (92%) had good analgesia without requiring supplemental medications during the first postoperative day using an infusion of 0.5% bupivacaine at 7mL/hour. Sixty-six patients (81.5%) remained satisfied with their analgesia over the following 4 days. Patients who experienced inadequate analgesia early in their course were thought to have leakage of anesthetic into the interpleural space. Subsequent decrements in analgesic efficacy were attributed to tachyphylaxis. The same authors modified the protocol to increase the infusion rate to a maximum of 10mL/hour.[49] This resulted in a significant improvement in pulmonary function over the control group, which required higher doses of intravenous rescue pain medications than the continuous intercostal infusion group.

### Complications of Intercostal Neural Blockade

The most common complications of intercostal nerve block are associated with the aberrant needle placement (pneumothorax, hemothorax, hemoptysis, hematoma, intravascular injection, neuritis, subarachnoid block, failed block) or problems associated with the injectate (allergic reaction, toxic reaction, epinephrine reaction, tissue necrosis, respiratory insufficiency).

The actual incidence of pneumothorax secondary to intercostal nerve block is quite small. A large, retrospective study reporting 50,097 intercostal nerve blocks in 4333 patients undergoing surgery or therapeutic nerve blocks revealed only four clinically significant pneumothoraces (0.092%) and no other significant complications.[50] The technique for intercostal neural blockade was similar to the posterior approach described by Nunn and Slavin.[46] There was some minor discomfort at the injection sites in 5% of patients. A prospective study by the same authors in 200 consecutive patients undergoing intercostal nerve block compared pre- and postinjection films to evaluate for pneumothorax.[51] There were only four pneumothoraces in a total of 2610 needle punctures, of which three pneumothoraces were attributed to the actual surgical procedure itself and not performance of the blocks. In the largest retrospective study with more than 100,000 needle punctures, Moore[52] reported an incidence of pneumothorax of 0.073% without any other serious complications. It is important to note that residents still in training performed most of these blocks.

There are sporadic case reports of other types of complications. Hematoma has occurred in a heparinized patient.[53] Bilateral intercostal nerve blocks have resulted in postoperative respiratory failure in patients with preoperative pulmonary compromise.[54,55] Motor blockade and the loss of accessory respiratory muscle function were the hypothesized etiologic mechanisms. In a study looking at the efficacy of continuous epidural versus intercostal analgesia, one intercostal catheter led to rib osteomyelitis which had to be treated surgically.[42]

Intraoperative intercostal nerve block performed by the surgical team has resulted in total spinal anesthesia. Presumably, this serious complication occurred because of the proximity of the injections to spinal nerve roots.[56,57] Paravertebral neural block has also occurred with attempted intercostal nerve block during surgery.[58]

Total spinal anesthesia has occurred during performance of percutaneous intercostal nerve blocks.[59] Dissection of the injectate through the endoneurium in continuity with the pia mater was the presumed etiologic mechanism. Retrograde spread could also occur through the dural cuff, which surrounds the peripheral nerves at the perineurium.

Intrapulmonary injection is a risk, especially when there has been an alteration in the pulmonary anatomy secondary to previous surgery. Acute bronchospasm from intrapulmonary injection of 8% phenol has been reported.[60] The characteristic odor of phenol was detected in the patient's exhaled air.

In addition to the issue of epidural blockade with continuous intercostal neural blockade, there is concern regarding misplacement of the catheter. The actual technique of catheter placement is somewhat imprecise, lacking a definitive end point. Mowbray et al.[21] performed intercostal catheterization in 22 patients scheduled for thoracotomy or median sternotomy. At the time of surgery, it was found that only 12 catheters (54.5%) were actually placed correctly in the intercostal space. There was also a report of neuritis with catheter placement. Catheter dislodgment and interpleural or intravenous catheter migration can occur.

Relative contraindications to intercostal blockade include patient refusal, history of allergic reaction to injectates, coagulopathy, and infection at the proposed site of injection.

## Interpleural Analgesia

Because interpleural analgesia is rarely performed in modern times, our discussion of this technique will be brief.

Interpleural analgesia has been evaluated for multiple uses, including surgery of the upper abdomen, flank and thoracic wall,[61,62] chronic regional pain syndrome,[63] multiple rib fractures,[4] and chronic pancreatitis.[64,65] The literature is ambivalent as to the ultimate efficacy of interpleural blockade. Direct comparison has been made to intercostal neural blockade and the latter technique was deemed to be superior.[66,67] Interpleural analgesia was compared with thoracic epidural analgesia after minimally invasive coronary artery bypass surgery and was found to be a safe and effective alternative.[68]

The block is easy to perform when clear landmarks are present, and usually involves the placement of a continuous catheter for infusion. The technique can be performed percutaneously. Alternatively, it may be performed intraoperatively under direct vision. The seated or lateral decubitus position (side to be blocked uppermost) can be used. After prepping the insertion site with appropriate sterile technique, the needle is placed at the superior border of the rib to avoid the neurovascular bundle. Because the paravertebral gutter is the eventual target for the catheter, a posterior approach is beneficial. The angle of the rib correlates to the widest aspect of the intercostal space, which may provide the best location for placement of the catheter.

The needle is advanced until it is felt to "pop" through the fascial layer of the parietal pleura. Entry into the pleural space is evidenced by visual techniques (Figure 7-10) which rely on entrance of fluid into the interpleural space with negative inspiratory interpleural pressure.[61] A saline-filled syringe, a column of saline in a syringe without a plunger,[69] and a hanging drop[70] have all been used to visually confirm entry. A multiport catheter should be easily advanced 5–10 cm through the epidural needle. If the catheter does not advance smoothly, either pleural adhesions or misplacement of the catheter is present. In spontaneously breathing patients, air will always be entrained when a needle and/or catheter are placed into the pleural space. Thus, it is important to minimize the total time of needle and catheter placements.

Once the catheter is in place, the patient should be positioned so the local anesthetic injected will pool in the paravertebral gutter. The amount of local anesthetic injected can vary from 10 mL[71] to 30 mL,[72] and most will select an intermediate volume (20 mL of 0.25%–0.5% bupivacaine with epinephrine).

The mechanism of blockade is believed to be a "retrograde" intercostal blockade at multiple levels.[73] Local anesthetic diffuses from the interpleural space to the intercostal nerves and paravertebral spaces where it pools (Figure 7-11). The area of spread for a given volume is greater in the supine position compared with the lateral position.[74]

Complications associated with interpleural block are related to all phases of the procedure: needle and catheter placement, injection of local anesthetic, and infection as a result of indwelling catheter. It is possible to cause direct damage to neurovascular structures if the needle is angled toward the inferior margin of the rib during placement.

Because of the nature of the technique, which involves the passage of a needle through the pleura, entrainment of small amounts of air occur during catheter

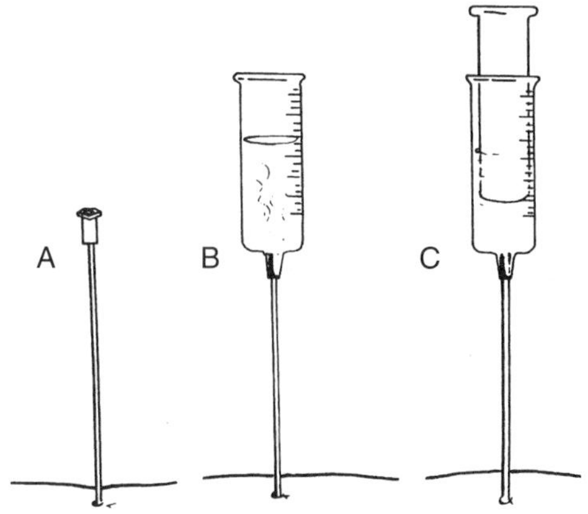


**FIGURE 7-10.** Visual techniques using fluid aspiration by negative interpleural pressure to recognize entry into the interpleural space. **(A)** Hanging drop. **(B)** A saline column in a syringe without a barrel. **(C)** A saline-filled glass syringe. (Reprinted from Ferrante FM, VadeBoncouer TR. Postoperative Pain Management. New York: Churchill Livingstone; 1993, with permission from Elsevier.)

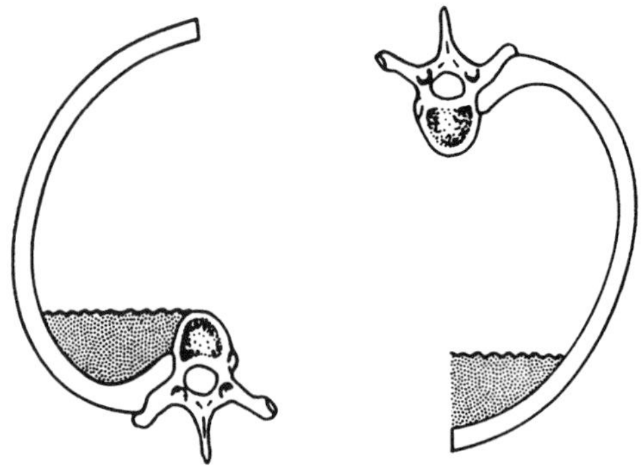


**FIGURE 7-11.** Gravity and volume are important factors in distributing interpleural anesthetic to the targeted nerves. The position of the patient is critical to obtaining and maintaining an effective block in the desired dermatomal distribution. The patient must be positioned so that the instilled local anesthetic pools in the paravertebral gutter of the desired levels. (Reprinted from Ferrante FM, VadeBoncouer TR. Postoperative Pain Management. New York: Churchill Livingstone; 1993, with permission from Elsevier.)

placement, and practically all patients (by definition) develop a pneumothorax (although usually less than 5% of lung volume).[75] Stromskag et al.[75] reviewed the incidence of significant pneumothorax in 703 patients, demonstrating an incidence of 2%. Most of these were asymptomatic. The potential for significant pneumothorax or bronchopleural fistula occurs in patients with adhesions or bullae or in patients on positive pressure ventilation. Tension pneumothorax has been reported and attributed to a loss of resistance technique.[76]

In a series of 21 patients, an interpleural catheter was placed under general anesthesia before thoracotomy. When the catheters were viewed after thoracotomy, 10 catheters were misplaced (seven were within the lung parenchyma). There were eight cases of lung damage, and three pneumothoraces (two tension). Thus, the authors concluded that interpleural catheterization can be dangerous.[76]

Additional complications mentioned in the literature include local anesthetic toxicity,[77] unilateral Horner's syndrome,[78] and phrenic nerve blockade.[79]

Contraindications to interpleural blockade include preexisting pleural effusions or hemothorax, because the fluid will make diffusion of the local anesthetic unpredictable and diminish the efficacy of the block. Infection at the insertion site or within the pleural cavity is an absolute contraindication to this technique. Finally, in any patient with a chest tube connected to continuous suction, the full dose of local anesthetic will not be administered. In fact, one study found that up to 30%–40% of an administered dose of bupivacaine was found in the thoracostomy drainage.[80]

All things considered, it seems unreasonable to expose patients to these aforementioned risks when other, often more effective means of anesthesia and analgesia are available.

## Conclusion

Paravertebral, intercostal nerve blocks and interpleural analgesia can all provide short- or long-term anesthesia and analgesia in a unilateral, dermatomal distribution in the thoracic and abdominal regions. When performed correctly, all can provide good results. However, each technique has specific circumstances under which it should and should not be performed. Careful attention to every technical detail is mandatory. One should also be fully cognizant of the side effects and complications of each procedure. Good planning and careful attention to all technical details will aid in the successful performance of these techniques and at the same time minimize complications.

## References


1. Concha M, Dagnino J, Cariaga M, Aguilera J, Aparicio R, Guerrero M. Analgesia after thoracotomy: epidural fentanyl/bupivacaine compared with intercostals nerve block plus intravenous morphine. J Cardiothorac Vasc Anesth 2004;18(3):322–326.
2. Taylor R, Massey S, Stuart-Smith K. Postoperative analgesia in video-assisted thoracoscopy: the role of intercostal blockade. J Cardiothorac Vasc Anesth 2004;18(3):317–321.
3. Karmakar MK, Critchley LAH, Ho AM-H, Gin T, Lee TW, Yim APC. Continuous thoracic paravertebral infusion of bupivacaine for pain management in patients with multiple fractured ribs. Chest 2003;123:424–431.
4. Karmakar MK, Ho AM-H. Acute pain management of patients with multiple fractured ribs. J Trauma 2003;54:615–625.
5. Osinowo OA, Zahrani M, Softah A. Effect of intercostal nerve block with 0.5% bupivacaine on peak expiratory flow rate and arterial oxygen saturation in rib fractures. J Trauma 2004;56:345–347.
6. Gilbert J, Hultman J. Thoracic paravertebral block: a method of pain control. Acta Anaesthesiol Scand 1989;33:142–145.
7. Johnson LR, Rocco AG, Ferrante FM. Continuous subpleural-paravertebral block in acute thoracic herpes zoster. Anesth Analg 1988;67:1105–1108.
8. Kairaluoma PM, Bachmann MS, Korpinen AK, Rosenberg PH, Pere PJ. Single-injection paravertebral block before general anesthesia enhances analgesia after breast cancer surgery with and without associated lymph node biopsy. Anesth Analg 2004;99(6): 1837–1843.
9. Naja MZ, Ziade MF, Lonnqvist PA. Nerve-stimulator guided paravertebral blockade vs. general anaesthesia for breast surgery: a prospective randomized trial. Eur J Anaesthesiol 2003;20(11):897–903.
10. Koorn R, Tenhundfeld-Fear KM, Miller C, Boezaart A. The use of cervical paravertebral block as the sole anesthetic for shoulder surgery in a morbid patient: a case report. Reg Anesth Pain Med 2004;29(3):227–229.
11. Boezaart AP, de Beer JF, Nell M. Early experience with continuous cervical paravertebral block using a stimulating catheter. Reg Anesth Pain Med 2003;28(5):406–413.
12. Naja MZ, Ziade MF, Lonnqvist PA. General anaesthesia combined with bilateral paravertebral blockade (T5-6) vs. general anaesthesia for laparoscopic cholecystectomy: a prospective, randomized clinical trial. Eur J Anaesthesiol 2004;21(6):489–495.
13. Weltz CR, Klein SM, Arbo JE, Greengrass RA. Paravertebral block anesthesia for inguinal hernia repair. World J Surg 2003;27(4):425–429.
14. Ho AM-H, Karmakar MK, Cheung M, Lam GCS. Right thoracic paravertebral analgesia for hepatectomy. Br J Anaesth 2004;93(3):458–461.
15. Matthews PJ, Govenden V. Comparison of continuous paravertebral and extradural infusions of bupivacaine for pain relief after thoracotomy. Br J Anaesth 1989;62:204–205.
16. Tenicela R, Pollan SB. Paravertebral-peridural block technique: a unilateral thoracic block. Clin J Pain 1990;6(3):227–234.
17. Engberg G. Relief of postoperative pain with intercostal blockade compared with the use of narcotic drugs. Acta Anaesthesiol Scand 1978;suppl 70:36–38.
18. Engberg G. Respiratory performance after upper abdominal surgery. A comparison of pain relief with intercostal blocks and centrally acting analgesics. Acta Anaesthesiol Scand 1985;29:427–433.
19. Purcell-Jones G, Pither CE, Justins DM. Paravertebral somatic nerve block: a clinical, radiographic, and computed tomographic study in chronic pain patients. Anesth Analg 1989;68:32–39.
20. Conacher ID, Kokri M. Postoperative paravertebral blocks for thoracic surgery. A radiological appraisal. Br J Anaesth 1987;59:155–161.
21. Mowbray A, Wong KKS, Murray JM. Intercostal catheterization: an alternative approach to the paravertebral space. Anaesthesia 1987;42:958–961.

22. Cheema S, Richardson J, McGurgan P. Factors affecting the spread of bupivacaine in the adult thoracic paravertebral space. Anaesthesia 2003;58:684–711.
23. Conacher ID. Resin injection of thoracic paravertebral spaces. Br J Anaesth 1988;61: 657–661.
24. Naja MZ, Ziade MF, El Rajab M, El Tayara K, Lonnqvist PA. Varying anatomical injection points within the thoracic paravertebral space: effect on spread of solution and nerve blockade. Anaesthesia 2004;59:459–463.
25. Asato F, Goto F. Radiographic findings of unilateral epidural block. Anesth Analg 1996;3:519–522.
26. Wooley EJ, Vandam LD. Neurological sequelae of brachial plexus nerve block. Ann Surg 1959;149(1):53.
27. Moore DC. Regional Block: A Handbook for Use in the Clinical Practice of Medicine and Surgery. 4th ed. Springfield, IL: Charles C Thomas; 1965:200.
28. Shaw WM. Medial approach for paravertebral somatic nerve block. JAMA 1952;148(9): 742–744.
29. Eason MJ, Wyatt R. Paravertebral thoracic block – a reappraisal. Anaesthesia 1979;34: 638–642.
30. Naja Z, Lonnqvist PA. Somatic paravertebral nerve blockade: incidence of failed block and complications. Anaesthesia 2001;56:1184–1188.
31. Garutti I, Hervias M, Barrio JM, Fortea F, de la Torre J. Subdural spread of local anesthetic agent following thoracic paravertebral block and cannulation. Anesthesiology 2003;98(4):1005–1007.
32. Sharrick NE. Postural headache following thoracic somatic paravertebral nerve block. Anesthesiology 1980;52:360–362.
33. Selander D, Shuner K-G, Lundborg G. Peripheral nerve injury due to injection needles used for regional anesthesia. Acta Anaesthesiol Scand 1977;21:182–188.
34. Moore DC, Hain RF, Ward A, Bridenbaugh DL. Importance of the perineural spaces in nerve blocking. JAMA 1954;156(1):1050–1054.
35. Selander D, Sjostrand J. Longitudinal spread of intraneurally injected local anesthetics: an experimental study of the initial neural distribution following intraneural injections. Acta Anaesthesiol Scand 1978;22:622–634.
36. Angerer AL, Su Hu, Head JR. Death following the use of Efocaine: report of a case. JAMA 1954;153(4):329–330.
37. Brittingham TE, Berlin LN, Wolff HG. Nervous system damage following paravertebral block with Efocaine: report of three cases. JAMA 1953;154(4):608–609.
38. Shapiro SK, Norman DD. Neurologic complications following the use of Efocaine. JAMA 1953;152(7):608–609.
39. Jurgens PE. A study of Efocaine. Anesthesiology 1955;16:615, 622.
40. McKnight CK, Marshall M. Monoplatythela and paravertebral block. Anaesthesia 1984; 39:1147.
41. Finucane BT, Terblanche OC. Prolonged duration of anesthesia in a patient with multiple sclerosis following paravertebral block. Can J Anaesth 2005;52(5):493–497.
42. Debreceni G, Molnar Z, Szelig L, Molnar TF. Continuous epidural or intercostal analgesia following thoracotomy: a prospective randomized double-blind clinical trial. Acta Anaesthesiol Scand 2003;47:1091–1095.
43. Roviaro GC, Varoli F, Fascianella A, et al. Intrathoracic intercostal nerve block with phenol in open chest surgery: a randomized study with statistical evaluation of respiratory parameters. Chest 1986;90(1):64–67.
44. Maiwand MO, Makey AR, Rees A. Cryoanalgesia after thoracotomy: improvement of technique and review of 600 cases. J Thorac Cardiovasc Surg 1986;92:291–295.
45. Tucker GT, Moore DC, Bridenbaugh PO, Bridenbaugh LD, Thompson GE. Systemic absorption of mepivacaine in commonly used regional block procedures. Anesthesiology 1972;37:277.
46. Nunn JL, Slavin G. Posterior intercostal nerve block for pain relief after cholecystectomy: anatomical basis and efficacy. Br J Anaesth 1980;52:253–259.
47. O'Kelly E, Garry B. Continuous pain relief for multiple fractured ribs. Br J Anaesth 1981; 53:989–991.
48. Sabanathan S, Beckford-Smith PJ, Pradhan GN, et al. Continuous intercostal nerve block for pain relief after thoracotomy. Ann Thorac Surg 1988;46:425–426.

49. Sabanathan S, Mearns AJ, Beckford-Smith PJ, et al. Efficacy of continuous extrapleural nerve block on post-thoracotomy pain. Br J Surg 1990;77:221–225.
50. Moore DC, Bridenbaugh DL. Intercostal nerve block in 4333 patients. Anesth Analg 1962;41(1):1–11.
51. Moore DC, Bridenbaugh DL. Pneumothorax: its incidence following intercostal nerve block. JAMA 1962;182:1005–1008.
52. Moore DC. Intercostal nerve block for postoperative somatic pain following surgery of thorax and upper abdomen. Br J Anaesth 1975;47:284–286.
53. Nielsen CH. Bleeding after intercostal nerve block in a patient anticoagulated with heparin. Anesthesiology 1989;71:162–164.
54. Cory PC, Mulroy MF. Postoperative respiratory failure following intercostal block. Anesthesiology 1981;54:418–419.
55. Casey WF. Respiratory failure following intercostal nerve blockade. Anaesthesia 1984;39:351–354.
56. Gallo JA Jr, Lebowitz PW, Battit GE, Bruner JMR. Complications of intercostal nerve blocks performed under direct vision during thoracotomy: a report of two cases. J Thorac Cardiovasc Surg 1983;86(4):628–630.
57. Gauntlett IS. Total spinal anesthesia following intercostal nerve block. Anesthesiology 1986;65(1):82–84.
58. Berrisford RG, Sabanathan SS. Direct access to the paravertebral space at thoracotomy. Ann Thorac Surg 1990;49:854.
59. Friesen D, Robinson RH. Total spinal anesthesia – a complication of intercostal nerve block. Kans Med 1987;88(3):84–85.
60. Atkinson GL, Shupak RC. Acute bronchospasm complicating intercostal nerve block. Anesth Analg 1989;68:400–401.
61. Reiestad F, Stromskag KE. Interpleural catheter in the management of postoperative pain. A preliminary report. Reg Anaesth 1986;11:89–91.
62. El-Naggar MA. Bilateral intrapleural regional analgesia for postoperative pain control: a dose-finding study. J Cardiothorac Anesth 1989;3(5):574–579.
63. Reiestad F, McIlvaine WB, Kvalheim L, et al. Interpleural analgesia in treatment of upper extremity reflex sympathetic dystrophy. Anesth Analg 1989;69:671–673.
64. Reiestad F, McIlvaine WB, Kvalheim L, et al. Successful treatment of chronic pancreatitis with interpleural analgesia. Can J Anaesth 1989;36(6):713–716.
65. Durrani Z, Winnie AP, Ikuta P. Interpleural catheter analgesia for pancreatic pain. Anesth Analg 1988;67:479–481.
66. Blake DW, Donnan G, Novella J. Interpleural administration of bupivacaine after cholecystectomy: a comparison with intercostal nerve block. Anaesth Intensive Care 1989;17:269–274.
67. Bachmann-Mennenga B, Boscoping J, Kuhn DFM, et al. Intercostal nerve block, interpleural analgesia, thoracic epidural block or systemic opioid application for pain relief after thoracotomy? Eur J Cardiothorac Surg 1993;7:12–18.
68. Mehta Y, Swaminathan M, Mishra Y, Trehan N. A comparative evaluation of intrapleural and thoracic epidural analgesia for postoperative pain relief after minimally invasive direct coronary artery bypass surgery. J Cardiothorac Vasc Anesth 1998;12(2):162–165.
69. Ben-David B. The falling column: a new technique for interpleural catheter placement. Anesth Analg 1990;71:212.
70. Squier RC, Morrow JS, Roman R. Hanging drop technique for intrapleural analgesia. Anesthesiology 1989;70:882.
71. Brismar B, Pettersson N, Tokics L, et al. Postoperative analgesia with intrapleural administration of bupivacaine-adrenaline. Acta Anaesthesiol Scand 1987;31:515–517.
72. El-Naggar MA, Schaberg FJ Jr, Phillips MR. Intrapleural regional analgesia for pain management in cholecystectomy. Arch Surg 1989;124:568–570.
73. Riegler FX, VadeBoncouer TR, Pelligrino DA. Interpleural anesthetics in the dog: differential somatic neural blockade. Anesthesiology 1989;71:744–750.
74. Stromskag KE, Hauge O, Steen PA. Distribution of local anesthetics injected into the interpleural space, studied by computerized tomography. Acta Anaesthesiol Scand 1990;34:323–326.
75. Stromskag KE, Minor B, Steen PA. Side effects and complications related to interpleural analgesia: an update. Acta Anaesthesiol Scand 1990;34:473–477.

76. Symreng T, Gomez MN, Johnson B, et al. Intrapleural bupivacaine – technical considerations and intraoperative use. J Cardiothorac Anesth 1989;3(2):139–143.
77. El-Naggar MA, Bennet B, Raad C, Yogartnam G. Bilateral intrapleural intercostal nerve block. Anesth Analg 1988;67:S57.
78. Parkinson SK, Mueller JB, Rich TJ, Little WL. Unilateral Horner's syndrome associated with interpleural catheter injection of local anesthetic. Anesth Analg 1989;68:61–62.
79. Lauder GT. Interpleural analgesia and phrenic nerve paralysis. Anaesthesia 1993;48:315–316.
80. Ferrante FM, Chan VW, Arthur R, Rocco AG. Interpleural analgesia after thoracotomy. Anesth Analg 1991;72:105–109.

# 8 Complications of Brachial Plexus Anesthesia

Brendan T. Finucane and Ban C.H. Tsui

In 1884, Carl Köller[1] discovered the local anesthetic properties of cocaine while working with Sigmund Freud. This was one of the most important discoveries in the history of medicine. In that very same year, Halsted[2] performed the first documented case of brachial plexus anesthesia at Johns Hopkins hospital when he injected the brachial plexus in the supraclavicular region under direct vision. The first percutaneous approach to the brachial plexus was performed by Hirschel[3] in 1911, when he injected local anesthetic drugs into the axillary sheath. In that same year, Kulenkampff[4] described the classic supraclavicular approach to the brachial plexus. Axillary approaches to the brachial plexus have always been more popular than supraclavicular techniques, perhaps because the risks seemed to be fewer.

More than 120 years have elapsed since brachial plexus anesthesia was first performed and since that time there have been numerous anecdotal reports of complications. In preparation for this update of the first edition, the author has searched the literature for the past 8 years, in an attempt to report the most common and most serious complications of brachial plexus anesthesia. Although it has only been 8 years since the first edition of this book was published, some interesting developments have taken place in the intervening period. One of the most important new developments has been the progression of new technology which will seriously impact how we practice regional anesthesia in the future. The debate about the use of nerve stimulation versus paresthesiae continued for almost 30 years. In today's practice, more than 90% of anesthesiologists use nerve stimulation. However, it did take a long time to convince the artisans of regional anesthesia that the application of nerve stimulation to regional anesthesia had something useful to offer. It seemed that there was some reluctance to abandon the art of regional anesthesia in favor of new technology. Nerve stimulation was the first step in the conversion of regional anesthesia from an art to a science.

One of the most exciting new advances in regional anesthesia in recent years has been the introduction of ultrasound. One of the first reports about the application of ultrasound in regional anesthesia was published in 1989 by Ting and Sivagnanratnam.[5] Since that time, there has been a growing number of reports in the world literature on this exciting application to regional anesthesia. It is only a matter of time before this technology will become mainstream in regional anesthesia. Brachial plexus anesthesia is one of the most challenging techniques in regional anesthesia and ultrasound has great potential to improve our success rate with this technique. When this happens, regional anesthesia will be a true science. The reason that the classic approach (supraclavicular) did not survive the test of time was that the potential for pneumothorax was an ever-present risk. The application of ultrasound in regional anesthesia may rejuvenate the classic approach to the brachial plexus, because with advances in this technology we will be better able to see the nerve trunks, the blood vessels, the pleura, and the approaching needle. For years we have been blindly inserting needles toward neural targets relying solely on our knowledge of anatomy. The introduction of nerve stimulation has been very helpful in that it provided some objective evidence that our needles were in the vicinity of the target nerve. With ultrasound, we can actually see the neural targets, the vascular structures, the advancing needle in real time, and the actual spread of local anesthetic solution following the injection. This is indeed enormous progress. By combining these two technologies, we can achieve very close to 100% success with these techniques provided we have sufficient time for the local anesthetic to work. There are at least two reports in the literature demonstrating the value of ultrasound techniques for supraclavicular blocks. Kopral et al.[6] demonstrated the safety and efficacy of ultrasound-guided supraclavicular blocks in 20 patients scheduled for upper extremity surgery. More recently, Williams et al.[7] performed ultrasound-guided supraclavicular blocks in 40 patients undergoing upper extremity surgery. They compared the ultrasound technique with nerve stimulation and showed that the ultrasound technique was performed successfully in half the time required to perform the nerve stimulation technique. None of the patients in the ultrasound group required general anesthesia to complete the surgery. We prefer to combine both technologies (ultrasound and nerve stimulation) when performing brachial plexus blocks. Ultrasound allows us to see the advancing needle approach the target nerve or trunk. Nerve stimulation allows one to identify which nerve we are approaching and if indeed it is a nerve. Ultrasound technology is indeed a great advance in regional anesthesia; however, we still have some difficulty accurately identifying structures and the advancing needle is not that easy to see in many cases. A number of regional anesthesia experts practicing ultrasound have already abandoned neurostimulation upon discovering the value of ultrasound. We are not quite ready to do that yet.

In this updated chapter, we will confine our discussion to single-injection, brachial plexus anesthesia in adults. Continuous techniques will be dealt with in Chapter 15.

## General Considerations

Not all patients are suitable candidates for brachial plexus anesthesia. Contraindications to regional anesthesia, regardless of technique, have already been alluded to in many chapters of this text. These include: patient refusal, excessive anxiety, mental illness, infection at the site of injection, clotting abnormalities, gross anatomic distortion, an uncooperative surgeon, an unskilled anesthesiologist, and an unfavorable environment.

Preoperative evaluation should be performed on all patients, preferably in advance of the scheduled surgery in elective cases. Patients should be fasting whenever possible, and brachial plexus anesthesia should not necessarily be chosen to avoid an obvious airway problem or full stomach.

Supraclavicular techniques should be avoided if possible in patients with advanced lung disease because of the risk of ipsilateral phrenic nerve paresis and pneumothorax. Brachial blocks, regardless of approach, should be used cautiously in patients with nerve injury, and, if selected in these circumstances, documentation of the neurologic deficits should be performed before the block.

Patients scheduled for brachial plexus anesthesia should be transported to the operating suite well in advance of the scheduled surgical procedure. Ideally, brachial blocks should be performed in a holding area, to allow ample time for the local anesthetic to work. Even under ideal circumstances, brachial blocks require at least 30 minutes setup time or "soak" time. The moment a patient enters the operating room, the momentum shifts in favor of performing surgery and few surgeons have the patience to wait for a block to work. The anesthesiologist should discuss the site of surgery with the surgeon in advance and select the most appropriate injection site for the procedure (e.g., interscalene for shoulder and upper arm surgery; axillary for elbow, forearm, and hand surgery).

The anesthesiologist should always be accompanied by an assistant when performing brachial plexus anesthesia, because when complications occur, a second pair of hands is essential. The minimal acceptable monitoring while performing brachial plexus anesthesia includes vital signs, electrocardiogram, and pulse oximetry (Chapter 1).

Brachial plexus anesthesia usually requires multiple injections of local anesthetics and most patients benefit from sedation. Sedation, when chosen, should be used judiciously and slowly. Combinations of opioids and benzodiazepines usually suffice. Profound sedation is undesirable because paresthesias may be difficult to discern, the risk of intraneural injection may be increased, and the adequacy of the intervention may be difficult to assess.

One must always be prepared to induce general anesthesia at a moment's notice while performing brachial plexus anesthesia. Therefore, all the necessary drugs and equipment required should be immediately at hand. It is very important to assess the adequacy of anesthesia before allowing the surgeon to proceed. Absence of pinprick sensation at the site of surgery does not automatically guarantee surgical anesthesia. The most practical way to assess the adequacy of surgical anesthesia is to ask the surgeon to apply the "Allis test" in the geographic area of the incision and then to objectively observe the patient's reaction. If the patient reacts adversely, one should intervene by asking the surgeon to refrain or to inject local anesthetic at the site of the incision. General anesthesia may be required in some cases. Inadequate surgical anesthesia during regional anesthesia has resulted in litigation.[8] Supplemental peripheral nerve blocks, if necessary, should be performed well in advance of the surgical incision, because they also take time to work.

One should never let one's ego stand in the way when a block is not working. This is not a time to question the patient's veracity. If a patient appears to be experiencing pain, do not hesitate to intervene immediately by asking the surgeon to stop operating. Then a decision should be made to infiltrate with local anesthesia or to induce general anesthesia: patient comfort should always be a priority.

There seems to be a subconscious tendency to decrease the level of vigilance over patients undergoing regional anesthesia. Patients undergoing regional anesthesia become hypoxic, hypercarbic, hypertensive, hypotensive, develop arrhythmias, aspirate, and even die; thus, the same degree of vigilance is required as for general anesthesia (Chapter 1).

## Complications Common to All Approaches to the Brachial Plexus

### *Local Anesthetic Toxicity*

Local anesthetic toxicity is a recognized complication of major conduction anesthesia. The incidence of toxicity is greater with brachial plexus techniques than most others, because larger than usual doses of local anesthetics are used and the injections are made in and around large vascular channels in the head, neck, and axillary regions. Toxicity occurs most frequently following accidental intravascular injections and rarely following absorption of injected solutions from peripheral sites (Chapter 6). Kozody et al.[9] demonstrated that seizures may occur when doses of bupivacaine as small as 2.5 mg are directly injected into the vertebral artery.

Epidemiologic information about the incidence of local anesthetic toxicity following regional anesthesia is quite sparse. The most up-to-date information comes from

TABLE 8-1. Overall Seizure Rates

| Anesthetic | Total no. of procedures | Total no. of seizures | Seizure rate/1000 procedures | 95% CI for seizure rate/1000 procedures* |
|---|---|---|---|---|
| Caudal† | 1,295 | 9 | 6.9 | 3.2–13.2 |
| Brachial‡ | 7,532 | 15 | 2.0 | 1.1–3.3 |
| Axillary | 6,620 | 8 | 1.2 | 0.5–2.4 |
| Interscalene | 659 | 5 | 7.6 | 2.5–17.7 |
| Supraclavicular | 253 | 2 | 7.9 | 1.0–28.6 |
| Epidural§ | 16,870 | 2 | 0.1 | 0.01–0.4 |

*95% CI calculated using Poisson approximation.
†Including only patients ≥18 years of age.
‡Brachial blocks can be further classified by type: axillary, interscalene, and supraclavicular. The total number of procedures for each type was projected using the 15 seizure procedures and a random sample of 300 nonseizure procedures.
§Excluding epidurals used only for postoperative analgesia.

Auroy et al.[10] who provided us with information on this topic from a large series of patients undergoing regional anesthesia in France. They reported 23 cases of seizures in 103,730 cases. The highest incidence of seizures was observed in patients undergoing peripheral nerve blocks [16/21,278 with a 95% confidence interval (CI) varying between 0.3–4.1]. Brown et al.[11] in the Mayo Clinic published a report focusing on the seizure rate following brachial plexus anesthesia and reported an incidence of 15 seizures in a series of 7532 cases. They also showed that the risk of seizures was at least six times greater with supraclavicular techniques (Table 8-1).

In a much smaller series, Plevak et al.[12] showed that the incidence of seizures following brachial plexus anesthesia was 1.4%.

Clinicians tend to base the dose of local anesthetic required for brachial plexus anesthesia on body weight. There is a poor correlation between weight and plasma levels of local anesthetics following brachial plexus anesthesia (Figure 8-1).[13] Furthermore, age does not seem to influence plasma levels of local anesthetics (Figure 8-2).[14] Winnie et al.[15] have suggested that height is a more useful guide on which to base dose. The size of the upper extremity is probably the most relevant parameter to use;

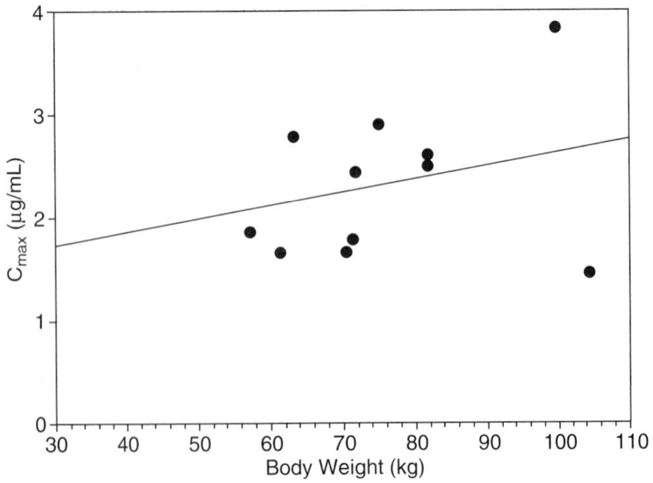


**FIGURE 8-1.** Correlation between maximum plasma concentration ($C_{max}$) after lidocaine 10 mg/kg and body weight.

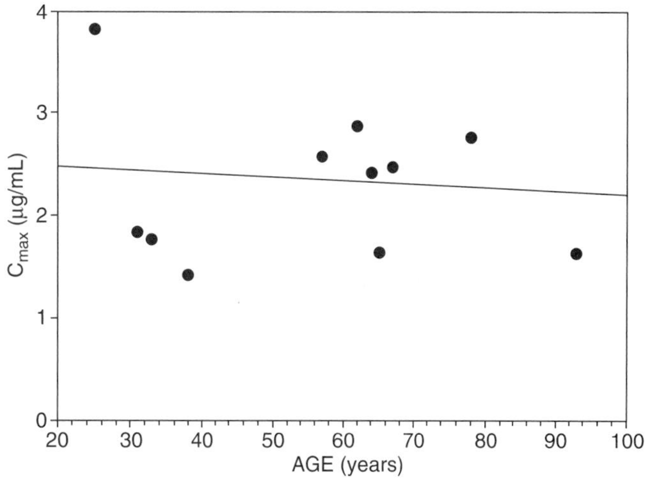


**FIGURE 8-2.** Correlation between $C_{max}$ and age after lidocaine.

however, it is practically difficult to determine the capacity of the sheath based on the limb size.

The maximum recommended, safe dose of lidocaine for regional anesthesia in adults is 300 mg using plain solutions and 500 mg for epinephrine-containing solutions.[16] In reality, much larger doses can be safely injected. This topic has been the source of considerable confusion for clinicians for years and the current recommendations about local anesthetic dosage do not have a scientific basis. Rosenberg et al.[17] addressed this topic thoroughly in a recent review. One of the most important factors influencing absorption of local anesthetics from the tissues is the site of injection (Figure 8-3).[18] Absorption of local anesthetics from the brachial plexus sheath is quite slow compared with absorption from the intercostal space. The addition of epinephrine also greatly influences absorption. Cockings et al.[19] showed that 750 mg of lidocaine can be safely administered in the axillary region in adults. Finucane and Yilling[20] showed that 750 mg of mepivacaine with epinephrine can be safely injected into the axillary region of adults (Figure 8-4). Urmey et al.[21] safely administered 800 mg of lidocaine with epinephrine into the interscalene groove. Pälve et al.[22] showed that 900 mg of lidocaine with epinephrine was safely administered to patients in the axillary region using the transarterial technique. Plasma levels of local anesthetics were well below those that usually cause symptoms or signs of toxicity in all of these reports. The largest dose of local anesthetic administered for brachial plexus blocks was reported by Büttner et al.[23] who administered approximately 5000 mg of mepivacaine to patients in a 24-hour period, during continuous axillary blocks. It should not surprise us that patients tolerate these large doses of local anesthetics, when one considers that cardiologists routinely administer 100-mg boluses of lidocaine followed by up to 250 mg per hour intravenously to patients to treat ventricular arrhythmias. Although there is no correlation between plasma level and the weight of patients following a given dose, it is wise to use milligrams/kilogram when dealing with patients who weigh 50 kg or less. The obvious question one must ask is why do we need to administer such large dose of local anesthetic drugs for brachial blocks? The reason is that brachial blocks have a very slow onset, especially when injected in the axillary region and when single-injection techniques are used. In summary, larger doses than those traditionally recommended can be safely administered for brachial plexus anesthesia. However, all injections of local anesthetic should be injected slowly and deliberately, with frequent aspirations and observation of the patient, and no more than 5 mL of the local anesthetic solution should be administered at any one time.

Caution must be exercised when injecting local anesthetics in patients with liver disease because the ability to metabolize local anesthetics is impaired. The $t_{1/2}$ alpha

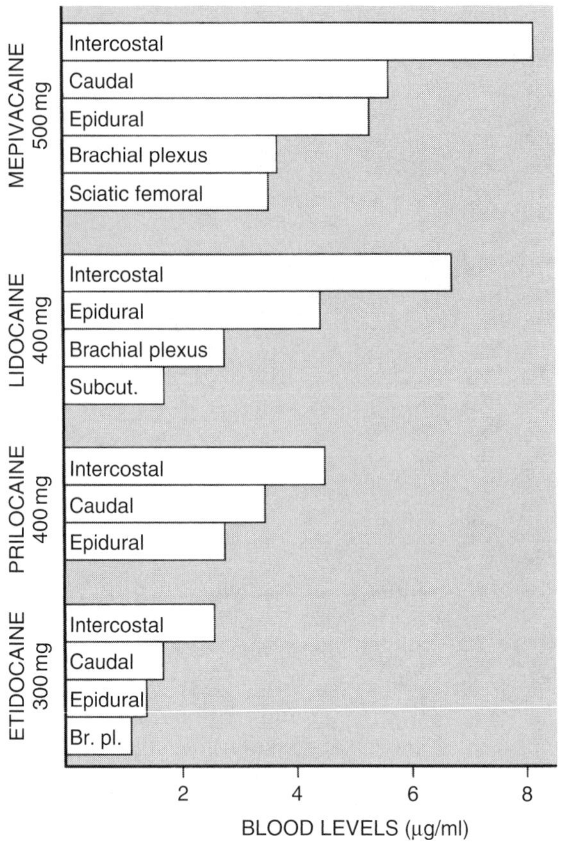


**FIGURE 8-3.** Comparative peak blood levels of several local anesthetic agents after administration into various anatomic sites. (Reprinted from Covino and Vassallo,[18] p 97. Copyright 1976, with permission from Elsevier.)

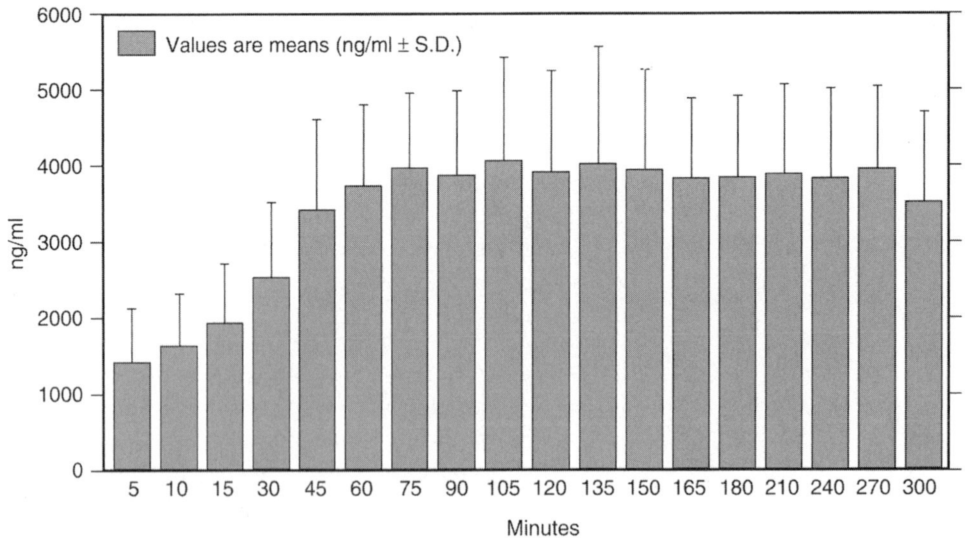


**FIGURE 8-4.** Mean plasma mepivacaine levels following axillary injection of mepivacaine with epinephrine 10.5 mg/kg over a 31-minute period. (From Finucane and Yilling.[20] Copyright 1989, with permission from Lippincott Williams & Wilkins.)

for lidocaine in healthy patients is 1.4 hours after an intravenous injection and increases to 7.3 hours in patients with active hepatitis.[24] Factors that interfere with hepatic blood flow may also influence metabolism of local anesthetics, e.g., age, cardiac failure, and drug therapy (cimetidine and propranolol).[24] The clearance of ropivacaine is reduced by 60% in patients with end-stage liver disease compared with healthy volunteers[25]; despite this, plasma concentrations remain within the normal range. This may be related to an increased volume of distribution at steady state. Alpha$_1$-acid glycoprotein (AAG) continues to be synthesized even in the presence of end-stage liver disease. Serious liver disease is often associated with altered renal and cardiac function, which may further impair the pharmacokinetic response of patients. Single-injection techniques, using recommended doses of local anesthetics, are safe in patients with hepatic dysfunction. However, if repeat injections of local anesthetics or continuous techniques are required, the dose of local anesthetics must by significantly reduced (10%–50%) because of a greatly reduced clearance of both the parent product and its metabolites.

Renal function is also an important factor influencing local anesthetic toxicity. The half-life of lidocaine and its primary metabolite, monoethylene glycine xylidine, is not influenced by renal failure. However, the secondary metabolite, glycine xylidine, is heavily dependent on renal function for excretion, and glycine xylidine causes central nervous system toxicity when it accumulates. Gould and Aldrete[26] performed brachial plexus anesthesia in a patient with chronic renal failure on five separate occasions using bupivacaine. They reported bupivacaine toxicity on two occasions out of five. The patient was acidotic and hyperkalemic on both of those occasions. The authors suggested that toxicity occurred because the quantity of free bupivacaine was increased in the presence of acidosis. Other investigators have shown that the concentration of AAG is increased in chronic renal failure and that binding of bupivacaine is increased, resulting in a lower concentration of free bupivacaine and a lower risk of toxicity. Tuominen et al.[27] measured AAG levels in patients with normal renal function following continuous brachial plexus block and showed that they were also increased. Uremic patients frequently have an increased cardiac output which enhances uptake of local anesthetics from the site of action.[28] Studies have shown a rapid uptake of ropivacaine and bupivacaine following brachial plexus anesthesia in uremic patients, and clearance of these compounds and their metabolites is also reduced.[29,30] The dose of local anesthetic should be reduced by 10%–20% in uremic patients even with single-injection techniques, especially when large doses of drugs are usually required. If repeat injections of local anesthetics are required (within 5 half-lives) or continuous techniques are being used, the dose should also be reduced by 10%–20%.

The pharmacokinetics of local anesthetics are also influenced at both extremes of age. However, we will confine our discussion in this chapter to the elderly. A number of changes take place in neural structures as we age. First, blood flow to neural tissue diminishes as we age because of a diminished cardiac output and a progressive decrease in blood flow to all tissues, secondary to arterial disease.[31] Furthermore, axonal function deteriorates and the amount of fat in neural tissue diminishes. There are also some changes in nerve morphology in the elderly[32,33]; consequently, elderly patients are more sensitive to the blocking effects of local anesthetics. The onset of action is faster, duration of neural blockade is prolonged, and clearance is increased. However, plasma levels of local anesthetics, after a single injection, are not increased.[34] For these reasons, the usual doses of local anesthetics are not required in the elderly. If repeat doses or continuous infusions are required, the dose should be reduced by 10%–20% in patients aged 70 years or older.

Occasionally, we are called upon to do a brachial plexus block on a patient who is pregnant. Because larger doses of local anesthetics are required for brachial plexus anesthesia, one should be familiar with the changes in sensitivity to local anesthetics in patients who are pregnant. Progesterone sensitizes the axon to local anesthetics during pregnancy.[35] The uptake of local anesthetics is increased because of increased cardiac output during late pregnancy.[36] Patients who are pregnant have a reduced degree of protein binding to the longer-acting local anesthetics; therefore, there is more free drug available in the plasma.[37] For all of these reasons, pregnant patients seem to be at greater risk of cardiac toxic effects of the longer-acting local anesthetics. Local anesthetics should be used cautiously during pregnancy. The dose of local anesthetic should be curtailed if possible, even with single-injection techniques. Avoid long-acting agents if large quantities of local anesthetic are required. Epinephrine can be safely added to local anesthetics during pregnancy.[38]

Ropivacaine is the first enantiomerically pure, local anesthetic to be synthesized and was recently approved for clinical use in many countries worldwide. Ropivacaine is similar to bupivacaine in many ways and is less toxic in animals.[39] Ropivacaine has been compared with bupivacaine for brachial plexus anesthesia in double-blind studies and there were no major differences noted.[40] If a long-acting local anesthetic is required, and if large doses or infusions of local anesthetic are being used, it would make good sense to use ropivacaine, because it is less toxic and more rapidly cleared from the circulation.[41]

Ropivacaine has been available for use in regional anesthesia for about 10 years and as expected there have been some sporadic reports of systemic toxic reactions associated with its use. Ropivacaine is not necessarily enhanced by the addition of epinephrine, therefore it is not usually added to this local anesthetic. Ropivacaine is a potent local anesthetic and the addition of epinephrine to it may alert one to the possibility of an unintentional, intravascular injection. Toxic reactions to ropivacaine seem to be no different from those to most local anesthetics and cardiac toxic reactions seem to be easier to treat than those to bupivacaine.[42] Müller et al.[43] reported a grand mal seizure after an accidental intravascular injection of 20 mL of ropivacaine 0.5%. The patient did not exhibit any signs of cardiac toxicity and was readily treated using standard guidelines. Epinephrine was not added to the solution.

In summary, the risk of local anesthesia toxicity is increased following brachial plexus anesthesia and especially following supraclavicular injections. Most toxic reactions result from accidental intravascular injections and can be avoided by slow deliberate injections, of no more than 5 mL of local anesthetic at any one time, with frequent aspirations and careful observation of patients. Epinephrine is a very useful marker for early detection of accidental intravascular injections and is strongly recommended, especially when using potent local anesthetics. Doses much larger than those recommended can be safely administered into the brachial plexus sheath, provided reasonable precautions are taken.

### *Nerve Injury Following Brachial Plexus Anesthesia*

Nerve injury following brachial plexus anesthesia has been a recognized complication since the early days of the technique (Chapter 7).

Kulenkampff[44] advised that in order to avoid injury to the brachial plexus "that ideally only a very fine needle should be used." In 1954, Bonica,[45] another master of these techniques, made the following statement about nerve injuries: "While it is true that promiscuous, repeated and rough probing of the nerves may cause neurologic sequelae, gently touching the nerve with the needle point does not cause any clinically apparent damage. . . ."

Even after 120 or more years of experience with brachial plexus techniques, we still do not have a good handle on either the incidence of these injuries or, indeed, the mechanism. In a recent report from the Closed Claims Study in the United States, there were 670 claims for nerve injury of a total of 4183 claims.[46] Nerve injuries were the second most frequent injury reported in the Closed Claims Study, accounting for 16% of all injuries going to litigation. Ulnar nerve injury was the most frequent nerve injury following anesthesia and, ironically, the incidence of ulnar nerve injury was far higher following general than regional anesthesia (85%).

Recent data on the incidence of nerve injury following brachial plexus anesthesia are sparse. Auroy et al.[10] published the largest prospective study on nerve injury related to regional anesthesia in recent years. The incidence of serious nerve injury related to peripheral nerve block was quite low. There were only four serious peripheral nerve injuries in a total of 21,278 cases. Two-thirds of the patients who reported serious nerve injuries experienced either paresthesias or pain on injection during the procedure. Plevak et al.[12] reported an incidence of 2.2% in a series of 716 cases and Selander et al.[47] reported an incidence of 1.9% in a series of 533 cases. Löfström and Sjöstrand[48] reviewed the literature on this topic going back to 1949 and showed that the incidence of brachial plexus injury was higher following supraclavicular techniques, and their explanation for this was that the "paresthesia method" was the sole method of verifying accurate needle placement with supraclavicular techniques, whereas paresthesias were not required to verify accurate needle placement in the axillary region. The authors' suggestion that the paresthesia method may be injurious to nerves sparked considerable controversy, especially among proponents of the paresthesia method, and this topic is still the subject of many debates and the controversy will continue. Moore,[49] who is a well-known master of regional anesthesia techniques, takes credit for the phrase "no paresthesia, no anesthesia," and has inspired many generations of anesthesiologists to adhere to this dictum. In reality, it is very difficult to prove that the act of deliberately seeking a paresthesia is injurious to nerves. Intuitively, it makes sense that if one encroaches upon a nerve with a cutting needle, the risk of damage increases. The prospective study by Selander et al.[47] failed to demonstrate scientifically that there was an increased incidence of injury following the use of paresthesias. Selander et al.[50] also suggested that the bevel configuration of the needle used influences the incidence and degree of trauma to nerves in both intact and isolated nerve preparations. They demonstrated that sharp-cutting needles are far more injurious to nerves than blunt needles. Rice and McMahon,[51] more than a decade later, challenged Selander et al.'s conclusions, and although they demonstrated a lower overall incidence of nerve trauma after using blunt-beveled needles, they did show that when injuries occurred secondary to blunt-beveled needles, the damage was more serious. This matter is discussed in much greater detail in Chapter 7. We should strive to use the smallest-gauge needle possible when performing local anesthesia techniques, especially when targeting specific nerves. Excessive pressures generated during injections can cause serious damage regardless of the bevel configuration, and we cannot ignore observations in Auroy's study that paresthesias and pain on injection are harbingers of injury to peripheral nerves. This explains the rationale for avoiding regional anesthesia in anesthetized patients.

Fortunately, most injuries attributable to needle damage cause self-limiting neuropraxias, which resolve in 1–3 months. Serious permanent injuries are rare. One must not assume that all neurologic injuries following regional anesthesia are directly attributable to the anesthetic management. Most serious neurologic injuries are unrelated to anesthetic interventions. Patients occasionally present with covert neurologic injury which only becomes evident in the postoperative period. Nerves are sometimes injured at surgery either accidentally or even deliberately. Improperly applied tourniquets may cause nerve injuries. The incidence of "tourniquet paralysis" has been reported to be as high as 1:8000 procedures.[52] Ideally, the tourniquet pressure should never exceed 150 mm Hg above that of the usual systolic blood pressure and the tourniquet should be deflated within 90–120 minutes if possible. Hidou et al.[53] reported a case of serious tourniquet-related injury after the application of a tourniquet for upper limb surgery for 45 minutes, in a healthy patient. Malposition of the limb during surgery or after surgery may also cause injury. Brachial neuritis[54] is a rare condition that may lead to diagnostic confusion when it occurs in the postoperative period following a brachial block. It is usually preceded by severe pain and is followed by weakness and atrophy of shoulder muscles. Sensory disturbances occur in two-thirds of the cases. The incidence is about 1:100,000. Most cases are preceded by a flu-like illness.

Overall recovery may take up to 2 years. It is most important to take a full history and perform a thorough neurologic examination and request relevant consultation when dealing with nerve injuries. One of the lessons learned from the Closed Claims Study in the United States is that even though appropriate standards of care are met while performing regional anesthesia, plaintiffs' lawyers are very successful in swaying juries to find fault with physicians (Chapter 23). Anesthesia care was judged to be appropriate in 66% of nerve injury cases in the Closed Claims Study.[46]

Forearm and hand surgery is frequently performed on an ambulatory basis. When brachial plexus blocks are performed in these patients, they should be warned about unknowingly injuring the anesthetized limb (e.g., resting the anesthetized limb against a heated radiator or over the back of a chair). They should also be specifically warned about lying on the anesthetized extremity. Ideally, patients should be given written instructions about the inherent dangers of injuring an anesthetized limb following anesthesia and surgery.

Brachial plexus anesthesia should be used with caution in patients with known neurologic damage, especially when the neurologic disease is ongoing.

Löfström and Sjöstrand[48] have shown that deliberate intraneural injection of local anesthetics results in a high incidence of neuropraxia and the injury is not solely the result of needle trauma. Considerable damage may also result from the pressure generated during the injection.

Local anesthetic drugs may also be toxic to nerves. Selander et al.[55] demonstrated in an in vitro study that the incidence of nerve damage increased when epinephrine was added to local anesthetics and the incidence was also influenced by the concentration of the local anesthetic used, especially if the blood/nerve barrier was damaged. This observation has not been demonstrated in clinical practice. Topical application of local anesthetic drugs to nerves (in vitro) does not cause injury, but intrafascicular injection does.

Patients who sustain nerve injuries usually do not develop symptoms immediately and the problem usually becomes evident during the first week postoperatively.

The controversy surrounding the use of paresthesias will continue. There is no proof that deliberate elicitation of paresthesias results in nerve injury. Intuitively, it makes sense to avoid contact with nerves, especially if reliable alternative methods to achieve successful anesthesia exist. If patients experience severe pain on injection, one should stop immediately and reposition the needle. Avoid brachial blocks in comatose patients or in those who cannot communicate. Be very selective about using regional anesthesia in patients with existing neurologic injury or in those in whom neurologic disease is suspected. Avoid concentrated local anesthetics (lidocaine >1.5%). Avoid long needles, and Kulenkampff's[44] advice back in 1928 that, ". . . ideally only a very fine needle should be used" is as good today as it was more than 75 years ago.

For a more complete discussion on peripheral nerve injury following regional anesthesia, refer to Chapter 7.

### *Failure of Brachial Plexus Anesthesia*

Of all the regional techniques routinely performed, the highest incidence of failure occurs following brachial plexus anesthesia. Failure rates for spinal or epidural anesthesia, in experienced hands, are usually no more than 5%–10%. However, it is not unusual to report failure rates between 20% and 30% with brachial plexus anesthesia. Table 8-2 includes success rates from several series of axillary blocks going back more than 25 years. Although not well documented, it seems that success rates are higher with supraclavicular approaches.

Why are failure rates so high with brachial blocks? There are a number of reasons. Most regional techniques require only a single injection. Single injections of local anesthetic work very well in the supraclavicular region where the nerve trunks are very closely clustered together. In contrast to this, a single injection of local anesthetic

TABLE 8-2. Success Rates with Axillary Brachial Blocks

| Author | Year | No. | % |
|---|---|---|---|
| Selander[56] | 1977 | 137 | 80 |
| Vester-Anderson et al.[57] | 1984 | 240 | 91 |
| Goldberg et al.[58] | 1987 | 59 | 76 |
| Cockings et al.[19] | 1987 | 100 | 99 |
| Baranowski and Pitheer[59] | 1990 | 100 | 70 |
| Stan[60] | 1995 | 1000 | 89 |

into the axilla results in a very slow onset of anesthesia because the nerves are quite separate from one another and perhaps the axillary sheath offers some impediment to uptake by the nerves. It may take up to an hour for the local anesthetic to reach all four major nerves of the upper extremity and may not reach the musculocutaneous nerve at all because that nerve lies outside the axillary sheath in the axilla. We now have the tools to allow us, with much greater certainty, to inject local anesthetic drugs within the sheath. Therefore, we will see fewer and fewer failures attributed to inaccurate placement of local anesthetics. To achieve a rapid onset axillary block, we need to block each individual nerve. Even when local anesthetic drugs are accurately placed, we are limited by the latency of the local anesthetic.

Over the years, a number of different methods have been used to enhance onset of local anesthetics. One of the simplest ways to enhance onset of action of local anesthetics is to increase the quantity of local anesthetic; however, in doing so, we also increase the risk of toxicity and other complications. If we study the intrinsic properties of local anesthetics, we observe that local anesthetic drugs with a low $pK_a$ and a high lipid solubility have a more rapid onset of action.[18] Etidocaine possesses both of these properties and, therefore, is associated with a very rapid onset of action.

Alkalinization of local anesthetics has been less convincing when used for brachial plexus anesthesia[61–63]; furthermore, there are some disadvantages and risks, e.g., cost, contamination, and the potential for error in preparation.

Carbonation has also been tested with equally equivocal results.[64] Hyaluronidase convincingly enhances onset of retrobulbar blocks, but these positive results have not been seen with brachial blocks.[65,66] Compounding local anesthetics has not added much more benefit than would be achieved by increasing the milligram dose of one or other local anesthetic. One study showed quite a dramatic effect on onset by heating the local anesthetic to 37°C.[67] The onset of action was reduced by about 55% in the major nerves. Cooling local anesthetics[68] has also been recommended and seems to work quite well. However, patients complain of considerable discomfort when cold solutions are injected perineurally (personal communication, B. Tsui, 2005).

Lavoie et al.[69] have shown that the incidence of success is proportional to the number of nerves blocked (using nerve stimulation). One of the most important strategies to use is to selectively block those nerves that provide sensory innervation within the boundaries of the skin incision.

Partridge et al.[70] have provided a very useful diagram showing the distribution of major nerve trunks around the axillary artery (Figure 8-5). From this diagram, one can see that the radial nerve is consistently posterior to the axillary artery, right in the epicenter of the axillary sheath. This favorable position of the radial artery may explain why Stan et al.[60] reported such a high success rate with the transarterial approach. The median nerve is positioned superoposteriorly, and the ulnar nerve inferoanteriorly in most subjects. Therefore, if the intended skin incision encroached on the nerve endings of the median and ulnar nerves, one would selectively block both of these nerves first and, subsequently, block the radial and or musculocutaneous nerve.

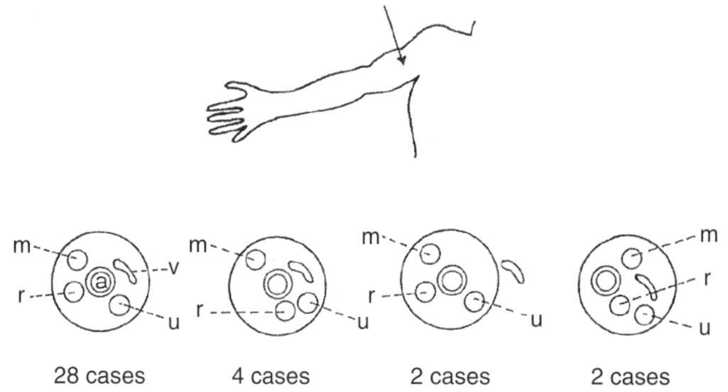


**FIGURE 8-5.** Variable anatomy of the axillary sheath. Displayed are drawings of the most common arrangements of components of the neurovascular bundle in 36 dissections from 18 cadavers. Cross-sections were taken at the point labeled with an arrow. Approximate positions of the median (m), radial (r), and ulnar (u) nerves are shown relative to the axillary artery (a) and vein (v). (From Partridge et al.[70] Copyright 1987, with permission from Lippincott Williams & Wilkins.)

The musculocutaneous nerve seems to be quite difficult to block in the axillary region. If the musculocutaneous nerve is the primary target nerve, one may selectively block this nerve high in the axilla, or attempt to block it by injecting directly into the coracobrachialis muscle. Alternatively, Yamamoto et al.[71] have shown a high incidence of musculocutaneous nerve block when the median nerve is the primary target.

The ulnar nerve occasionally eludes the spread of local anesthetic following an interscalene injection. This problem can be circumvented by selectively blocking the ulnar nerve in the axilla as well. This modification of technique is referred to as the axis block.[72]

Single-injection techniques seem to work well in the supraclavicular region but not so in the axillary region, especially if there are time constraints.

Multiple-injection techniques can be achieved using the paresthesia method, nerve stimulation, transarterial method, and just plain infiltration in and around the axillary artery. The multiple-injection technique can be a problem if one relies on nerve stimulation because it is sometimes difficult to elicit a motor response when performing the second or third injection, because the local anesthetic has already spread to adjoining nerves. Bouaziz et al.[73] described a midhumeral approach to the brachial plexus that allows one to readily stimulate all four major nerves, which are widely separated in the midhumeral region.

In summary, brachial plexus anesthesia is associated with a high failure rate. The reasons for failure include: failure to enter the sheath, an inadequate volume and/or milligram dose of local anesthetic, failure to inject the local anesthetic close to the nerve, and perhaps most importantly, an inadequate amount of "soak time." It is generally agreed that the main limiting factor mitigating against success is time. A number of strategies are recommended, including organizational changes, enhancement techniques, and technical approaches. Single-injection techniques seem to work well in the supraclavicular region and multiple-injection techniques are preferable in the axillary region. Finally, large doses and volumes of local anesthetics are recommended when single-injection techniques are used, especially in the axillary region. Application of some of these strategies should enhance success rates.

Sometimes we become so obsessed with the importance of success in many of life's pursuits, including regional anesthesia, that we lose sight of the most important issues. The paradigm shift from inpatient to ambulatory surgery has had an enormous impact on the practice of regional anesthesia. The emphasis on "turnover" and "throughput," the short exposure we have to discuss issues such as regional anesthesia with patients, has had a very negative impact on the practice of regional anesthesia and, especially, brachial plexus anesthesia. We have solved this problem in our institution by using ultrasound-guided supraclavicular brachial plexus blocks in combination with nerve stimulation. We use combinations of lidocaine 2% and bupivacaine 0.5%. We use combinations of remifentanil and propofol in large doses initially to facilitate surgery during the early phase while the local anesthetic is penetrating the neural targets. Using this approach, patients are ready for surgery in 20 minutes. We complete five hand surgeries using supraclavicular blocks in a typical day using this approach.

### *Inadvertent Injection of the Wrong Solution*

Inadvertent injection of the wrong solution usually involves intravenous injections. Fortunately, the number of reports of accidental injections of the wrong solution into the brachial plexus sheath are few. Tuohy and MacEvilly[74] described a case in which thiopental was accidentally injected into the axillary sheath. Fifteen milliliters of 2.5% thiopental was injected, after which the patient complained of mild pain. The error was then discovered and an axillary block was performed using 40mL of lidocaine 1% with adrenaline. Forty milliliters of 0.9% NaCl was also injected into the axillary space to dilute the thiopental. A stellate ganglion block was also performed on the ipsilateral side using bupivacaine 0.25% 15mL. All regional blocks were successful; however, surgery was postponed. The patient had continuing pain in the axilla on recovery from the blocks, but there were no long-term sequelae.

Patterson and Scanlon[75] reported a case of an inadvertent injection of an antibiotic into the interscalene groove in an 18-year-old male patient. Ironically, the patient was admitted to hospital after traumatic amputation of the left thumb. An interscalene block was performed to improve blood flow and provide postoperative pain relief. A 20-gauge cannula was inserted into the interscalene groove to facilitate additional injections of local anesthetic. When the patient was on the ward, a house officer was called to administer flucloxacillin 500mg intravenously. He inadvertently injected the antibiotic into the interscalene groove. The patient complained of pain and tingling during the injection, and when the error was discovered, 20mL of 0.9% NaCl was mixed with 20mL of bupivacaine 0.25% and injected into the sheath to dilute any remaining antibiotic. There were no long-term sequelae reported. This error was made even though painstaking efforts were taken to prevent such a happening. These cases are sobering reminders that one can never be too careful when administering medications and the presence of a cannula does not automatically mean that the cannula is in a venous channel.

## Complications of Supraclavicular Techniques

The potential for serious complications following brachial plexus anesthesia seems to be greater with supraclavicular techniques. A review of the literature reveals that the number of anecdotal reports of complications is greater following supraclavicular techniques even though the axillary approach is used more frequently. The advent of ultrasound should greatly reduce the risk of pneumothorax and increase success rates with this technique.

### *Pneumothorax*

Pneumothorax has been a dreaded complication of supraclavicular techniques since Kulenkempff[4] first described the classic supraclavicular approach in 1911. The risk of pneumothorax has deterred many anesthesiologists from using the supraclavicular approach and is the most likely reason that axillary approaches are more popular. Any technique that requires the insertion of a needle in the direction of the lung carries with it the risk of pneumothorax. Tall, thin patients seem to be at greater risk and the risk is greater on the right side because the cupola of the lung is higher on the right side. Winnie[76] carefully studied the anatomy of the brachial plexus in the supraclavicular region in the 1970s and noted the intimate relationship the plexus had with the interscalene muscles. As a result of these observations, he popularized the interscalene approach to the brachial plexus. Pneumothorax may occur following the interscalene approach to the brachial plexus; however, the risk is lower than that following the classic supraclavicular approach. Through Winnie's enthusiastic teaching, there has been a renewed interest in supraclavicular techniques during the past 30 years. The true incidence of pneumothorax is difficult to determine and varies to some degree with the approach selected. Brand and Papper[77] reported an incidence of 6.1% in a large teaching hospital using the classic Kulenkampff technique. DeJong[78] found radiologic evidence of pneumothorax in 25% of patients following supraclavicular techniques. The incidence of symptomatic pneumothorax is much less than that. Ward[79] reported a 3% incidence of symptomatic pneumothorax following the interscalene technique. Hickey et al.[80] found no symptomatic pneumothoraces in 156 patients following the subclavian perivascular approach. The majority of upper extremity surgeries are now performed on ambulatory patients who are usually discharged home within a few hours of surgery.

When supraclavicular techniques are used in an ambulatory setting, patients should be warned about the risk of and appraised of the symptoms and signs of pneumothorax. Patients who develop chest pain, dyspnea, or cyanosis after discharge should be instructed to go to the nearest emergency room.

An episode of coughing or sudden inspiratory effort while performing the block may indicate that the pleura has been penetrated and the lung punctured. Symptoms and signs may not develop for hours and patients may not become symptomatic until a 20% pneumothorax is present. A chest tube is usually required when the degree of collapse is 25% or greater. General anesthesia may be required when brachial blocks fail. Positive pressure ventilation with $N_2O/O_2$ in the presence of a small pneumothorax may lead to tension pneumothorax with rapid deterioration in vital signs. Therefore, a high index of suspicion should always be present when general anesthesia is required after a failed supraclavicular block, and of course nitrous oxide should always be avoided in these cases.

Manara[81] described an unusual case of intrapleural injection of local anesthetic during attempted supraclavicular block. The patient developed anesthesia of the chest wall and eventually upper extremity anesthesia. The patient did not develop symptoms or signs of pneumothorax.

Brown et al.[82] described a new supraclavicular approach entitled the "Plumb-bob" technique (Figure 8-6). The following is a brief description of this technique:

> With the patient lying in the supine position, a mark is made on the skin at a point just above where the clavicular head of the sternomastoid meets the clavicle. A needle is inserted at this point in the parasagittal plane with the needle directed at right angles to the plane of the floor. The needle is redirected cephalad in repeated stages until paresthesiae are elicited or until an angle of 30° cephalad is reached. If paresthesiae are not found, the needle is redirected up to 30° in a caudal direction.

Using cadaver, magnetic resonance imaging data, and clinical application in more than 110 patients, Brown has convincingly demonstrated that the "Plumb-bob" method is safe (0% pneumothorax) and effective. Further experiences with this technique in larger numbers of patients will allow us to assess its true value in clinical practice.

In summary, a technique that requires the insertion of a needle in the supraclavicular region, directed toward the lung, carries with it the risk of pneumothorax. Patients should be warned in advance of this risk, and ambulatory patients should be given careful instructions on how to proceed should symptoms develop. Supraclavicular techniques should be used only when indicated. Axillary techniques satisfy the anesthesia demands of most upper extremity surgery, with the exception of the shoulder down to the midhumeral region.

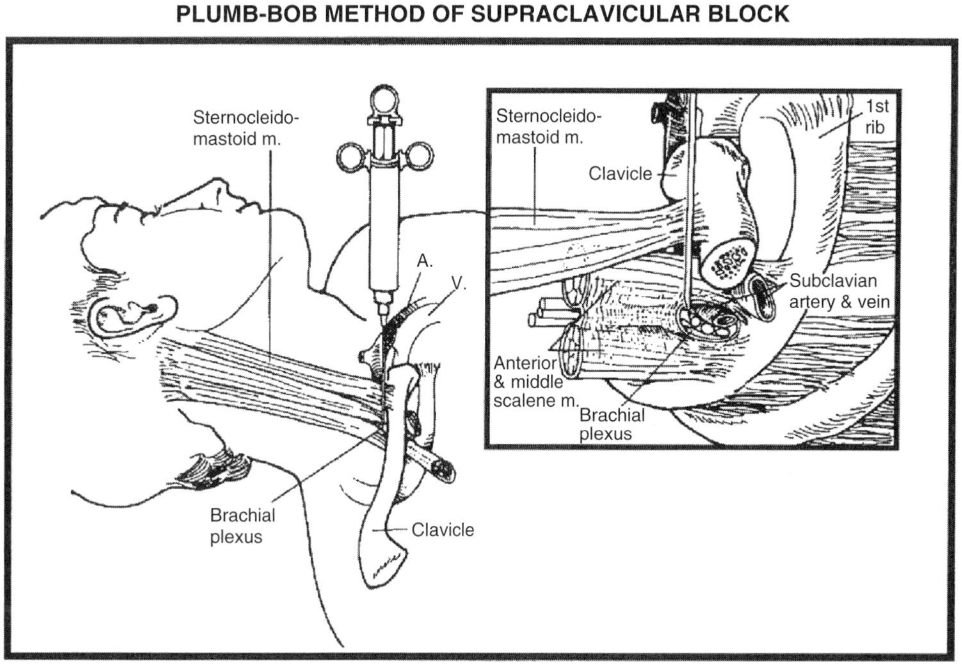


**FIGURE 8-6.** Plumb-bob technique. (From Brown et al.[82] Copyright 1993, with permission from Lippincott Williams & Wilkins.)

## *Phrenic Nerve Paresis*

Ipsilateral phrenic nerve paresis has been reported sporadically since Kulenkampff first described the supraclavicular technique.

In 1979, Knoblanche[83] demonstrated a 67% incidence of ipsilateral phrenic nerve paresis in a small series of patients using an image intensifier following interscalene block. X-rays were taken within 3 hours of supraclavicular brachial plexus block. Knoblanche concluded that the phrenic nerve was blocked peripherally.

In 1981, Farrar et al.[84] demonstrated that the incidence of ipsilateral phrenic nerve paresis varied between 36% and 40% regardless of the supraclavicular technique chosen. This was a retrospective study involving more than 368 cases. X-rays were taken preoperatively and 4 hours after injection of local anesthetic. Farrar et al. concluded that the phrenic nerve was being blocked at the root level as opposed to peripherally.

Urmey et al.[85] studied the incidence of ipsilateral hemidiaphragmatic paresis in 13 patients following interscalene block, using ultrasonography. Data were collected before the block was performed and at 2, 5, 10 minutes and then hourly until normal function was restored. They reported changes in the Sniff and Müller maneuvers within 5 minutes. They also showed that ipsilateral hemidiaphragmatic paralysis occurred in all patients and persisted for 5 hours. Urmey et al. also studied the effect of reducing the mass of local anesthetic on the incidence of phrenic nerve paresis and demonstrated that the incidence was still 100%.

Pere et al.[86] studied the effects of ipsilateral hemidiaphragmatic paralysis on respiratory function in a small series of patients following continuous interscalene block. They demonstrated that all patients had reduced forced vital capacity, forced expiratory volume, and peak expiratory flow. Urmey and McDonald[87] also studied pulmonary function and attempted to quantify the deficit in respiratory function. They corroborated Pere et al.'s findings and showed that forced vital capacity and forced expiratory volume decreased by 27% and 26%, respectively.

Fujimura et al.[88] also evaluated the effects of hemidiaphragmatic paralysis on respiratory function following interscalene block in a small series (10 patients). There were no major changes in pulmonary function studies; however, $Pa_{O_2}$ decreased significantly. The clinical significance of this decrease in $Pa_{O_2}$ was questionable.

We must reevaluate the use of supraclavicular techniques in certain groups of patients in light of this new information. Clearly, supraclavicular techniques should be avoided in patients with advanced pulmonary disease and bilateral supraclavicular techniques are absolutely contraindicated. However, there are anecdotal reports of patients, devoid of respiratory disease, who became symptomatic following interscalene block. Kayerker and Dick[89] described two such cases. The first case was a 42-year-old woman who presented for a right carpal tunnel release. She was healthy apart from mild diabetes. She became symptomatic following interscalene injection of 50mL of 0.375% bupivacaine. X-ray revealed marked elevation of the hemidiaphragm but no pneumothorax. The second patient was a 39-year-old woman with chronic renal failure scheduled for creation of an arteriovenous fistula. She was also a diabetic. She experienced respiratory difficulty following a similar dose of 0.375% bupivacaine. Neither of these patients required major intervention but were symptomatic for several hours. Hood and Knoblanche[90] also described a case of respiratory distress following a supraclavicular brachial plexus block. This patient also had renal failure and radiologic studies revealed ipsilateral hemidiaphragmatic paralysis and the case was postponed.

Ward[79] described two cases of dyspnea in young patients following interscalene block. Both had radiologic evidence of unilateral phrenic nerve block and were healthy patients aged 19 and 27. The symptoms abated when the block wore off. These two cases represent a 6% incidence of symptomatic phrenic nerve paresis in Ward's series. Rau et al.[91] published a report of significant dyspnea in an obese patient following an interscalene block.

There is, without question, a very high incidence of ipsilateral hemidiaphragmatic paralysis following supraclavicular brachial plexus block, which seems to be of no consequence in the vast majority of healthy patients. These techniques clearly should be avoided in patients with advanced lung disease. Ironically, these were the very cases in whom brachial plexus anesthesia was considered to be safest in the past. The interscalene approach requires the insertion of a needle diagonally toward the sixth cervical nerve root; therefore, one might expect a higher incidence of ipsilateral phrenic nerve paresis when using this technique. One cannot assume that the incidence of this complication is the same with all supraclavicular approaches. Neal et al.[92] studied the incidence of hemidiaphragmatic paresis and respiratory function following supraclavicular blocks in eight healthy volunteers and demonstrated that the overall incidence of paresis was 50% following 30mL of lidocaine 1.5% with epinephrine. None of these volunteers reported respiratory symptoms. However, until we have more data on this topic, it would be prudent to avoid all supraclavicular techniques in patients with moderate to severe impairment of lung function. There is also some suggestion that the volume and quantity of local anesthetic chosen for supraclavicular blocks may influence the incidence of hemidiaphragmatic paresis. Al-Kaisy et al.[93] performed interscalene blocks on 11 healthy volunteers using either 10mL of 0.25% or 0.5% bupivacaine. They observed pulmonary function in these volunteers for 90 minutes after the injection of bupivacaine and noted that respiratory function was significantly impaired in the volunteers who received the stronger concentration of bupivacaine. Most of us who perform interscalene blocks for shoulder surgery do so to provide good pain relief in the postoperative period. The duration of action of bupivacaine at any concentration will be significantly curtailed if only 10mL of solution is used. It would seem that few patients develop symptoms following unilateral hemidiaphragmatic paresis. However, we should inform patients that they may become symptomatic and, of course, it should not be necessary to say this, but bilateral interscalene blocks are never indicated.

In contrast to all of these reports demonstrating the potential negative impact of ipsilateral phrenic nerve paresis on respiratory function, Betts and Eggan[94] reported a case of unilateral pulmonary edema in a patient who had had an interscalene block for right-sided shoulder surgery. The patient had a combined regional/general technique and developed laryngeal spasm upon emergence. Unilateral pulmonary edema developed on the left side. Negative pressure developed on the left side and did not develop on the right side because diaphragmatic action was impaired on that side.

In summary, ipsilateral phrenic nerve paresis is quite common following all supraclavicular approaches to the brachial plexus. The majority of healthy patients do not experience any symptoms. The duration of action of this impairment depends on the dose and the individual properties of the local anesthetic used. Supraclavicular approaches to the brachial plexus should be avoided in patients with significant lung disease.

### *Neurologic Injury Following Supraclavicular Brachial Plexus Block*

Fortunately, serious neurologic injury following any approach to the brachial plexus is rare. Candido et al.[95] recently reported their experience with neurologic injury following interscalene blocks in a series of 693 patients for shoulder and upper arm surgery. Follow-up was performed in 660 of these patients in 4 weeks. Eighty patients reported neurologic symptoms during the 4-week follow-up period. Symptoms cleared up in 24 of these patients within 48 hours and these were not considered serious symptoms. Thirty-one of these neurologic deficits were linked with the interscalene blocks, including one brachial plexopathy. All the symptoms related to interscalene block resolved spontaneously within 4 weeks except the brachial plexopathy. Independent risk factors for neurologic sequelae related to interscalene block were paresthesias or pain or bruising at the needle insertion site within 24 hours. Surgery performed in the sitting position and bruising at the interscalene block insertion site were considered to be risk factors not related to interscalene block.

Further review of the literature revealed a small number of case reports of neurologic injury following supraclavicular techniques. Barutell et al.[96] described a motor deficit in the distribution of C7, C8, T1 following interscalene brachial plexus block. While performing the block, the patient experienced a sharp paresthesia and marked pain on injection. This warning sign was not heeded, and following an injection of 8 mL of local anesthetic, the patient became hoarse and lost consciousness and required intubation. The patient recovered about 1 hour later and the following day had paralysis of the extensor and flexor muscles of her fingers. Subsequent electromyogram revealed total denervation of C8 and T1, with no improvement 2 months later. The authors concluded that the neurologic deficit was caused by needle damage to the roots of C8 and T1. An 8.8-cm needle was used and the clinician failed to heed the warning sign of severe pain on injection. Lim and Pereira[97] described a case of brachial plexus injury following supraclavicular block. It was difficult to determine the etiology of injury in this case. Electromyogram studies revealed that the injury was likely the result of focal demyelination at the level of the cords. The patient recovered after about 8 weeks. A multidose vial of lidocaine 1% combined with 0.1% W/V chlorocresol preservative was used in this case. The patient did experience a paresthesia during the procedure but no major discomfort during injection. The deficit experienced by this patient was predominantly motor. The authors concluded that the deficit was likely attributable to needle or injection trauma.

Bashein et al.[98] described a case of persistent phrenic nerve paresis following interscalene block. Within 30 minutes of a 50-mL injection of bupivacaine 0.5% with epinephrine into the interscalene groove, the patient developed a generalized seizure and subsequently presented with ipsilateral phrenic nerve paresis which did not improve with time. The authors concluded that this injury was likely attributable to needle trauma of the phrenic nerve peripherally. There has been at least one additional report of a case of phrenic nerve paralysis in recent years. Robaux et al.[99] described a case of persistent phrenic nerve paresis following an uneventful interscalene block. The patient was a 60-year-old man in good general health presenting for shoulder surgery. A Stimuplex HNS 11, short-beveled needle (B. Braun) was used. The phrenic nerve was transiently stimulated during attempts at performing the block. A combination of ropivacaine 0.75% and clonidine was used. The patient recovered uneventfully initially but returned to the hospital 10 days later with shortness of breath. The chest X-ray showed a marked elevation of the hemidiaphragm consistent with paresis of the phrenic nerve. The patient had significant respiratory dysfunction a year later. Electromyography revealed absence of compound action potentials, suggesting that the phrenic nerve was completely interrupted or extensively demyelinated. Although the precise mechanism of injury could not be elucidated on the basis of electromyography, the authors concluded that needle trauma was the likely cause of this injury.

Passannante[100] reported a case of spinal anesthesia and permanent neurologic deficit in a 53-year-old patient following interscalene block for shoulder surgery. The block was performed using a 3-inch insulated needle and the patient was anesthetized when the block was performed. The mechanism of injury is speculative but likely the result of intraneural injection of local anesthetic at the root level. Finally, Winnie et al.[15] described an anecdotal report of a patient who developed a Brown-Séquard syndrome following attempted interscalene block with a spinal needle.

Brockway et al.[101] described a case of prolonged anesthesia following a supraclavicular brachial plexus block. Thirty milliliters of bupivacaine 0.42% was injected using nerve stimulator. The patient did not experience paresthesiae or pain on injection. Full function was restored in 40 hours. It is difficult to explain why the block was so protracted. The likely reason for this protracted block was unusually accurate placement of the local anesthetic.

In summary, permanent neurologic injury is rare following supraclavicular techniques. Lessons to be learned from the cases described above should be heeded:

1. Avoid needles that are more than 1–1/2 inches long.
2. Persistent pain on injection infers intraneural injection and should be a signal to discontinue the injection.
3. Avoid brachial plexus anesthesia in unconscious patients because of their inability to report paresthesias or pain on injection.
4. Avoid high concentrations of local anesthetics.
5. Avoid excessive injection pressures.

### *Central Neural Blockade Following Supraclavicular Techniques*

Central neural blockade may occur following routine supraclavicular brachial plexus anesthesia. Fortunately, this complication is rare. Winnie et al.[15] suggested three possible mechanisms for this complication. First, the local anesthetic may be directly deposited in the subarachnoid, epidural, or subdural space by advancing a needle toward the central neuraxis. Anatomists have demonstrated that the dural cuff may extend as far as 8cm beyond the intervertebral foramen. Therefore, it is possible to puncture the dura during a supraclavicular block. Finally, intraneural injection of local anesthetics peripherally move in a retrograde manner and reach the spinal cord and subarachnoid space. Shanta[102] has demonstrated that the epineurium is an extension of the dura and the perineurium an extension of the pia. Rapid onset of spinal anesthesia following attempted supraclavicular block is likely attributable to dural puncture. Slower onset of spinal anesthesia may be explained by retrograde spread of local anesthetics into the substance of the spinal cord, or subperineurial spread. Central neural blockade, although rare, is more likely to occur following interscalene injection of local anesthetics.

Kumar et al.[103] described two cases of epidural block following the interscalene approach to the brachial plexus in 1971. This was one of the first reports of this complication since Winnie's description of the interscalene approach. Dyspnea developed in both patients after about 20 minutes, probably because of bilateral phrenic nerve paresis.

Both patients required assisted ventilation for a period of time and recovered fully within 4 hours. The authors were of the opinion that this complication was likely due to an epidural injection because of the slow onset and maintenance of consciousness.

In 1973, Ross and Scarborough[104] described a case of total spinal anesthesia following an interscalene block in a 16-year-old boy. A 2-inch needle was used. Following a 30-mL injection of local anesthetic, the patient became unconscious and the classic signs of total spinal anesthesia were noted (apnea, papillary dilation, absent corneal reflexes, and hypotension). The patient recovered fully in 2 hours without sequelae. The most likely explanation for this complication was subarachnoid injection of the local anesthetic.

In 1976, Edde and Deutsch[105] described a case of total spinal anesthesia following an interscalene block. Immediately after the needle was withdrawn from the interscalene groove, the patient had a cardiopulmonary arrest with electrocardiogram evidence of ventricular fibrillation. Following resuscitation, it was noted that he had all the signs of total spinal anesthesia. The patient recovered fully without sequelae. The authors used a 6-cm needle and ruled that the most likely cause of the cardiac arrest was total spinal anesthesia.

McGlade[106] described a case of total spinal anesthesia in a 17-year-old male following an interscalene block using 28 mL of lidocaine 1.5% with epinephrine. The patient rapidly became apneic and developed other signs of total spinal anesthesia; however, he rapidly regained his ability to breathe, suggesting the possibility of a subdural injection.

Baraka et al.[107] described a case of total spinal anesthesia following the parascalene approach to the brachial plexus. This patient experienced agonizing pain during the injection, and after 5 mL of local anesthetic was injected, the needle was repositioned. The patient became apneic, hypotensive, and rapidly lost consciousness and had complete relaxation of the masseter muscles and vocal cords. The authors attributed these symptoms to an intraneural injection of local anesthetic with central spread to the subarachnoid space.

Dutton and Eckhardt[108] report a case of total spinal anesthesia in a 30-year-old patient following an interscalene block. A 2.5-cm, short-beveled, 22-gauge needle was used. A total of 40 mL of a mixture of bupivacaine 0.5% and lidocaine 2% was used. The patient moved suddenly after a significant portion of the local anesthetic was injected and the remainder of the injection was completed. The patient rapidly became apneic and unresponsive and was immediately intubated. The cardiovascular system remained relatively stable during this episode. Spontaneous breathing resumed in 2 hours following with the patient was extubated but reintubation was required because of further respiratory embarrassment. The patient recovered soon thereafter without permanent sequelae.

The symptoms and signs reported in this case were very typical of those occurring following a subarachnoid injection. It is likely that the needle entered the subarachnoid space when the patient moved suddenly.

Norris et al.[109] reported a case of delayed onset spinal anesthesia following interscalene brachial plexus blockade. These authors did not provide details about the length of needle used for the block but did mention that forearm paresthesias were obtained at a depth of 2 cm. They then proceeded to slowly inject 30 mL of a mixture of bupivacaine 0.5% and carbonated lidocaine 2%. During the initial injection, they reported a paresthesia in the contralateral arm which they attributed to cycling of the blood pressure cuff. A dense block of the upper extremity ensued. A surgical incision over the radial head was performed 12 minutes after the injection. Upon completion of surgery 50 minutes later, the patient moved herself onto the stretcher. Sixty-five minutes after the initial injection, the patient experienced weakness in the contralateral arm and had difficulty moving her head. Examination at that time revealed a dense bilateral motor and sensory block extending from C2 to T4. Her vital signs were stable and she had no difficulty breathing. The block gradually extended to the lumbar region after 110 minutes. The block regressed to the cervicothoracic dermatomes after 4 hours and 20 minutes, during which time the patient was completely stable. The patient was admitted for observation overnight and was discharged the following morning. She was readmitted 40 hours later because of a severe postdural puncture headache. She was discharged 3 days later and had no further sequelae. It is quite difficult to explain what happened in this case. The contralateral paresthesia observed at the initial injection obviously was significant in retrospect, but if indeed the needle was in the subarachnoid space, the subsequent injection of the 30mL of local anesthetic would have resulted in a total spinal. Perhaps the needle was repositioned after the initial paresthesia was reported and only a very small quantity of local was injected into the subarachnoid space. Patients are usually quite heavily sedated during regional anesthesia and therefore the extent of the block may not have been fully observed until the patient was asked to move upon completion of the procedure.

Majid et al.[110] reported a case of total spinal anesthesia following a posterior approach to the brachial plexus. They used a 100-mm, 21-gauge Stimuplex, short-beveled needle (B. Braun). Following an injection of 18mL of 0.5 % bupivacaine, the patient developed a rapid, flaccid paralysis of all extremities and became apneic yet remained conscious and he had a moderate decrease in blood pressure (80/40mmHg). The patient was anesthetized and the procedure was completed. Following a 2-hour procedure, the patient awoke and was able to breathe spontaneously. This was another example of an excessively long needle being used. It is likely that the needle deviated toward the central neuraxis, and judging by the rapidity of the symptoms and signs, the needle must have entered the subarachnoid space.

There have been several other cases of bilateral cervical and thoracic anesthesia following interscalene block that do not fit the typical description of epidural injections. Some of these cases present only with sensory anesthesia, others with varying degrees of motor and sensory anesthesia. The most likely explanation for these atypical cases is seepage of local anesthetic into the epidural space following interscalene block.

Anesthesiologists performing this technique should be aware of the potential for subarachnoid, subdural, epidural, intraneural, or intravascular injection. The length of the needle used for interscalene block should not usually exceed 3.8cm (1.5 inches) and the needle should never be introduced perpendicularly toward the central neuraxis. Difficult injection and persistent painful ipsilateral or contralateral paresthesiae may indicate that the needle is in the central neuraxis, and if there is any doubt about needle placement it should be repositioned before injecting local anesthetic. Both the volume and concentration of local anesthetics may influence the incidence of this complication. Volumes of local anesthetic in excess of 30mL have been used in most cases of abnormal spread following interscalene block. Interscalene blocks are in effect paravertebral blocks and we are aware that spread into the adjoining epidural space occurs in 80% of cases. Concentrations of local anesthetic greater than 1.5% lidocaine or its equivalent should also be avoided. Finally, interscalene blocks and indeed all brachial blocks should be avoided in unconscious patients, if possible.

Upon reading a series of case reports of central neural spread of local anesthetics following attempted interscalene block, one may get the impression that this is a common occurrence. The senior author of the chapter has not observed one case of total spinal anesthesia following an interscalene block in 35 years of practice in teaching hospitals; therefore, this is not a common occurrence. However, one must always be prepared to deal with this emergency should it occur.

### *Horner's Syndrome*

Horner's syndrome is a common accompaniment of all supraclavicular approaches to the brachial plexus. It is difficult to label it as a complication because it is quite harmless other than causing unilateral nasal stuffiness. Uninformed enthusiastic clinicians may diagnose "red eye" in patients following supraclavicular block. Occasionally, patients with blunt head trauma present with upper extremity injuries. Regional anesthesia is often a good option in these patients. Horner's syndrome may present some diagnostic dilemmas in some of these cases; therefore, supraclavicular techniques should be avoided for this reason.[111] The incidence of Horner's syndrome varies considerably (18.5%–98%)[80] and is no indication of the success or failure of a block. Patients should be informed of this side effect because it is associated with some temporary distortion of the facies.

Sukhani et al.[112] reported a case of persistent Horner's syndrome following an interscalene block. The patient was a middle-aged woman who was concerned about the distortion in her appearance, especially the ptosis, and requested treatment. The patient was initially treated with neosynephrine drops which proved unsatisfactory and surgery was recommended. The patient declined surgery and her condition improved with time. Fortunately, this is a rare complication.

### *Recurrent Laryngeal Nerve Palsy*

Hoarseness is an occasional complication of interscalene and subclavian perivascular techniques, and is most likely caused by ipsilateral recurrent laryngeal nerve block. Ward[79] reported an incidence of 3% and Ramamurthy[80] an incidence of 1.5%. This complication is usually of little consequence other than an annoyance to patients, but again is a reminder to avoid bilateral interscalene blocks.

Rollins et al.[113] reported an unusual case of airway obstruction following a subclavian perivascular block. The patient was a 71-year-old woman with squamous cell carcinoma of the tongue presenting for a right-sided open reduction and internal fixation of a fractured humerus. She had had a previous neck dissection and partial glossectomy on the left side. She had a difficult airway for other reasons also. The plan was to perform a subclavian perivascular block followed by a fiberoptic-assisted intubation. The patient developed respiratory difficulties shortly after the block was performed. It was subsequently noted that the patient had left vocal cord paresis before the performance of the block. The likely cause of the airway difficulty was a right-sided recurrent laryngeal nerve block which in addition to a left-sided recurrent laryngeal paresis led to complete airway obstruction. Plit et al.[114] reported a very similar case in which an elderly patient presented for shoulder arthroplasty. She had had a thyroidectomy 35 years previously for carcinoma. The patient developed hoarseness and respiratory obstruction following an interscalene block and subsequently required a tracheostomy. These two cases illustrate the danger of supraclavicular blocks in patients who have had major neck surgery in the past.

### *Bronchospasm*

There have been some isolated cases of bronchospasm following interscalene block. The mechanism is not well understood. Thiagarajah et al.[115] suggested that blockade of the sympathetics to the bronchi may cause bronchospasm because of unopposed action of the parasympathetics. However, this explanation Shah and Hirschman[116] pointed out that the lungs are sparsely innervated by sympathetic nerves and if bronchospasm was caused by this mechanism, unilateral bronchospasm would occur. Bronchospasm occurs occasionally following spinal and epidural anesthesia also, and although the mechanism of bronchospasm is not well understood, one should be aware of this complication in patients who have asthma.

### *Other Complications of Supraclavicular Techniques*

Hematoma formation occasionally occurs following supraclavicular techniques and is usually of no consequence. Ramamurthy[80] reported a 22% incidence of subclavian puncture and a recognizable hematoma in 1.4% of cases. Ward[79] reported a 3%

incidence in a series of 34 cases and Brand and Papper[77] reported a 1.2% incidence in a series of 230 cases.

Durrani and Winnie[117] reported a case of "locked in syndrome" following a probable intraarterial injection of local anesthetic following an interscalene block.

Mani et al.[118] reported an unusual case of bleeding and hemopneumothorax in a patient who was heparinized following an otherwise uneventful subclavian perivascular block.

Siler et al.[119] reported an unusual case of carotid bruit following an interscalene block which dissipated within a few hours of the block. It was suggested that injection of the local anesthetic encroached upon the lumen of the carotid artery during performance of the block. There were no permanent sequelae.

### *Auditory Impairment Associated with Interscalene Block*

Rosenberg et al.[120] described a case of ipsilateral deafness in a 24-year-old patient during continuous interscalene block. Rosenberg subsequently performed audiometry on 20 patients following interscalene block. Three patients reported hearing impairment on the day of surgery which was restored the following day. Sympathetic blockade may have been implicated, although patients in the series with Horner's syndrome did not have hearing impairment.

In summary, the risk of complications following supraclavicular approaches to the brachial plexus is clearly not rare. The majority of these complications have a direct impact on pulmonary function. For this reason, supraclavicular techniques should be avoided in patients with significant impairment of pulmonary function. The risk of central neural blockade seems to be higher following the interscalene approach. Long, large-gauge needles should be avoided. Volumes of local anesthetic should not exceed 40mL and concentrations greater than 1.5% lidocaine or its equivalent should be avoided. The needle should be repositioned if significant pain is experienced on injection, and for this reason, these techniques should be avoided in comatose patients.

## Complications Following the Axillary Approach to the Brachial Plexus

The axillary approach to the brachial plexus continues to be the most popular technique selected by anesthesiologists for forearm and hand surgery. Axillary blocks are also very effective for elbow surgery,[121] but this fact was only recently realized. The main reasons that the axillary approach is so popular are that it is easy to perform, easy to teach, and the risk of complications is lower than the supraclavicular approach. However, the axillary approach is not devoid of complications. In common with supraclavicular techniques, local anesthetic toxicity, nerve injury, and failure are the most common complications. There are also some very specific complications unique to the axillary approach.

### *Vascular Complications*

The axillary artery is the main landmark used by anesthesiologists to identify the nerves of the axillary plexus and, as such, may be accidentally or deliberately penetrated. The transarterial approach to the axillary plexus is considered to be one of the most reliable methods with a very high success rate. The transarterial method is now accepted as a standard method of inducing successful axillary block. However, there are some risks associated with this technique. The technique requires penetration of the artery at two points; therefore, the risk of hematoma formation is real. There are a few anecdotal reports of loss of circulation to the upper extremity following the transarterial approach. The pulse usually returns when the sympathetic block sets in. Merrill et al.[122] described a similar case of temporary vascular insufficiency in

TABLE 8-3. Complications Following Transarterial Axillary Block

| Complication | No. | % | N |
|---|---|---|---|
| Vascular spasm | 10 | 1 | 1000 |
| Hematoma | 2 | 0.2 | 1000 |
| Systemic toxicity | 2 | 0.2 | 1000 |
| Persistent paresthesia | 2 | 0.2 | 1000 |

a 49-year-old patient undergoing hand surgery. The authors concluded that vasospasm was the most likely cause of the problem. The most up-to-date information about the transarterial approach comes from Stan et al.[60], who published their experience with this technique in 1000 consecutive cases. They reported a successful block in 88.8% of patients. Ten percent required supplementation and only 1.2 required general anesthesia. The incidence of complications was very low (Table 8-3). This is the largest published series of cases performed using the transarterial approach and offers strong support to the safety of this interesting approach to axillary blocks.

In 1984, Restelli et al.[123] described a more serious problem of insufficient venous drainage following a routine axillary block. The transarterial approach was not used in this case but instead the paresthesia method was used. The patient returned a month later with severe pain and swelling in the arm and hand. Surgical exploration of the axilla revealed an aneurysm of the axillary vein which was repaired with good results. This complication was most likely caused by subadventitial injection with subsequent hematoma and aneurysm of the vein wall.

Ott et al.[124] described a serious case of vascular insufficiency following a routine axillary block. The patient was an obese 16-year-old who had an uneventful surgery, but returned 2 weeks later with vascular insufficiency and an 8-cm thrombus was removed from the axillary artery following arteriotomy. A saphenous vein graft was required to repair the artery. One should emphasize that the transarterial approach was not used in this case.

Radiologists perform percutaneous angiography using the axillary artery and have reported nerve injury following hematoma formation and they stressed the importance of prompt surgical exploration when neural deficits occur. This may not be much consolation to the anesthesiologist who must wait until motor and sensory function returns after a block.[125] It is likely that radiologists use much larger needles and multiple punctures, thus hematoma formation is more common. Despite the very high success rates and low complication rate reported with the transarterial approach, deliberate penetration of the axillary artery at two points is not without risk. However, serious complications have been reported in the absence of arterial violation. Blunt needles may be more damaging to blood vessels than sharp ones. Perhaps the best advice is to use fine-caliber needles whenever possible.

## Conclusion

This is an attempt to provide a comprehensive review of complications following brachial plexus anesthesia reported during the past 30 years or so. Although the overall incidence of complications following brachial plexus anesthesia is low, the proportion of complications following supraclavicular methods is much higher than that reported following axillary blocks; e.g., the incidence of seizure activity following interscalene or subclavian perivascular methods is at least six times that of the axillary approach.

Many of the complications of supraclavicular methods have an impact on pulmonary function; therefore, supraclavicular methods should be avoided in patients with even moderate pulmonary dysfunction. In a sense, there should always be a clear-cut indication for selecting supraclavicular methods because of the risk of pulmonary complications. The incidence of neurologic complications is higher following supraclavicular approaches.

Most of the serious complications of brachial plexus anesthesia are avoidable. Local anesthetic drugs must be injected slowly and patients must be observed carefully for signs of local anesthetic toxicity. The addition of epinephrine to local anesthetics is a useful marker for detecting accidental intravascular injections.

Persistent pain on injection of local anesthetics is a clear warning of an intraneural injection. Large-gauge and long needles should be avoided and brachial blocks should be avoided in comatose patients.

Finally, brachial plexus anesthesia is not yet an exact science. Ultrasound-guided needle insertion is rapidly converting regional anesthesia from an art to a science. There has been renewed interest in regional anesthesia as a result of this great advance. Brachial plexus block has been a great challenge to anesthesiologists for more than 100 years. We can expect success rates close to 100% in the near future. However, complications will still occur. We must select patients carefully. We must seek informed consent. We must select the safest approach. We must use an appropriate dose of local anesthetic. We must minimize patient discomfort and we must know when to abandon our efforts when we are not being successful.

## References


1. Köller C. History of cocaine as a local anesthetic. JAMA 1941;117:1284–1285.
2. Halsted WS. Surgical papers. In: Burket WC, ed. 1st ed. Baltimore: Johns Hopkins Press; 1925.
3. Hirschel G. Anasthesierung des plexus brachialis bei operationen an der oberen extremitat. Muenchener Medizinische Wochenschrift 1911;58:1555–1556.
4. Kulenkampff D. Anesthesia of the brachial plexus [German]. Zentralb Chir 1911; 38:1337–1340.
5. Ting PL, Sivagnanratnam V. Ultrasonographic study of the spread of local anesthetic during axillary brachial plexus block. Br J Anaesth 1989;63:326–329.
6. Kopral S, Krafft P, Eibenberger K, et al. Ultrasound-guided supraclavicular approach for regional anesthesia of the brachial plexus. Anesth Analg 1994;78:503–507.
7. Williams SR, Chouinard P, Arcind G, et al. Ultrasound guidance speeds execution and improves quality of supraclavicular block. Anesth Analg 2003;97:1518–1523.
8. Kroll DA, Caplan RA, Posner K. Nerve injury associated with anaesthesia. Anaesthesiology 1990;73:202–207.
9. Kozody B, Ready LB, Barsa JE, et al. Dose requirement of local anaesthetic to produce grand mal seizure during stellate ganglion block. Can Anaesth Soc J 1982;29:489–491.
10. Auroy Y, Narchi P, Messiah A, et al. Serious complications related to regional anesthesia: results of a prospective survey in France. Anesthesiology 1997;87:479–486.
11. Brown DL, Ransom DM, Hall JA, et al. Regional anaesthesia and local anesthetic – induced systemic toxicity: seizure frequency and accompanying cardiovascular changes. Anesth Analg 1995;81:321–328.
12. Plevak DJ, Lindstromberg JW, Danielson DR. Paresthesia vs non-paresthesia – the axillary block [abstract]. Anaesthesiology 1983;59:A216.
13. Finucane BT, Zaman N, Kashkari I, et al. The dose of lidocaine selected for axillary blocks should not be based on body weight in adults [abstract]. Can J Anaesth 1998:A 47B.
14. Finucane BT, Zaman N, Tawfik S, et al. Influence of age on the uptake of lidocaine from the axillary space [abstract]. 4th American-Japanese Congress. San Francisco; 1997.
15. Winnie AP, Hakansson L, Buckhoj P. Plexus Anaesthesia Perivascular Techniques of Brachial Plexus Block. Philadelphia: WB Saunders; 1983.
16. Canadian Pharmaceutical Association. Compendium of Pharmaceuticals and Specialties CPS. 29th ed. Toronto; 1994.
17. Rosenberg PH, Veering PD, Urmey WF. Maximum recommended doses of local anesthetics: a multifactorial concept. Reg Anesth Pain Med 2004;29:564–575.

18. Covino BG, Vassallo HG. Local Anesthetics: Mechanisms of Action and Clinical Use. New York: Grune & Stratton; 1976.
19. Cockings E, Moore PL, Lewis RC. Transarterial brachial plexus blockade using high doses of 1.5% mepivacaine. Reg Anesth 1987;12:159–164.
20. Finucane BT, Yilling F. Safety of supplementing axillary brachial plexus blocks. Anesthesiology 1989;70:401–403.
21. Urmey WF, Stanton J, Sharrock NE. Interscalene block. Effects of dose volume and mepivacaine concentrations on anesthesia and plasma levels [abstract]. Reg Anesth 1994;19:34.
22. Pälve H, Kirvela O, Olin H, et al. Maximum recommended doses of lidocaine are not toxic. Br J Anaesth 1995;74:704–705.
23. Büttner J, Klose R, Argo A. Serum levels of mepivacaine – HC1 during continuous axillary plexus block: a prospective evaluation of 1,133 cases. Reg Anesth 1989;14:124–127.
24. Covino BG, Scott DB. Handbook of Epidural Anesthesia and Analgesia. New York: Grune & Stratton; 1985.
25. Jokinen M. Effects of drug interactions and liver disease on the pharmacokinetics of ropivacaine [PhD thesis]. University of Helsinki, Finland; 2003.
26. Gould DB, Aldrete JA. Bupivacaine cardiotoxicity in a patient with renal failure. Acta Anaesthesiol Scand 1983;27:18–21.
27. Tuominen M, Haasio J, Hekali R, et al. Continuous interscalene brachial plexus block. Clinical efficacy, technical problems and bupivacaine plasma concentration. Acta Anaesthesiol Scand 1989;33:84–88.
28. Norio K, Mäkisalo H, Isonemi H, et al. Are diabetic patients in danger at renal transplantation? An invasive perioperative study. Eur J Anaesthesiol 2000;17:729–736.
29. Pere P, Salonen M, Jokinen M, et al. Pharmacokinetics of ropivacaine in uremic and nonuremic patients after axillary brachial plexus block. Anesth Analg 2002;96:563–569.
30. Wald-Oboussier G, Viell B, Biscoping J, et al. Die Wirkung von Bupavacain-HCL nach Supraklavikulärer Plexusblockade bei Patienten mit chronis cher Niereninsuffizienz. Reg Anaesth 1988;11:65–70.
31. Bowdle TA, Freund PR, Slattery JT. Age-dependent lidocaine pharmacokinetics during lumbar peridural anesthesia with lidocaine hydrocarbonate and lidocaine hydrochloride. Reg Anaesth 1986;11:123–127.
32. Kurokawa K, Mimori Y, Tanaka E, et al. Age-related change in peripheral nerve conduction: compound action potential duration and dispersion. Gerontology 1999;45: 168–173.
33. Igarashi T, Hirabayashi Y, Shimizu R, et al. The lumbar extradural structure changes with increasing age. Br J Anaesth 1997;78:149–152.
34. Finucane BT, Hammonds WD, Welch MB. Influence of age on the vascular absorption of lidocaine from the epidural space. Anesth Analg 1987;66:843–846.
35. Butterworth JF, Walker FO, Lysak SZ. Pregnancy increases median nerve susceptibility to lidocaine. Anesthesiology 1990;72:962–965.
36. Pihlajamäki K, Kanto J, Lindberg R, et al. Extradural administration of bupivacaine: pharmacokinetics and metabolism in pregnant and non-pregnant women. Br J Anaesth 1990;64:556–562.
37. Santos AC, Pederson H, Harmon TW, et al. Does pregnancy alter the systemic toxicity of local anesthetics? Anesthesiology 1989;70:991–995.
38. Brownridge P, Cohen SE, Ward ME. Neural blockade for obstetric and gynecologic surgery. In: Cousins MJ, Bridenbough PO, eds. Neural Blockade in Clinical Anesthesia and Management of Pain. Philadelphia: Lippincott-Raven; 1988:557–604.
39. Markham A, Faulds D. Ropivacaine. A review of its pharmacology and therapeutic use in regional anaesthesia. Drugs 1996;52:429–438.
40. Hickey R, Hoffman J, Ramamurthy S. A comparison of ropivacaine 0.5% and bupivacaine 0.5% for brachial plexus block. Anesthesiology 1991;74:639–642.
41. Lee A, Fagan D, Lamont M, et al. Disposition kinetics of ropivacaine in humans. Anesth Analg 1989;69:736–739.
42. Finucane BT. Ropivacaine cardiac toxicity – not as troublesome as bupivacaine. Can J Anaesth 2005;52:449–453.
43. Müller M, Litz RJ, Hubler M, Albrecht DM. Grand mal convulsion and plasma concentrations after intravascular injection of ropivacaine for axillary brachial plexus blockade. Br J Anaesth 2001;87:784–787.

44. Kulenkampff D. Brachial plexus anaesthesia: its indications, techniques and dangers. Ann Surg 1928;87:883–888.
45. Bonica JJ. The Management of Pain. 2nd ed. Philadelphia: Lea & Fabinger; 1954.
46. Cheney FW, Domino KB, Caplan RA, et al. Nerve injury associated with anaesthesia: a closed claims analysis. Anesthesiology 1999;90:1062–1069.
47. Selander D, Edshage S, Wolff T. Paresthesia or no paresthesia. Acta Anaesthesiol Scand 1979;23:27–33.
48. Löfström JB, Sjöstrand U. Local Anesthesia and Regional Blockade. Amsterdam: Elsevier; 1988.
49. Moore DC. Regional Block. 4th ed. Springfield, IL: Charles C. Thomas; 1975.
50. Selander D, Dhuner KG, Lundsborg G. Peripheral nerve injury due to injection needles used for regional anaesthesia. Acta Anaesthesiol Scand 1977;21:182–188.
51. Rice ASC, McMahon SB. Peripheral nerve injury caused by injection needles used in regional anesthesia: influence of bevel configuration studied in a rat model. Br J Anaesth 1992;69:433–438.
52. Middleton RW, Varian JP. Tourniquet paralysis. Aust NZ J Surg 1974;44:124–128.
53. Hidou M, Huraux C, Viry-Babel F, et al. Pneumatic tourniquet paralysis: a differential diagnosis after loco-regional anesthesia of the upper limb. J Chir 1992;129:213–214.
54. Fibuch EE, Mertz J, Geller B. Postoperative onset of idiopathic brachial neuritis. Anesthesiology 1996;84:455–457.
55. Selander D, Brattsand R, Lungborg G, et al. Local anesthetics: importance of mode of application, concentration and adrenaline for the appearance of nerve lesions. Acta Anaesthesiol Scand 1979;23:127–136.
56. Selander D. Axillary plexus block, paresthetic or perivascular. Anesthesiology 1987; 66:726–728.
57. Vester-Andersen T, Husum B, Lindeburg T, Borrits L, Gothgen I. Perivascular axillary block IV: blockade following 40, 50 or 60ml of mepivacaine 1% with adrenaline. Acta Anaesthesiol Scand 1984;28:99–105.
58. Goldberg ME, Gregg C, Larijani GE, et al. A comparison of three methods of axillary approach to the brachial plexus block for upper extremity surgery. Anesthesiology 1987;66:814–816.
59. Baranowski AP, Pitheer CE. A comparison of three methods of axillary brachial plexus anaesthesia. Anaesthesia 1990;45:362–365.
60. Stan T, Krantz MA, Soloman DL, et al. The incidence of neurovascular complications following axillary brachial plexus block, using a transarterial approach. Reg Anesth 1995;20:486–492.
61. Difazio CA, Carron H, Grosslight KA, et al. Comparison of pH adjusted lidocaine solutions for epidural anesthesia. Anesth Analg 1986;65:760–763.
62. Hilgier M. Alkalinization of bupivacaine for brachial plexus block. Reg Anesth 1985;10:59–61.
63. Morison DH. Alkalinization of local anaesthetics. Can J Anaesth 1995;42:1076–1078.
64. McClure JH, Scott DB. Comparison of bupivacaine HCL and carbonated bupivacaine in brachial plexus block by the interscalene technique. Br J Anaesth 1981;53:523–526.
65. Keeler JF, Simpson JH, Ellis FR. Effect of addition of hyaluronidase to bupivacaine during axillary brachial plexus block. Br J Anaesth 1992;68:68–73.
66. Rosenquist RW, Berman S, Finucane BT. Hyaluronidase and axillary brachial plexus block: effect on latency and plasma levels of local anesthetics [abstract]. Reg Anesth 1989;14:50.
67. Heath PJ, Brownlee GS, Herrick MJ. Latency of brachial plexus block. Anaesthesia 1990;40:297–301.
68. Butterworth JF, Walker FO, Neal JM. Cooling potentiates lidocaine inhibition of median nerve sensory fibers. Anesth Analg 1990;70:507–511.
69. Lavoie J, Marlin R, Tetrault JP. Axillary plexus block using a peripheral nerve stimulator: single or multiple injections. Can J Anaesth 1992;39:583–587.
70. Partridge BL, Katz J, Beninschke K. Functional anatomy of the brachial plexus sheath: implications for anaesthesia. Anesthesiology 1987;66:743–747.
71. Yamamoto K, Tsubokawa T, Shibata K, Kobayashi T. Area of paresthesia as determinant of sensory block in axillary brachial plexus block. Reg Anesth 1995;20:493–497.
72. Urmey WF. Combined axillary–interscalene (axis) brachial plexus block for elbow surgery [abstract]. Reg Anesth 1993;18:88.

73. Bouaziz H, Narchi P, Mercier FJ, et al. Comparison between conventional axillary block and a new approach at mid-humeral level. Anesth Analg 1997;84:1058–1061.
74. Tuohy SA, MacEvilly MA. Inadvertent injection of thiopentone to brachial plexus sheath. Br J Anaesth 1982;54:355–357.
75. Patterson KW, Scanlon P. An unusual complication of brachial plexus sheath cannulation. Br J Anaesth 1990;65:542–543.
76. Winnie AP. Interscalene brachial plexus block. Current researches. Anesth Analg 1970;49:455–466.
77. Brand L, Papper EM. A comparison of supraclavicular and axillary techniques or brachial plexus blocks. Anesthesiology 1961;22:226–229.
78. DeJong RH. Local anesthetics: adverse effects. Springfield, IL: Charles C. Thomas; 1977:254.
79. Ward ME. Interscalene approach to brachial plexus. Anaesthesia 1974;29:147–157.
80. Hickey R, Garland TA, Ramamurthy S. Subclavian perivascular block: influence of location of paresthesia. Anesth Analg 1989;68:767–771. Reg Anesth 1983.
81. Manara AR. Brachial plexus block, unilateral thoraco-abdominal blockade following the supraclavicular approach. Anaesthesia 1987;42:757–759.
82. Brown LD, Cahill DR, Bridenbaugh LD. Supraclavicular nerve block: anatomic analysis of a method to prevent pneumothorax. Anesth Analg 1993;76:530–534.
83. Knoblanche GE. Incidence and etiology of phrenic nerve block in association with supraclavicular brachial plexus block. Anaesth Intensive Care 1979;4:346–349.
84. Farrar MD, Scheybani M, Nolte H. Upper extremity block effectiveness and complications. Reg Anesth 1981;6:133–134.
85. Urmey WF, Talts KH, Sharrock ME. 100% incidence of hemidiaphragmatic paresis associated with interscalene brachial plexus anesthesia diagnosed by ultra sonography. Anesth Analg 1991;72:498–503.
86. Pere P, Pitkanen M, Rosenberg P. Continuous interscalene brachial plexus block decreases diaphragmatic motility and ventilatory function. Acta Anaesthesiol Scand 1992;36:53–57.
87. Urmey WF, McDonald M. Hemidiaphragmatic paresis during interscalene brachial plexus block: effect on pulmonary function and chest wall mechanics. Anesth Analg 1992;74:352–357.
88. Fujimura N, Anamba H, Tsunoda K, et al. Effect of hemi diaphragmatic paresis caused by interscalene brachial plexus block on breathing, patterns chest wall mechanics and arterial blood gases. Anesthesiology 1995;81:962–966.
89. Kayerker UN, Dick MD. Phrenic nerve paralysis following interscalene brachial plexus block. Anesth Analg 1983;62:536–537.
90. Hood J, Knoblanche G. Respiratory failure following brachial plexus block. Anaesth Intensive Care 1979;7:285–286.
91. Rau RH, Chan YL, Chuang HI. Dyspnea resulting from phrenic nerve paralysis after interscalene block in an obese male. Acta Anaesthesiol Sin 1997;35:113–118.
92. Neal JM, Moore JM, Kopacz DJ, et al. Quantitative assessment of respiratory and sensory function after supraclavicular block. Anesth Analg 1998;86:1239–1244.
93. Al-Kaisy AA, Chan VWS, Perlas A. Respiratory effects of low dose bupivacaine interscalene block. Br J Anaesth 1999;82:217–220.
94. Betts A, Eggan JR. Unilateral pulmonary edema with interscalene block. Anesthesiology 1998;88:1113–1114.
95. Candido KD, Sukhani R, Doty R, et al. Neurologic sequelae after interscalene brachial plexus block for shoulder/upper arm surgery: the association of patient, anesthetic, and surgical factors to the incidence and the clinical course. Anesth Analg 2005;100: 1489–1495.
96. Barutell C, Videll F, Raich M, et al. Neurological complication following interscalene brachial plexus block. Anaesthesia 1980;35:365–367.
97. Lim EK, Pereira R. Brachial plexus injury following brachial plexus block. Anaesthesia 1984;39:691–695.
98. Bashein G, Thompson-Robertson H, Kennedy WF Jr. Persistent phrenic nerve paresis following interscalene brachial plexus block. Anesthesiology 1985;63:102–104.
99. Robaux S, Bouaziz H, Boisseau N, et al. Persistent phrenic nerve paralysis following interscalene brachial plexus block. Anesthesiology 2001;95:1519–1521.
100. Passannante PAN. Spinal anaesthesia and permanent neurologic deficit after interscalene block. Anesth Analg 1996;82:873–874.

101. Brockway MS, Winter AW, Wildsmith JA. Prolonged brachial plexus block with 0.42% bupivacaine. Br J Anaesth 1989;63:604–605.
102. Shantha TR, Evans JA. The relationship of epidural anesthesia to neural membranes and arachnoid villi. Anesthesiology 1972;37:543–557. Review. No abstract available.
103. Kumar A, Battit GE, Froese AB, et al. Bilateral cervical and thoracic epidural blockade complicating interscalene brachial plexus block – 2 cases. Anesthesiology 1971;35: 650–652.
104. Ross S, Scarborough CD. Total spinal anesthesia following brachial plexus block. Anesthesiology 1974;39:458.
105. Edde S, Deutsch S. Cardiac arrest after interscalene brachial plexus block. Anesth Analg 1977;56:446–447.
106. McGlade DP. Extensive central neural blockade following interscalene brachial plexus block. Anaesth Intensive Care 1992;20:514–516.
107. Baraka A, Hanna M, Hammoud R. Unconsciousness and apnea complicating parascalene brachial plexus block, possible subarachnoid block. Anesthesiology 1992;77: 1046–1047.
108. Dutton RP, Eckhardt WF III, Sunder N. Total spinal anesthesia after interscalene blockade of the brachial plexus. Anesthesiology 1994;80:939–941.
109. Norris D, Klahsen A, Milne B. Delayed bilateral spinal anesthesia, following interscalene block. Can J Anaesth 1996;43:303–305.
110. Majid A, van den Oever HL, Walstra GJ, Dzoljic M. Spinal anesthesia as a complication of brachial plexus block using the posterior approach. Anesth Analg 2002;94: 1338–1339.
111. Al-Khafaji JM, Ellias MA. Incidence of Horner's syndrome with interscalene brachial plexus block and its importance in the management of head injury. Anesthesiology 1986;64:127.
112. Sukhani CR, Barclay LJ, Aasen M. Prolonged Horner's syndrome after interscalene block: a management dilemma. Anesth Analg 1994;79:701–745.
113. Rollins M, McKay WR, Eshima RE. Airway difficulty after subclavian perivascular block. Anesth Analg 2003;96:1191–1192.
114. Plit ML, Chhajed PN, MacDonald P, et al. Bilateral vocal cord palsy following Interscalene brachial plexus block. Anaesth Intensive Care 2002;30:499–501.
115. Thiagarajah S, Moore E, Azar I, et al. Bronchospasm following interscalene brachial plexus block. Anesthesiology 1984;61:759–761.
116. Shah MB, Hirschman DA. Sympathetic blockade cannot explain bronchospasm following interscalene brachial plexus block. Anesthesiology 1985;62:847.
117. Durrani Z, Winnie AP. Brainstem toxicity with reversible "locked in syndrome" after interscalene brachial plexus block. Anesth Analg 1991;72:249–252.
118. Mani M, Ramamurthy N, Rao TLK, et al. An unusual complication of brachial plexus block and heparin therapy. Anesthesiology 1978;48:213–214.
119. Siler PL, Lief JS, Davis JS. A complication of interscalene brachial plexus block. Anesthesiology 1973;38:590–591.
120. Rosenberg PH, Lambert TS, Tarkkila T, et al. Auditory disturbance associated with interscalene brachial plexus block. Br J Anaesth 1995;74:89–91.
121. Schroeder LE, Horlocker TT, Schroeder DR. The efficacy of axillary block for surgical procedures about the elbow. Anesth Analg 1996;83:747–751.
122. Merrill DJ, Brodsky JB, Hentz RH. Vascular insufficiency following axillary block of the brachial plexus. Anesth Analg 1981;60:162–164.
123. Restelli L, Pingiroli D, Conoscente F, et al. Insufficient venous drainage following axillary approach to brachial plexus blockade. Br J Anaesth 1984;56:1051–1053.
124. Ott L, Neuberger L, Frey HP. Obliteration of the axillary artery after axillary block. Anaesthesia 1989;44:773–774.
125. Dudrick S, Masland W, Mishkin M. Brachial plexus injury following axillary artery puncture. Radiology 1967;88:271–273.

# 9 Complications Associated with Spinal Anesthesia

Pekka Tarkkila

Spinal anesthesia celebrated its first centennial in 1998 and still is one of the centerpieces of modern regional anesthesia. August Bier from Germany was the first to publish a report of the first successful spinal anesthesia with cocaine on his friend and assistant Hildebrandt. Since then, spinal anesthesia has gained worldwide popularity and an impressive safety record. However, the history of complications of spinal anesthesia is as old as the method itself.[1] The very first spinal anesthetics were followed by postdural puncture headaches (PDPHs) as Bier and Hildebrandt both developed a headache after their experiment that, at least with Bier himself, was posture related. The wine and cigars consumed during the celebration of a successful experiment may have augmented the development of headache.

In the early days of spinal anesthesia, it was claimed to be a very safe method of anesthesia and was used successfully even in operations on the head, neck, and thorax, with low mortality.[2] After initial great popularity, some tragic events occurred with spinal anesthesia, at a time when major advances were being made in inhalation anesthesia, that almost made this technique obsolete, at least in the United Kingdom. The most famous of these tragedies was the Woolley and Roe case in which two patients, in adjoining operating rooms, became paraplegic following spinal anesthesia for relatively minor procedures.[3] It is probable that this tragedy was caused by contamination of the spinal needles or syringes during the sterilization process.[4] In the 1950s, the reputation of spinal anesthesia was restored, mostly as a result of several reports from Vandam and Dripps[5] involving more than 10,000 patients. They showed that spinal anesthesia was a safe technique and only rarely caused serious morbidity and mortality.

With modern equipment and developed techniques, this old anesthesia method remains an important and cost efficient part of modern anesthesiology. With advanced knowledge of the mechanisms, this versatile anesthesia method can be adjusted according to our needs. In the last one or two decades, there have been many changes in the treatment of patients and spinal techniques. More and more operations are being performed on an ambulatory basis and spinal anesthesia methods have been adjusted to meet the demands of a busy environment. The focus of complications with these patients has changed accordingly. Mortality or major complications are not usually an issue with short-stay patients, but we should be able to provide them "fast track" anesthesia without side effects and with a high degree of patient satisfaction. However, we should be able to use spinal anesthesia safely for major operations in elderly patients with numerous comorbidities.

## Failure of Spinal Anesthesia

Failure of spinal anesthesia is one of the most embarrassing complications for the patient and the anesthesiologist. Spinal anesthesia, in contrast to many other regional anesthesia methods, has a clear end point indicating correct needle placement [free flow of cerebrospinal fluid (CSF) from the needle]. Despite this, there is, in common with other regional anesthesia techniques, a potential risk for failure. Correspondingly, even general anesthesia may be associated with failure, as patients can be aware of the surgical operation during anesthesia. Failure rates may be reduced by proper selection of patients, timing, and the skill of the anesthesiologist. The reasons for failure in spinal blocks are in most cases related to technical factors rather than to the anesthetic agent used.[6]

The incidence of failure with spinal anesthesia varies in different studies, ranging from 3% to 17%.[6–9] In some smaller studies, failure rates as high as 30% have been reported. Spinal anesthesia can be classified as a failure if the surgical operation cannot be performed without the addition of general anesthetic or an alternative regional block. The subarachnoid space may be impossible to locate or the needle may move during the injection of the anesthetic. The spinal puncture may be difficult to perform because of abnormal anatomy, obesity, or poor cooperation or pain experienced by the patient. One cannot give unambiguous instructions regarding when the spinal technique should be abandoned and the anesthesia plan changed. Regardless, if the spinal puncture does not succeed after several attempts and especially if many paresthesias have been attained, the anesthesiologist should change the planned anesthesia. Good clinical judgment and cooperation with the patient are essential to prevent complications associated with multiple punctures in close proximity to the spinal canal and nerve roots. Unfortunately, most often patients who are at risk for unsuccessful spinal anesthesia tend to be high-risk patients for general anesthesia as well.

The anesthesiologist should make the best possible effort to prevent unsuccessful spinal anesthesia by careful technique, which ensures free flow of CSF before injection of local anesthetic and good fixation of the spinal needle during the injection to prevent needle movement. In some cases, failure occurs despite free-flowing CSF from the needle hub, and this may be caused by the needle entering an arachnoid cyst that is not in direct communication with the subarachnoid space.

The Sprotte needle has been implicated in higher failure rates, and this may be because the side hole is large and elongated and located distal to the tip. However, in a prospective study comparing failure rates between Sprotte and Quincke needles, there was no difference noted.[10]

The use of low-dose spinal anesthesia for ambulatory surgery has gained popularity in recent years. Interestingly, the use of low-dose spinal anesthesia (bupivacaine less than 10mg) for day surgery has not increased the risk of failure if a proper technique has been used.[11–13] Usually, low-dose spinal anesthesia is used for surgery of the lower extremities, although it can be used also for bilateral anesthesia, such as for tubal ligation. With low-dose, selective or unilateral spinal anesthesia, the proper technique is even more important than with higher doses. The position of the patient (sitting, lateral decubitus position, prone) is essential with respect to baricity of local anesthetic. The maintenance of the selected position affects the spread of anesthesia. With conventional (larger) doses of local anesthetics, even a longer period of time spent in the lateral decubitus position does not prevent bilateral block.[14]

With hyperbaric bupivacaine and ropivacaine, the sensory level of analgesia can be modified with repositioning of the patient after local anesthetic injection. With isobaric bupivacaine, the sensory level of analgesia is difficult to predict and more difficult to modify after puncture. However, there is a tendency for a higher level when a higher lumbar interspace for spinal anesthesia is used.[15]

## Hemodynamic Complications

Cardiovascular side effects are common during spinal anesthesia, hypotension being the most common.[16,17] Decrease of blood pressure can be considered a normal physiologic effect of spinal anesthesia. In some cases, the decrease can be so severe that it can be considered a complication. There is no agreement at which level the low blood pressure should be treated. Clinical judgment is needed to decide when an individual patient needs treatment for a low blood pressure.

### *Hypotension*

The reported incidence of hypotension during spinal anesthesia varies from 0% to more than 50% in nonpregnant patients. Pregnant patients are more susceptible to hypotension with incidences ranging from 50% to more than 90%. The high variation among publications may be explained by different definitions of hypotension, varying patient materials, and different methods used to prevent hypotension. Systolic blood pressures less than 85–90 mm Hg or a decrease of more than 25%–30% from the preanesthetic value have been used to define hypotension.[16,17]

Hypotension during spinal anesthesia results principally from the preganglionic sympathetic blockade. Systemic vascular resistance decreases as a result of a reduction in sympathetic tone of the arterial circulation. This leads to peripheral arterial vasodilatation, the extent of which depends on the number of spinal segments involved. Other theories are proposed to explain hypotension during spinal anesthesia, among them: 1) direct depressive circulatory effect of local anesthetics, 2) relative adrenal insufficiency, 3) skeletal muscle paralysis, 4) ascending medullary vasomotor block, and 5) concurrent mechanical respiratory insufficiency.[18] Hypotensive effects of spinal anesthesia are exaggerated in advanced pregnancy because of aortocaval compression caused by the gravid uterus. Nerve fibers in pregnant patients are also more sensitive to the effect of local anesthetics[19], probably because of chronic exposure of progesterone altering the protein synthesis in nerve tissue.[20]

Risk factors for hypotension include older patients, patients with peak block height greater than or equal to T5, and patients undergoing combined spinal and general anesthesia.[16,17]

### *Bradycardia*

Loss of sympathetic input to the heart, leaving vagal, parasympathetic innervation unopposed, and a decrease in cardiac preload are the main reasons for bradycardia during spinal anesthesia. The extent of sympathetic blockade is not always comparable with the sensory level[21], and this may be the reason why cardiovascular complications do not always occur despite high sensory levels.[22] Younger patients and those with sensory levels above T6 are more susceptible to bradycardia during spinal anesthesia.[23] Baseline heart rates less than 60 beats/minute and current therapy with beta-adrenergic–blocking drugs also increase the risk factors for bradycardia.[17]

The decrease of venous return to the heart leads to decreased stretch to the right side of the heart leading to decreased heart rate (Bainbridge reflex). Also, a paradoxical form of the Bezold-Jarisch reflex has been thought to occur rarely during spinal anesthesia, leading to severe bradycardia and asystole.[24] During spinal anesthesia, a sudden decrease in ventricular volume (an empty ventricle) coupled with a vigorous ventricular contraction leads to activation of the mechanoreceptors, and subsequently increased vagal tone and decreased sympathetic activity as the heart perceives itself to be full. Other possible mechanisms of bradycardia during spinal anesthesia include excessive sedation, preexisting autonomic dysfunction, heart block, vasovagal reaction,[25] or athletic heart syndrome.[26]

**Treatment and Prevention of Hypotension and Bradycardia**

Preventive procedures before spinal anesthesia are more frequently used for pregnant patients because these subjects are more susceptible to the hypotensive effects of spinal anesthesia. A decrease in blood pressure lasting more than 2 minutes may have a deleterious effect on the neonate.[27]

Relative hypovolemia caused by spinal anesthesia may be successfully prevented either with sympathomimetic medication or by preloading with crystalloid or colloid. Even leg-wrapping has been used with good success in patients scheduled for cesarean delivery.[28] Crystalloid preload has often been used but it does not seem to lessen the cardiovascular complication frequency even with elderly patients in good health.[29] However, if the patient is preoperatively hypovolemic, the hypovolemia must be corrected before establishing the block.

The most common sympathomimetic drugs used in the prevention and treatment of hypotension are ephedrine (combined alpha and beta effects, with predominant beta-adrenergic effects) and etilefrine (which has combined alpha and beta effects). They can be both infused according to blood pressure response or given as boluses and have quite similar effects on patients. Methoxamine and phenylephrine (pure alpha-adrenergic agonists) are other sympathomimetics used. Ephedrine is mostly used for pregnant patients because it restores uterine blood flow despite the increase in maternal blood pressure.[30] Small increments of phenylephrine have also been considered safe for the fetus. The use of phenylephrine may be indicated if the increase in heart rate in the mother is not tolerated. Because bradycardia during spinal anesthesia is most often caused by decreased preload to the heart, restoring the blood pressure is the best treatment for bradycardia. Stimulating an empty heart with atropine may be deleterious, especially if the patient has coronary disease. Increased work load (tachycardia) increases the oxygen demand of the heart without increasing the oxygen supply.

Whenever serious hemodynamic instability occurs with spinal anesthesia, it is most likely attributable to some interference with the venous return. Therefore, one of the most important steps to take in treatment is to check the position of the patient and if not optimal place the patient in a position that will enhance venous return. One should also make sure that the surgeon is not interfering with the venous return during surgical manipulation. In the words of one of the great masters of spinal anesthesia, Professor Nicholas Greene, "The sine qua non of safe spinal anesthesia is maintenance of the venous return."

### *Nausea and Vomiting*

Nausea and vomiting are quite rare during spinal anesthesia and most often associated with hypotension. Therefore, nausea in these cases is alleviated in combination with the successful treatment of hypotension and does not need any specific treatment itself. The other suggested mechanisms for nausea during spinal anesthesia are cerebral hypoxia, inadequate anesthesia, and traction-related parasympathetic reflexes provoked by surgical manipulation. Female gender, opiate premedication, and sensory level of analgesia above Th6 have all been shown to be significant risk factors for nausea during spinal anesthesia.[23] A history of motion sickness has also been associated with nausea during spinal anesthesia.[17]

### *Cardiac Arrest*

In recent studies, the incidence of cardiac arrest during spinal anesthesia has been reported to be between 2.5–6.4 per 10,000 anesthesias.[31–33] Cardiac arrest is often associated with a perioperative event such as significant blood loss or cement placement during orthopedic surgery. It is often difficult to determine whether surgical, anesthesia, or patient factors are the most significant leading up to the problem.

Fortunately, the frequency of cardiac arrests has decreased significantly over the last two or three decades.[33] The reason for this decrease is not clear. The awareness of this potential complication may have increased after Caplan and colleagues[34] reported 14 cases of sudden cardiac arrests in healthy patients who had spinal anesthesia for minor operations. Also, the use of pulse oximetry has become a standard during spinal anesthesia, although no randomized studies have been or will be done to confirm the effectiveness of pulse oximetry with this respect. Patients should be monitored during spinal anesthesia as vigorously as during general anesthesia and side effects should be treated aggressively as soon as possible to prevent life-threatening complications. Cardiac arrest during neuraxial anesthesia has been associated with an equal or better likelihood of survival than a cardiac arrest during general anesthesia.[33]

## Urinary Retention

There is a high incidence of micturition difficulties postoperatively. Acute urinary retention can occur following all types of anesthesia and operative procedures. The etiology of postoperative urinary retention involves a combination of many factors, including surgical trauma to the pelvic nerves or to the bladder, overdistention of the bladder by large quantities of fluids given intravenously, postoperative edema around the bladder neck, and pain- or anxiety-induced reflex spasm of the internal and external urethral sphincters.[35,36] Urinary retention is more likely to occur after major surgery and with elderly male patients. Opiates and confinement to bed may also be likely explanations for the development of urinary retention after surgery. The type of anesthetic and the management of postoperative pain may have little effect on the occurrence of postoperative urinary dysfunction.[36]

Disturbances of micturition are common in the first 24 hours after spinal anesthesia. There is a higher frequency of these disturbances after bupivacaine than lidocaine spinal anesthesia.[37] After administration of spinal anesthesia with bupivacaine or tetracaine, the micturition reflex is very rapidly eliminated. Detrusor muscle contraction is restored to normal 7–8 hours after the spinal injection. On average, patients recover enough motor function to be mobilized 1–2 hours before the micturition reflex returns. Full skin sensation is usually restored at the same time or slightly before patients are able to micturate. To avoid protracted postoperative bladder symptoms, careful supervision of bladder function is of great importance in patients receiving spinal anesthesia with long-acting anesthetics.[38] A single episode of excessive bladder distention may result in significant morbidity. Overfilling of the bladder can stretch and damage the detrusor muscle, leading to atony of the bladder wall, so that recovery of micturition may not occur when the bladder is emptied. Patients at risk for urinary retention should be encouraged to void and provided a quiet environment in which to do so. They should be encouraged to sit, stand, or ambulate as soon as possible.[36] Expedient catheterization when needed and the prophylactic placement of indwelling catheters in patients with previous disturbances are recommended.[36,37]

### *Urinary Retention and Outpatient Surgery*

The reported frequency of urinary retention after intrathecal administration of opioids varies considerably. The risk for urinary retention is increased with higher doses of opioids or local anesthetics. Many patients who receive opioids intrathecally are catheterized because they are more likely to develop urinary retention postoperatively. However, 10–20 μg of fentanyl administered with small-dose bupivacaine for ambulatory surgery does not seem to increase the risk for urinary retention or prolong discharge times.[39–41] Small-dose or unilateral spinal anesthesia is associated with a lower risk for urinary retention than conventional methods.

During the past few years, the home discharge criteria have been changed. The routine requirement of voiding before discharge can be considered mandatory only for high-risk patients. These high-risk patients include those with preoperative difficulties in urinating, operations in the perineal area, older men, etc. All patients must receive oral and written instructions before discharge regarding when, where, and whom to contact in case of difficulty voiding. A follow-up phone call is recommended for all patients who are discharged before they have voided.

## Transient Neurologic Problems

### *Radiculopathy*

Damage to a nerve root can occur during identification of the subarachnoid space or during the insertion of a spinal catheter. Paresthesia with or without motor weakness is the presenting symptom, and although the majority of patients recover completely, a small number may be affected permanently. Although neurologic complications may present immediately postoperatively, some may require days or even weeks to emerge. Should neurologic dysfunction occur, early detection and intervention are required to promote complete neurologic recovery.[42] Documentation of critical data concerning spinal anesthetic technique, such as level of needle placement, needle type, and local anesthetic solution, is an important part of the anesthesia procedure. As demonstrated by the Closed Claims Study database, nerve damage is a major source of anesthetic liability. Therefore, the same consideration must be given to the documentation of prudent regional anesthetic practice as is given to its delivery.[43]

Auroy et al.[31] found, in their prospective, multicenter study of 40,640 spinal anesthetics and 30,413 epidural anesthetics, 19 cases of radiculopathy after spinal anesthesia and five cases of radiculopathy after epidural anesthesia. In 12 of the 19 cases of radiculopathy after spinal anesthesia and in all five cases of radiculopathy after epidural anesthesia, the needle insertion or drug injection was associated with paresthesia or pain. In all cases, the radiculopathy was in the same distribution as the associated paraesthesias.

Oblique lateral entry into the ligamentum flavum may direct the needle into the dural cuff region. This may result in direct trauma to a nerve root, with resultant unisegmental paresthesia; such a sign should warn the anesthesiologist not to persist with needle insertion in this position and not to attempt to thread a catheter.[44]

To avoid trauma to nerves, careful technique and accurate anatomic knowledge are mandatory. Low lumbar interspace for puncture should be chosen as the spinal cord terminates in normal adults, usually at L1 level although this is variable and it may be as low as L3. It has also been shown that the anesthesiologist quite often estimates the interspace for puncture incorrectly, although this has little clinical significance in most cases. Paresthesia during the insertion of a spinal needle is common with incidences varying between 4.5%–18%.[45–49] Fortunately, in most cases, no harmful effects occur following paresthesia. In one study, elicitation of a paresthesia during needle placement was identified as a risk factor for persistent paresthesia.[43] If a paresthesia is elicited during spinal needle advancement into the subarachnoid space, it is reasonable to draw the needle 0.5–1.0 mm before injecting the anesthetic, in order to avoid direct trauma to a single spinal nerve. One should never continue injecting anesthetic if the patient complains of pain during injection.

### *Backache*

Backache after spinal anesthesia is quite common and rarely a major issue. Incidences of approximately 20% have been described.[10] The long duration of operation is associated with higher incidence of back problems and the incidence is quite similar with spinal anesthesia as with general anesthesia. Relaxation of the back muscles leads to unusual strain and this can lead to postoperative back pain. A pillow under the lumbar area is a cheap and effective method to prevent at least some of the back problems.

If unusual back pain is encountered postoperatively, local infection and spinal hematoma should be excluded. Strict aseptic technique during the administration of spinal anesthesia should be used to prevent infectious complications. Local infection can be associated with tenderness, redness, and other usual signs of infection.

The increased use of low-molecular-weight heparins (LMWHs) for thromboprophylaxis has caused concern about the use of spinal anesthesia for these patients. Patients taking preoperative LMWH can be assumed to have altered coagulation, and needle placement should occur at least 10–12 hours after the LMWH dose. The decision to perform spinal anesthesia in a patient receiving antithrombotic therapy should be made on an individual basis, weighing the small, though definite, risk of spinal hematoma with the benefits of regional anesthesia for a specific patient. Alternative anesthetic and analgesic techniques exist for patients considered an unacceptable risk. It must also be remembered that identification of risk factors and establishment of guidelines will not completely eliminate the complication of spinal hematoma.[50]

Signs of cord compression, such as severe back pain, progression of numbness or weakness, and bowel and bladder dysfunction, warrant immediate radiographic evaluation because spinal hematoma with neurologic symptoms must be treated within 6–8 hours in order to prevent permanent neurologic injury.

### *Transient Neurologic Symptoms*

For almost 60 years, lidocaine has proven to be safe and reliable for spinal anesthesia in a hyperbaric 5% solution.[51,52] Hyperbaric lidocaine has been implicated as a causative agent in the cauda equina syndrome, associated with the use of spinal microcatheters.[53] The first report of transient neurologic symptoms (TNSs), termed initially transient radicular impairment or transient radicular irritation (TRI), after single-shot spinal anesthesia with hyperbaric 5% lidocaine was published by Schneider and colleagues[54] in 1993. This finding has later been confirmed by several other studies.[47,55–59]

#### **Definition**

TNSs are defined as back pain and/or dysesthesia radiating bilaterally to the legs or buttocks after total recovery from spinal anesthesia and beginning within 24 hours of surgery. Usually no objective signs of neurologic deficits can be demonstrated.[49,54,55] The pain is usually moderate and relieved by nonsteroidal antiinflammatory agents, but opioids are also often needed.[49,59] In some cases, the patients state that the transient neurologic pain is worse than their incisional pain.[59]

#### **Etiology**

The cause and etiology of TNSs have not yet been elucidated. Even the name of this syndrome is controversial and different suggestions appear in the literature every now and then. To avoid confusion, it is not reasonable to change the name of the syndrome until the etiology is clear.

It is surprising that this new syndrome was not recognized until the beginning of the 1990s. Lidocaine has been used since 1948 for spinal anesthesia in millions of patients without major central nervous system sequelae. The reason for a new syndrome may be either a change in methods or prior lack of recognition. One reason for the high number of reports of TNSs after spinal anesthesia may be that these symptoms are being sought more aggressively after the first case reports.

The practice of spinal anesthesia has changed radically in recent years. Use of premedication before spinal anesthesia has diminished. New, small-gauge Quincke and pencil-point spinal needles have been introduced for everyday use. Patients are now ambulated as soon as possible after surgery. It is not clear if any of these changes could be responsible for the establishment of TNSs.

The delayed recognition of this phenomenon may be attributable to a high underlying rate of nonspecific back pain. A heightened awareness of the potential for local anesthetic–induced neurotoxicity after the association of lidocaine and microcatheters with cauda equina syndrome and the recognition of a distinct pattern of symptoms may have a part in the recognition of these symptoms.[60]

### Identification of Risk Factors

Possible causes or contributing factors to TNSs include a specific local anesthetic toxicity, neural ischemia secondary to sciatic nerve stretching, spinal cord vasoconstriction, patient positioning, needle trauma, or pooling of local anesthetic secondary to small-gauge, pencil-point needles. Patient diseases or some other undefined patient factors predisposing them to neurologic abnormalities and infection should also be ruled out. Musculoskeletal disturbances in the back and leg symptoms cannot be totally excluded. TNS frequency was observed to be high with outpatient surgery and lithotomy position in one study.[61] However, in two randomized studies, early ambulation did not increase the risk for TNSs.[62,63]

After the initial report of TNSs with lidocaine, this syndrome has also been associated with other local anesthetics. The incidence of TNSs with 5% lidocaine has been between 10% and 37%.[45,47,59] The risk for TNSs is highest with lidocaine and also with mepivacaine and there seems to be approximately a seven times higher risk of developing TNSs after intrathecal lidocaine than after bupivacaine, prilocaine, or procaine.[64] It is thought that a local anesthetic toxic effect may be an important contributing factor in the development of TNSs after spinal anesthesia with concentrated solutions.[65,66] Because the toxicity is believed to be concentration related, a rational approach to the problem would be to look at the comparative efficacy of lower concentrations of lidocaine for spinal anesthesia. However, in clinical studies, decreasing the concentration of lidocaine from 5% to 2% did not prevent the development of TNSs.[47,59]

The incidence of TNSs after 4% mepivacaine for spinal anesthesia has been high and up to 30%.[49] Three randomized studies combined gave a similar incidence of TNSs with mepivacaine than with lidocaine.[64] The incidence of these symptoms with 0.5% tetracaine containing phenylephrine was 12.5%, but only 1.0% when 0.5% tetracaine without phenylephrine was used.[48] The incidence of TNSs after hyperbaric 0.5% or 0.75% bupivacaine was 0%–3%.[45,49,59,67] The duration of symptoms after bupivacaine spinal anesthesia was less than 12 hours compared with 12–120 hours after mepivacaine spinal anesthesia.[49] Prilocaine has also been associated with a low incidence of TNSs (between 0% and 4%).[64]

The dorsal roots of spinal nerves are positioned most posteriorly in the spinal canal[54] and therefore hyperbaric solution pools in this area when the patient is supine. Individual physical characteristics of patients may predispose to the development of transient radicular symptoms after spinal anesthesia. Anatomic configuration of the spinal column affects the spread of subarachnoid anesthetic solutions that move under the influence of gravity.[68] Both lumbar lordosis and thoracic kyphosis will differ among individuals, particularly with respect to the lowest point of the thoracic spinal canal.[69]

Sacral maldistribution of local anesthetic with pencil-point needles has been suggested to cause toxic peak concentrations of lidocaine. Maldistribution has been shown in spinal models when the side port of a Whitacre needle is directed sacrally (between 0% and 4%) and the speed of injection is slow. In contrast, the distribution from a sacrally directed Quincke needle was uniform even with slow injection rates,[56] well-distributed blocks, and with different types of spinal needles.[45,55,70] However, in clinical practice, TNSs have occurred following well-distributed blocks.

In addition to toxic effects of the local anesthetics, the lithotomy position during surgery has been thought to contribute to TNS.[54] The lithotomy position may contribute to TNSs by stretching the cauda equina and sciatic nerves, thus decreasing the vascular supply and increasing vulnerability to injury. During knee surgery, where the position of the operative leg is varied and nerve stretching may occur, there is an increased risk for TNSs. The incidence of TNSs is higher after knee arthroscopy compared with inguinal hernia repairs.[59]

Spinal cord vasoconstrictors may be implicated through either localized ischemia or prolonged spinal anesthesia because of decreased uptake of local anesthetic. Adding phenylephrine to tetracaine spinals increased the frequency of transient radicular symptoms.[48] Intrathecal tetracaine increases spinal cord blood flow and the effect can be reversed or prevented by epinephrine.[71] Lidocaine induces less vasodilatation in the spinal cord[72] and bupivacaine is a vasoconstrictor.[73] Epinephrine added to lidocaine did not increase the incidence of TNSs compared with lidocaine without epinephrine. However, different concentrations of lidocaine (5% with epinephrine and 2% without epinephrine) were used.[59] Preliminary animal data suggest that the concurrent administration of epinephrine enhances sensory deficits resulting from subarachnoid administration of lidocaine.[74] It is not clear whether animal data have clinical relevance for TNSs.

It has been speculated that profound relaxation of the supportive muscles of the lumbar spine may result in straightening of the lordotic curve, and even transient spondylolisthesis, when the patient is lying on the operating table. This may be responsible in part for the radiating back symptoms that can occur after intense motor block.[49]

Needle-induced trauma is typically unilateral and closely associated with needle insertion or local anesthetic injection. TNSs appear after otherwise uneventful spinal anesthetics and no correlation with paraesthesias and incidence of symptoms has been found.[45,48,49,55,59] Chemical meningitis or arachnoiditis is an improbable cause of these syndromes because there is no progression of symptoms and they usually resolve promptly without special treatment. However, results of one case report of magnetic resonance imaging (MRI) of two patients with TNSs after lidocaine spinal anesthesia showed enhancement of the cauda equina and the lumbosacral nerve roots that according to the authors may support the theory of a direct toxic effect of lidocaine. The MRI findings are suggestive of pial hyperemia or breakdown of the nerve root–blood barrier by a noninfectious inflammatory process.[75] No association with TNSs and patient sex, weight, or age has been found.[49,59]

Studies exploring a possible etiologic role of hyperosmolarity secondary to glucose suggests that it does not contribute to transient radicular symptoms.[46,48,65,76] Glucose can also promote maldistribution of local anesthetics and thus contribute indirectly to neural injury. However, a similar incidence of TNSs was found after spinal anesthesia with 5% hyperbaric lidocaine with epinephrine and 2% isobaric lidocaine without epinephrine.[59]

The site of local anesthetic action is in sodium channels, and therefore a logical step toward determining a mechanism for the local anesthetic neurotoxicity is in establishing whether ongoing blockade of sodium channels is causative for neurotoxicity. According to Sakura et al.,[77] the local anesthetic toxicity does not result from the blockade of sodium channels, and they suggest that the pursuit of a Na channel blocker not associated with TNSs is a realistic goal.

### Clinical Implications

The clinical significance of TNSs is still unclear. Although it is possible that TNSs represent the lower end of a spectrum of toxicity, their relationship to neurologic injury remains speculative at the present time[78], even more than 10 years after the discovery of this syndrome. There are not even any case reports that would indicate that TNSs are permanent or have not disappeared completely. Whether the use of lidocaine or mepivacaine should be continued for spinal anesthesia is controversial.

Adding epinephrine to lidocaine seems to potentiate persistent sensory impairment induced by subarachnoid lidocaine[75] and may explain cauda equina syndrome after single-shot spinal anesthesia.[70] There is no reason to add epinephrine to lidocaine because the solution can be substituted with bupivacaine.[60,78] It has been suggested that lidocaine should be used sparingly – if at all – in anesthetic procedures in which product pooling, nerve stretching, or both could compromise neural viability.[79] It may be wise to substitute lidocaine with bupivacaine or ropivacaine until the etiology and clinical significance of TNSs are determined. Decreasing the dose of bupivacaine makes it a suitable alternative for short-stay surgery.[59] However, there is still a place for a new nontoxic, effective, and short-acting local anesthetic.

### *Headache*

Nonspecific headache after spinal anesthesia can be more common than usually reported in the anesthesiology literature. Incidences of approximately 15%–20% have been described in recent publications.[80,81] Dehydration, fasting, and possibly associated hypoglycemia, deprivation from intake of caffeine, anxiety, and immobilization leading to muscle tension could explain the occurrence of nonspecific headache.[81] This headache is not pathognomonic for spinal anesthesia because similar incidences have been reported after general anesthesia for various operations. The treatment is symptomatic.

## Postdural Puncture Headache

PDPH used to be a common postoperative side effect of spinal anesthesia. With the development of thinner needles and needle tip design, this harmful complication has become rarer. But despite these positive developments, we still cannot promise our patients that they will not get this complication if spinal anesthesia is chosen for their anesthesia method.

### ***Definition***

PDPH is a typical headache that is usually bifrontal and occipital and is aggravated by upright posture and by straining. Nausea and vomiting are also common symptoms. The headache may first be experienced several hours to days after the dural puncture. It is relieved by lying down. The headache is different than any headache that the patient has had before (except possible previous PDPH). PDPH needs to be differentiated from tension/migraine headache, aseptic or infective meningitis, cortical vein thrombosis, or cerebral/epidural hematoma.

The pain is often associated with other symptoms that can be related with the nerve involved. Usually these symptoms resolve with the recovery from the headache. Auditory disturbances may occur secondary to eighth nerve dysfunction. These include unilateral or bilateral deafness that may go unnoticed if not specifically asked about from the patient. Traction on the abducens nerve can cause visual disturbances, diplopia being the most common symptom.

### ***Etiology***

The spinal dura mater extends from the foramen magnum to the second segment of the sacrum. It contains the spinal cord and nerve roots that pierce it. Usually after dural puncture the hole caused by the needle will close, but in some cases the hole remains open with subsequent loss of CSF through the hole. The dynamic relationship between dural and arachnoideal tear may have a role in the closure of the puncture hole. There is a clear relationship between the loss of CSF and the severity of the symptoms. According to present knowledge, the typical headache in the upright position is caused by the traction of the cerebral structures when the brain descends. Also, the compensatory cerebral vasodilatation due to loss of CSF can also cause headache.

Dura mater is a dense, connective tissue layer made up of collagen and elastic fibers that are running in a longitudinal direction at least in the superficial layer of the dura. However, light and electron microscopic studies of human dura mater have contested this classical description of the anatomy of the dura mater. Measurements of dural thickness have also demonstrated that the posterior dura varies in thickness, and that the thickness of the dura at a particular spinal level is not predictable within an individual or between individuals.[82] Dural perforation in a thick area of dura may be less likely to lead to a CSF leak than a perforation in a thin area, and may explain the unpredictable consequences of a dural perforation.

Despite the new knowledge about dural anatomy, cutting spinal needles should still be orientated parallel rather than at right angles to these longitudinal dural (and also arachnoideal) fibers (or spine) to reduce the number of fibers cut. The cut dural fibers, previously under tension, would then tend to retract and increase the longitudinal dimensions of the dural perforation, increasing the likelihood of a postspinal headache. Clinical studies have confirmed that postdural puncture headache is more likely when the cutting spinal needle is orientated perpendicular to (versus parallel) the direction of the dural fibers.[10,83]

As previously mentioned, the risk for the occurrence of PDPH may be highest if the puncture is aimed at the thinnest part of the dura. However, the anesthesiologist does not have any possibility to aim the spinal needle to the thicker part of the dura. There are some patient groups that are at a higher risk to develop PDPH than the others (Table 9-1). Especially, younger and obstetric patients and those who have had PDPH before have a higher risk for this syndrome. There are differing opinions about the effect of gender, as in some studies it did not have any effect and in some other studies even nonpregnant women have been more susceptible to PDPH. There are also some risk factors that the anesthesiologist can influence. If spinal anesthesia is chosen for a risk patient, proper technique should be used. Multiple punctures should be avoided. Thin spinal needles should be used. However, the smallest available spinal needles (29-gauge) are more difficult to use and more expensive than the thicker ones. The anesthesiologist should use the spinal needle that he or she is familiar with to avoid technical difficulties during the puncture. Modern 27-gauge, pencil-point needles are quite easy to use after some practice and may offer the optimal balance between ease of puncture and incidence of complications. With these modern needles, CSF appears in the needle hub so fast that it does not hamper the procedure. Thus, even routine use of the 27-gauge (0.41 mm) Whitacre spinal needle when performing spinal anesthesia has been recommended.[81]

### *Treatment*

The anesthetic literature contains numerous publications about different treatment options for PDPH, and more than 50 different remedies have been proposed for the

Table 9-1. Factors Influencing Likelihood of PDPH

| |
|---|
| Needle size |
| Age |
| Number of punctures |
| Bevel design |
| Pregnancy |
| Bevel orientation |
| Previous PDPH |
| Angle of approach |
| "Prep" solution |

treatment of this syndrome. Fortunately, time heals PDPH in almost every case within a couple of days. The most effective curative treatment is epidural blood patch (EBP), in which the patient's own blood is injected into epidural space.

The symptoms of PDPH are alleviated by assuming the horizontal position. However, prophylactic treatment by placing the patient horizontal for a period of time (e.g., 24 hours) after a dural puncture has no effect on the incidence or duration of a PDPH; it only delays the onset of the PDPH until the patient ambulates.[84]

Normal hydration of the patient should be maintained because dehydration can worsen the symptoms. Extra hydration has been suggested to help generate more CSF but does not alleviate the headache. Narcotic analgesics and, in some instances, non-steroidal antiinflammatory agents are often administered for symptomatic treatment of the headache.

Caffeine has been suggested as a mode of therapy to help constrict the vasodilated cerebral vessels with differing results. It is best administered early in the day so that patients can sleep at night. The dose of caffeine sodium benzoate is 500mg intravenously which can be repeated once 2 hours later if the first dose does not have the desired effect.

Boluses or infusions of epidural normal saline can help to transiently increase the epidural pressure, slowing the speed at which CSF leaks through the dural hole. This may speed the natural healing process. Bolus doses of 30–60mL given 6 hourly for four doses has been used. Alternatively, a continuous infusion at a rate of 1000mL administered over a 24-hour period has been used. Colloids have also been used but probably their effect does not differ from crystalloids. Although epidural saline or colloid can be a useful technique, higher success rates are achieved with EBPs and continuous epidural infusion or repetitive boluses necessitate that the patient stays at the hospital.

### *Epidural Blood Patch*

EBP has been shown to be the only curative treatment for PDPH that shortens effectively the duration of PDPH with high incidence of succession and low incidence of complications. Patient's autologous blood is injected into epidural space near the spinal puncture site to seal the hole and stop the CSF leak. EBP should be considered if the patient's PDPH is so severe that he or she is bedridden because of headache and consents to the procedure. Breast-feeding mothers with newborn babies should be offered EBP if PDPH hampers breast feeding and prevents them from enjoying the pleasures of recent motherhood.

The timing of EBP is controversial. Some authorities recommend a prophylactic blood patch if a dural tap is encountered during epidural puncture. However, not everyone gets PDPH even after dural puncture with a 16-gauge epidural needle. These patients would be exposed to an unnecessary procedure with potential side effects. Also, the results with prophylactic blood patches have not been convincing. The success rate has been higher if EBP has been administered 24 hours after the dural puncture instead of earlier.[85]

According to present theory, the rapid effect of EBP is caused by the volume effect of the blood in the epidural space. The blood compresses the dural canal and increases the CSF pressure and the headache is relieved. An MRI study has confirmed the tamponade effect of the 20-mL EBP, which is believed to be responsible for the immediate resolution of PDPH.[86] In the later stage, the blood is clotting into dura and the hole will close, preventing the further leakage of CSF. There are no good studies indicating how long the patients should be treated in the hospital after the EBP and what they can or cannot do to achieve best possible results. Our practice is to keep the patient supine for 30 minutes after the EBP. Thereafter, sitting and standing is tried. Patients are released from the hospital 1 hour after the procedure. They are advised to avoid any strain such as lifting during the first 24 hours after the EBP.

Thereafter, the patients can return to their normal activities. They can contact the hospital again if there are problems or the headache returns.

The contraindications to EBP are those that normally apply to epidurals (patient refusal, local infection, bleeding disorders, etc.). The anesthesiologist should interview the patient before EBP to find out if the symptoms are typical for PDPH. When in doubt, a neurologic opinion should be sought and perhaps a computed tomography scan or MRI taken to exclude other possible pathologic findings in the central neural system. Viral infection and malignancy are at least relative contraindications. There are not enough data to exclude the possibility that viruses or neoplastic cells introduced into the epidural space are potentially harmful to the patient.

The success rate with EBP has been approximately 70%–90%. In the first report by Gormley only 2–3 mL of blood was recommended.[87] Higher blood volumes seem to lead to higher success rate of EBP. Volumes between 15–20 mL have been used most often, although even 30-mL volume has been used without complications. Strict aseptic technique should be used during the procedure. The administrator of EBP should be experienced with epidural technique because a dural tap with a Tuohy needle makes things only worse. According to Szeinfeld and colleagues,[88] the blood spreads more in cephalad than caudad direction in the epidural space. Therefore, if the same interspace that was used for the lumbar puncture cannot be used, it may be wise to choose a lower one. Usually the patient feels a sensation of "fullness" during the injection. If there is persistent pain or paresthesia during the injection, the injection should be stopped. If the first EBP fails, the procedure can be repeated with a similar success rate. Usually, the PDPH is at least milder after EBP even if the headache returns. If two EBPs do not relieve the symptoms, even more caution than before should be used to exclude other reasons for headache.

### *Pruritus*

Pruritus may be a problem if intrathecal opioids are used in combination with local anesthetics. Fentanyl is used quite often in combination with low-dose local anesthetic in order to intensify the block without delaying the discharge. Sufentanil and morphine are used more often for postoperative analgesia of the inpatients. Most often, the pruritus is mild and does not need any treatment. In some cases, itching can become a real problem and needs rescue medication. A 5-HT antagonist ondansetron has been shown to alleviate the symptoms effectively.

### *Continuous Spinal Anesthesia*

Spinal catheters can be used for repeating dosing or continuous infusion of drugs into the subarachnoid space. Excessive block can be avoided with careful titration of the drugs into catheter. With more restricted block, there is smaller risk for cardiovascular complications such as hypotension and bradycardia. If the duration of surgery is long, additional doses of local anesthetics can be injected. The use of catheters can be extended also for postoperative analgesia.

In the beginning of the 1990s, 14 cases of cauda equina syndrome were reported in association with the use of small-gauge spinal catheters. This led to the withdrawal of the microcatheters from the market in the United States and Canada. The mechanism of these unhappy events was probably attributable to direct toxic effect of local anesthetic. Maldistribution or potential pooling of local administered through the catheters near the roots of cauda equina is the most likely explanation. Therefore, hyperbaric local anesthetics should be avoided with microcatheters. Injection of hyperbaric solution through a single-hole microcatheter may lead to neurotoxic concentrations of local anesthetic in CSF. The risk seems to increase when the catheter is directed caudad and glucose-containing solutions are injected. Unfortunately, it is impossible to predict the direction of a subarachnoid catheter despite attempts to direct it cranially at least with sharp-beveled needles.[89] More accurate positioning may be achieved by using directional puncture needles such as Sprotte or Tuohy needles. The catheter should not be advanced more than 2–3 cm into subarachnoid space.

Small-gauge spinal catheter systems with different techniques of dural perforation have been developed to reduce the risk of PDPH in continuous spinal anesthesia. Despite different catheter designs, the incidence of PDPH seems to be high with the risk patients. An incidence of 78% has been reported with the over-the-needle catheter technique.[90] Spinal cutaneous fistula is a rare but harmful complication of continuous spinal anesthesia. In one reported case, the fistula followed a 5-hour catheterization with an 18-gauge epidural nylon catheter. The fistula was closed with a single stitch, deep, at the puncture site.[91]

There are many technical problems associated with placement of small-diameter spinal catheters. Coiling and kinking of the catheters, catheter breakage, and failure to aspirate have been problems associated with these catheters. Over-the-needle devices have been associated with high failure rates.[92] Traumatic catheter placement can in worst case lead to spinal hematoma that fortunately is a rare but a potentially catastrophic complication of spinal catheterization.

Spinal catheters should be properly marked and the personnel that manage the patients should be aware of the proper use of spinal catheters and the possible complications associated with them. Injecting the wrong solution into subarachnoid space can cause disastrous complications for the patient.

Strict aseptic routine should be used during the insertion and use of spinal catheters. There are no prospective studies about the incidence of infective complications associated with the use of these catheters. Occasional case reports have been published about aseptic meningitis during continuous spinal analgesia. The preservatives have been suspected to be the cause of meningitis.[93] There are no data either about the safe time period that the spinal catheter can be used. In most studies, the spinal catheter had remained in situ for 1 or 2 postoperative days.

Catheter breakage can also occur during catheter withdrawal. During withdrawal of the catheter, the patient should be positioned preferably in the same position as during the insertion of the catheter. Excessive force should be avoided. Catheter removal is not acceptable during therapeutic levels of anticoagulation. The catheter must be checked after removal and if broken pieces are retained in the patient, they should be informed about the incident. It is recommended to leave possible broken pieces in situ if they do not cause problems such as CSF fistula.

## Conclusion

Spinal anesthesia is one of the oldest and most reliable techniques in anesthesia today and its use now spans three centuries. The circumstances surrounding its introduction are fascinating. The basic technique has changed very little in more than 100 years of use. We now have better needles, local anesthetics, and catheters. We now add opiates to our local anesthetic solutions which have many benefits but also add to the list of complications. The phenomenon of TRI or TNSs is fascinating and inexplicable. We have learned a great deal about the physiology of spinal anesthesia in the last 50 years thanks to outstanding contributions made by Sir Robert Macintosh and Professor Nicholas Greene. It is very likely that anesthesiologists will still be performing spinal anesthesia 100 years from now. We owe a debt of gratitude to Bier and Hildebrandt for the gift of spinal anesthesia.

## References

1. Bier AKG, von Esmarch JFA. Versucheúber cocainisiring des rúckenmarkes. Dtsch Z Chir 1899;51:361–369.

2. Babcock WW. Spinal anesthesia: an experience of twenty-four years. Am J Surg 1928;5: 571–576.
3. Cope RW. The Woolley and Roe case. Anaesthesia 1954;9:249–270.
4. Maltby JR, Hutter CD, Clayton KC. The Woolley and Roe case. Br J Anaesth 2000; 84:121–126.
5. Vandam LD, Dripps RD. Long-term follow-up of patients who received 10,098 spinal anesthetics. IV. Neurological disease to traumatic lumbar puncture during spinal anesthesia. JAMA 1960;172:1483–1487.
6. Tarkkila P. Incidence and causes of failed spinal anesthetics in a university hospital: a prospective study. Reg Anesth 1991;16:48–51.
7. Levy JH, Islas JA, Ghia JN, et al. A retrospective study of the incidence and causes of failed spinal anesthetics in a university hospital. Anesth Analg 1985;64:705–710.
8. Manchikanti L, Hadley C, Markwell SJ, et al. A retrospective analysis of failed spinal anesthetic attempts in a community hospital. Anesth Analg 1987;66:363–366.
9. Munhall RJ, Sukhani R, Winnie A. Incidence and etiology of failed spinal anesthetics in a university hospital: a prospective study. Anesth Analg 1988;67:843–848.
10. Tarkkila PJ, Heine H, Tervo R-R. Comparison of Sprotte and Quincke needles with respect to post dural puncture headache and backache. Reg Anesth 1992;17:283–287.
11. Kuusniemi KS, Pihlajamäki KK, Pitkänen MT. A low dose of plain or hyperbaric bupivacaine for unilateral spinal anesthesia. Reg Anesth Pain Med 2000;25:605–610.
12. Fanelli G, Borghi B, Casati A, et al. Unilateral bupivacaine spinal anesthesia for outpatient knee arthroscopy. Italian Study Group on Unilateral Spinal Anesthesia. Can J Anaesth 2000;47:746–751.
13. Korhonen AM, Valanne JV, Jokela RM, et al. Influence of the injection site (L2/3 or L3/4) and the posture of the vertebral column on selective spinal anesthesia for ambulatory knee arthroscopy. Acta Anaesthesiol Scand 2005;49:72–77.
14. Esmaoglu A, Boyaci A, Ersoy O, et al. Unilateral spinal anaesthesia with hyperbaric bupivacaine. Acta Anaesthesiol Scand 1998;42:1083–1087.
15. Tuominen M, Taivainen T, Rosenberg PH. Spread of spinal anaesthesia with plain 0.5% bupivacaine: influence of the vertebral interspace used for injection. Br J Anaesth 1989; 62:358–361.
16. Tarkkila P, Kaukinen S. Complications during spinal anesthesia: a prospective study. Reg Anesth 1991;16:101–106.
17. Carpenter RL, Caplan RA, Brown DL, et al. Incidence and risk factors for side effects of spinal anesthesia. Anesthesiology 1992;76:906–916.
18. Greene NM. Physiology of Spinal Anesthesia. Baltimore: Williams & Wilkins; 1981: 112–115.
19. Datta S, Lambert DH, Gregus J, et al. Differential sensitivities of mammalian nerve fibers during pregnancy. Anesth Analg 1983;62:1070–1072.
20. Bader AM, Datta S, Moller RA, et al. Acute progesterone treatment has no effect on bupivacaine-induced conduction blockade in the isolated rabbit vagus nerve. Anesth Analg 1990;71:545–548.
21. Malmqvist L-A, Bengtsson M, Björnsson L et al. Sympathetic activity and haemodynamic variables during spinal analgesia in man. Acta Anaesthesiol Scand 1987;31:467–473.
22. Cook PR, Malmqvist L-A, Bengtsson M, et al. Vagal and sympathetic activity during spinal analgesia. Acta Anaesthesiol Scand 1990;34:271–275.
23. Tarkkila PJ, Isola J. Identification of patients in high risk of hypotension, bradycardia and nausea during spinal anesthesia with a regression model of separate risk factors. Acta Anaesthiol Scand 1992;36:554–558.
24. Mackey DC, Carpenter RC, Thompson GE, et al. Bradycardia and asystole during spinal anesthesia: a report of three cases without mortality. Anesthesiology 1989;70:866–868.
25. Leynardier F. Les accidents des anesthetiques locaux. Rev Prat Med Gen 1991;5: 1081–1086.
26. Kreutz JM, Mazuzan JE. Sudden asystole in a marathon runner: the athletic heart syndrome and its anesthetic implications. Anesthesiology 1990;73:1266–1268.
27. Corke BC, Datta S, Ostheimer GW, et al. Spinal anaesthesia for caesarean section. The influence of hypotension on neonatal outcome. Anaesthesia 1982;37:658–662.
28. Bhagwanjee S, Rocke DA, Rout CC, et al. Prevention of hypotension following spinal anesthesia for elective caesarean section by wrapping of the legs. Br J Anaesth 1990; 65:819–822.

29. Coe AJ, Revanäs B. Is crystalloid preloading useful in spinal anaesthesia in the elderly? Anaesthesia 1990;45:241–243.
30. Jouppila P, Jouppila R, Barinoff T, et al. Placental blood flow during cesarean section performed under subarachnoid blockade. Br J Anaesth 1984;56:1379–1383.
31. Auroy Y, Narchi P, Messiah A, et al. Serious complications related to regional anesthesia. Results of a prospective study in France. Anesthesiology 1997;87:479–486.
32. Auroy Y, Benhamou D, Bargues L, et al. Major complications of regional anesthesia in France: The SOS Regional Anesthesia Hotline Service. Anesthesiology 2002;97: 1274–1280.
33. Kopp SL, Horlocker TT, Warner ME, et al. Cardiac arrest during neuraxial anesthesia: frequency and predisposing factors associated with survival. Anesth Analg 2005;100: 855–865.
34. Caplan RA, Ward RJ, Posner K, et al. Unexpected cardiac arrest during spinal anesthesia. A closed claim analysis of predispositive factors. Anesthesiology 1988;68:5–11.
35. Tammela T, Kontturi M, Lukkarinen O. Postoperative urinary retention. I. Incidence and predisposing factors. Scand J Urol Nephrol 1986;20:197–201.
36. Pertek JP, Haberer JP. Effects of anaesthesia on postoperative micturition and urinary retention [French]. Ann Fr Anesth Reanim 1995;14:340–351.
37. Lanz E, Grab BM. Micturition disorders following spinal anaesthesia of different durations of action (lidocaine 2% versus bupivacaine 0.5%) [German]. Anaesthetist 1992;41: 231–234.
38. Axelsson K, Möllefors K, Olsson JO, et al. Bladder function in spinal anaesthesia. Acta Anaesthesiol Scand 1985;29:315–321.
39. Kuusniemi KS, Pihlajamäki KK, Pitkänen MT, et al. The use of bupivacaine and fentanyl for spinal anesthesia for urologic surgery. Anesth Analg 2000;91:1452–1456.
40. Korhonen AM, Valanne JV, Jokela RM, et al. Intrathecal hyperbaric bupivacaine 3 mg + fentanyl 10 μg for outpatient knee arthroscopy with tourniquet. Acta Anaesthesiol Scand 2003;47:342–346.
41. Jankowski CJ, Hebl JR, Stuart MJ, et al. A comparison of psoas compartment block and spinal and general anesthesia for outpatient knee arthroscopy. Anesth Analg 2003;97: 1003–1009.
42. Renck H. Neurological complications of central nerve blocks. Acta Anaesthesiol Scand 1995;39:859–868.
43. Horlocker T, McGregor DG, Matsushige DK, et al. A retrospective review of 4767 consecutive spinal anesthetics. Central nervous system complications. Anesth Analg 1997;84: 578–584.
44. Cousins MJ, Bromage PR. Epidural neural blockade. In: Cousins MJ, Bridenbaugh PO, eds. Neural Blockade. 2nd ed. Philadelphia: JB Lippincott; 1988:253.
45. Hampl K, Schneider M, Ummenhofer W, et al. Transient neurologic symptoms after spinal anesthesia. Anesth Analg 1995;81:1148–1153.
46. Hampl K, Schneider M, Thorin D, et al. Hyperosmolarity does not contribute to transient radicular irritation after spinal anesthesia with hyperbaric 5% lidocaine. Reg Anesth 1995; 20:363–368.
47. Hampl K, Schneider M, Pargger H, et al. Transient neurologic symptoms after spinal anesthesia with 2% and 5% lidocaine. Anesth Analg 1996;83:1051–1054.
48. Sakura S, Sumi M, Sakaguchi Y, et al. The addition of phenylephrine contributes to the development of transient neurologic symptoms after spinal anesthesia with 0.5% tetracaine. Anesthesiology 1997;87:771–778.
49. Hiller A, Rosenberg PH. Transient neurological symptoms after spinal anaesthesia with 4% mepivacaine and 0.5% bupivacaine. Br J Anaesth 1997;79:301–305.
50. Horlocker TT, Wedel DJ, Benzon H, et al. Regional anesthesia in the anticoagulated patient: defining the risks. Reg Anesth Pain Med 2004;29:S1–S11.
51. Dahlgren N, Törnebrandt K. Neurological complications after anaesthesia. A follow-up of 18,000 spinal and epidural anaesthetics performed over three years. Acta Anaesthesiol Scand 1995;39:872–880.
52. Phillips OC, Ebner H, Nelson AT, et al. Neurologic complications following spinal anesthesia with lidocaine: a prospective review of 10,440 cases. Anesthesiology 1969;30: 284–289.
53. Rigler ML, Drasner K, Krejcie T, et al. Cauda equina syndrome after continuous spinal anesthesia. Anesth Analg 1991;72:275–281.

54. Schneider M, Ettlin T, Kaufmann M, et al. Transient neurologic toxicity after hyperbaric subarachnoid anesthesia with 5% lidocaine. Anesth Analg 1993;76:1154–1157.
55. Tarkkila P, Huhtala J, Tuominen M. Transient radicular irritation after spinal anaesthesia with hyperbaric 5% lignocaine. Br J Anaesth 1995;74:328–329.
56. Beardsley D, Holman S, Gantt R, et al. Transient neurologic deficit after spinal anesthesia: local anesthetic maldistribution with pencil point needles? Anesth Analg 1995;81: 314–320.
57. Pinczower GR, Chadwick HS, Woodland R, et al. Bilateral leg pain following lidocaine spinal anaesthesia. Can J Anaesth 1995;42:217–220.
58. Rodriguez-Chinchilla R, Rodriguez-Pont A, Pintanel T, et al. Bilateral severe pain at L3-4 after spinal anaesthesia with hyperbaric 5% lignocaine. Br J Anaesth 1996;76:328–329.
59. Pollock JE, Neal JM, Stephenson CA, et al. Prospective study of the incidence of transient radicular irritation in patients undergoing spinal anesthesia. Anesthesiology 1996;84: 1361–1367.
60. Carpenter RL. Hyperbaric lidocaine spinal anesthesia: do we need an alternative? [editorial] Anesth Analg 1995;81:1125–1128.
61. Freedman JM, Li D, Drasner K, et al. Transient neurologic symptoms after spinal anesthesia. An epidemiologic study of 1863 patients. Anesthesiology 1998;89:633–641.
62. Lindh A, Andersson AS, Westman L. Is transient lumbar pain after spinal anaesthesia with lidocaine influenced by early mobilisation? Acta Anaesthesiol Scand 2001;45: 290–293.
63. Silvanto M, Tarkkila P, Mäkela ML, et al. The influence of ambulation time on the incidence of transient neurologic symptoms after lidocaine spinal anesthesia. Anesth Analg 2004;98:642–646.
64. Zaric D, Christiansen C, Pace NL, et al. Transient neurologic symptoms after spinal anesthesia with lidocaine versus other local anesthetics: a systematic review of randomized, controlled trials. Anesth Analg 2005;100:1811–1816.
65. Lambert LA, Lambert DH, Strichartz GR. Irreversible conduction block in isolated nerve by high concentrations of local anesthetics. Anesthesiology 1994;80:1082–1093.
66. Bainton C, Strichartz GR. Concentration dependence of lidocaine-induced irreversible conduction loss in frog nerve. Anesthesiology 1994;81:657–667.
67. Tarkkila P, Huhtala J, Tuominen M, Lindgren L. Transient radicular irritation after bupivacaine spinal anesthesia. Reg Anesth 1996;21:26–29.
68. Greene N. Distribution of local anesthetic solutions within the subarachnoid space. Anesth Analg 1985;64:715–730.
69. Hirabayashi Y, Shimizu R, Saitoh K, et al. Anatomical configuration of the spinal column in the supine position. I. A study using magnetic resonance imaging. Br J Anaesth 1995; 75:3–5.
70. Gerancher J. Cauda equina syndrome following a single spinal administration of 5% hyperbaric lidocaine through a 25-gauge Whitacre needle. Anesthesiology 1997;87: 687–689.
71. Kozody R, Palahniuk RJ, Cumming MO. Spinal cord blood flow following subarachnoid tetracaine. Can J Anaesth 1985;32:23–29.
72. Kozody R, Swartz J, Palahniuk RJ, et al. Spinal cord blood flow following sub-arachnoid lidocaine. Can J Anaesth 1985;32:472–478.
73. Kozody R, Ong B, Palahniuk RJ, et al. Subarachnoid bupivacaine decreases spinal cord blood flow in dogs. Can J Anaesth 1985;32:216–222.
74. Hashimoto K, Nakamura Y, Hampl KF, et al. Epinephrine increases the neurologic potential of intrathecally administered local anesthetic in the rat [abstract]. Anesthesiology 1996;85:A770.
75. Avidan A, Gomori M, Davidson E. Nerve root inflammation demonstrated by magnetic resonance imaging in a patient with transient neurologic symptoms after intrathecal injection of lidocaine. Anesthesiology 2002;97:257–258.
76. Sakura S, Chan VWS, Ciriales R, et al. The addition of 7.5% glucose does not alter the neurotoxicity of 5% lidocaine administered intrathecally in the rat. Anesthesiology 1995; 82:236–240.
77. Sakura S, Bollen AW, Ciriales R, et al. Local anesthetic neurotoxicity does not result from blockade of voltage-gated sodium channels. Anesth Analg 1995;81:338–346.
78. Drasner K. Lidocaine spinal anesthesia: a vanishing therapeutic index? Anesthesiology 1997;87:469–472.

79. de Jong R. Last round for a "heavyweight"? [editorial] Anesth Analg 1994;78:3–4.
80. Flaatten H, Felthaus J, Larsen R, et al. Postural post-dural puncture headache after spinal and epidural anaesthesia. A randomised, double-blind study. Acta Anaesthesiol Scand 1998;42:759–764.
81. Santanen U, Rautoma P, Luurila H, et al. Comparison of 27-gauge (0.41-mm) Whitacre and Quincke spinal needles with respect to post-dural puncture headache and non-dural puncture headache. Acta Anaesthesiol Scand 2004;48:474–479.
82. Reina MA, de Leon-Casasola OA, Lopez A, et al. An in vitro study of dural lesions produced by 25-gauge Quincke and Whitacre needles evaluated by scanning electron microscopy. Reg Anesth Pain Med 2000;25:393–402.
83. Lybecker H, Moller JT, May O, et al. Incidence and prediction of postdural puncture headache. A prospective study of 1021 spinal anesthesias. Anesth Analg 1990;70:389–394.
84. Kaukinen S, Kaukinen L, Kannisto K, et al. The prevention of headache following spinal anesthesia. Ann Chir Gynaecol 1981;70:107–111.
85. Loeser EA, Hill GE, Bennet GM, et al. Time vs. success rate for epidural blood patch. Anesthesiology 1978;49:147–148.
86. Vakharia SB, Thomas PS, Rosenbaum AE, et al. Magnetic resonance imaging of cerebrospinal fluid leak and tamponade effect of blood patch in postdural puncture headache. Anesth Analg 1997;84:585–590.
87. Gormley JB. Treatment of post spinal headache. Anesthesiology 1960;21:565–566.
88. Szeinfeld M, Ihmeidan IH, Moser MM, et al. Epidural blood patch: evaluation of the volume and spread of blood injected into epidural space. Anesthesiology 1986;64:820–822.
89. Standl T, Beck H. Radiological examination of the intrathecal position of the microcatheters in continuous spinal anaesthesia. Br J Anaesth 1993;71:803–806.
90. Gosch UW, Hueppe M, Hallschmid M, et al. Post-dural puncture headache in young adults: comparison of two small-gauge spinal catheters with different needle design. Br J Anaesth 2005;94:657–661.
91. Hullander M, Leivers D. Spinal cutaneous fistula following continuous spinal anesthesia. Anesthesiology 1992;76:139–140.
92. Puolakka R, Pitkänen MT, Rosenberg PH. Comparison of three catheter sets for continuous spinal anesthesia in patients undergoing total hip or knee arthroplasty. Reg Anesth Pain Med 2000;25:584–590.
93. Kasai T, Yaegashi K, Hirose M, et al. Aseptic meningitis during combined continuous spinal and epidural analgesia. Acta Anaesthesiol Scand 2003;47:775–776.

# 10 Complications of Epidural Blockade

Ciaran Twomey and Ban C.H. Tsui

Epidural anesthesia was first reported by Sicard and Cathelin in France, in 1901.[1] Whereas continuous techniques were pioneered by Hingson et al.[2] and Tuohy,[3] Dawkins[4] and Bromage[5] established lumbar epidural anesthesia as the gold standard for the management of labor pain. As these techniques evolved, undesirable effects became apparent; those that were repeatedly seen were judged to be side effects of the technique, and were accepted as an expected and predictable part of practice. Less common, more serious outcomes may be considered complications; these events may result in significant morbidity or mortality if left unchecked. Anesthesiologists should take great care to identify those patients at risk of developing serious complications, and must make risk–benefit evaluations in determining the suitability of a particular technique. In some cases in which the absolute risk may be difficult to quantify, and the outcome may be potentially catastrophic, the practitioner may exclude an entire subset of the patient population (e.g., the anticoagulated patient and the risk of epidural hematoma). There are a multitude of factors that can lead to adverse epidural usage outcomes. Safety in clinical practice is a complex system, which is beyond description within the confines of this paragraph. However, careful patient selection and adherence to established guidelines form the cornerstones of complication prevention.

Recent research has focused on the usage of ultrasound and epidural stimulation techniques to aid accurate placement of the epidural catheter. Although some may consider these new techniques cumbersome or unnecessary, they are valuable teaching tools, and are promising developments that have the potential to improve the success and safety of epidural anesthesia. Time will tell which of these techniques will become widely accepted and, more importantly, will reduce the incidence of epidural complications. This chapter reviews these new relevant developments and focuses on the clinical aspects of epidural complications in terms of their incidence, prevention, and management.

## New Developments in Epidural Placement

### *Ultrasound*

Ultrasound allows the real-time visualization of anatomic structures and offers the potential to guide epidural needle and catheter placement. Ultrasound is useful for guiding peripheral nerve block placement in adult patients;[6,7] however, its application in central neuraxial blockade in adults and children remains limited, and its use is not as yet widespread.

Real-time ultrasound imaging of the lumbar spine is a simple procedure, and there is some evidence that it can aid the placement of lumbar epidural catheters and the performance of combined spinal-epidural anesthesia.[8,9] Ultrasound use improves the learning curve of obstetric lumbar epidural catheter placement for anesthesia trainees.[10] In patients with anticipated difficult epidural localization, it is helpful in estimating lumbar epidural depth, and facilitates ease of placement.[11,12] Although ultrasound imaging has been used to guide lumbar needle placement, it may be of limited value in the thoracic region, particularly in older children and adults when visualization of the spinal cord and relevant structures is sought.[13,14] Calcification of the posterior vertebral bodies in children older than 6 months prevents reliable imaging of the spinal cord.[13] At the present time, ultrasound guidance is helpful in the lumbar region for most patients, whereas its use for thoracic epidural placement is of value only in infants and small children because their vertebrae are not fully ossified.

### *Epidural Stimulation Test*

Whereas peripheral nerve and spinal cord stimulation techniques have been in use for many years, it is only recently that electrical epidural stimulation has been used to confirm and guide catheter placement in the epidural space. The epidural stimulation test confirms epidural catheter placement through stimulation of the spinal nerve roots (not the spinal cord) with a low-amplitude electrical current conducted through normal saline via an electrically conducting catheter.[15] The stimulating catheter setup requires the cathode lead of the nerve stimulator to be connected to the epidural catheter via an electrode adapter, while the anode lead is connected to an electrode on the patient's skin as a grounding site. To avoid misinterpretation of the stimulation response (e.g., local muscle contraction thought to be epidural stimulation), the ground electrode should be placed on the lower extremity for thoracic epidurals and on the upper extremity for lumbar epidurals. Correct placement of the epidural catheter tip (1–2 cm from the nerve roots) is indicated by a motor response elicited with a current between 1–10 mA.[15,16] Any motor response observed with a significantly lower threshold current (<1 mA) may suggest that the catheter is in the subarachnoid or subdural space, or is in close proximity to a nerve root.[17,18] In these rare cases, a motor response is elicited with a significantly lower threshold current because the stimulating catheter may be very close (<1 cm) to the nerve roots or because it may be in direct contact with highly conductive cerebrospinal fluid (CSF).

#### **Safety of Electrical Stimulation**

Electrical stimulation has been applied to neural structures for neurophysiologic evaluation and pain control for many years,[19–23] and has proven to be safe. The safety of the epidural stimulation test is not completely known, but it is anticipated that the risk of a brief intermittent electrical stimulation used in this setting would be lower than the risk of chronic epidural stimulation used in long-term pain management. In addition, epidural stimulation uses milliamperages within the range used for patients with chronic pain disorders (4–30 mA)[24] and for intraoperative monitoring during spinal surgery (2–40 mA).[25–27] Although no known complications or patient discomfort have resulted from the epidural stimulation test, it has been recommended to keep the current below 15 mA and the stimulation time as brief (<minutes) as possible.[15,16,28,29] In particular, the current output must be carefully increased from zero and stopped once motor activity is visible to ensure that all motor responses, even those elicited with low current (<1 mA), are detected. The nerve stimulator must be sensitive to allow a gradual increase in current output to at least 10 mA.

## Clinical Applications

Electrical epidural stimulation is a recently available tool for clinician usage which has significant impact on three of the most hazardous complications associated with epidural use: systemic toxicity, subarachnoid placement, and subdural placement. A comparison of features of the standard test dose (lidocaine with 1:200,000 epinephrine) and the epidural stimulation test is summarized in Table 10-1.

## Systemic Toxicity

It is because inadvertent intravascular catheter placement goes unrecognized that the effects of local anesthetic toxicity are observed. An obstetric study[30] has shown that repeated injections of local anesthetic into a properly placed epidural catheter results in impairment of nerve conduction and requires a gradual increase in the amplitude of electrical current to produce a positive motor response to the stimulation test. Absence of this trend after repeated doses of local anesthetic suggests that the injected local anesthetic may be rapidly disappearing from the epidural space, as is the case with intravascular placement. This hypothesis was confirmed in an obstetric patient who remained uncomfortable, and had no sensory change following significant amounts of local anesthetic (12mL of bupivacaine 0.25% followed by 12mL of bupivacaine 0.125%).[17] Stimulation at 5mA confirmed that the catheter was still in the epidural space, and that there was a minimum amount of local anesthetic present, most likely because it was entering the systemic circulation. This suspicion was confirmed when typical symptoms and signs of intravascular placement (metallic taste and increased heart rate) were observed following a standard test dose. After reinsertion of the epidural catheter, the stimulation test was repeated with a positive response at 5mA. Five minutes after the test dose, a subsequent stimulation test showed a positive response at 8mA; this occurrence suggested nonintravascular epidural placement. Similar observations were confirmed clinically when a patient developed an appropriate sensory block while remaining comfortable. Although there are only a few reported cases of intravascular catheter detection, the epidural stimulation test has the potential to detect intravascular catheter placement, and should not be overlooked.

Table 10-1. Standard Test Dose Versus Epidural Stimulation Test

| Catheter location | Test dose | Epidural stimulation test |
|---|---|---|
| Subarachnoid | Hypotension/total spinal | *Positive unilateral/bilateral motor response (<1mA)* |
| Subdural | ? | *Diffuse motor response in many segments (<1mA)* |
| Epidural space | | |
| Against nerve root | ? | *Unilateral motor response (<1mA)* |
| No intravascular | ? | *Positive motor response (1–10mA), occasionally up to 15mA; threshold current increased after local anesthetic injected* |
| Intravascular | ↑ Heart rate<br>↑ Blood pressure<br>Electrocardiogram changes | *Remain or return to baseline positive motor response (1–10mA) even after local anesthetic injection* |
| Subcutaneous | ? | *Negative response* |

*Source:* Tsui BC, Finucane BT. Epidural stimulator catheter. Tech Reg Anesth Pain Manag 2002; 6:150–154.

### Subarachnoid Placement

Not only do muscle twitches elicited by low-current stimulation detail the position of the catheter in the epidural space, but the threshold current for motor response can also predict intrathecal placement.[15,17,31] When a catheter is situated properly within the epidural space, muscle twitches should be elicited with a current much greater than 1 mA. However, if any motor response is detected at a current less than 1 mA, subarachnoid placement should be suspected; this was confirmed in a patient with positive CSF aspiration through the epidural catheter.[15,32] In this case, bilateral motor responses were seen at a current of 0.4 mA, suggesting close proximity of the catheter tip to the nerves.[15] Another case report describes two confirmed cases of subarachnoid placement with the observation of a low current and bilateral motor response (with 0.2 and 0.3 mA, respectively), which is consistent with this hypothesis.[17] Epidural stimulation is a useful tool to identify subarachnoid catheter placement when uncertainty exists, and may prevent the serious sequelae of local anesthetic drug (including the standard test dose) injection into the subarachnoid space.

### Subdural Placement

Identification of subdural placement using the epidural stimulation test is described.[18] Subdural catheter placement was suspected during a quality-assurance project checking all epidural catheters postoperatively using the stimulation test. A diffuse motor response in the right anterior chest wall, paravertebral muscles, and a bilateral motor response in the legs were observed with 0.3 mA during the epidural stimulation test. Subdural placement was subsequently confirmed radiologically. Similarly, this unusual response with low current (0.3 mA) in an inadvertent subdural placement has also been recently described by Lena and Martin[33] when performing the epidural stimulation test. In this case report, the epidural catheter was confirmed to be in subdural space by computed tomographic scan imaging.

One feature of subdural catheter placement is that fluid injected into this space can spread a considerable distance. The injected fluid is separated from the spinal nerves by the relatively thin arachnoid and pia mater. During the epidural stimulation test described, the electrical impulse was conducted through the injected fluid into the subdural space. Thus, a diffuse motor response involving multiple segments occurs at a low current (<1 mA) when a catheter is in the subdural space. The diffuse spread of injected fluid in the subdural space conducts electricity to multiple nerve roots. Further studies are needed to validate the sensitivity and specificity for detection of subdural placement.

## Complications of Epidural Placement

### *Direct Needle Trauma*

As a needle or catheter is advanced into the epidural space, direct trauma to the spinal cord, the conus medullaris, and spinal nerve roots can occur, resulting in sensory loss, and less frequently a motor deficit. Some patients recover completely, yet the injury may persist in a small minority of patients. The incidence of this complication is very low, and much of the data available to us comes from retrospective sources. In a prospective, multicenter study, Auroy et al.[34] found five cases of radiculopathy following 30,413 epidurals. In each of these patients, pain or paresthesia was noted on needle insertion or drug administration, and the radiculopathy was in the same distribution as the associated paresthesias.

To avoid nerve trauma, careful technique and accurate anatomic knowledge are advised.[35] Whereas epidural placement in the anesthetized child is considered safe, similar placement in the adult population remains controversial. Recent case reports highlight the potential for neurologic trauma when placing an epidural in the anesthetized patient.[36–38] The use of the epidural stimulation catheter allows the pediatric anesthetist to place lumbar or thoracic epidurals from the caudal space, minimizing the risk of needle-mediated nerve injury.[29] When placing an epidural in the awake cooperative adult, needle advancement should be stopped if the patient complains of pain. In most adults, the spinal cord terminates at the L1 vertebral body; however, in some it may terminate above or below this landmark. The ability of the clinician to correctly identify lumbar spinous interspaces has been questioned by Broadbent and coworkers[39] using magnetic resonance imaging. In this study, only 29% of the interspaces were correctly identified, 51% of the time clinicians were at a higher vertebral level than anticipated, and the spinal cord terminated below L1 in 19% of subjects. Oblique lateral entry into the ligamentum flavum may direct the needle into the dural cuff region, resulting in potential nerve trauma with resultant unisegmental paresthesia. This should alert the clinician against persisting with further needle insertion or catheter threading.[40]

Paresthesia associated with spinal cord injury can occur at the time of needle placement but it also has been reported to develop only at the time of injection or secondary to irritation, edema, or hematoma.[41,42] In addition, pain is more common in extraaxial lesions affecting the nerve roots or blood vessels that are innervated by sensory neurons mediating pain.[43] In contrast, because there are no pain receptors within the spinal cord (or the brain), intraaxial lesions may be painless;[43] this allows percutaneous cervical cordotomy to be performed in awake patients.[44,45] During the procedure, the cervical cord is typically punctured multiple times with a 22-gauge needle electrode, and yet the patient generally describes neither pain nor paresthesia.[46] In addition, pain reported from dural puncture is rare in clinical practice. Thus, anesthesiologists should be reminded that they should not simply assume paresthesia will always be reported as a needle encroaches upon the spinal cord. Although electrical stimulation during epidural needle advancement provides an additional monitoring technique,[32,47] there is still no clear evidence that direct thoracic epidural placement can be performed without risk in either awake or anesthetized patients.

The management of postoperative neurologic sequelae requires the cooperation of the anesthetist, surgeon, and neurologist. As well, the advice of the radiologist and neurosurgeon may also be sought. Although it is easy to blame an adverse neurologic outcome on the presence of an epidural, it should be borne in mind that other factors can lead to demonstrable nerve injury. These include undiagnosed preexisting neurologic disorders; ligation of nutrient spinal cord vessels during abdominal surgery; injury to the femoral nerve during pelvic surgery, or to the lateral cutaneous nerve of thigh during retraction close to the inguinal ligament; or, pressure on the fibular head leading to neuropraxia of the lateral popliteal nerve. If an adverse outcome occurs, an attempt to localize the lesion by history and examination should be made. Bilateral symptoms associated with pain should alert one to the possibility of neuraxial pathology. Injury at the nerve roots affects both posterior and anterior rami. Preservation of sensation over the paraspinous muscles suggests a more distal injury. Investigations should include blood cultures and coagulation studies. Immediate magnetic resonance imaging is the gold standard for outruling central lesions. Electromyography can be used to determine the site of injury and the degree of axonal loss, although it can take up to 3 weeks after injury for changes to appear via electromyography.

### *Hematoma*

Epidural hematoma after neuraxial anesthesia is a rare event. Bleeding from an epidural vein may occur on needle or catheter insertion, but it is usually self-limiting. Neurologic symptoms and signs attributable to an epidural hematoma are atypical in the presence of normal coagulation; the true incidence is unknown, but is estimated to occur less than 1 in 150,000 cases of neuraxial anesthesia.[48] Vandermeulen et al.[49]

reviewed 61 case reports between 1906 and 1994 and found that two-thirds of cases had a hemostatic abnormality. Early diagnosis and intervention are essential to preventing any long-term adverse outcomes.

In recent years, new anticoagulant and antiplatelet drugs have been introduced giving rise to new challenges in the management of the anticoagulated patient undergoing neuraxial blockade. The American Society of Regional Anesthesia has released guidelines in response to this evolving shift in medical practice;[48] the following is a summary of these recommendations published in May 2003:

> Subcutaneous deep venous thrombosis prophylaxis with low-dose heparin is not a contraindication to epidural placement. The risk of bleeding may be reduced by delaying heparin administration until after the block. Patients who have had heparin for 4 days or more can develop thrombocytopenia, and should have their platelet count measured before catheter placement or removal. There is no evidence that a "bloody" or difficult epidural placement increases the risk of hematoma development.

Patients receiving preoperative low-molecular-weight heparin (LMWH) should be considered to have an altered coagulation state. Epidural placement should be avoided for 10–12 hours after the last dose. Higher doses such as enoxaparin 1 mg/kg require delays of epidural placement of at least 24 hours. Postoperative dosing with LMWH is safe in the context of an epidural catheter provided a dosing schedule is followed:

1. Twice daily dosing. The first dose of LMWH is administered no earlier than 24 hours postoperatively, and only when surgical hemostasis is established. Indwelling catheters should be removed at least 2 hours before the initiation of LMWH prophylaxis.
2. Single daily dosing. The first LMWH dose should be administered 6–8 hours postoperatively. The second dose should occur no earlier than 24 hours after the first. Catheter removal should occur at least 10–12 hours after the last LMWH dose, and subsequent dosing should be delayed for a further 2 hours.

Warfarin therapy should be stopped 4–5 days before surgery in order to allow factors II, VII, IX, and X to return to normal levels. The use of medications that affect other parts of the clotting cascade further increases the bleeding risk. Catheters should not be removed when the international normalized ratio (INR) is >1.5, and this INR value correlates with factor activity of about 40%. The analgesic regimen should be tailored to allow routine neurologic testing which should continue for 24 hours after catheter removal, and longer than 24 hours if the INR was >1.5 at the time of removal.

Patients taking nonsteroidal antiinflammatory drugs are at no greater risk of developing hematomas following neuraxial blockade. Recommendations for patients taking ticlopidine, clopidogrel, and GP IIb/IIIa antagonists are based on surgical and interventional cardiology/radiology data. Preoperatively, ticlopidine and clopidogrel should be stopped at 14 and 7 days respectively. GP IIb/IIIa antagonists are contraindicated within 4 weeks of surgery. After administration, normal platelet aggregation occurs in 24–48 hours in the case of abciximab, and 4–8 hours in the case of eptifibatide and tirofiban. Close neurologic monitoring is warranted should these drugs be administered within the perioperative period.

There are limited data available on the newer anticoagulants. However, spontaneous intracranial bleeding has been reported with thrombin inhibitor use. There is no information available about the risks of developing a spinal hematoma in patients receiving thrombin inhibitors such as argatroban and the hirudin derivatives. The risks with fondaparinux, a factor Xa inhibitor, are unknown.

Back pain with lower limb weakness and sensory deficit should alert the clinician to the presence of a central compressing lesion. Bowel and bladder incontinence may be an associated finding. Painless evolution of this complication has been reported, and early warning signs may be masked by the administration of local anesthetic via an epidural catheter and the presence of a urinary catheter. Magnetic resonance imaging confirms the diagnosis, and rapid surgical intervention within 12 hours is indicated.

## *Infection*

Epidural abscess formation, although rare, is a serious, potentially devastating complication. Kane's retrospective review of 50,000 epidurals found no case of abscess formation,[50] whereas Moen et al.[51] reported 12 cases from an estimated 250,000 patients following epidural use. Of these, only three were healthy, whereas the others had infection risk factors including diabetes, cancer, alcohol abuse, and steroid use. Six of the patients received their epidural for analgesia following trauma, and of these, five were thoracic epidurals for thoracic trauma. The authors speculated that the overrepresentation of thoracic trauma patients might in part be attributable to a lesser hygienic standard being observed, where placement likely occurred outside the "cleaner" environment of the operating suite.

Local infection at the needle entry site is considered a contraindication to regional anesthesia. Debate continues as to whether systemic or localized infection distal to the entry sight carries significant risk, and the concern is that the catheter may act as a secondary focus for infection. Interestingly, Jakobsen et al.[52] reported no complications in 69 patients who had catheters in situ for an average of 9 days and who required repeated surgery for abscess and infected wounds. Darchy et al.[53] studied 75 intensive care patients who received epidural analgesia for a median of 4 days. Twenty-seven had signs of local inflammation (erythema or local discharge); of these, nine had local (catheter site) infections, and four had epidural catheter infections (local inflammation and positive epidural catheter culture). *Staphylococcus epidermidis* was the most frequently cultured organism found in this study. As a result of the findings, the authors recommended daily catheter site inspection and removal of the catheter when both erythema and local discharge were present.

Although the immunocompromised patient may carry a greater risk of developing infective complications with epidural use, extensive experience with patients who have human immunodeficiency virus (HIV) has countered early fears surrounding regional anesthesia in this population. The routine use of epidural analgesia and anesthesia for these patients is widely practiced. Regional anesthesia is particularly beneficial for the HIV carrier population, because it eliminates delayed metabolism of systemic opioids caused by protease inhibitors.[54] Patients with autoimmune deficiency syndrome (AIDS) often have neurologic manifestations of their disease, and the prevalence of peripheral neuropathy increases as the disease progresses,[55] affecting 2% of those with CD4 counts $>500/mm^3$, and up to 30% among those with AIDS. Attention should be given to assessing the preoperative neurologic status, because this allows the clinician to correctly attribute postblock neurologic sequelae to the true underlying cause.

Factors that contribute to the low incidence of epidural space infections are meticulous aseptic technique, monitoring of the infection site, antibiotic prophylaxis, and bacterial filter use. Although both lidocaine and bupivacaine are bactericidal in high concentration, this property is much reduced at the concentrations frequently used in clinical practice.[56]

Epidural abscess presentation can be variable, but the cardinal signs and symptoms involve back pain with localized tenderness and fever. With the presence of an epidurally induced abscess, a leucocytosis can be expected and may occur several days or months after needle and catheter insertion. After the formation of an epidural abscess, the patient can develop progressive weakness which may lead to paraplegia if untreated. Meningitis may develop if the patient has endured a lumbar puncture in this setting. The most common pathogen involved in abscess formation is *S. aureus*, which should act as a standard for guiding antibiotic treatment until definitive culture results are available. As with an epidural hematoma, prompt surgical consultation is warranted for abscess development.

In pediatric patients, there is some concern regarding catheter infection with prolonged use of caudally placed catheters, because of the proximity of the sacral hiatus to the rectum. Although studies have not found clinical evidence of greater infection rates with the caudal approach to catheter placement, bacterial colonization has been reported to be increased with this technique. *S. epidermidis* was the predominant microorganism colonized on the skin and catheters of lumbar and caudal epidurals; gram-negative bacteria were also found on the tips of the caudal catheter.[57] Although the overall infection rate associated with caudal epidural catheters seems to be quite low, tunneling caudal catheters or simply fixing the catheter with occlusive dressing in an immediate cephalad direction has been recommended to reduce the risk of contamination by stool and urine.[29,58]

### *Total Spinal and Subdural Anesthesia*

Total spinal anesthesia occurs when an excessive dose of local anesthetic is injected into the subarachnoid space, usually as a result of accidental delivery of an epidural dose. A high spinal may be seen when a small epidural dose or a large spinal dose of local anesthetic enters the subarachnoid space. Obstetric patients are particularly vulnerable because the engorged epidural venous plexus reduces spinal CSF volume and predisposes this population to cephalad local anesthetic spread. Total spinal anesthesia is rarely seen in the nonobstetric patient, as observed by Dawkins[4] who reported an incidence of 0.2% total spinal anesthesia in 48,000 patients. To prevent total spinal anesthesias from occurring, it is essential to use careful technique when aspiring and the epidural test dose should be utilized; furthermore, subsequent incremental dosing may guard against this complication. The use of electrical stimulation has shown to be a useful and reliable real-time technique to confirm epidural catheter placement[15,28–30,59] (see above).

With a high spinal, the patient may complain of numbness in the hands or have difficulty breathing; if this occurs, the situation can usually be managed with reassurance, careful use of sedation, and treatment of hypotension. Respiratory function should be closely monitored with pulse oximetry and measures of adequate airflow such as the ability to vocalize or to blow out a match (the match test).[60] The potency of sedative agents is increased in the presence of a high spinal,[61–63] and one should be prepared to intervene in the event of serious respiratory compromise. Total spinal anesthesia is a true medical emergency because patients become profoundly hypotensive, apneic, and unconscious with pupillary dilatation. Resuscitation with endotracheal intubation, mechanical ventilation, and vasopressor therapy is frequently required, and recovery may take anywhere between 30 minutes and 3 hours depending on the agent used and dose administration. Cerebrospinal lavage via an epidural catheter being accidentally placed in the subarachnoid space has been used to successfully treat a total spinal in a 14-year-old; in this case, the patient underwent recovery within 30 minutes.[64]

Dawkins[4] also describes a condition referred to as "massive epidural" as being characterized by an extensive block following an epidural injection of local anesthetics which results in apnea after approximately 20 minutes without cardiovascular collapse. The recovery phase after massive epidural seems to be slower than that following total spinal anesthesia. The massive epidural condition is not yet a well-defined entity and there are no reports of this occurrence in recent medical literature; it may be suggested that a "massive epidural" is another example of the subdural spread of local anesthetic drugs.

### *Subdural Injections of Local Anesthetic Drugs*

The subdural space is a potential region between the dura and the arachnoid which extends from the level of the second sacral vertebra up to the floor of the third ventricle; the subdural space differs from the epidural space in that it is both extra- and intracranial. This space envelops the cranial and spinal nerves for a short distance, being widest in the cervical area. The incidence of subdural injections of local anesthetic drugs is reported to range from 0.1% to 0.8%,[65] occurring more frequently after epidural injections;[66] however, it may also be an explanation for the occasional failed spinal anesthesia when pencil-point needles with side apertures are used. The design of a pencil-point needle with side apertures makes it possible for the opening to exist partially in the subarachnoid and the subdural spaces.[67] To determine the diagnosis of a subdural catheter placement, the injection of radio opaque dyes is traditionally used to confirm the placement of the catheter via a typical dye patterning. Furthermore, the epidural stimulation test is a new alternative diagnostic test that may offer an alternative in detecting subdural catheter placement.[18,33]

Subdural injections are more likely to occur in patients who have had previous back surgery or a dural puncture at the same or adjoining interspace. The practice of rotating the Tuohy needle upon entering the epidural space has been implicated as a cause of subdural placement but there are no firm data to support this allegation. Clinically, subdural injection of local anesthetic drugs should be suspected when motor or sensory changes do not follow the expected pattern. Subdural injections result in very slow onset of motor and sensory anesthesia and extensive and/or patchy sensory block.[33] Patients may also complain of respiratory difficulties and may appear obtunded. The degree of cardiovascular depression may vary but hypotension is usually not severe; however, rapid onset of cardiovascular depression with concurrent loss of consciousness can result within 2 minutes, and cardiorespiratory arrest has been reported in the obstetric setting.[68] Treatment resultant of the adverse events present due to subdural injections is very supportive as patients often require intubation, ventilation, and sedation. Post-symptom recovery is normally lengthy in time with estimated recovery time taking up to 6 hours.

### *Systemic Toxicity*

There has been a dramatic decrease in the incidence of systemic toxic reactions to local anesthetics following epidural anesthesia within the past 30 years. Dawkins[4] reported a 0.2% incidence of toxicity in a retrospective analysis of 48,292 cases of epidural anesthesia in 1969; this series included thoracic, lumbar, and sacral epidurals. More recently, Brown et al.[69] reported a 0.01% incidence of toxicity following lumbar epidural anesthesia in a retrospective study of 16,870 cases and a 0.69% incidence of toxicity following caudal epidural anesthesia in a series of 1295 cases. Auroy et al.,[34] in their prospective study of more than 30,000 patients, found a similar incidence of seizure activity of 0.01% following epidural anesthesia. This 20-fold reduction in toxic reactions following epidural anesthesia during the past 30 years is in part explained by significant changes in regional anesthesia practice, and the influence of regional anesthesia societies in North America and Europe. Single-injection epidural techniques, which were frequently implemented 30 years ago, are now rarely used. Spinal anesthesia is the worldwide favored technique for cesarean deliveries. Presently, there is a greater emphasis on using test doses of local anesthetics, and the administration of small incremental doses. The bupivacaine cardiac toxicity problem reported in the early 1980s drew attention to the dangers of rapid injections of large doses of local anesthetics and is a relevant example of the necessity for accuracy when administering test doses. A widespread change in practice after this point is evident in the subsequent findings of Auroy et al.,[34] which failed to associate bupivacaine with cardiac arrests.

Central nervous excitation and cardiovascular manifestations of systemic toxic responses following epidural anesthesia almost always occur as a result of accidental intravascular injections. Local anesthetics are amphiphilic molecules, having both lipophilic and hydrophilic properties. They enter a variety of cellular compartments, and have the potential to interact with a wide variety of molecules including ionotropic signaling pathways (sodium, potassium, and calcium ion channels), and also influence adrenergic and lysophosphatide signaling systems, cardiac bioenergetic, and mitochondrial dynamics.[70]

Before seizures develop resultant of systemic toxicity, the patient may complain of light-headedness, tinnitus, blurred vision, and tongue numbness. With increasing plasma concentrations of local anesthetic, muscle twitching and drowsiness may occur before the onset of generalized tonic-clonic convulsions. The presence of central nervous system (CNS) depressant medication may modify the clinical prodrome of a toxic reaction, masking some of the early warning signs.

The cardiovascular system is more resistant than the CNS to the toxic effects of local anesthetics. Local anesthetics affect both electrical and mechanical cardiac activity. As a toxic cardiovascular system response evolves, tachycardia and hypertension may occur, followed by bradycardia and hypotension.

Early recognition of intravascular injection has been the subject of much interest in the research community. Methods investigated to detect intravascular injection include dye injection detected by pulse oximetry,[71] and epinephrine and isoproterenol administration.[72] Increased heart rate and systolic blood pressure in addition to T wave changes are considered sensitive and specific end points in response to an intravascular injection of a test dose containing epinephrine. A single injection of 15 mg of epinephrine produces a heart rate increase of >10 bpm, a blood pressure increase >15 mmHg, and a decrease in T wave amplitude of 25%.[73] In the sedated patient, changes in heart rate may not be as reliable as T wave and blood pressure changes.[74] Elderly patients and those taking β-blockers are less sensitive to β-adrenergic stimulation.

Incremental administration of the local anesthetic, frequent aspiration, and close observation of heart rate, systolic blood pressure, and T wave changes are sensible precautions that should be undertaken to minimize the impact of accidental intravascular injection. The epidural stimulation test has been used to detect intravascular catheter placement[17] (see above). The advantage of this real-time stimulation test is that intrathecal placement can be ruled out before the administration of a potentially harmful test dose. A test dose of lidocaine and epinephrine should still be administered to detect inadvertent intravascular placement. However, when combined with the epidural stimulation test, the test dose can be given in confidence with a reduced risk of causing a total spinal.

Initial treatment for systemic toxicity is of a supportive nature. Hypoxia, hypercapnia, and acidosis exacerbate bupivacaine toxicity.[75,76] Endotracheal intubation and ventilation to correct acidosis and hypoxia, chest compressions, and cardioversion and defibrillation to restore organ perfusion should be instituted as necessary. Because reduced cardiac contractility is a core element in this condition, it is thought that maintenance of coronary perfusion with the administration of epinephrine and norepinephrine improves outcome.[77] Because epinephrine can exacerbate dysrhythmias, alternative therapeutic avenues that are less dysrhythmogenic have been investigated, including the use of vasopressin[78,79] and phosphodiesterase inhibitors such as milrinone and amrinone.[80] Effective resuscitation in this setting is difficult, and cardiopulmonary bypassing has been successfully used.[81] In the past, bretylium has been advocated as a resuscitation drug in this setting, but because it is no longer manufactured, it has no role in today's modern anesthetic practice. Recent interest has been generated by the reports by Weinberg et al.[82,83] of improved hemodynamics and survival in animal models of bupivacaine toxicity with the administration of intravenous lipid emulsion; however, the mechanism by which this occurs is unclear. In this situation, lipid emulsion may remove local anesthetic molecules from binding sites that are responsible for the profound cardiovascular depression that is part of bupivacaine toxicity. Propofol, which is formulated in lipid, may reduce susceptibility to local anesthetic toxicity, yet its negative inotropic effects may mitigate against its use as an antidote in the face of cardiovascular collapse.[84] Further evaluation needs to be done before either lipid or propofol can become recommended elements of the resuscitation paradigm.

### *Postdural Puncture Headache*

Postdural puncture headache (PDPH) is a widely discussed and published topic in regional anesthesia; it is also one of the most common complications of epidural and spinal anesthesia. This topic is also discussed in some depth in Chapters 9, 13, and 14, however from different perspectives; therefore, we elected to allow this duplication because there are subtle differences in each discussion.

Advances in needle design and gauge as well as a better understanding of the physiologic mechanism of PDPH have dramatically reduced the incidence of PDPH associated with spinal anesthesia, even in the obstetric population.[85] However, the incidence of PDPH following epidural anesthesia in obstetric patients remains unchanged, with headaches ranging from 0% to 2.6% of cases.[85] The incidence of PDPH is also inversely related to the experience of the practitioner, because the more experienced practitioner has better technique, resulting in fewer mistakes made than the recently graduated anesthesiologist who has less clinical experience. The incidence of PDPH has been reported to be as high as 70% when frequently used 16- or 17-gauge Tuohy needles inadvertently puncture through the dura.[85]

The first reference to PDPH came a day after Bier described the first spinal anesthetic in 1898.[86] Hildebrandt and Bier were appropriately jubilant after their important discovery and celebrated with wine and cigars; both men suffered greatly from headaches as a result. The headache Bier experienced was clearly postural in nature; it is likely his headache was caused by CSF leakage. Vandam and Dripps[87] published a report on PDPH in 1956 involving more than 10,000 patients; in this study, the syndrome of PDPH and decreased intracranial pressure were noted by citing the incidence of the various symptoms and signs of headache (11% of patients experiencing complications develop PDPH), ocular disturbances (0.4% of those experiencing PDPH), and auditory difficulties (0.4% of PDPH cases).

Although the actual mechanism causing PDPH is still unclear, a clear relationship is defined regarding the development of PDPH and the loss of CSF. As CSF leaks out, the brain is no longer cushioned and as a result of the leaking CSF, the relative weight of the brain increases, thereby stretching pain-sensitive structures. This explains the postural component to the syndrome, as the headache worsens when the patient is in the upright position. The postural component of the headache is the key feature of PDPH, and the diagnosis should be questioned if such symptoms are absent when diagnosing. The pain of the PDPH is relayed through various nerve endings in the venous sinuses, the dura at the base of the brain, and the dural and cerebral arteries. The typical pain of PDPH is frontal in nature and is relayed through the trigeminal nerve. Traction on the infratentorial structures causes a different set of symptoms including occipital and neck pain and spasming of the cervical muscles; pain experienced during PDPH is relayed mainly through the glossopharyngeal, vagus, and cervical nerves.[88]

Another possible explanation for PDPH is that the loss of CSF produces a compensatory venodilation. The Monroe-Kelly doctrine states that the total volume of the elements of the intracranial cavity (blood, CSF, and brain tissue) remains constant.[85] The consequence of CSF loss is vasodilatation which compensates for the loss of volume within the intracranial cavity. Headache experienced by patients following CSF leak may in part be attributable to intracranial vasodilatation. The beneficial effect of cerebral vasoconstrictor drugs including caffeine, theophylline, and sumatriptan supports a vascular etiology for PDPH.

Visual disturbances occurred in 0.4% of PDPH cases in the study by Vandam and Dripps,[87] in which it was noted that those who received spinal anesthetics developed decreased intracranial pressure. Diplopia is the most common ocular symptom resultant of decreased intracranial pressure and is caused by traction on the abducens nerve (sixth cranial nerve), which has the longest course within the intracranial cavity. Today the incidence of diplopia is probably less than 0.4% of total PDPH cases. Auditory symptoms, attributable to eighth nerve dysfunction, may also occur occasionally, presenting with unilateral or bilateral deafness. The incidence of auditory loss correlates with the size and type of needle used[89,90] and has been documented to be relieved by epidural blood patching.[91] The effect on hearing is resultant of the change in CSF pressure, which is transmitted to circulating endocochlear lymph in the semicircular canals,[92] and results in a temporary condition similar to the hydrops of Ménière's disease. Further associated symptoms of PDPH include dizziness, nausea, and vomiting. Although these symptoms normally resolve with treatment, Wemama et al.[93] have reported a case of permanent unilateral vestibulocochlear dysfunction following spinal anesthesia.

A number of factors are reported to influence the incidence of PDPH, and this information is based on previous clinical case reports and studies; among these factors, there is a strong link between onset of headache and needle gauge, age, gender, pregnancy, bevel design, and bevel orientation. Dura consists of a mixture of elastic collagen and elastin fibers contained in a viscous intercellular ground substance;[94] it is primarily a longitudinally oriented structure, and its greatest tensile strength and stiffness exist in the longitudinal orientation. Dura also has relaxation properties characteristic of viscoelastic materials. When a needle penetrates the dura, the size of the defect will depend on the number of elastin fibers cut, and also on the tendency of those cut fibers to recoil in opposing directions, creating a crescent-shaped defect. As the gauge of the needle increases, more elastic fibers are cut. Fink[95] examined the dura of elderly cadavers and found less viscoelastic material and more fibrous connective tissue. Young patients are at greatest risk of PDPH because their greater dural elasticity maintains a patent defect compared with the less elastic dura of the elderly. Norris et al.[96] demonstrated the importance of bevel orientation in relation to the incidence of PDPH following penetration of the dura with an epidural needle. Lybecker et al.[97] suggested that bevel orientation may be even more important than needle gauge and was unable to show any difference in PDPH when using 22- and 25-gauge needles, provided the bevel was vertically oriented. Ready et al.[98] have suggested that an oblique direction of the needle will reduce the incidence of PDPH. The arachnoid is closely adherent to the dura, and when a needle is advanced perpendicularly, the holes made by the bevel in the dura and arachnoid regions are directly in line with one another. When a needle is directed obliquely, the dural puncture does not line up with that in the arachnoid layer, thus obstructing CSF leakage.

Vandam and Dripps[87] reported that the incidence of PDPH was increased in both pregnant and nonpregnant women as compared with the male patient population. Lybecker and colleagues[97] later found no difference between the incidence of PDPH experienced by males and nonpregnant females. The higher incidence experienced during pregnancy may be explained on the basis of increased intraabdominal pressure. The incidence of PDPH is highest between 18 and 30 years of age, and is least experienced by children younger than 13 years and adults older than 60 years. With the widespread application of epidural anesthesia in obstetric anesthesia, it is not surprising that the obstetric patient is at particular risk of dural puncture and subsequent headache because of their gender and young age.

Gurmarnik[99] has proposed that when povidone-iodine is used as the preparatory solution, it may enter the subarachnoid space in minute quantities and stimulate a chemical reaction, thus limiting CSF leak. Patients with a headache before lumbar puncture, those who have a history of PDPH, and patients who are already dehydrated are more likely to experience PDPH than those who do not fall into these categories.

### Treatment of PDPH

Obviously, the most effective way to treat PDPH is preventing this problem in the first place. The principal factor responsible for the development of PDPH is the size of the dural perforation. Although spinal needles have undergone numerous modifications in recent years, the most common epidural needle used is the 16- or 17-gauge Tuohy needle. It has been suggested that fatigue from sleep deprivation or continuous night work can be a confounding factor in producing the higher incidence of inadvertent dural puncture.

After inadvertent dural puncture with a Tuohy needle during epidural catheter placement, some have suggested that placement of the epidural catheter through the puncture hole may reduce the incidence of PHDH; this has been suggested because catheter punctures cause inflammatory reaction that seals the puncture hole. Because this epidural catheter is in the intrathecal space, extreme caution should be exercised to treat this catheter as a spinal catheter in avoiding possible neurologic complication and infection.[85]

Conservative measures such as bed rest and oral hydration remain popular therapies for PDPH, despite the dearth of evidence to support them. Bed rest may postpone the occurrence of the headache, yet it does not prevent the onset.[100] Obstetric patients should be encouraged to mobilize soon after delivery, so that PDPH, if present, can be diagnosed and treated while in the hospital. Intrathecal placement of the epidural catheter following accidental dural puncture in the obstetric setting is common practice in some centers.[101] It is thought that the presence of the epidural catheter generates an inflammatory response, leading to early closure of the dural defect.[102]

Mild headaches may be treated with intravenous fluids, caffeine, and theophylline; methylxanthines may block cerebral adenosine receptors that lead to cerebral vasoconstriction. Camann et al.[103] demonstrated the efficacy of caffeine in 40 postpartum patients. A single oral dose of caffeine is safe, less expensive than intravenous caffeine, and offers temporary relief. Caffeine is a potent CNS stimulant and should be avoided in women who have pregnancy-induced hypertension, because it may lower the seizure threshold.[104] When considering the use of caffeine as treatment for mild headache, it is of worth to realize that the cerebral vasoconstrictive properties of caffeine are transient, and the headache may return after 48 hours.

Sumatriptan is a serotonin type 1-d receptor agonist, and has been used for cluster headaches and migraine; as well, it has been used to successfully treat PDPH.[105] Cosyntropin, the synthetic form of adrenocorticotropic hormone, has been used for treating PDPH; this pharmaceutical is thought to work by stimulating CSF production and β-endorphin output.[106]

### Epidural Blood Patch

The epidural blood patch (EBP) was introduced by Gormley[107] in 1960 and is known to be the most effective treatment for PDPH. Gormley observed that patients who bled during myelography had a lower incidence of PDPH, and when he himself subsequently developed PDPH, Gormley requested an injection of autologous blood into his epidural space with the positive result of alleviation of his headache. In 1970, DiGiovanni and Dunbar's[108] report of the successful use of epidural blood patching in 41 of 45 patients led to its popularization. This form of treatment is indicated when conservative measures have failed, the headache is severe, or it is likely to extend the hospital stay. The success rate for a first EBP is 85%, and 98% after a second patching.

DiGiovanni et al.[109] suggested that epidural blood patching acts as a gelatinous tamponade, and when injected, the blood generates sufficient pressure to lift the brain; these authors have suggested that blood acts as a sealant, plugging the hole created by the needle, thus preventing further CSF leakage. Magnetic resonance images displaying the lumbar region after blood patching show a mass effect that compresses the thecal sac and conus. The blood spreads 3–5 spinal segments from the injection site, mostly in the cephalad direction. The mass effect persists beyond 3 hours, and clot resolution occurs in 7 hours.[110] Symptoms are frequently relieved within minutes of the procedure, and this response supports the counter pressure theory.

Szeinfeld et al.[111] studied the dynamics of an epidural injection of blood using tagged red cells. Blood was injected into the lumbar region until patients complained of discomfort in the back, buttocks, or legs. The mean volume of blood required to result in this lower physical discomfort was 14.8 mL; this study demonstrated that the blood injectate extended over nine segments, in which six were in the cephalad direction, and three in the caudad direction.

When performing an EBP, great care should be taken to maintain a sterile field, and the epidural space should be identified in the usual manner. To undergo EBP, an assistant draws 15–20 mL of autologous blood aseptically, which should be analyzed for cultures. The administration of blood should be done at a rate of 1 mL/3 seconds. The end point of injection occurs when the patient complains of back, neck, or buttock pain. Much less blood is required for blood patching in the midthoracic region than in the lumbar region, usually in the order of 5–10 mL. To ensure adequate healing, the patient should remain recumbent for 1–2 hours after a blood patch and may resume ambulation thereafter; the patient should refrain from any strenuous activity for several days.

Complications from EBP are rare, but can be serious. Transient bradycardia, lumbovertebral syndrome, and facial palsy have been reported.[112–115] One case of cauda equina syndrome has been reported in a patient who was subjected to six blood patches; the patient made a full recovery following evacuation.[116]

EBP has also been successfully performed in children. A caudal blood patch has been performed in a 4-year-old child[117] and a lumbar EBP has been performed in a 7-year-old child.[118] The case reported by Kowbel et al.[117] involved a 4-year-old who developed a subarachnoid cutaneous fistula following repeated lumbar punctures for chemotherapy. In this situation, the epidural blood patching was performed by passing an epidural catheter via the caudal canal, and by injecting 8 mL of blood. Furthermore, there has been one case reported of cervical dural puncture treated successfully with a lumbar epidural blood patch.[119]

Blood patches have been safely performed in HIV-positive patients. HIV crosses the blood-brain barrier and infects the CNS early in the clinical course. EBP is unlikely to introduce HIV into the CNS.[100]

### Prophylactic EBP

Prophylactic blood patching is controversial and has supporters and detractors.[120,121] The effectiveness of using EBP as a prophylactic depends on the proximity of the catheter tip to the dural tear. Although blood patching is a relatively safe procedure, there are some risks associated with its use, and patients do not always get a headache following dural puncture, even with a large-gauge needle. Aldrete and Brown[122] describe a case of intrathecal hematoma and arachnoiditis after prophylactic blood patching through a catheter.

### Variations on the EBP

Epidural saline treatment has been used for PDPH, but is less effective than EBP. Successful use of prolonged saline infusion has been reported in patients with failed EBP.[123,124] Fibrin glue, a pooled plasma product, has been used to treat CSF leak in cancer patients,[125] and also in PDPH cases following spinal anesthesia in which two EBPs had failed.[126] Dextran-40 has also been used to treat PDPH because it undergoes delayed absorption from the epidural space because of its high viscosity and molecular weight.[127]

## Side Effects of Epidural Placement

### *Hypotension*

Hypotension is a common physiologic change associated with neuraxial blockade. Its presence predicts block success, but as a side effect, if left untreated or poorly managed, hypotension can lead to serious morbidity or death. Hypotension results from preganglionic sympathetic blockading, and leads to a reduction in systemic vascular resistance and cardiac output. Systemic vascular resistance decreases as a result of a reduction in sympathetic tone, the extent of which is related to the number of spinal segments blocked. Cardiac output is altered by changes in heart rate and stroke volume. The reduction in stroke volume is the result of a decrease in preload and contractility, which is load dependent. If the block involves the cardiac sympathetic nerve supply, bradycardia and reduced contractility can be expected.

Epidural placement for analgesia with concurrent administration of general anesthesia is a commonplace technique used in anesthesiology; however, concern exists regarding the chance that the combined cardiovascular depressive effects of the epidural and the general anesthetic may predispose the patient to an adverse outcome. Borghi et al.[128] evaluated the frequency of hypotension and bradycardia during general anesthesia, combined epidural–general anesthesia, and in epidural anesthesia alone in a population of 210 patients undergoing hip arthroplasty. In this study, hypotension was observed in 18% of patients during the induction of the epidural block. The induction of general anesthesia in the presence of an epidural block was associated with a fourfold increase in the odds of developing hypotension compared with general anesthesia without an epidural, and a twofold increase in these odds when compared with epidural anesthesia alone. One criticism of this study is that the local anesthetic dose administered was the same whether the patient received a general anesthetic or not. Many practitioners would discriminate between epidural analgesia with general anesthesia and epidural anesthesia, and would adjust the dosing regimen accordingly.

High thoracic epidural anesthesia has the potential to block cardiac afferent and efferent fibers which originate at the first to fifth thoracic levels. Interest has evolved concerning the potential positive effects of cardiac sympathetic blockade in patients with coronary artery disease – dilation of coronary vessels, reduced heart rate, and decreased myocardial oxygen demand.[129]

The presence of hypotension prompts the clinician to intervene with fluid or pressor administration in order to restore the systemic blood pressure to acceptable levels. Wright and Fee[130] examined the effect of prophylactic administration of intravenous fluid, ephedrine, and methoxamine on cardiovascular responses to both epidural and combined epidural and general isoflurane anesthesia in 45 adult patients undergoing knee arthroplasty. Systolic blood pressure was significantly greater after ephedrine administration than after fluid preloading or methoxamine administration. An increase in plasma volume triggered by epidural-induced hypotension has been observed, with movement from the interstitial to the intravascular space.[131] A larger percentage of fluid administered is retained by hypotensive than normotensive patients[132], resulting in hemodilution. Holte et al.'s[133] recent study showed that it was not the epidural that leads to changes in blood volume, but rather the infusion of fluid that affects blood volume. Hydroxyethyl starch and ephedrine have similar hemodynamic effects and may be the preferred option for patients in whom excess fluid administration is undesirable.

Significant changes in blood pressure are uncommon in pediatric patients after the proper administration of epidural analgesia (Chapter 13). A high sympathetic single-shot caudal block to T6 caused no significant changes in heart rate, cardiac index, or blood pressure in children.[134,135] Even when thoracic epidural blockade is combined with general anesthesia, cardiovascular stability is usually maintained in otherwise healthy pediatric patients. Hypotension should prompt anesthesiologists to immediately rule out a total spinal and/or intravascular injection leading to local anesthetic toxicity and cardiovascular collapse.

### Respiratory Complications

Several studies have examined high thoracic epidurals in both healthy people and in those with chronic obstructive airway disease. Peak expiratory flows, forced vital capacity, forced expiratory volume in 1 second, and maximum expiratory pressures are reduced[136,137] in those with this disorder. Kochi et al.[138] investigated the effect of high thoracic epidural anesthesia on the hypercapnic ventilatory response and ventilation pattern. Duration of inspiration, rib cage excursion and its contribution to tidal volume decreased significantly, whereas mean inspiratory flow rate and minute ventilation increased; end-tidal $P_{CO_2}$ and the tidal excursion of the abdomen were unchanged, and hypercapnic ventilatory response decreased significantly. Lumbar and high thoracic region–induced epidurals do not interfere with the ventilatory response to hypoxemia.[139] Gruber et al.[140] demonstrated the safety of thoracic epidural anesthesia with bupivacaine 0.25% in patients with severe chronic obstructive pulmonary disease. The potential for phrenic (C3–C5) palsy is low with an epidural block, except during inadvertent blockade following an interscalene brachial plexus block.[141]

Cervical epidural anesthesia has been used for upper limb, parathyroid, and carotid surgeries.[142–144] Bonnet et al.[142] reported respiratory difficulties in 3 of 394 patients undergoing carotid endarterectomy using 15 mL 0.5% bupivacaine or 0.37%–0.40% bupivacaine plus fentanyl (50–100 μg). Many case series, although smaller in number than this study published by Bonnet et al., have not reported respiratory difficulties to be a significant problem.[143,144] Capdevila et al.[145] reported that both 0.25% and 0.375% cervical epidural bupivacaine impaired diaphragmatic excursion, tidal volume, forced vital capacity, and hand grip strength in patients having postoperative hand rehabilitation, and did not recommend the technique for this purpose.

### Failure of Epidural Anesthesia

Anesthesiologists recognize entry into the subarachnoid space by the tactile sensation produced and the visual element of inserting the epidural catheter. Entry into the epidural space is purely tactile, and the end point of entry is subject to misinterpretation. There are false losses of resistance, and quite often the only proof that the needle was correctly positioned is that the resulting block is effective. False losses of resistance are more frequently encountered in obese patients in whom anatomy may be ill defined. Sharrock[146] has suggested that false loss of resistance may also occur in the elderly who have a high incidence of cyst formation within the interspinous ligaments.

The introduction of a catheter into the epidural space introduces an additional number of reasons for the failure of epidural anesthesia. The inability to pass a catheter into the epidural space frequently indicates that the needle is not in the epidural space. Catheters may become occluded with blood, or the catheter may kink, take a unilateral course, break, or become knotted, all of which can contribute to the failure of epidural anesthesia. The presence of a midline epidural band is well established[147] and may explain why difficulty may be encountered when threading the catheter through the Tuohy needle.

An important distinction that should be made during epidural catheter threading is that of complete failure versus a partial blockade/failure. Epidural local anesthetic dosing for anesthesia may approach the maximum safe limit, preventing significant further administration of local anesthetic. Thus, a failed epidural may prompt the clinician to pursue an alternative course of anesthesia. Matching the dermatomal level of the catheter tip to that of the surgical site will yield greater success. The epidural stimulation catheter has been used in children to verify accurate epidural tip placement,[29] ensuring that the dermatomes involved in the surgical procedure are selectively blocked. Testing minimal doses of local anesthetic is important to consider for maximal analgesic effect.

The partially working epidural is frequently encountered when undergoing anesthesia for cesarean deliveries; reported rates for failure are in the order of 2%–13.1%.[148] A poorly functioning epidural should be identified early before the decision to proceed to cesarean delivery is made. In an emergency situation, the anesthetist has a number of options available to rescue the situation; such options include spinal or general anesthesia, supplemental epidural or caudal injections, and local infiltration anesthesia. Intraoperative discomfort and visceral pain may occur in up to 50% of cesarean patients.[149]

A block to the T4 level is considered optimal in most cesarean patients; however, debate exists concerning the best modality with which to test the upper level of the block. Loss of pinprick and cold sensation are popular testing options, but may have poor predictive value.[150,151] The loss of touch is considered by some to best equate with surgical anesthesia as an effective test.[152]

Surgical factors that increase the likelihood of intraoperative discomfort include exteriorization of the uterus, and round ligament stretching, both of which overcome the analgesia provided during an apparently adequately dense nerve block. Subdiaphragmatic blood or amniotic fluid may cause back, chest, or shoulder discomfort. Intervention by the clinician should involve direct communication to the patient involving reassurance and an explanation of why the patient is experiencing these sensations; as well, pharmacologic management is necessary depending on the patient's level of distress. Intravenous ketamine in 10- to 20-mg increments and small doses of fentanyl or benzodiazepines are considered safe, although some advise waiting to administer these pharmaceuticals until the umbilical cord is clamped.[148] Nitrous oxide has been used in the treatment of patients,[153] but this may be associated with contributing to airway difficulties. If the mentioned rescue efforts fail, general anesthesia should be considered with special attention to preoxygenation and potential airway difficulties.

### *Nausea and Pruritus*

Nausea and pruritus are common side effects seen with the administration of epidural opioids, and have reported incidences of 30%–65% for postoperative nausea and vomiting (PONV)[154–156] and 80% for pruritus.[157] Pruritus is thought to be multifactorial in nature, and is speculated to operate via an "itch center" in the CNS, medullary dorsal horn activation, and antagonism of inhibitory transmitters.[158] Pruritus is a dose-dependent phenomenon, where its onset involves possible mediators including C fibers in the skin, serotonin (5-HT3) receptors, and prostaglandins. The obstetric population seems to be at greater risk for developing pruritus. Antihistamines, opioid antagonists (naloxone and nalbuphine), propofol, nonsteroidal antiinflammatory drugs, and 5-HT3 receptor antagonists have been used as both preventive and therapeutic measures to treat this bothersome condition.

PONV is a complex, multifactorial problem. Epidural administration of local anesthetics alone carries a low risk of causing the occurrence of PONV.[159] Factors including surgery, age, and gender influence the reported incidence of PONV associated with epidural anesthesia.[160] Within 5–15 minutes of epidural administration, peak plasma opioid concentrations can reach levels similar to those seen following an intramuscular injection.[161] In patients receiving epidural morphine, there have been no differences in PONV onset or duration when different doses up to 5 mg were administered,[162] whereas higher doses have been shown to lead to both an increase and a decrease in reported PONV.[160] Epidural fentanyl and meperidine do not seem to influence PONV in the same way that morphine does, as reported where fewer PONV cases have been documented with the use of fentanyl and meperidine after orthopedic surgery when compared with morphine.[163] Dexamethasone has been shown to be a superior antiemetic for PONV-associated epidural morphine when compared with metoclopramide[164] and 5-HT3 receptor antagonists.[165]

### *Urinary Retention*

Postoperative urinary retention (POUR) is common after major surgery with a reported incidence of 20%–68% after abdominoperineal resection, 16%–80% after radical hysterectomy, 20%–25% after anterior resection, and 10%–20% after proctocolectomy.[166] POUR is a multifactorial problem and involves elements including age, pain, bladder outlet obstruction, detrusor-inhibiting medication, pelvic autonomic nerve damage, and inhibition of sympathetic reflexes. A single episode of bladder overdistention can result in significant POUR morbidity. Overfilling of the bladder can stretch and damage the detrusor muscle, leading to atony of the bladder wall, so that recovery of micturition may not occur when the bladder is emptied. However, the excessive use of an indwelling catheter can lead to urinary tract infection, urethral stricture, prolonged hospital stay, or death.[167,168]

Epidural use for postoperative pain management is usually reserved for patients undergoing major surgery, where urinary catheter placement may be performed for reasons other than anticipated postoperative urinary retention. Stenseth and colleagues[169] found an incidence of 42% for POUR in 1085 uncatheterized patients having epidural morphine for a variety of major surgeries. Epidural morphine relaxes the detrusor muscle with a corresponding increase in the maximal bladder capacity; epidurally injecting morphine gives a localized effect, whereas intramuscular and intravenous morphine have no effect on detrusor contraction. This is further supported by the fact that detrusor changes occur 15–30 minutes after epidural morphine administration, and are reversed by intravenous naloxone, suggesting that spinal opioid receptors have an important role.[170] Other epidural opioids such as fentanyl, meperidine, and methadone may also contribute to POUR, but contribute to a lesser degree than that observed with morphine.[163,171]

In addition to bladder catheterization, treatment options for opioid-mediated POUR may include intravenous naloxone administration.[172] Nalbuphine is an opioid mixed agonist/antagonist and has been used to restore detrusor function without reversing the analgesic effects of epidural morphine.[173] Short-term (24 hours) urinary catheterization for major surgery involving morphine epidural analgesia may help prevent the morbidities associated with both POUR, and longer-term catheterization.[174]

### *Backache*

Backache is a common complaint following epidural anesthesia and its incidence ranges between 2%–30% of patients.[4,175] The causal relationship between epidural anesthesia and backache has been suggested by some studies,[176,177] and refuted by others.[178,179] The etiology of backache is multifactorial in nature; drug use, abnormal posture, muscle relaxation, and in obstetric cases, exaggerated lumbar lordosis and the process of undergoing labor have been implicated as causes.[100] In a retrospective study, MacArthur and colleagues[176] looked at 11,701 parturients; of the 1634 women who reported backache, 1132 (69%) had experienced it for more than 1 year. In this study, a significant association was found between backache and epidural anesthesia (relative risk = 1.8); 903 of 4766 women (18.9%) who had had epidural anesthesia reported this symptom, compared with 731 of the 6935 women (10.5%) who had not undergone epidural anesthesia. However, prospective data refute the findings of MacArthur et al., as noted by Breen et al.[178], who interviewed 1185 women and found that of the 1042 (88%) for which follow-up data were available, the incidence of postpartum back pain in those who received epidural anesthesia was equivalent to those who did not (44% versus 45%). Multiple logistic regression revealed that postpartum back pain was associated with a history of back pain, younger age, and greater weight. Russell[151] demonstrated that newly onset postpartum back pain is not associated with regional anesthesia. Among the women in Russell's study who received either 0.125% bupivacaine or 0.0625% bupivacaine, the incidence of new long-term back pain was 7.6% when compared with controls, and there was no difference found between the groups. Women seeking analgesia for labor should be reassured that back pain following epidural analgesia is minimal and is usually limited to the early postpartum period.

In 1987, 2-chloroprocaine was marketed by Astra Zeneca in a new formulation (Nesacaine-MPF) involving disodium ethylenediaminetetraacetic acid (EDTA) as a chelating agent, for epidural and caudal use. Reports linking this new formulation with backache emerged,[180,181] and gave way to a possible explanation that the EDTA could cause hypocalcemic tetany of the paraspinous muscles. The drug now comes preservative-free, and is bottled in dark-glass bottles to prevent light-induced disintegration. Despite the elimination of EDTA from this pharmaceutical, backache continues to be reported with its use.[182]

Backache following epidural placement should not be ignored, because it can be a cardinal symptom of a space-occupying lesion within the spinal canal. Complications such as an epidural hematoma and abscess, although rare, can have catastrophic outcomes if unrecognized and untreated.

## Conclusion

Drug delivery via an epidural catheter is a safe and effective method for providing analgesia for lower extremity, abdominal, and thoracic procedures, as well as for managing labor pain. In the perioperative setting, effective pain relief by applying epidural analgesia has numerous benefits, including earlier ambulation, rapid weaning from mechanical ventilation, reduced time spent in a catabolic state, and lowered circulating stress hormone levels.[183] Although serious complications are uncommon, patients should be informed about common side effects, such as urinary retention and pruritus, and should be counseled concerning the risks of major neurologic complication such as paralysis. Newer technologies such as the use of ultrasound and the stimulating epidural catheter may increase the safety and ease of catheter placement. For the individual patient, the risks and benefits of epidural analgesia should be carefully considered, and the Hippocratic axiom "primum non nocere" should be kept in mind.

*Acknowledgments*

The authors thank those who wrote the chapter "Complications of Central Neural Blockade" for the previous edition – Drs. S. Gupta, P. Tarkkila, and B. Finucane – for providing an invaluable template from which this chapter was fashioned.

## References

1. Cathelin F, Sicard J. Discovery of epidural anesthesia. Surv Anesthesiol 1979;23:271.
2. Hingson RA, Ferguson CH, Palmer LA. Advances in spinal anesthesia. Ann Surg 1943; 118:971.
3. Tuohy EB. Continuous spinal anesthesia: a new method utilizing a ureteral catheter. Surg Clin North Am 1945;25:834.
4. Dawkins CJ. An analysis of the complications of extradural and caudal block. Anaesthesia 1969;24:554–563.
5. Bromage PR. Epidural analgesia. In: Bromage PR, ed. Epidural Analgesia. Philadelphia: WB Saunders; 1978:14.

6. Chan VW, Perlas A, Rawson R, Odukoya O. Ultrasound-guided supraclavicular brachial plexus block. Anesth Analg 2003;97:1514–1517.
7. Chan VW. Applying ultrasound imaging to interscalene brachial plexus block. Reg Anesth Pain Med 2003;28:340–343.
8. Grau T, Leipold RW, Conradi R, et al. Efficacy of ultrasound imaging in obstetric epidural anesthesia. J Clin Anesth 2002;14:169–175.
9. Grau T, Leipold RW, Fatehi S, et al. Real-time ultrasonic observation of combined spinal-epidural anaesthesia. Eur J Anaesthesiol 2004;21:25–31.
10. Grau T, Bartusseck E, Conradi R, et al. Ultrasound imaging improves learning curves in obstetric epidural anesthesia: a preliminary study. Can J Anaesth 2003;50:1047–1050.
11. Grau T, Leipold RW, Horter J, et al. Paramedian access to the epidural space: the optimum window for ultrasound imaging. J Clin Anesth 2001;13:213–217.
12. Grau T, Leipold RW, Conradi R, Martin E. Ultrasound control for presumed difficult epidural puncture. Acta Anaesthesiol Scand 2001;45:766–771.
13. Chawathe MS, Jones RM, Gildersleve CD, et al. Detection of epidural catheters with ultrasound in children. Paediatr Anaesth 2003;13:681–684.
14. Chen CP, Tang SF, Hsu TC, et al. Ultrasound guidance in caudal epidural needle placement. Anesthesiology 2004;101:181–184.
15. Tsui BC, Gupta S, Finucane B. Confirmation of epidural catheter placement using nerve stimulation. Can J Anaesth 1998;45:640–644.
16. Tsui BC, Guenther C, Emery D, Finucane B. Determining epidural catheter location using nerve stimulation with radiological confirmation. Reg Anesth Pain Med 2000; 25:306–309.
17. Tsui BC, Gupta S, Finucane B. Detection of subarachnoid and intravascular epidural catheter placement. Can J Anaesth 1999;46:675–678.
18. Tsui BC, Gupta S, Emery D, Finucane B. Detection of subdural placement of epidural catheter using nerve stimulation. Can J Anaesth 2000;47:471–473.
19. Hoppenstein R. Percutaneous implantation of chronic spinal cord electrodes for control of intractable pain: preliminary report. Surg Neurol 1975;4:195–198.
20. Krainick JU, Thoden U, Riechert T. Spinal cord stimulation in post-amputation pain. Surg Neurol 1975;4:167–170.
21. North RB, Kidd DH, Zahurak M, et al. Spinal cord stimulation for chronic, intractable pain: experience over two decades. Neurosurgery 1993;32:384–394.
22. North RB. Spinal cord stimulation for chronic, intractable pain. Adv Neurol 1993;63: 289–301.
23. Richardson RR, Nunez C, Siqueira EB. Histological reaction to percutaneous epidural neurostimulation: initial and long-term results. Med Prog Technol 1979;6:179–184.
24. Sherwood AM. Biomedical engineering aspects of spinal cord stimulation. Appl Neurophysiol 1981;44:126–132.
25. Komanetsky RM, Padberg AM, Lenke LG, et al. Neurogenic motor evoked potentials: a prospective comparison of stimulation methods in spinal deformity surgery. J Spinal Disord 1998;11:21–28.
26. Nagle KJ, Emerson RG, Adams DC, et al. Intraoperative monitoring of motor evoked potentials: a review of 116 cases. Neurology 1996;47:999–1004.
27. Pereon Y, Bernard JM, Fayet G, et al. Usefulness of neurogenic motor evoked potentials for spinal cord monitoring: findings in 112 consecutive patients undergoing surgery for spinal deformity. Electroencephalogr Clin Neurophysiol 1998;108:17–23.
28. Tsui BC, Seal R, Koller J, et al. Thoracic epidural analgesia via the caudal approach in pediatric patients undergoing fundoplication using nerve stimulation guidance. Anesth Analg 2001;93:1152–1155.
29. Tsui BC, Wagner A, Cave D, Kearney R. Thoracic and lumbar epidural analgesia via the caudal approach using electrical stimulation guidance in pediatric patients: a review of 289 patients. Anesthesiology 2004;100:683–689.
30. Tsui BC, Gupta S, Finucane B. Determination of epidural catheter placement using nerve stimulation in obstetric patients. Reg Anesth Pain Med 1999;24:17–23.
31. Tsui BC, Wagner A, Finucane B. The threshold current in the intrathecal space to elicit motor response is lower and does not overlap that in the epidural space: a porcine model. Can J Anaesth 2004;51:690–695.
32. Tsui BC, Wagner AM, Cunningham K, et al. Threshold current of an insulated needle in the intrathecal space in pediatric patients. Anesth Analg 2005;100:662–665.

33. Lena P, Martin R. Subdural placement of an epidural catheter detected by nerve stimulation. Positionnement sous-dural d'un catheter epidural detecte par stimulation nerveuse et confirme par tomographie. Can J Anaesth 2005;52:618–621.
34. Auroy Y, Narchi P, Messiah A, et al. Serious complications related to regional anesthesia: results of a prospective survey in France. Anesthesiology 1997;87:479–486.
35. Wong CA. Neurologic deficits and labor analgesia. Reg Anesth Pain Med 2004;29: 341–351.
36. Bromage PR, Benumof JL. Paraplegia following intracord injection during attempted epidural anesthesia under general anesthesia. Reg Anesth Pain Med 1998;23:104–107.
37. Kao MC, Tsai SK, Tsou MY, et al. Paraplegia after delayed detection of inadvertent spinal cord injury during thoracic epidural catheterization in an anesthetized elderly patient. Anesth Analg 2004;99:580–583.
38. Rose JB. Spinal cord injury in a child after single-shot epidural anesthesia. Anesth Analg 2003;96:3–6.
39. Broadbent CR, Maxwell WB, Ferrie R, et al. Ability of anaesthetists to identify a marked lumbar interspace. Anaesthesia 2000;55:1122–1126.
40. Cousins MJ, Veering BT. Epidural neural blockade. In: Cousins MJ, Bridenbaugh PO, eds. Neural Blockade in Clinical Anesthesia and Management of Pain. 3rd ed. Philadephia: Lippincott-Raven; 1998;243–320.
41. Hamandi K, Mottershead J, Lewis T, et al. Irreversible damage to the spinal cord following spinal anesthesia. Neurology 2002;59:624–626.
42. Simon SL, Abrahams JM, Sean GM, et al. Intramedullary injection of contrast into the cervical spinal cord during cervical myelography: a case report. Spine 2002;27: E274–E277.
43. Kandel ER, Schwartz JH, Jones RM. The perception of pain. In: Kandel ER, Schwartz JH, Jessel TM, eds. Principles of Neural Science. New York: McGraw Hill, Health Professions Division; 2000:472–491.
44. Jackson MB, Pounder D, Price C, et al. Percutaneous cervical cordotomy for the control of pain in patients with pleural mesothelioma. Thorax 1999;54:238–241.
45. Lahuerta J, Bowsher D, Lipton S, Buxton PH. Percutaneous cervical cordotomy: a review of 181 operations on 146 patients with a study on the location of "pain fibers" in the C-2 spinal cord segment of 29 cases. J Neurosurg 1994;80:975–985.
46. Pounder D, Elliott S. An awake patient may not detect spinal cord puncture. Anaesthesia 2000;55:194.
47. Tsui BC, Emery D, Uwiera RR, Finucane B. The use of electrical stimulation to monitor epidural needle advancement in a porcine model. Anesth Analg 2005;100: 1611–1613.
48. Horlocker TT, Wedel DJ, Benzon H, et al. Regional anesthesia in the anticoagulated patient: defining the risks (the second ASRA Consensus Conference on Neuraxial Anesthesia and Anticoagulation). Reg Anesth Pain Med 2003;28:172–197.
49. Vandermeulen EP, Van Aken H, Vermylen J. Anticoagulants and spinal-epidural anesthesia. Anesth Analg 1994;79:1165–1177.
50. Kane RE. Neurologic deficits following epidural or spinal anesthesia. Anesth Analg 1981; 60:150–161.
51. Moen V, Dahlgren N, Irestedt L. Severe neurological complications after central neuraxial blockades in Sweden 1990–1999. Anesthesiology 2004;101:950–959.
52. Jakobsen KB, Christensen MK, Carlsson PS. Extradural anaesthesia for repeated surgical treatment in the presence of infection. Br J Anaesth 1995;75:536–540.
53. Darchy B, Forceville X, Bavoux E, et al. Clinical and bacteriologic survey of epidural analgesia in patients in the intensive care unit. Anesthesiology 1996;85:988–998.
54. Hughes SC. HIV and anesthesia. Anesthesiol Clin North Am 2004;22:379–404.
55. Verma A. Epidemiology and clinical features of HIV-1 associated neuropathies. J Peripher Nerv Syst 2001;6:8–13.
56. Feldman JM, Chapin-Robertson K, Turner J. Do agents used for epidural analgesia have antimicrobial properties? Reg Anesth 1994;19:43–47.
57. Kost-Byerly S, Tobin JR, Greenberg RS, et al. Bacterial colonization and infection rate of continuous epidural catheters in children. Anesth Analg 1998;86:712–716.
58. Bubeck J, Boos K, Krause H, Thies KC. Subcutaneous tunneling of caudal catheters reduces the rate of bacterial colonization to that of lumbar epidural catheters. Anesth Analg 2004;99:689–693.

59. Tsui BC, Bateman K, Bouliane M, Finucane B. Cervical epidural analgesia via a thoracic approach using nerve stimulation guidance in an adult patient undergoing elbow surgery. Reg Anesth Pain Med 2004;29:355–360.
60. Ben-David B, Rawa R. Complications of neuraxial blockade. Anesthesiol Clin North Am 2002;20:669–693.
61. Ben-David B, Vaida S, Gaitini L. The influence of high spinal anesthesia on sensitivity to midazolam sedation. Anesth Analg 1995;81:525–528.
62. Tverskoy M, Shagal M, Finger J, Kissin I. Spinal anesthesia and midazolam hypnotic requirements. Anesth Analg 1996;83:198–199.
63. Tverskoy M, Shifrin V, Finger J, et al. Effect of epidural bupivacaine block on midazolam hypnotic requirements. Reg Anesth 1996;21:209–213.
64. Tsui BC, Malherbe S, Koller J, Aronyk K. Reversal of an unintentional spinal anesthetic by cerebrospinal lavage. Anesth Analg 2004;98:434–436.
65. Lubenow T, Keh-Wong E, Kristof K, et al. Inadvertent subdural injection: a complication of an epidural block. Anesth Analg 1988;67:175–179.
66. Reynolds F, Speedy HM. The subdural space: the third place to go astray. Anaesthesia 1990;45:120–123.
67. Mollmann M, Holst D, Enk D, et al. Subdural intra-arachnoid spread of local anesthetics. A complication of spinal anesthesia [German]. Anaesthesist 1992;41:685–688.
68. Wills JH. Rapid onset of massive subdural anesthesia. Reg Anesth Pain Med 2005;30: 299–302.
69. Brown DL, Ransom DM, Hall JA, et al. Regional anesthesia and local anesthetic-induced systemic toxicity: seizure frequency and accompanying cardiovascular changes. Anesth Analg 1995;81:321–328.
70. Weinberg GL. Current concepts in resuscitation of patients with local anesthetic cardiac toxicity. Reg Anesth Pain Med 2002;27:568–575.
71. Laurito CE, Chen WX. Biological dyes may improve the safety of local anesthetics. J Clin Anesth 1998;10:176–177.
72. Tanaka M, Kimura T, Goyagi T, et al. Evaluating hemodynamic and T wave criteria of simulated intravascular test doses using bupivacaine or isoproterenol in anesthetized children. Anesth Analg 2000;91:567–572.
73. Tanaka M, Nishikawa T. A comparative study of hemodynamic and T-wave criteria for detecting intravascular injection of the test dose (epinephrine) in sevoflurane-anesthetized adults. Anesth Analg 1999;89:32–36.
74. Tanaka M, Sato M, Kimura T, Nishikawa T. The efficacy of simulated intravascular test dose in sedated patients. Anesth Analg 2001;93:1612–1617.
75. Heavner JE, Dryden CF Jr, Sanghani V, et al. Severe hypoxia enhances central nervous system and cardiovascular toxicity of bupivacaine in lightly anesthetized pigs. Anesthesiology 1992;77:142–147.
76. Rosen MA, Thigpen JW, Shnider SM, et al. Bupivacaine-induced cardiotoxicity in hypoxic and acidotic sheep. Anesth Analg 1985;64:1089–1096.
77. Heavner JE, Pitkanen MT, Shi B, Rosenberg PH. Resuscitation from bupivacaine-induced asystole in rats: comparison of different cardioactive drugs. Anesth Analg 1995;80: 1134–1139.
78. Krismer AC, Hogan QH, Wenzel V, et al. The efficacy of epinephrine or vasopressin for resuscitation during epidural anesthesia. Anesth Analg 2001;93:734–742.
79. Mayr VD, Raedler C, Wenzel V, et al. A comparison of epinephrine and vasopressin in a porcine model of cardiac arrest after rapid intravenous injection of bupivacaine. Anesth Analg 2004;98:1426–1431.
80. Neustein S, Sampson I, Dimich I, et al. Milrinone is superior to epinephrine as treatment of myocardial depression due to ropivacaine in pigs. Can J Anaesth 2000;47:1114–1118.
81. Long WB, Rosenblum S, Grady IP. Successful resuscitation of bupivacaine-induced cardiac arrest using cardiopulmonary bypass. Anesth Analg 1989;69:403–406.
82. Weinberg G, Ripper R, Feinstein DL, Hoffman W. Lipid emulsion infusion rescues dogs from bupivacaine-induced cardiac toxicity. Reg Anesth Pain Med 2003;28:198–202.
83. Weinberg GL, VadeBoncouer T, Ramaraju GA, et al. Pretreatment or resuscitation with a lipid infusion shifts the dose-response to bupivacaine-induced asystole in rats. Anesthesiology 1998;88:1071–1075.
84. Groban L, Butterworth J. Lipid reversal of bupivacaine toxicity: has the silver bullet been identified? Reg Anesth Pain Med 2003;28:167–169.

85. Turnbull DK, Shepherd DB. Post-dural puncture headache: pathogenesis, prevention and treatment. Br J Anaesth 2003;91:718–729.
86. Faccenda KA, Finucane BT. Complications of regional anaesthesia. Incidence and prevention. Drug Saf 2001;24:413–442.
87. Vandam LD, Dripps RD. Long-term follow-up of patients who received 10,098 spinal anesthetics: syndrome of decreased intracranial pressure (headache and ocular and auditory difficulties). J Am Med Assoc 1956;161:586–591.
88. Horlocker TT. Complications of spinal and epidural anesthesia. Anesthesiol Clin North Am 2000;18:461–485.
89. Fog J, Wang LP, Sundberg A, Mucchiano C. Hearing loss after spinal anesthesia is related to needle size. Anesth Analg 1990;70:517–522.
90. Sundberg A, Wang LP, Fog J. Influence of hearing of 22G Whitacre and 22G Quincke needles. Anaesthesia 1992;47:981–983.
91. Lybecker H, Andersen T, Helbo-Hansen HS. The effect of epidural blood patch on hearing loss in patients with severe postdural puncture headache. J Clin Anesth 1995; 7:457–464.
92. Marchbanks RJ, Reid A. Cochlear and cerebrospinal fluid pressure: their interrelationship and control mechanisms. Br J Audiol 1990;24:179–187.
93. Wemama JP, Delecroix M, Nyarwaya JB, Krivosic-Horber R. Permanent unilateral vestibulocochlear dysfunction after spinal anesthesia. Anesth Analg 1996;82: 406–408.
94. Patin DJ, Eckstein EC, Harum K, Pallares VS. Anatomic and biomechanical properties of human lumbar dura mater. Anesth Analg 1993;76:535–540.
95. Fink BR. Postspinal headache. Anesth Analg 1990;71:208–209.
96. Norris MC, Leighton BL, DeSimone CA. Needle bevel direction and headache after inadvertent dural puncture. Anesthesiology 1989;70:729–731.
97. Lybecker H, Moller JT, May O, Nielsen HK. Incidence and prediction of postdural puncture headache. A prospective study of 1021 spinal anesthesias. Anesth Analg 1990; 70:389–394.
98. Ready LB, Cuplin S, Haschke RH, Nessly M. Spinal needle determinants of rate of transdural fluid leak. Anesth Analg 1989;69:457–460.
99. Gurmarnik S. Skin preparation and spinal headache. Anaesthesia 1988;43:1057–1058.
100. Munnur U, Suresh MS. Backache, headache, and neurologic deficit after regional anesthesia. Anesthesiol Clin North Am 2003;21:71–86.
101. Baraz R, Collis RE. The management of accidental dural puncture during labour epidural analgesia: a survey of UK practice. Anaesthesia 2005;60:673–679.
102. Kuczkowski KM, Benumof JL. Decrease in the incidence of post-dural puncture headache: maintaining CSF volume. Acta Anaesthesiol Scand 2003;47:98–100.
103. Camann WR, Murray RS, Mushlin PS, Lambert DH. Effects of oral caffeine on postdural puncture headache. A double-blind, placebo-controlled trial. Anesth Analg 1990;70: 181–184.
104. Bolton VE, Leicht CH, Scanlon TS. Postpartum seizure after epidural blood patch and intravenous caffeine sodium benzoate. Anesthesiology 1989;70:146–149.
105. Carp H, Singh PJ, Vadhera R, Jayaram A. Effects of the serotonin-receptor agonist sumatriptan on postdural puncture headache: report of six cases. Anesth Analg 1994; 79:180–182.
106. Kshatri AM, Foster PA. Adrenocorticotropic hormone infusion as a novel treatment for postdural puncture headache. Reg Anesth 1997;22:432–434.
107. Gormley JB. Treatment of post spinal headache. Anesthesiology 1960;21:565.
108. DiGiovanni AJ, Dunbar BS. Epidural injections of autologous blood for postlumbar-puncture headache. Anesth Analg 1970;49:268–271.
109. DiGiovanni AJ, Galbert MW, Wahle WM. Epidural injection of autologous blood for postlumbar-puncture headache. II. Additional clinical experiences and laboratory investigation. Anesth Analg 1972;51:226–232.
110. Beards SC, Jackson A, Griffiths AG, Horsman EL. Magnetic resonance imaging of extradural blood patches: appearances from 30min to 18h. Br J Anaesth 1993;71: 182–188.
111. Szeinfeld M, Ihmeidan IH, Moser MM, et al. Epidural blood patch: evaluation of the volume and spread of blood injected into the epidural space. Anesthesiology 1986;64: 820–822.

112. Andrews PJ, Ackerman WE, Juneja M, et al. Transient bradycardia associated with extradural blood patch after inadvertent dural puncture in parturients. Br J Anaesth 1992;69:401–403.
113. Palmer JH, Wilson DW, Brown CM. Lumbovertebral syndrome after repeat extradural blood patch. Br J Anaesth 1997;78:334–336.
114. Perez M, Olmos M, Garrido FJ. Facial nerve paralysis after epidural blood patch. Reg Anesth 1993;18:196–198.
115. Seeberger MD, Urwyler A. Lumbovertebral syndrome after extradural blood patch. Br J Anaesth 1992;69:414–416.
116. Tekkok IH, Carter DA, Brinker R. Spinal subdural haematoma as a complication of immediate epidural blood patch. Can J Anaesth 1996;43:306–309.
117. Kowbel MA, Comfort VK. Caudal epidural blood patch for the treatment of a paediatric subarachnoid-cutaneous fistula. Can J Anaesth 1995;42:625–627.
118. Roy L, Vischoff D, Lavoie J. Epidural blood patch in a seven-year-old child. Can J Anaesth 1995;42:621–624.
119. Colonna-Romano P, Linton P. Cervical dural puncture and lumbar extradural blood patch. Can J Anaesth 1995;42:1143–1144.
120. Cheek TG, Banner R, Sauter J, Gutsche BB. Prophylactic extradural blood patch is effective. A preliminary communication. Br J Anaesth 1988;61:340–342.
121. Palahniuk RJ, Cumming M. Prophylactic blood patch does not prevent post lumbar puncture headache. Can Anaesth Soc J 1979;26:132–133.
122. Aldrete JA, Brown TL. Intrathecal hematoma and arachnoiditis after prophylactic blood patch through a catheter. Anesth Analg 1997;84:233–234.
123. Baysinger CL, Menk EJ, Harte E, Middaugh R. The successful treatment of dural puncture headache after failed epidural blood patch. Anesth Analg 1986;65:1242–1244.
124. Stevens RA, Jorgensen N. Successful treatment of dural puncture headache with epidural saline infusion after failure of epidural blood patch. Case report. Acta Anaesthesiol Scand 1988;32:429–431.
125. Gerritse BM, van Dongen RT, Crul BJ. Epidural fibrin glue injection stops persistent cerebrospinal fluid leak during long-term intrathecal catheterization. Anesth Analg 1997;84:1140–1141.
126. Crul BJ, Gerritse BM, van Dongen RT, Schoonderwaldt HC. Epidural fibrin glue injection stops persistent postdural puncture headache. Anesthesiology 1999;91: 576–577.
127. Reynvoet ME, Cosaert PA, Desmet MF, Plasschaert SM. Epidural dextran 40 patch for postdural puncture headache. Anaesthesia 1997;52:886–888.
128. Borghi B, Casati A, Iuorio S, et al. Frequency of hypotension and bradycardia during general anesthesia, epidural anesthesia, or integrated epidural-general anesthesia for total hip replacement. J Clin Anesth 2002;14:102–106.
129. Meissner A, Rolf N, Van Aken H. Thoracic epidural anesthesia and the patient with heart disease: benefits, risks, and controversies. Anesth Analg 1997;85:517–528.
130. Wright PM, Fee JP. Cardiovascular support during combined extradural and general anaesthesia. Br J Anaesth 1992;68:585–589.
131. Hahn RG. Increased haemodilution in hypotension induced by epidural anaesthesia. Acta Anaesthesiol Scand 1993;37:357–360.
132. Hahn RG. Haemoglobin dilution from epidural-induced hypotension with and without fluid loading. Acta Anaesthesiol Scand 1992;36:241–244.
133. Holte K, Foss NB, Svensen C, et al. Epidural anesthesia, hypotension, and changes in intravascular volume. Anesthesiology 2004;100:281–286.
134. Dalens B, Hasnaoui A. Caudal anesthesia in pediatric surgery: success rate and adverse effects in 750 consecutive patients. Anesth Analg 1989;68:83–89.
135. Tsuji MH, Horigome H, Yamashita M. Left ventricular functions are not impaired after lumbar epidural anaesthesia in young children. Paediatr Anaesth 1996;6:405–409.
136. McCarthy GS. The effect of thoracic extradural analgesia on pulmonary gas distribution, functional residual capacity and airway closure. Br J Anaesth 1976;48:243–248.
137. Sundberg A, Wattwil M, Arvill A. Respiratory effects of high thoracic epidural anaesthesia. Acta Anaesthesiol Scand 1986;30:215–217.
138. Kochi T, Sako S, Nishino T, Mizuguchi T. Effect of high thoracic extradural anaesthesia on ventilatory response to hypercapnia in normal volunteers. Br J Anaesth 1989;62: 362–367.

139. Sakura S, Saito Y, Kosaka Y. Effect of extradural anaesthesia on the ventilatory response to hypoxaemia. Anaesthesia 1993;48:205–209.
140. Gruber EM, Tschernko EM, Kritzinger M, et al. The effects of thoracic epidural analgesia with bupivacaine 0.25% on ventilatory mechanics in patients with severe chronic obstructive pulmonary disease. Anesth Analg 2001;92:1015–1019.
141. Scammell SJ. Case report: inadvertent epidural anaesthesia as a complication of interscalene brachial plexus block. Anaesth Intensive Care 1979;7:56–57.
142. Bonnet F, Derosier JP, Pluskwa F, et al. Cervical epidural anaesthesia for carotid artery surgery. Can J Anaesth 1990;37:353–358.
143. Michalek P, David I, Adamec M, Janousek L. Cervical epidural anesthesia for combined neck and upper extremity procedure: a pilot study. Anesth Analg 2004;99: 1833–1836.
144. Nystrom UM, Nystrom NA. Continuous cervical epidural anesthesia in reconstructive hand surgery. J Hand Surg [Am] 1997;22:906–912.
145. Capdevila X, Biboulet P, Rubenovitch J, et al. The effects of cervical epidural anesthesia with bupivacaine on pulmonary function in conscious patients. Anesth Analg 1998;86: 1033–1038.
146. Sharrock NE. Recordings of, and an anatomical explanation for, false positive loss of resistance during lumbar extradural analgesia. Br J Anaesth 1979;51:253–258.
147. Gallart L, Blanco D, Samso E, Vidal F. Clinical and radiologic evidence of the epidural plica mediana dorsalis. Anesth Analg 1990;71:698–701.
148. Portnoy D, Vadhera RB. Mechanisms and management of an incomplete epidural block for cesarean section. Anesthesiol Clin North Am 2003;21:39–57.
149. Alahuhta S, Kangas-Saarela T, Hollmen AI, Edstrom HH. Visceral pain during caesarean section under spinal and epidural anaesthesia with bupivacaine. Acta Anaesthesiol Scand 1990;34:95–98.
150. Bourne TM, deMelo AE, Bastianpillai BA, May AE. A survey of how British obstetric anaesthetists test regional anaesthesia before caesarean section. Anaesthesia 1997;52: 901–903.
151. Russell IF. Levels of anaesthesia and intraoperative pain at caesarean section under regional block. Int J Obstet Anesth 1995;4:71–77.
152. Russell IF. The futility of using sharp pinprick (or cold) to assess spinal or epidural anesthesia for cesarean delivery. Reg Anesth Pain Med 2001;26:385–387.
153. Wong CA, Norris MC. Acute situations: obstetrics. In: Raj PP, ed. Textbook of Regional Anesthesia. New York: Elsevier, 2002;25:471–504.
154. Chaney MA. Side effects of intrathecal and epidural opioids. Can J Anaesth 1995;42: 891–903.
155. Tzeng JI, Wang JJ, Ho ST, et al. Dexamethasone for prophylaxis of nausea and vomiting after epidural morphine for post-caesarean section analgesia: comparison of droperidol and saline. Br J Anaesth 2000;85:865–868.
156. Wang JJ, Ho ST, Liu YH, et al. Dexamethasone decreases epidural morphine-related nausea and vomiting. Anesth Analg 1999;89:117–120.
157. Jeon Y, Hwang J, Kang J, et al. Effects of epidural naloxone on pruritus induced by epidural morphine: a randomized controlled trial. Int J Obstet Anesth 2005;14:22–25.
158. Szarvas S, Harmon D, Murphy D. Neuraxial opioid-induced pruritus: a review. J Clin Anesth 2003;15:234–239.
159. Emanuelsson BM, Persson J, Alm C, et al. Systemic absorption and block after epidural injection of ropivacaine in healthy volunteers. Anesthesiology 1997;87: 1309–1317.
160. Borgeat A, Ekatodramis G, Schenker CA. Postoperative nausea and vomiting in regional anesthesia: a review. Anesthesiology 2003;98:530–547.
161. Sjostrom S, Hartvig P, Persson MP, Tamsen A. Pharmacokinetics of epidural morphine and meperidine in humans. Anesthesiology 1987;67:877–888.
162. Lanz E, Kehrberger E, Theiss D. Epidural morphine: a clinical double-blind study of dosage. Anesth Analg 1985;64:786–791.
163. Gedney JA, Liu EH. Side-effects of epidural infusions of opioid bupivacaine mixtures. Anaesthesia 1998;53:1148–1155.
164. Tzeng JI, Hsing CH, Chu CC, et al. Low-dose dexamethasone reduces nausea and vomiting after epidural morphine: a comparison of metoclopramide with saline. J Clin Anesth 2002;14:19–23.

165. Wang JJ, Tzeng JI, Ho ST, et al. The prophylactic effect of tropisetron on epidural morphine-related nausea and vomiting: a comparison of dexamethasone with saline. Anesth Analg 2002;94:749–753.
166. Wein AJ. Neuromuscular dysfunction of the lower urinary tract and its management. In: Walsh PC, ed. Campbell's Urology. Philadelphia: WB Saunders; 2002:954.
167. Givens CD, Wenzel RP. Catheter-associated urinary tract infections in surgical patients: a controlled study on the excess morbidity and costs. J Urol 1980;124:646–648.
168. Platt R, Polk BF, Murdock B, Rosner B. Mortality associated with nosocomial urinary-tract infection. N Engl J Med 1982;307:637–642.
169. Stenseth R, Sellevold O, Breivik H. Epidural morphine for postoperative pain: experience with 1085 patients. Acta Anaesthesiol Scand 1985;29:148–156.
170. Rawal N, Mollefors K, Axelsson K, et al. An experimental study of urodynamic effects of epidural morphine and of naloxone reversal. Anesth Analg 1983;62:641–647.
171. Lytle SA, Goldsmith DM, Neuendorf TL, Lowry ME. Postoperative analgesia with epidural fentanyl. J Am Osteopath Assoc 1991;91:547–550.
172. Rawal N, Mollefors K, Axelsson K, et al. Naloxone reversal of urinary retention after epidural morphine. Lancet 1981;2:1411.
173. Malinovsky JM, Lepage JY, Karam G, Pinaud M. Nalbuphine reverses urinary effects of epidural morphine: a case report. J Clin Anesth 2002;14:535–538.
174. Basse L, Werner M, Kehlet H. Is urinary drainage necessary during continuous epidural analgesia after colonic resection? Reg Anesth Pain Med 2000;25:498–501.
175. Brown EM, Elman DS. Postoperative backache. Anesth Analg 1961;40:683–685.
176. MacArthur C, Lewis M, Knox EG, Crawford JS. Epidural anaesthesia and long term backache after childbirth. BMJ 1990;301:9–12.
177. Russell R, Groves P, Taub N, et al. Assessing long term backache after childbirth. BMJ 1993;306:1299–1303.
178. Breen TW, Ransil BJ, Groves PA, Oriol NE. Factors associated with back pain after childbirth. Anesthesiology 1994;81:29–34.
179. Russell R, Dundas R, Reynolds F. Long term backache after childbirth: prospective search for causative factors. BMJ 1996;312:1384–1388.
180. Fibuch EE, Opper SE. Back pain following epidurally administered Nesacaine-MPF. Anesth Analg 1989;69:113–115.
181. Levy L, Randel GI, Pandit SK. Does chloroprocaine (Nesacaine MPF) for epidural anesthesia increase the incidence of backache? Anesthesiology 1989;71:476.
182. Drolet P, Veillette Y. Back pain following epidural anesthesia with 2-chloroprocaine (EDTA-free) or lidocaine. Reg Anesth 1997;22:303–307.
183. Peutrell JM, Lonnqvist PA. Neuraxial blocks for anaesthesia and analgesia in children. Curr Opin Anaesthesiol 2003;461–470.

# 11 Complications of Other Peripheral Nerve Blocks

Guido Fanelli, Andrea Casati, and Daniela Ghisi

This chapter will discuss peripheral nerve blocks (PNBs) of the lower extremity. There are relatively few reports about complications associated with the use of PNBs in general and also about the mechanisms of injury after nerve blockade and methods to prevent them.

There is a general agreement about the benefits of PNBs, including preservation of consciousness, hemodynamic stability, postsurgery analgesia, early discharge of the patient, and limited sensory and motor blockade. Lower extremity blocks are very useful techniques to be familiar with and apply, because they provide excellent postoperative pain relief and have a very low incidence of complications, varying between 0%–5%.[1]

A complication is an undesired event subsequent to a medical treatment that may or may not be reversible, has different grades of severity, and is not always preventable. It differs from an adverse reaction, which may be defined as an undesired event ranging from a simple discomfort to damage limiting daily activities of the patient, but generally preventable.

PNBs of the lower extremity have never been as widely taught or used as other techniques of regional anesthesia. This may be attributable to the impossibility of anesthetizing the entire lower extremity with a single injection. Furthermore, injections required to perform a block of the lower extremity are generally deeper than those required for upper extremity block.[2]

Over the past decade, several developments have led to a growing interest in PNBs of the lower extremity; these changes in clinical practice are mainly the result of reports of new complications associated with central neuraxial techniques, e.g., transient neurologic symptoms associated with spinal anesthesia, an increased risk of epidural hematoma with the introduction of new antithromboembolic prophylaxis regimens, and to the positive effects on rehabilitation outcomes associated with continuous lower extremity PNBs.[2] PNBs are often incorrectly blamed for nerve injuries that are more likely caused by tourniquet pressure, surgical intervention, or poor positioning of the patient.

## Epidemiology of Complications of Peripheral Nerve Blocks of the Lower Extremity

A great deal of literature has been devoted to the techniques of regional anesthesia. The clearest picture of regional anesthesia complications comes from the ASA Closed Claims Project database.[3] The ASA Closed Claims analysis permits a structured evaluation of adverse anesthetic outcomes collected from the closed anesthesia malpractice insurance claim files.

In the 1990s, 308 claims in the United States were associated with regional anesthesia, versus 642 associated with general anesthesia. In this decade, the percentage of claims for patient death (10%) continues its steady decrease from more than 20% in the 1970s to 13% in the 1980s.[4]

In the same decade, we also observed a significant increase in the percentage of claims arising from pain management in nonoperative settings,[5] where anesthetic blocks accounted for 84% of the ASA Closed Claims Project database (neuraxial blocks 55%, sympathetic blocks 16%, axial nerve blocks 15%, other blocks 9%).[4]

Another study from the ASA Closed Claims Project database evaluated injuries associated with regional anesthesia in the 1980s and 1990s in surgical settings: PNBs accounted for 13% of all regional anesthesia claims; death or brain damage was associated with 11% of peripheral block claims and included mostly interscalene, axillary, and intravenous regional blocks. Damaging events in these claims were related mostly to block technique, wrong dose or wrong drug, inadequate ventilation, delayed absorption of local anesthetic, and difficult intubation. Permanent nerve damage was associated with 29% of PNB claims (according to frequency: brachial plexus damage, median nerve, ulnar, radial, femoral/sciatic) and temporary injury with 58% of claims.[6] Auroy et al.[7] have studied complications of regional anesthesia over 30 geographical regions, including overseas French departments. Every hospital or private clinic was surveyed during 3 consecutive days, from February 1, 1996 to January 31, 1997. The aim of this survey was to identify three types of information: main characteristics of patients undergoing anesthesia, anesthesia (urgent or elective, starting and ending time, general or regional anesthesia, airway management, pharmacologic agents), and procedure. The annual rate of anesthetic procedures in the whole population was 13.5 anesthesia procedures per 100 inhabitants, and the number of anesthetic procedures for surgery was 9.5/100. Regional anesthesia was performed in 21% of cases, and in 2% of cases a combined technique of regional and general anesthesia with intravenous or volatile agents was performed. Orthopedic surgery was the most common surgery, accounting for the majority of regional anesthesia procedures. The two major findings of this study were that anesthesia has both increased and changed since 1980: the number of anesthetic procedures increased by 120% from 1980 to 1996 in France, and there was a consistent growth in the number of anesthetics performed in the elderly. There was an increase in the number of regional anesthetics performed.

There was a 16-fold increase in the use of plexus/nerve blocks reported since the 1980s. In the French survey from Clergue and colleagues,[8] 21,278 PNBs were performed in the 5-month period of the study: they estimated the potential for serious complications per 10,000 PNBs and found 0–2.6 deaths, 0.3–4.1 cardiac arrests, 0.5–4.8 neurologic injuries, 3.9–11.2 seizures, and 0.5–4.8 radiculopathy.

In a more recent analysis in 2002 from Auroy et al.,[9] of a total of 158,083 regional blocks performed in the 10-month period of the study, anesthesiologists reported 56 serious complications related to regional anesthesia. The study estimated an incidence of major complications after the 394 posterior lumbar plexus blocks higher than expected and higher than that reported with other PNBs (25.4/10,000 cardiac arrests, 50.8/10,000 respiratory failures, 25.4/10,000 seizures, and 25.4/10,000 deaths).

Apart from specific considerations, the study estimated that the total incidence of severe complications after regional blocks to be lower than 5/10,000. It is rare for serious cardiac and neurologic complications to occur in association with regional anesthesia. Published information primarily involves retrospective studies or case reports[7]; moreover, large numbers of patients are required to compare the incidence and characteristics of serious critical events.

There is a paucity of reports of complications specifically attributable to PNBs of the lower extremity, which is really evident if compared with reports about PNBs of the upper extremity. Nevertheless, according to some authors, this is likely related to their less common application, rather than to the inherent safety of the techniques.[2] According to Ben-David[4] in his overview about complications of neuraxial and PNBs, we should consider four categories: first, psychogenic reactions such as anxiety and agitation, vasovagal reactions, severe bradycardia, hypotension, loss of consciousness, and even seizures. These problems can be prevented with the judicious use of sedation, together with carefully monitoring the patient. The second group of coincident complications includes those injuries occurring during anesthetic block completely unrelated or indirectly related to the block itself. The third group of complications is those resulting from trauma from the technique itself, and finally, we must consider untoward effects of the local anesthetic and adjuvant drugs themselves. These two latter categories comprise the most frequent complications of both peripheral and neuraxial regional anesthesia.

We have evaluated two large groups of complications related to PNBs: the first includes the intrinsic complications directly attributable to the anesthetic technique itself; the second category includes extrinsic complications not strictly related to the PNB performed.

In the first category we include:

1. Nerve injury
2. Systemic toxicity
3. Hematoma and its relation to deep vein thrombosis prophylaxis
4. Infection

In the second category, we consider complications that can occur after surgery and that might be caused by surgery itself and not by the anesthetic technique:

1. Stretching of the nerves because of patient positioning
2. Ischemic nerve injury because of tourniquet pressure
3. Surgical factors leading to neuropathy

We also stress another important theme about complications of lower extremity PNBs, and that is the risk of failure in performing these blocks. This is a very important part of this discussion for both expert practitioners and those learning the techniques.

## Failure in Performing Peripheral Nerve Blocks of the Lower Extremity

Failure of anesthesia is not strictly a complication of PNBs. However, it can lead to serious complications.[10] Over the years, the use of regional anesthesia has been confronted with the need to produce an adequate level and degree of blockade in an acceptable period of time with a safe dose of local anesthetic. The nerve blockade has to be complete, must have a desired duration of action, and must be reproducible.[11] The purpose of any regional anesthetic technique is to deposit a quantity of local anesthetic close enough to the nerve to block nerve transmission in that nerve. In anesthetic practice, this is usually performed percutaneously.[12] Because we usually use a blind approach, the success rate varies.

The failure rate with PNBs depends on the type of block performed: a success rate greater than 95% is frequently reported for ophthalmic anesthesia,[10] whereas a failure rate of up 30% is reported with brachial plexus anesthesia[13](Chapter 8).

In view of the risk of failure of regional anesthesia, the anesthesiologist is always expected to have an alternative plan of anesthesia including general anesthesia. The efficacy of PNBs is estimated to range from 70% to 85%. There are a number of methods available to increase success rates with PNBs, including electrical nerve stimulation (ENS) techniques, multiple injection techniques, percutaneous electrode guidance (PEG) techniques, and imaging techniques (ultrasonography).

## *ENS, Multiinjection Technique, PEG*

Not all nerve fibers within a peripheral nerve will be stimulated by a given electric current. In general, the Aα motor fibers and the smaller C fibers subserving touch and pain respond at different current levels: the motor fibers can be stimulated with a lower intensity of current. This means that if a nerve is stimulated at just above its threshold, the effect will be twitching in the muscles that it supplies without pain or sensation in the dermatome. This phenomenon is the basis for the use of ENS in regional anesthesia.[12]

In the past, PNBs were usually performed using paresthesias, blind approaches, or transarterial methods, but these methods were associated with a high risk of intraarterial injection of drugs, pseudoaneurysm, and hemorrhage. If the act of eliciting a paresthesia represents traumatic contact with nerve fibers, it may be wise to avoid it. There is some evidence in the literature that most cases of nerve injury following spinal anesthesia and all cases after epidural and PNBs were associated with paresthesias during needle placement or pain during injection[7]; however, this matter is still controversial and contradictory data exist.

One important advantage of the nerve stimulator technique is that it is an objective method of confirming the needle–nerve contact. This is not true when using the paresthesia method, which is purely subjective.[1] The use of a nerve stimulator may reduce the potential risk for posttraumatic nerve complications, hemorrhage, and toxicity. It increases the specificity of peripheral nerve blockade and the reliability of the technique. According to many authors, the major benefits of using a nerve stimulator is that patients have a clearer understanding of your goals as opposed to the paresthesia method. Nevertheless, a study from Auroy and colleagues[9] in 2002 reported the occurrence of neurologic complications even after the use of a nerve stimulator for PNBs.

It has been suggested that the use of ENS alerts one to the proximity of the needle to the nerve, thereby reducing the chance of traumatic injury to the nerve. Despite this theory, there are reports of permanent nerve injury, including spinal cord injury following electrostimulation-guided nerve block.

In particular, caution should be exercised when stimulation is obtained with currents lower than 0.2 mA. According to Hadžić,[1] stimulation with such low current intensity is often associated with paresthesia on injection, perhaps suggesting an intraneural placement of the needle. In this scenario, it is recommended to withdraw the needle until a motor response is obtained at a current of 0.2–0.5 mA.

A multiple-injection technique, using electrical stimulation methods, has also been suggested to reduce the failure rate in PNBs. The rationale for this technique is that if there are many nerves to be blocked, it is possible to block them one by one. As Fanelli[14] observed, nerve stimulators allow a multiple injection technique by eliciting different muscular twitches during block placement. This technique provides effective PNBs with volumes of local anesthetic solution markedly less than those usually reported, without increasing the risk for nerve injury.[15] Use of a multiple injection technique with a nerve stimulator may increase the safety of PNBs by reducing the required volumes of local anesthetic solution, as well as the volume of anesthetic injected at each site.[16]

In 1999, Fanelli and colleagues[15] collected information from 28 departments of anesthesia in Italy that routinely used nerve stimulator and multiple injection techniques when performing PNBs. The study involved either upper or lower limb blockade. They excluded patients with a history of neuropathy, diabetes, or those who required surgical procedures involving nerve structures. The results showed no case of systemic adverse reaction and a failure rate similar in the three groups with a mean value of approximately 7%. The success rate reported was greater than 90%, and higher than that previously reported.[17]

Although it has been demonstrated that the multiple injection technique allows both a faster onset time and a greater success rate, most anesthesiologists are concerned about the theoretical risk of needle trauma or intraneural injection. This observational study by Fanelli, involving a multiinjection technique, demonstrated an incidence of local neurologic injury equal to that reported by Selander et al.[18] using a single injection technique (1.9%, >500 blocks). Fanelli et al.[15] concluded that the withdrawal and redirection of the needle was not associated with an increased incidence of nerve injury.

The third technique mentioned is PEG, or percutaneous electrode guidance. This is a noninvasive technique for prelocation of peripheral nerves to facilitate peripheral plexus or nerve block.

### *Imaging Techniques: Ultrasound Guidance*

Blind insertion of needles to block neural targets is known to result in complications. The use of ENS does not guarantee success of PNBs. The rationale for the use of imaging techniques such as ultrasonography in regional anesthesia is that one can see the advancing needle approaching the nerve. Furthermore, one can also see the spread of local anesthetic solution during the injection and make adjustments if necessary.[19]

The use of ultrasound guidance in regional anesthesia was first reported by La Grange et al.[20] in 1978: they performed supraclavicular brachial plexus blocks with the help of a Doppler ultrasound blood-flow detector. According to Greher et al.[21] and Peterson,[22] ultrasound will be the guidance technique of the future, even if the transition from the conventional technique of nerve stimulation will take another 10 years or even longer to complete. Over the past decade, Marhofer and colleagues[19] have studied the use of ultrasound guidance in order to significantly improve the quality of PNBs and to reduce complications such as intravascular injection and intraneuronal injection.

The potential advantages of ultrasonography in regional anesthesia may be direct visualization of nerve, direct visualization of anatomic structures, direct and indirect visualization of the spread of the local anesthetic, avoidance of side effects, avoidance of painful muscular contractions during nerve stimulation (in cases of fractures), reduction of the dose of local anesthetic, faster sensory onset time, longer duration of blocks, and improved quality of block.

Marhofer et al.[19] have performed more than 4000 nerve blocks under direct ultrasound guidance in a period of 10 years, and they found that the success rate improved up to 100% with significant improvements obtained in terms of sensory and motor onset times.

What type of equipment do we need to effectively use ultrasonography in regional anesthesia? It is evident that the higher the frequency, the higher the resolution, but the smaller the penetration depth. Most nerve block applications require frequencies in the range of 10–14 MHz.[19]

Peripheral nerves can appear both as hypoechoic and hyperechoic sonographic images when using ultrasound guidance.[23,24] This different appearance depends on the size of the nerve, the sonographic frequency used, and the angle of approach of the ultrasound beam. Marhofer et al.[19] performed most of the ultrasound-guided peripheral blocks on a transversal scan: the nerves appeared as multiple round or oval hypoechoic areas encircled by a relatively hyperechoic horizon (the fascicles of the nerves) in a hypoechoic background (connective tissue between neuronal structures). Tendons appear as multiple hyperechoic continuous lines, which gives them a fibrillar pattern (this is why peripheral nerves are said to have a fascicle pattern, instead); that is how they can be distinguished from nerves. The smallest fascicles cannot be visualized by ultrasound. The fascicular pattern is typical of large peripheral nerves and not of small nerves such as the superior laryngeal nerve.

Most peripheral nerves can be visualized over their entire course; only bony structures or large vessels can limit the visualization of nerves by ultrasound. During the performance of PNBs, the needle itself generates a dorsal acoustic shadow which can be identified as a hypoechoic structure. Once the needle is optimally placed, the local anesthetic can be observed spreading under direct sonographic visualization. The transverse approach allows one to maintain the same approach used when performing PNBs with nerve stimulation and also allows one to use the shorter insertion pathway compared with the longitudinal probe approach.

If guided by nerve stimulation, the three-in-one block has a failure rate of up to 20% when using nerve stimulation.[25] This block is ideally suited for ultrasound guidance with a high-frequency ultrasonographic probe (10MHz or even more). The puncture is performed 1cm distal to the probe. This technique can significantly improve the success rate of the 3-in-1 block. It reduces onset time, improves the quality of all three blocks, avoids complications,[26] and reduces the quantity of local anesthetic required.[27]

The reported incidence of success rate of lumbar plexus block never exceeds 80% irrespective of the approach used.[28] The ideal ultrasonographic frequency for this block is 5MHz according to Kirchmair et al.[29], who collected 20 volunteers and succeeded in visualizing the lumbar paravertebral region but not the lumbar plexus. Using additional computed tomographic scans on cadavers, they demonstrated that the needle could be accurately placed in the psoas compartment in 98% of cases.[30] Despite these good results, psoas compartment blocks are difficult to perform under ultrasound guidance because of the relative depth of the plexus.[29] A good success rate can be achieved with sciatic nerve block when the block is performed with ENS (87%–97%),[31,32] presumably because of its large dimension. Ultrasound guidance can reduce the risk of intraneural puncture, increase the success rate, allow the anesthetist to detect the sciatic nerve bifurcation, and allow the block of the posterior femoral cutaneous nerve.[19] The first problem with this approach is that the sciatic nerve has anisotropic behavior so that the beam has to be perpendicular to the nerve. The nerve is embedded in muscles which reduce the quality of the ultrasonographic image. In the popliteal region, a 5- to 12-MHz linear probe can be used to aid in its visualization. Ultrasound-guided imaging should be performed in the subgluteal region, where the nerve is relatively close to the skin surface. The distal branches can also be visualized distal to the head of the fibula; in addition, high-frequency linear probes can be used to visualize other subcutaneous branches.[19]

Some preliminary experiences have also been reported in children (Chapter 13). In this patient population, PNBs are usually performed under general anesthesia[33]; therefore, ultrasound is especially welcome as a guidance technique in this patient group. Children can be managed with high-frequency linear ultrasound probes because their nerves are very close to the skin. Ultrasound guidance has been routinely used in children by Marhofer et al.[19] for ilioinguinal nerve block, three-in-one block, sciatic block, femoral block, and brachial plexus block with good results.

## Intrinsic Complications

### *Nerve Injury*

For practical purposes, we can define a nerve injury as a clinical, anatomic, or laboratory finding consistent with damage to discrete elements of the peripheral nervous system.[34] According to Liguori,[35] the importance and severity of a nerve injury depends on three factors: first, the severity and quality of the sensory or motor deficit (from dysesthesia to severe pain, numbness and weakness interfering with daily activities); second, the duration of clinical symptoms (from transient phenomena for most nerve injuries to long-term or permanent injuries); third, the patient in whom the nerve injury occurs.

The incidence of nerve injury has been evaluated by many authors.[7,15,36–41] Liguori[35] noted that the wide range in the incidence of nerve injury reported depends on how accurate the anesthesiologist's investigation is, whether the study is prospective or retrospective, and the timing of the follow-up. The range varies from 0.004%[7] to 14%[40]: the closer investigators look at nerve injury after surgery, the more frequently problems are encountered. Although there are relatively few reports on anesthesia-related nerve injury associated with the use of PNBs, it may be that the incidence is underestimated. The less frequent clinical application of lower extremity PNBs may be the reason that there are even fewer reports of anesthesia-related nerve injury associated with lower extremity PNBs.[2]

Neurologic complications after lower extremity PNBs can be the consequence of the anesthetic technique itself including needle trauma, local anesthetic neurotoxicity, ischemic injury secondary to pressure and volume of local anesthetic or added vasoconstrictors, hematoma, or vascular injury. However, injuries can also be related to intraoperative factors, including surgical trauma and positioning, tourniquet injury, and postoperative factors, including swelling and positioning.

According to some authors, the first way to minimize the chance of causing a nerve injury is to maintain an awake and alert patient when performing PNBs, no matter what technique is used.[42] Nevertheless, judicious use of sedation can help the anesthesiologist in performing the block, allows better patient acceptance, and will allow the patient to warn the anesthesiologist when they experience paresthesias or pain on injection. Obviously, this goal cannot be achieved in pediatric patients.

Some case reports suggest that pain may be absent as a warning sign in pending nerve injury. However, the combination of premedication with sedatives and analgesics, along with the neuronal blocking properties of local anesthetics, may render pain on injection as the sole indicator of intraneural injection unreliable.[1]

Injuries to peripheral nerves after intrafascicular injection of therapeutic and other agents are well documented. Nerve injury following intraneural injection varies from minimal damage to severe axonal and myelin degeneration, depending on the agent injected and dose of the drug used. Nonetheless, several studies have documented that regardless of the agent used, intrafascicular injection is the main determinant of nerve injury. Experimental evidence suggests that such injections may be associated with a resistance to needle advancement and an increased pressure on injection of local anesthetic.[1]

Local anesthetics are innocuous when injected perineurally in appropriate quantities and concentrations, whereas high concentrations are known to permanently damage neural tissue in some cases. Kalichman et al.[43] demonstrated a concentration-dependent increase in neural edema, lipid inclusions, fiber injury, and Schwann cell injury using extraneural injection of various local anesthetic agents on rat sciatic nerve. Intraneural injection of local anesthetics, particularly when associated with epinephrine, can produce significant nerve injury. Concurrent injury, ischemia, or disease may also predispose to neurotoxic injury.[44,45]

There is no evidence in the literature that a prolonged duration of blockade or a continuous block can worsen the nerve damage caused by the local anesthetic.[46] Local anesthetic toxicity also extends to muscles and includes focal myonecrosis with regeneration occurring over several weeks.[47] Myotoxicity is enhanced by the use of epinephrine.[48]

According to Faccenda and Finucane,[10] substances added to local anesthetics may also cause local toxicity; e.g., a change in the preservative of chloroprocaine resulted in several cases of cauda equina in 1970s in the United States, EDTA (ethylenediaminetetraacetic acid) added to the same compound caused severe back pain in some patients following epidural anesthesia, and 5% hyperbaric lidocaine has been linked with transient neurologic symptoms following spinal anesthesia.

As Hadžić describes,[1] neurologic injuries resulting from an intraneuronal injection may be related to several factors, including direct needle trauma with perforation of the perineurium and other nerve sheaths, physical disruption of the nerve fibers, and disruption of the neuronal microvasculature, with the consequent intraepineural or intrafascicular hematoma and nerve ischemia. Because the perineurium is a tough and resistant tissue layer, an injection into this compartment or a fascicle can cause a prolonged increase in endoneurial pressure, exceeding the capillary perfusion pressure. This pressure in turn may result in endoneural ischemia. The addition of a vasoconstrictor and the application of a tourniquet over the site of nerve blockade will inevitably result in an additional decrease in blood supply to the nerve. The combination of all these factors contributes to neuronal ischemia and increases the risk of neurologic injury. However, in patients undergoing lower extremity surgery, the addition of epinephrine to the local anesthetic solution used in combined femoral and sciatic nerve blocks was not shown to be a risk factor for the development of post–nerve block dysfunction.[15]

There is no clear-cut algorithm for the management of a postoperative nerve injury. According to Liguori,[35] symptoms are often first noted and referred by surgeons during the first postoperative visit; these symptoms are usually blamed as consequences of the regional anesthetic technique. For the majority of these patients complaining about complications, a single call by the anesthesiologist is enough to reassure the patient. Most frequently, residual dysesthesias and hypoesthesias are reported and in these cases simple reassurance is all that is required.

Symptoms of neurologic injury resolve in 4–6 weeks in 92%–97% of patients and in more than 99% in 1 year.[39,40] If symptoms interfere with daily activities or persist beyond a few weeks, neurologic consultation and testing should be considered.[35]

According to Hadžić,[1] these are the measures to take into account to prevent nerve injuries:

1. Aseptic technique: Most nerve block techniques are merely percutaneous injections. However, infections are known to occur and can result in significant disability. Because this complication is almost entirely preventable, every effort should be made to strictly adhere to aseptic technique.
2. Short bevel insulated needles: The short bevel design helps prevent nerve penetration. Insulated needles are now widely available and result in much more precise needle placement when nerve stimulator is used. A contrary opinion is expressed in Chapter 5.
3. Needles of appropriate length for each block procedure. In addition, needles of appropriate length can be advanced with far greater precision than excessively long needles.
4. Needle advancement: During needle localization, advance and withdraw the needle slowly. Keep in mind that nerve stimulators deliver a current of very short duration (usually 1–2 Hz) and no current is delivered between the pulses. Fast insertion and withdrawal of the needle may result in failure to stimulate the nerve because the needle may pass nearby, or even through, the nerve between the stimuli without eliciting nerve stimulation.
5. Fractionated injections: Inject smaller doses and volumes of local anesthetics (3–5 mL) with intermittent aspiration to avoid inadvertent intravascular injection. Always observe the patient during the injection of local anesthetic because negative aspiration of blood is not always present with an intravenous injection. This approach may allow detection of the signs of local anesthetic toxicity before the entire dose is injected.
6. Accuracy of the nerve stimulator: Always make sure that the nerve stimulator is operational, delivering the specified current, and that the leads are properly connected to the patient and the needle.
7. Avoidance of forceful, fast injections: Forceful, fast injections are more likely to result in channeling of local anesthetic to the unwanted tissue layers, lymphatic vessels, or small veins that may have been cut during needle advancement. Such injections may result in massive channeling of the local anesthetic into the systemic circulation, with the consequent risk of severe central nervous system and cardiac

toxicity. Forceful, fast injections under excessive pressure may also carry more risk of intrafascicular injection. Limit the injection speed to 15–20mL/minute.

8. Avoidance of injection under high pressure: Intrafascicular needle placement results in higher resistance (pressure) to injection because of the compact nature of the neuronal tissue and its connective tissue sheaths. Always use the same syringe and needle size to develop a "feel" during the injection. As a rule, when injection of the first milliliter of local anesthetic proves difficult, the injection should be abandoned and the needle completely withdrawn. Check for patency before reinserting.

9. Avoidance of paresthesia on injection: Severe pain or discomfort on injection may signify intraneuronal placement of the needle and should be avoided. This should not be confused with a normal mild "paresthesia-like" symptom, frequently reported by patients when the needle is placed in the immediate vicinity to the nerve. Keep in mind that published case reports suggest that the absence of pain on injection alone does not guarantee that the needle is not placed intraneurally. Absence of pain and abnormal resistance to injection should be documented in the anesthetic record after each block procedure.

10. Choose your local anesthetic solution wisely: Always choose a shorter-acting (and less toxic) local anesthetic for short procedures in which long-lasting postoperative analgesia is not required. Local anesthetic toxicity is the most common complication with neuronal blockade, and it is much safer when this occurs with chloroprocaine or lidocaine than with bupivacaine.

11. Blocks in anesthetized patients: Blocks in anesthetized patients should be avoided or at least be an uncommon practice. When it is necessary to place blocks in anesthetized patients, this should be done only by practitioners with substantial experience with the planned technique. Such cases should *never* be considered "teaching" and one should carefully note the reasons for doing the block in these circumstances.

12. Repeating blocks after a failed block: It should be avoided whenever possible. When indicated, it should be done only by those with substantial experience in the planned technique.

## *Systemic Toxicity (Chapter 4)*

Although the use of large quantities of local anesthetic solutions improves the success rate and predictability of PNBs, it may also increase the risk of local anesthetic-related systemic toxicity. The risk of systemic toxicity is reduced when the minimum effective dose of local anesthetic is used. The clinical relevance of this assumption further increases when a combination of different nerve blocks is used as in lower limb procedures.[16]

The potential for systemic local anesthetic toxicity would seem to be much higher for lower extremity PNBs compared with other regional techniques: for instance, combined femoral and sciatic nerve blocks require large doses of local anesthetic to effectively anesthetize the entire lower extremity.[2] However, there are only a few case reports of local anesthetic toxicity associated with these blocks and some authors report no cases of systemic toxicity after PNBs of the lower extremity. Fanelli and colleagues[15] evaluated 2175 femoral sciatic combined blocks, with no systemic toxic reactions reported.

The safety of lower extremity PNBs seems to vary depending on the individual nerve block. There are no cases of systemic toxicity following popliteal sciatic block, whereas there are several reports of severe toxicity following lumbar plexus blocks and proximal sciatic blocks.[9,49–52]

In a study by Auroy and colleagues,[7] seizures were reported in 23 patients among 103,730 who underwent regional anesthesia in the 5-month period of the study, but up to 16 seizures were PNB related and all were preceded by minor auditory symptoms and complaints of metallic taste. In this study, seizures occurred more frequently after PNBs than after other techniques and occurred five times more frequently than with epidural anesthesia. In those patients who experienced seizures, a larger volume of lidocaine 2% or bupivacaine 0.5% was injected for PNBs than for epidural (41 ± 14 versus 15 ± 4mL).

The incidence of seizures associated with regional anesthesia ranges between 1/1000 to 4/1000, but few reports are available. Brown et al.[53] collected cases of seizures related to brachial plexus blocks, epidural anesthesia, and caudal regional anesthetics from 1985 to 1992 and their series included 25,627 patients. Seizures occurred in 26 patients. The frequency of seizures associated with the use of regional anesthesia varied significantly among anesthetic types, with caudal > brachial > epidural, with bupivacaine as the most frequent agent related to seizures. None of the 26 patients who had seizures required hemodynamic support more intense than intravenous ephedrine or atropine, coupled with delivery of supplemental oxygen and controlled ventilation. None of these patients required epinephrine or antiarrhythmic therapy; furthermore, none of these patients required an extra length of stay in the postanesthesia care unit, compared with patients undergoing similar procedures.

Auroy et al.[9] in 2002 reported one case of irreversible cardiac arrest after a posterior lumbar plexus block in a series of 158,083 regional blocks. This patient had a T2 sensory level and bilateral mydriasis was noted immediately before the arrest. They were aware that intrafascicular proximal spread of the local anesthetic can occur proximally toward the spinal cord and result in neuraxial blockade. This is a particular concern with block techniques that involve needle placement at the level of nerve roots, especially paravertebral blocks and psoas compartment block. Auroy and colleagues recommended that these cases required the same level of vigilance as that required for neuraxial block because of the high risk of complications. Details about diagnosis and management of systemic toxicity following local anesthetic injections are covered in detail in other chapters in this text (Chapters 4 and 8).

## Hematoma

It has been noticed[2] that the psoas compartment approach to the lumbar plexus, the obturator nerve block, the parasacral, and classical approaches to sciatic nerve involve deep needle penetration. Vascular puncture during femoral nerve block placement has been reported to be as frequent as 5.6%.[54] However, few complications have been reported as a consequence of unintentional vascular puncture while performing femoral nerve block.[55]

Several investigators have documented hematoma as a complication occurring after psoas compartment block. To reach the lumbar plexus, the needle must transverse multiple muscles and other tissue layers. Moreover, lumbar plexus block is often used to provide anesthesia and analgesia in patients undergoing total hip replacement.[56] This kind of surgery requires and justifies prolonged thromboprophylactic treatment. The combination of anticoagulant administration together with blind needle puncture required for this block presents significant risk factors for the development of a hematoma.

In 2003, Weller and colleagues[57] described two cases of delayed retroperitoneal hematoma after lumbar plexus block. In one of these cases, the hematoma was diagnosed on postoperative day 4 even though it was evident that vessel trauma had occurred during catheter placement; in the other case, no apparent vessel trauma was noted during needle placement, but clinical symptoms of retroperitoneal hematoma occurred on postoperative day 3. Also, Aveline and Bonnet[58] in 2004 reported a similar case. They attempted to perform a lumbar plexus block in a patient. They advanced the needle in a cephalad direction twice after its insertion and, because they were unable to achieve the required end point, neither the aspiration test nor the injection was performed. The anesthetic technique was then changed to a fascia iliaca compartment block, but on postoperative day 17, a computed tomographic scan showed a retroperitoneal hematoma where the first block had been attempted.

In a previous case from Klein et al.[59] in 1997, a patient reported the same complication after lumbar plexus block. The patient was receiving enoxaparin at the time of anesthetic procedure and the block was performed successfully after several attempts. In the two cases reported by Weller et al.[57] and in the case reported by Aveline and Bonnet,[58] enoxaparin was administered 8 hours, 40 hours, and 14 hours, respectively, after placing the block. This means that the patients were not anticoagulated while receiving the block; however, they did receive anticoagulant therapy in the rehabilitation period and this contributed to the occurrence of hematoma.

These cases demonstrate the risk of significant, concealed bleeding from needle placement in an area that cannot be observed when anticoagulation is initiated after nerve block. In the case reports by Weller and colleagues,[57] the signs of substantial occult bleeding from lumbar plexus block were anemia and back pain without apparent neurologic deficits. Both patients required blood transfusion and prolonged hospitalization.

### *Infection*

Infectious complications may occur with any regional anesthetic technique. However, those associated with neuraxial anesthesia are of greater concern because of their potentially devastating sequelae. Aromaa et al.[60] collected information on 170,000 epidural and 550,000 spinal blocks, and reported an overall incidence of infection after epidural and spinal anesthesia of 1.1/100,000 blocks. Nevertheless, Wang et al.[61] estimated the risk of epidural abscess after epidural analgesia as 1/1930 and of persistent neurologic deficit as 1/4343. The frequency of infection associated with PNBs still remains undefined to our knowledge. Some reports refer to bacteremia or localized infection after continuous PNBs,[62–64] but there is no report about long-term infectious complications or dysfunctions[65] and there are no case reports of infection after lower extremity PNBs performed with single injection.

Cuvillon et al.[64] reported on the incidence of bacterial complications associated with the use of continuous femoral nerve blocks. They evaluated 208 patients; 57% had positive bacterial colonization of the catheter at 48 hours postoperatively. Three patients had transitory symptoms of bacteremia that resolved with removal of the catheter, but no long-term complications occurred in these cases. Two case reports of psoas abscess requiring drainage and intravenous antibiotic therapy have been described in patients who received a continuous femoral nerve block.[63,66]

The suspected mechanism of infection after PNBs and, more widely, regional anesthesia is mostly the invasion by skin bacteria through a needle track, contaminated syringes, contaminated catheter hubs, or contaminated local anesthetics, hematogenous spread from distant foci, or breaches in sterile technique.[67]

Skin disinfection is crucial to prevent infection, although there is not yet a wide consensus on how to provide such an optimal skin antisepsis. Second, the role of antibiotic therapy is still controversial: it is still unknown whether concurrent antibiotic therapy is protective against clinically significant infections. However, anecdotal evidence still suggests this is true, especially during periods of extended neuraxial and peripheral catheterization.[65] Further investigations will be necessary to establish definitive recommendations regarding perineural catheter use and antibiotic administration. Handwashing still remains the single, most important component in antisepsis: gloves are not to be considered as a replacement for handwashing.[68]

According to Hebl and Horlocker,[65] while we wait for more detailed recommendations and guidelines, it seems that the advice our mothers gave us when we were small was true: "Wash your hands, scrub behind your ears, cover your mouth when you sneeze, and always wear clean clothes . . . because you never know"!

## Extrinsic Complications

### *Stretching of the Nerves Because of Patient Positioning*

PNBs are often blamed for causing nerve injury; however, neuropathy after abdominal or lower extremity surgery is not an uncommon event.[2] Postoperative neurologic complications may actually be more common after general and neuraxial anesthesia than after PNBs. Such injuries were thought to be caused mostly by compression or stretching of the nerves or plexuses during patient positioning after general anesthesia, whereas injuries to the lumbosacral plexus primarily occur after central neuraxial blockade. Cheney et al.[69] evaluated sciatic nerve injury claims in the Closed Claims analysis: 50% of claims were associated with the lithotomy or frog-leg operative positioning. Warner et al.[70] observed nerve injury to the obturator, lateral femoral cutaneous, and sciatic nerves associated with the lithotomy position. Gruson and Moed[71] found an association between deep hip flexion or extension in total hip arthroplasty (THA) and repair of acetabular fracture and femoral nerve palsy. The same finding has been reported by Slater and colleagues.[72] According to Warner et al.[70] and Slater et al.,[72] positioning nerve injuries are consistently related to the length of surgery.

### *Ischemic Nerve Injury Because of Tourniquet Pressure*

In a study from Fanelli et al.,[15] the tourniquet inflation pressure was more predictive of postoperative neurologic dysfunction than the anesthetic technique used: tourniquet neuropathy is due to an increased risk of transient nerve injury, especially when comparing tourniquet pressures lower than 400 mmHg with those higher than 400 mmHg. Current recommendations for tourniquet use during surgery include the maintenance of a pressure no higher than 150 mmHg above the systolic pressure and deflation of the tourniquet every 90–120 minutes.[73] Even following these recommendations, post-tourniquet neuropathy has been reported.[74,75]

### *Surgical Factors Leading to Neuropathy*

Femoral neuropathy has been reported in association with operations that require deep pelvic exposure, such as acetabular fracture repair.[71] The incidence of nerve injury after ankle arthroscopy is 17%, according to Barber and colleagues[76]: The injury, in this kind of surgery, often involves the peroneal nerve because of its proximity to the dorsal arthroscopy portal.[77] Joint distension, excessive traction, extravasation of fluid during surgery, and the clinician's experience using the arthroscope are all factors associated with a higher risk of neuropathy specifically attributable to the surgical technique itself.

## Residency Training Programs: How Training Influences the Use of Peripheral Nerve Blocks in Clinical Practice

The advantages of PNBs have resulted in a diffuse and growing interest in regional anesthesia. The many qualities of these techniques include increasing patient satisfaction, answering to the actual growing demand for cost-effective anesthesia, and assuring a favorable postoperative recovery profile.[78] Despite these advantages, there is a wide perception that PNBs are infrequently used in clinical practice over general and neuraxial anesthesia, especially PNBs of the lower extremity.[79]

From 1990 to 1994, Hadžić et al.[79] reviewed all the abstracts presented at five consecutive American Society of Anesthesia meetings: only 0.8% of these abstracts focused on PNBs and only 0.2% focused on PNBs of the lower extremity; in the same period, reviewing the abstracts presented at American Society of Regional Anaesthesia meetings, only 3.5% addressed the lower extremity PNBs.

Does the literature interest reflect clinical practice of regional anesthesia and, more specifically, the use of PNBs of the lower extremity? According to Hadžić et al.,[79] in the United States the majority of anesthesiologists performed at least some regional anesthesia techniques during the same period of the literature cited; nevertheless, half of them performed less than five PNBs per month. Even among those who consider regional anesthesia a substantial part of their clinical practice, the same trend persists. Regarding the major conduction blocks of lower and upper extremity usually performed, it has been noted that femoral, sciatic, or popliteal blocks represent just a small part of the clinical practice if compared with the use of PNBs of the upper extremity.

The possible explanation for this disparity is that lower extremity PNBs may be considered more technically demanding than upper extremity PNBs and multiple blocks are required to provide complete conduction block of the lower extremity. Moreover, neuraxial anesthesia is almost always an alternative option for regional anesthesia of the lower limb, whereas no other choice is available for regional anesthesia of the upper extremity. This may be the reason why even the majority of anesthesiologists who provide anesthesia in the ambulatory setting often prefer neuraxial anesthesia over PNBs of the lower extremity.

To discover the possible explanation of the phenomenon, we have to analyze the environmental factors that can influence the anesthetists' choice about PNBs of the lower extremity, first of all considering their exposure to PNBs techniques during residency training programs.

Even during the past decades of the 1970s and 1980s, surveys have already shown that regional anesthesia would be the anesthesiologists' first preference for their surgical patients, especially in emergent situations.[80,81] More recent surveys have repeatedly shown that this attitude continued and escalated in the 1990s.[78] Nevertheless, this preference does not always influence clinical practice and teaching programs as we could expect.

It is a public perception that the number of blocks performed by a resident anesthetist and the proficiency acquired during training are both strictly related to the use of a particular technique in clinical practice.[82] Maybe because of this tight association between resident education and clinical practice, large discrepancies among training programs were noted over the last decades in the United States. It has been noted that at least some anesthesiology teaching programs have failed in their teaching of regional anesthesia.[83]

Kopacz and Bridenbaugh[84] reported that the average resident in training in the United States used regional anesthesia in 30% of cases, and general anesthesia or minimal anesthetic concentration in 70% of cases; this means a significant increase in the use of regional anesthesia since 1980, but wide disparities between programs and individuals still remained all over the United States (the wide range goes from 3% to 60%).

Since the 1990s, numerous educational changes have occurred in training programs and several techniques have also been invented or reborn in regional anesthesia (midhumeral brachial plexus block, combined spinal–epidural, lateral popliteal nerve block, paravertebral block, psoas compartment block).[85] Because every change in practice is usually expected to have a positive or negative influence on the teaching of regional anesthesia, once more Kopacz[85] in 2002 tried to answer the question: "Is resident exposure to regional anesthesia currently sufficient to provide adequate training of these techniques?"

Considering the indications stated in 1990 by the residence review committee (RRC) for Anaesthesiology of the American Directory of Graduate Medical Education Program (ADGME) about the educational requirements of anesthesiology training programs, 90% of residents reach the requirements for spinal and epidural anesthesia, whereas the greatest deficiency occurs in the area of PNBs: approximately 40% of residents report having inadequate exposure.[85]

Looking more specifically at the type of regional anesthesia where residency programs have failed, PNBs of the lower extremity were the most undertaught. For instance, femoral and sciatic blocks were infrequently used, maybe because of the more experience needed to attain a high degree of success, despite their accepted reliability.[83]

According to Buffington et al.,[82] practitioners interviewed about their use of regional anesthesia reported that what really changes from residency to practice is the type of block performed: spinal and axillary blocks almost doubled, whereas the use of epidural and sciatic/femoral blocks decreased.

Nevertheless, it is clear that high users in practice had been high users in residency. Chelly et al.[86] observed that residents in programs with a specific PNB rotation are exposed to a greater number of PNB techniques than those who do not have such a rotation included in their curriculum.

To discover what could make the anesthetist choose that specific technique for his patients, Buist[87] collected questionnaires from practitioners in the United Kingdom in the 1990s. Most respondents to Buist's study cited better postoperative analgesia as the main advantage of regional anesthesia, then lower morbidity, more rapid recovery, and suitability for day cases; others most frequently quoted included the suitability of regional anesthesia for patients with lung disease and the reduction in blood loss when regional anesthesia is used. Extra time required to establish the block, poor patient acceptance, low success rate, fear of nerve damage, and lack of surgeon compliance were the disadvantages cited by anesthesiologists.[87]

As a consequence, training programs cannot be the only influence in the practice of regional anesthesia. Residents should also be taught how to control environmental factors in addition to the technical steps of performing a block, because time pressure, surgeon attitude, patient compliance, and logistical requirements discourage the use of regional techniques in practice.[82]

## References


1. Hadžić A. www.NYSORA.com. New York School of Regional Anesthesia.
2. Enneking FK, Chan V, Greger J, Hadžić A, Lang SA, Horlocker TT. Lower extremity peripheral nerve blockade: essentials of our understanding. Reg Anesth Pain Med 2005; 30(1):4–35.
3. Cheney FW. High severity injuries associated with RA in the 1990s. Am Soc Anesthesiol Newslett 2001;65:6–8.
4. Ben-David B. Complications of regional anaesthesia. Anesthesiol Clin North Am 2002; 20:427–429.
5. Fitzgibbon DR. Liability arising from anaesthesiology-based pain management in the nonoperative setting. Am Soc Anesth Newslett 2001;65:12–15.
6. Lee LA, Posner KL, Domino KB, Caplan RA, Cheney FW. Injuries associated with regional anaesthesia in the 1980s and 1990s. A closed claims analysis. Anesthesiology 2004;101:143–152.
7. Auroy Y, Narchi P, Messiah A, Litt L, Rouvier B, Samii K. Serious complications related to regional anaesthesia: results of a prospective survey in France. Anesthesiology 1997; 87(3):479–486.
8. Clergue F, Auroy Y, Pequignot F, Jougla E, Lienhart A, Laxenaire MC. French survey of anesthesia in 1996. Anesthesiology 1999;91(5):1509–1529.
9. Auroy Y, Benhamou D, Bargues L, et al. Major complications of regional anesthesia in France: the SOS regional anesthesia hotline service. Anesthesiology 2002;97(5): 1274–1280.
10. Faccenda K, Finucane BT. Complications of regional anaesthesia. Drug Saf 2001;24(6): 413–442.

11. DiFazio CA. Adjuvant techniques to improve the success of regional anesthesia, mixtures. In: Raj PP, ed. Clinical Practice of Regional Anesthesia. New York: Churchill-Livingstone; 1991:154–160.
12. Pitcher C. Adjuvant techniques to improve the success of regional anesthesia, nerve stimulation. In: Raj PP, ed. Clinical Practice of Regional Anesthesia. New York: Churchill-Livingstone; 1991:161–169.
13. Baranowsky AP, Pither CE. A comparison of three methods of axillary brachial plexus anaesthesia. Anaesthesia 1990;45:362–365.
14. Fanelli G. Peripheral nerve block with electric nerve stimulation. Minerva Anestesiol 1992;58:1025–1026.
15. Fanelli G, Casati A, Garancini P, Torri G. Nerve stimulator and multiple injection technique for upper and lower limb blockade: failure rate, patient acceptance and neurologic complications. Anesth Analg 1999;88(4):847–852.
16. Casati A, Fanelli G, Beccaria P, Magistris L, Albertin A, Torri G. The effects of single or multiple injections on the volume of 0.5% ropivacaine required for femoral nerve blockade. Anesth Analg 2001;93:183–186.
17. Goldberg ME, Gregg C, Larijani GE, Norris MC, Marr AT, Seltzer JL. A comparison of three methods of axillary approach to brachial plexus blockade for upper extremity surgery. Anesthesiology 1987;66:814–816.
18. Selander D, Edshage S, Wolff T. Paresthesia or no paresthesia? Acta Anaesthesiol Scand 1979;23:27–33.
19. Marhofer P, Greher M, Kapral S. Ultrasound guidance in regional anaesthesia. Br J Anaesth 2005;94(1):7–17.
20. La Grange P, Foster PA, Pretorius LK. Application of the Doppler ultrasound bloodflow detector in supraclavicular brachial plexus block. Br J Anaesth 1978;50: 965–967.
21. Greher M, Retzl G, Niel P, Kamholz L, Marhofer P, Kapral S. Ultrasonographic assessment of topographic anatomy in volunteers suggests a modification of the infraclavicular vertical brachial block. Br J Anaesth 2002;88:632–636.
22. Peterson MK. Ultrasound guided nerve blocks. Br J Anaesth 2002;88:621–624.
23. Fornage BD. Peripheral nerves of the extremity: imaging with ultrasound. Radiology 1988;167:179–182.
24. Steiner E, Našel C. Sonography of peripheral nerves: basic principles. Acta Anaesthesiol Scand 1998;42(suppl 112):46–48.
25. Thierney E, Lewis G, Hurtig JB, Johnson D. Femoral nerve block with bupivacaine 0.25 per cent for postoperative analgesia after open knee surgery. Can J Anaesth 1987; 34:455–458.
26. Marhofer P, Schrögendorfer K, Koinig H, Kapral S, Weinstabl C, Mayer N. Ultrasonographic guidance improves sensory block and onset time of three-in-one blocks. Anesth Analg 1997;85:854–857.
27. Marhofer P, Schrögendorfer K, Wallner T, Koinig H, Mayer N, Kapral S. Ultrasonographic guidance reduces the amount of local anesthetic for 3-in-1 blocks. Reg Anesth Pain Med 1998;23:584–588.
28. Parkinson SK, Mueller JB, Little WL, Bailey SL. Extent of blockade with various approaches to the lumbar plexus. Anesth Analg 1989;68:243–248.
29. Kirchmair L, Entner T, Wissel J, Morrigl B, Kapral S, Mitterschiffthaler G. A study of the paravertebral anatomy for ultrasound-guided posterior lumbar plexus block. Anesth Analg 2001;93:477–481.
30. Kirchmair L, Entner T, Kapral S, Mitterschiffthaler G. Ultrasound guidance for the psoas compartment block: an imaging study. Anesth Analg 2002;94:706–710.
31. Davies MJ, McGlade DP. One hundred sciatic nerve blocks: a comparison of localisation techniques. Anaesth Intensive Care 1993;21:76–78.
32. Morris GF, Lang SA, Dust WN, Van der Wal M. The parasacral sciatic nerve block. Reg Anesth 1997;22:223–228.
33. Marhofer P, Greher M, Kapral S. Ultrasound guidance in regional anaesthesia. Br J Anaesth 2005;94:7–17.
34. Kroll DA, Caplan RA, Posner K, et al. Nerve injury associated with anesthesia. Anesthesiology 1990;73:202–207.
35. Liguori GA. Complications of regional anesthesia. Nerve injury and peripheral neural blockade. J Neurosurg Anesthesiol 2004;16:84–86.

36. Schroeder LE, Horlocker TT, Schroeder DR. The efficacy of axillary block for surgical procedures about the elbow. Anesth Analg 1996;83:747–751.
37. Horlocker TT, Kufner RP, Bishop AT, et al. The risk of persistent paresthesia is not increased with repeated axillary block. Anesth Analg 1999;88:382–387.
38. Stan TC, Krantz MA, Solomon DL, et al. The incidence of neurovascular complications following axillary brachial plexus block using a transarterial approach. Reg Anesth 1995; 20:486–492.
39. Urban MK, Urquart B. Evaluation of brachial plexus anesthesia for upper extremity surgery. Reg Anesth 1994;19:175–182.
40. Borgeat A, Ekatodramis G, Kalberer F, et al. Acute and non acute complications associated with interscalene block and shoulder surgery. A prospective study. Anesthesiology 2001;95:875–880.
41. Hartung HJ, Rupprecht A. The axillary brachial plexus block: a study of 178 patients. Reg Anaesth 1989;12:21–24.
42. Benumoff JL. Permanent loss of cervical spinal cord function associated with interscalene block performed under general anesthesia. Anesthesiology 2000;93:1541–1544.
43. Kalichman MW, Powell HC, Myers RR. Quantitative histologic analysis of local anesthetic-induced injury to rat sciatic nerve. J Pharmacol Exp Ther 1989;20: 406–413.
44. Selander D, Brattsand R, Lundborg G, et al. Local anesthetics: importance of mode of application, concentration, and adrenaline for the appearance of nerve lesions – an experimental study of axonal degeneration and barrier damage after intrafascicular injection or topical application of bupivacaine (Marcain). Acta Anaesthesiol Scand 1979; 23:127–136.
45. Selander D, Mansson LG, Karlsson L, Svanvik J. Adrenergic vasoconstriction in peripheral nerves of the rabbit. Anesthesiology 1985;62:6–10.
46. Ben-David B. Complications of peripheral blockade. Anesthesiol Clin North Am 2002; 20:695–707.
47. Komorowski TE, Shepard B, Okland S, Carlson BM. An electron microscopic study of local anesthetic-induced skeletal muscle fibre degeneration and regeneration in the monkey. J Orthop Res 1990;8:495–503.
48. Yagiela JA, Benoit PW, Buoncristiani RD, et al. Comparison of myotoxic effects of lidocaine with epinephrine in rats and humans. Anesth Analg 1981;60:471–480.
49. Pham-Dang C, Beaumont S, Floch H, Bodin J, Winer A, Pinaud M. Acute toxicity accident following lumbar plexus block with bupivacaine [French]. Ann Fr Anesth Reanim 2000; 19:356–359.
50. Breslin DS, Martin G, Macleod DB, D'Ercole F, Grant SA. Central nervous system toxicity following the administration of levobupivacaine for lumbar plexus block: a report of two cases. Reg Anesth Pain Med 2003;28:144–147.
51. Mullanu C, Gaillat F, Scemama F, Thibault S, Lavand'homme P, Auffray JP. Acute toxicity of local anesthetic ropivacaine and mepivacaine during combined lumbar plexus and sciatic block for hip surgery. Acta Anesthesiol Belg 2002;53:221–223.
52. Petitjeans F, Mion G, Puidupin M, Tourtier JP, Hutson C, Saissy JM. Tachycardia and convulsions induced by accidental intravascular ropivacaine injection during sciatic block. Acta Anaesthesiol Scand 2002;46:616–617.
53. Brown DL, Ransom DM, Hall JA, Leicht CH, Schroeder DR, Offord KP. Regional anesthesia and local anesthetic induced systemic toxicity: seizure frequency and accompanying cardiovascular changes. Anesth Analg 1995;81:321–328.
54. Cuvillon P, Ripart J, Lalourcey L, et al. The continuous femoral nerve block catheter for postoperative analgesia: bacteria colonization, infectious rate and adverse effects. Anesth Analg 2001;93:1045–1049.
55. Jöhr M. A complication of continuous femoral nerve block [German]. Reg Anaesth 1987; 10:37–38.
56. Capdevila X, Barthelet Y, Biboulet P, Ryckwaert Y, Rubenovitch J, D'Athis F. Effects of perioperative analgesic technique on the surgical outcome and duration of rehabilitation after major knee surgery. Anesthesiology 1999;91:8–15.
57. Weller RS, Gerancher JC, Crews JC, Wade KL. Extensive retroperitoneal hematoma without neurologic deficit in two patients who underwent lumbar plexus block and were later anticoagulated. Anesthesiology 2003;98:581–585.

58. Aveline C, Bonnet F. Delayed retroperitoneal haematoma after failed lumbar plexus block. Br J Anaesth 2004;93(4):589–591.
59. Klein SM, D'Ercole F, Greengrass RA, Warner DS. Enoxaparin associated with psoas hematoma and lumbar plexopathy after lumbar plexus block. Anesthesiology 1997;87: 1576–1579.
60. Aromaa U, Lahdensuu M, Cazanitis DA. Severe complications associated with epidural and spinal anaesthesias in Finland 1987–1993. A study based on patient insurance claims. Acta Anaesthesiol Scand 1997;41:445–452.
61. Wang LP, Hauerberg J, Schmidt JF. Incidence of spinal epidural abscess after epidural analgesia. Anaesthesiology 1999;91:1928–1936.
62. Bergamnn BD, Hebl JR, Kent J, Horlocker TT. Neurologic complications of 405 consecutive continuous axillary catheters. Anesth Analg 2003;96:247–252.
63. Adam F, Jaziri S, Chauvin M. Psoas abscess complicating femoral nerve block catheter. Anesthesiology 2003;99:230–231.
64. Cuvillon P, Ripart J, Lalourcey L, et al. The continuous femoral nerve block catheter for postoperative analgesia: bacterial colonization, infectious rate and adverse effects. Anesth Analg 2001;93:1045–1049.
65. Hebl JR, Horlocker TT. You're not as clean as you think! The role of asepsis in reducing infectious complications related to regional anesthesia. Reg Anesth Pain Med 2003; 28(5):376–379.
66. Bernstein IT, Hansen BJ. Iatrogenic psoas abscess. Case report. Scand J Urol Nephrol 1991;25:85–86.
67. Sato S, Sakuragi T, Dan K. Human skin flora as a potential source of epidural abscess. Anesthesiology 1996;85:1276–1282.
68. Saloojee H, Steenhoff A. The health professional's role in preventing nosocomial infections. Postgrad Med J 2001;77:16–19.
69. Cheney FW, Domino KB, Caplan RA, Posner KL. Nerve injury associated with anesthesia: a closed claims analysis. Anesthesiology 1999;90:1062–1069.
70. Warner MA, Warner DO, Harper CM, Schroeder DR, Maxson PM. Lower extremity neuropathies associated with lithotomy positions. Anesthesiology 2000;93:938–942.
71. Gruson KI, Moed BR. Injury of the femoral nerve associated with acetabular fracture. J Bone Joint Surg [Am] 2003;85A:428–431.
72. Slater N, Singh R, Senasinghe N, Gore R, Goroszeniuk T, James D. Pressure monitoring of the femoral nerve during total hip replacement: an explanation for iatropathic palsy. J R Coll Surg Edinb 2000;45:231–233.
73. Finsen V, Kasseth AM. Tourniquets in forefoot surgery: less pain when placed at the ankle. J Bone Joint Surg [Br] 1997;79:99–101.
74. Schurman DJ. Ankle block anesthesia for foot surgery. Anesthesiology 1976;44: 348–352.
75. Lichtenfeld NS. The pneumatic ankle tourniquet with ankle block anesthesia for foot surgery. Foot Ankle 1992;13:344–349.
76. Barber FA, Click J, Britt BT. Complications of ankle arthroscopy. Foot Ankle 1990;10: 263–266.
77. Ferkel RD, Heath DD, Guhl JF. Neurological complications of ankle arthroscopy. Arthroscopy 1996;12:200–208.
78. Shevde K, Panagopoulos G. A survey of 800 patients' knowledge attitudes and concerns regarding anesthesia. Anesth Analg 1991;73:190–198.
79. Hadžić A, Vloka JD, Kuroda MM, Koorn R, Birnbach DJ. The practice of peripheral nerve blocks in the United States: a national survey. Reg Anesth Pain Med 1998; 23(3):241–246.
80. Katz J. A survey of anesthetic choice among anesthesiologists. Anesth Analg 1973;52: 373–375.
81. Broadman LM, Mesrobian R, Ruttimann U, McGill WA. Do anesthesiologists prefer a regional or a general anesthetic for themselves? [abstract] Reg Anesth 1985;11:57.
82. Buffington CW, Ready LB, Horton WG. Training and practice factors influence the use of regional anesthesia. Implications for resident education. Reg Anesth 1985;10: 2–6.
83. Bridenbaugh LD. Are anesthesia resident programs failing regional anesthesia? Reg Anesth 1982;7:26–28.

84. Kopacz DJ, Bridenbaugh LD. Are anesthesia residency training programs failing regional anesthesia? The past, present and future. Reg Anesth 1993;18:84–87.
85. Kopacz DJ, Neal JM. Regional anesthesia and pain medicine: residency training – the year 2000. Reg Anesth Pain Med 2002;27(1):9–14.
86. Chelly JE, Greger J, Gebhard R, Hagberg CA, Al-Samsam T, Khan A. Training of residents in peripheral nerve blocks during anaesthesiology residency. J Clin Anesth 2002; 14(8):584–588.
87. Buist RJ. A survey of the practice of regional anaesthesia. J R Soc Med 1990;83: 709–712.

# 12 Complications of Intravenous Regional Anesthesia

Dominic A. Cave and Barry A. Finegan

Intravenous regional anesthesia (IVRA) of the limb was first described by Bier in 1908.[1] The original technique involved the surgical exposure of, and direct injection of local anesthetic into, an antecubital vessel, of an exsanguinated and isolated upper limb, thereby rendering the tissue below the applied tourniquet insensitive to pain. IVRA is a simple and effective method of providing anesthesia to peripheral tissues that anatomically have a blood supply which can be occluded by a pneumatic cuff. The technique in use today consists of the placement of a catheter in a suitable vein before exsanguination of the surgical site by gravity or compression, the inflation of a pneumatic double tourniquet, and the injection of a local anesthetic into the venous system of the isolated limb. Serious IVRA-related complications are rare and can be classified as drug and tourniquet related.[2]

## Drug-Related Complications

In IVRA, drugs are injected directly into a contained vascular space. The integrity of this compartment is dependent on the ability of a pneumatic occlusion cuff, applied externally, to occlude the venous system. Systemic complications arising from drugs used in IVRA can occur when this occlusion fails. Failure of occlusion can occur because of inadvertent deflation of the cuff, cuff failure, an increase in venous pressure within the occluded tissue to a value greater than cuff pressure, or where there is an intact interosseous circulation that bridges the cuff. In each of the aforementioned circumstances, drug-related complications result from the inadvertent spillage of drug into the general circulation. Drug is also released into the systemic circulation with deflation of the cuff at the end of the procedure and under certain circumstances this can also lead to complications.

A number of different classes of drugs have been used in IVRA with varying degrees of success including local anesthetics, opioids, NMDA (N-methyl D-aspartate) inhibitors, neuromuscular blocking agents, and sympatholytic compounds.

The drugs used, and therefore the drugs capable of causing complications, can be classified into two groups, the primary agents and the adjuvant agents.

### *Primary Agents*

The primary agents used for IVRA are the local anesthetics. In North America, lidocaine is the predominant choice, whereas in Europe prilocaine is a popular choice.

## Local Anesthetics

### *Mechanism of Action*

Local anesthetics inhibit action potential propagation within neuronal tissue by binding to receptors in $Na^+$ channels located on the nerve cell membrane. $Na^+$ channels have widespread cellular distribution, providing a significant potential for unintended sites of action and associated clinical complications. The major clinically relevant locations of extra-neuronal $Na^+$ channels susceptible to local anesthetic (LA) blockade are those found in cardiac and central nervous system (CNS) tissue.[3,4]

Normal functioning of the $Na^+$ channel is required for appropriate $Ca^{++}$ entry and egress across the myocardial cell membrane, which in turn is essential for the preservation of normal ventricular contractility and propagation of the cardiac action potential in pacemaker tissue. Local anesthetics exert negative inotropic effects on ventricular myocytes, the degree of contractile depression correlating with the potency of the LA.[5–7] In contrast, alterations in cardiac electrophysiology are less predictable, are more dependent on $Na^+$ channel kinetics, and can occur in the absence of a marked reduction in contractility.[5,8,9]

CNS toxicity of local anesthetic solutions is more predictable than cardiac toxicity and correlates relatively closely with the potency of the drug selected.[10] It is important to note that CNS and cardiac toxicity vary between local anesthetics, and that local anesthetics are not a homogenous group in regard to the complications they may produce.

### *Lidocaine*

Lidocaine IVRA is safe and effective and is associated with a rapid onset (4.5 ± 0.3 minutes) of anesthesia after injection and termination of analgesia (5.8 ± 0.5 minutes) once the tourniquet is deflated.[11] Release of the tourniquet 5 minutes after the administration of 2.5 mg/kg of 0.5% lidocaine resulted in no signs of cardiovascular or CNS toxicity; however, symptoms of tinnitus were noted between 20 and 70 seconds after deflation.[12] Approximately 70% of lidocaine remains within the tissues of the previously isolated limb following tourniquet release, the remainder entering the general circulation in the subsequent 45 minutes.[13] Release of tissue-bound lidocaine is increased if the limb is exercised, emphasizing the importance of keeping the previously anesthetized limb quiescent immediately after tourniquet deflation.

The cardiovascular safety of lidocaine is attributable to the characteristics of its interaction with the sodium channel in the conduction system. Lidocaine does not accumulate significantly at the $Na^+$ channel at therapeutic plasma concentrations,[13–17] and rapidly binds to (time constant <500 ms) and dissociates from (time constant = 154 ms) the channel, preventing toxic accumulation of the drug.[18] Consequently, electrophysiologic disturbances do not occur at heart rates less than 150 bpm.[7] Excessive plasma lidocaine levels are associated with peripheral vasodilatation and reduced contractility which is manifest as hypotension, particularly in the volume-depleted patient.

### *Bupivacaine*

Bupivacaine was first used for IVRA in the 1970s with Ware[19] reporting its use in 50 cases without major complication. The use of bupivacaine in IVRA was initially met with enthusiasm because it offered a more prolonged period of pain relief after the tourniquet release than lidocaine. However, it was not long after Ware's report that the first reports began to come to light of serious problems associated with the use of bupivacaine in IVRA, with seven deaths occurring between 1979 and 1983.[20–22] Bupivacaine binds to activated $Na^+$ channels at low plasma concentrations (0.2 mg/mL) displaying fast on/slow off kinetics (time constant of 1.467 seconds) facilitating accumulation of bupivacaine at the $Na^+$ channel, at heart rates as slow as 60 bpm.[18] This provides a significant risk of electrophysiologic disturbance, including ventricular fibrillation resistant to conventional therapy, on the release of a bolus of bupivacaine into the circulation when the tourniquet is deflated at the end of IVRA.

### *Levobupivacaine*

A study by Atanassoff et al.[23] in 2002 demonstrated in eight volunteers that onset of sensory block was delayed with levobupivacaine (12.5 versus 1.5 minutes) and pinprick sensation return was delayed after tourniquet release (15 versus 4.5 minutes) when compared with lidocaine. They also reported >50% incidence of CNS symptoms on tourniquet release with lidocaine, and a 0% incidence with levobupivacaine. No cardiac adverse events were observed, but the numbers involved are too small to draw any firm conclusions. Levobupivacaine has been compared with bupivacaine in a sheep model. The numbers of animals studied were few, but although convulsions were produced with both drugs, the ventricular dysrhythmias produced by levobupivacaine were relatively more benign and no sheep died during the levobupivacaine infusion.[24]

### *Ropivacaine*

Ropivacaine (0.2%) has a favorable CNS profile relative to lidocaine.[25] Ropivacaine 0.375% provided superior analgesia in the first 2 hours after surgery versus lidocaine 0.5% with no reported local anesthetic side effects.[26] In a direct comparison in a dog model among bupivacaine, levobupivacaine, ropivacaine, and lidocaine, the most frequent cause of collapse was cardiac depression, with arrhythmias being more common in the bupivacaine-treated animals.[27] Resuscitation was successful in 100% of the lidocaine dogs, 90% of the ropivacaine group, 70% of the L-bupivacaine group, and 50% of the bupivacaine group. Most concerning, there was no difference between the unbound plasma concentration of bupivacaine and L-bupivacaine at collapse, whereas the concentration for ropivacaine required to produce collapse was significantly higher. This suggests that ropivacaine might be a better choice than L-bupivacaine or bupivacaine, but that none of these drugs are ideal for IVRA.

### *Prilocaine*

Prilocaine is metabolized by the liver. Dose-related formation of methemoglobin occurs 4–8 hours after prilocaine administration.[28–30] As a result, prilocaine is not used for IVRA in North America. However, significant methemoglobinemia has *not* been reported when prilocaine has been used in IVRA. The large experience with prilocaine in Europe without reported adverse effect brings into question the choice to limit its use in North America. The main advantage of prilocaine over lidocaine is a reduction in the incidence of symptoms of CNS toxicity. Prilocaine 0.5% upper limb IVRA is associated with onset of analgesia in 11.0 ± 6.8 minutes and termination of analgesia after tourniquet deflation in 7.2 ± 4.6 minutes.[31] Prilocaine IVRA is extremely safe.[32] Bartholomew and Sloan[33] reviewed a series of 45,000 IVRA blocks and reported no serious side effects and no deaths related to the use of prilocaine in IVRA. Prilocaine IVRA is equally effective in terms of anesthesia to lidocaine IVRA.[34]

### *Chloroprocaine*

Chloroprocaine is rapidly metabolized by ester hydrolysis to nontoxic metabolites and theoretically should be a very safe local anesthetic to use in IVRA. Local ester hydrolysis should produce a very low risk of release of a toxic concentration of local anesthetic into the general circulation. Unfortunately, chloroprocaine formulated with preservative is damaging to the vascular endothelium[35] and elicits severe pain on injection. The use of chloroprocaine with preservative in IVRA is contraindicated. There has been limited but successful performance of IVRA with preservative-free solutions of chloroprocaine.[36] However, venous irritation, even with preservative-free solutions, remains a problem.[37]

### *Articaine*

Articaine has been used in dentistry since the 1970s. It is an amide local anesthetic with a thiophene rather than a benzene ring. It is metabolized to inactive articainic acid by plasma carboxyesterase and this adds to its safety. It is short acting and has a similar onset of analgesia to prilocaine, and is faster than lidocaine. Both its CNS and cardiovascular side effect profiles seem to be favorable.[38] Despite all these apparent benefits, it has not come into widespread use. This may be attributable to the propensity of articaine to cause an erythematous rash in the area where the drug is injected.

### *Mepivacaine*

An interesting development has been the investigation of mepivacaine for IVRA. Mepivacaine in a dose of 5mg/kg was compared with lidocaine in a small (n = 42) double-blind study.[39] Mepivacaine provided better intraoperative analgesia than lidocaine with no difference in side effects. Of note, mepivacaine levels after deflation were less than expected for the dose injected, but they also did not decrease significantly over the following hour, unlike lidocaine levels.

### *Ketamine*

Ketamine is an NMDA antagonist with local anesthetic qualities which has been studied as a sole agent for IVRA. Whereas it provided some, although inadequate, pain relief during IVRA, it was associated with the occurrence of hallucinations on tourniquet release and in some cases the loss of consciousness.[40,41] Ketamine is not a suitable drug as the sole agent for IVRA. However, ketamine when used in combination with local anesthetics has been shown to be very effective in reducing the incidence of tourniquet pain. When ketamine is used in IVRA for this purpose, the recommended dose is 0.1mg/kg and there are no CNS symptoms when used in this dosage.[42]

## Sympatholytic Drugs

The intravenous regional administration of guanethidine and reserpine inhibits sympathetic nervous system outflow in the isolated area.[43] Sympatholytic therapy is used in the treatment of reflex sympathetic dystrophy, causalgia, chronic regional pain syndrome,[44,45] rheumatoid arthritis,[46] frostbite,[47] and to improve blood flow in tissue flap procedures.[48] Despite widespread use of this technique and many anecdotal accounts of its success, randomized, controlled trials have not supported this optimistic conclusion in the area of chronic pain syndrome management.[49] The original work took place in the early 1970s, but it was not until the 1990s that a true double-blind study was conducted. The results of this study found that the placebo medication (in this case normal saline) was an effective therapy, and that there was no benefit in adding guanethidine in treating chronic pain syndromes.

Guanethidine acts at the terminal portion of the nerve fiber and interferes with the normal release and storage of norepinephrine.[50] Guanethidine evokes pain on intravenous injection and consequently it is usually coadministered with a local anesthetic. There is some limited evidence suggesting that repeated doses of guanethidine can permanently reduce norepinephrine reuptake and induce nerve end retraction, the latter being associated with a widening of the synaptic gap.[51] The major systemic complication of guanethidine intravenous regional sympathetic block is the frequent occurrence of hypotension, which can be prolonged in nature and in susceptible patients can be associated with apnea and angina.[52–54]

### *Adjuvant Agents*

The ideal IVRA agent would be simple, safe, give excellent intraoperative analgesia, both at the surgical site and at the tourniquet, and provide prolonged postoperative pain relief. It should also provide the best possible surgical conditions. From the discussion above it can be seen that no single agent achieves this aim, as yet. The only way to attempt to provide these conditions is to use adjunctive agents. Many drugs have been studied in this role (see comprehensive review by Choyce and Peng[55]).

#### Opioids

The aim of opioid administration in IVRA is to prolong analgesia after cuff deflation and, although many have been studied, including fentanyl, morphine, sufentanil, and meperidine, none have proven to have any clear advantage over the administration of a local anesthetic alone. Indeed, the coadministration of an opioid in IVRA is associated with an increased incidence of unpleasant side effects, especially nausea and vomiting, after cuff deflation.[56,57] Opioids administered as sole agents for IVRA are not therapeutically effective.

#### Neuromuscular Blocking Drugs

The administration of neuromuscular blocking drugs including atracurium (2 mg) and pancuronium (0.5 mg) with local anesthetics in upper limb IVRA improves surgical conditions in adults undergoing fracture reduction.[58,59] There have been no reported complications from using adjuvant neuromuscular blocking drugs in IVRA. Atracurium is probably the best choice if regional muscle relaxation is required, given the role of Hoffman degradation in its elimination from the body. The use of neuromuscular blocking agents alone cannot be recommended.

#### Nonsteroidal Antiinflammatory Drugs

Ketorolac has been extensively studied as an adjuvant in IVRA. Reuben et al.[60] found that the addition of 60 mg of ketorolac to local anesthetics improved intraoperative analgesia and reduced the intensity of pain in the first hour after deflation and the demand for analgesics in the first postoperative day. This dose of ketorolac raises some concerns, and Steinberg et al.[61] conducted a dose finding study which showed a linear dose response up to 20 mg and then no additional benefit. There were no reported side effects of ketorolac use.

Tenoxicam and acetyl-salicylate at a dose of 20 and 90 mg, respectively, are also effective adjuvants, although the duration of postoperative analgesia is shorter than that reported for ketorolac.[62,63] It seems reasonable, if no contraindications exist, to use nonsteroidal antiinflammatory drugs as adjuvants in IVRA.

#### Alpha-2 Agonists

Clonidine, in a dose of 1 μg/kg added to the IVRA solution, has been shown in a double-blind study to prolong the time to request for first postoperative analgesia significantly (460 versus 115 minutes) and reduce overall analgesic requirements in the first 24 hours.[64] Clonidine has also been shown to decrease tourniquet pain.[65] However, the reduction in the severity of tourniquet pain and the prolongation of postanalgesia by clonidine may only be replacing one set of complications for another. At doses of 2 μg/kg, hypotension and sedation have been noted on tourniquet release.[66]

Dexmedetomidine is about eight times more selective for $\alpha_2$ receptor than clonidine. A dose of 0.5 μg/kg is associated with reported improvements in the onset time of sensory and motor blockade, intraoperative analgesic requirements, onset of tourniquet pain, and duration of postoperative analgesia (564 versus 129 minutes).[67]

In contrast to high-dose clonidine, no side effects were observed. These data are very promising and dexmedetomidine may well become a valuable and standard adjuvant in IVRA.

### Anticholinesterases

Neostigmine has been found to improve anesthesia in some regional techniques; however, the evidence for its benefit in IVRA is unclear.[68]

## Tourniquet-Related Complications

Tourniquets have a long history of use in medicine. They have two basic functions: 1) isolation of the limb from the systemic circulation, as when preventing blood loss in limb trauma or in the isolated arm technique for monitoring anesthetic awareness, and 2) isolation of the systemic circulation from the limb as in IVRA. The shared feature of both scenarios is the loss of oxygenated blood supply to the limb that has the tourniquet applied. There is consequently the possibility of significant harm even in the case of a properly applied and fully functioning tourniquet.

An intact tourniquet is essential for the establishment and maintenance of IVRA. Inadvertent deflation of the tourniquet or the presence of a vascular communication across an intact tourniquet can lead to serious local anesthetic-related complications. Loss of limb isolation can result in both neurologic and, in extreme cases, cardiovascular collapse if the systemic vascular concentration of the local anesthetic exceeds the safe range. Consequently, the tourniquet, manometer, and inflation equipment should undergo regular maintenance to minimize the risk of equipment failure. Before each use, the competency of the tourniquet should be visually assessed. Where automated dual-cuff devices are used, it is essential that staff are trained in the appropriate use of the equipment and are familiar with the technique of IVRA. Equipment malfunction or misuse is an important and avoidable cause of morbidity in IVRA.[69,70] An intact and properly functioning cuff has a number of common side effects or complications associated with it. Local pressure effects usually evoke discomfort and pain in patients. Prolonged tourniquet time is associated with an increase in systemic blood pressure, often into the hypertensive range.

The presence of an intact tourniquet does not completely prevent drugs injected into the isolated limb from entering the systemic circulation.[71,72] Location of the tourniquet has a role. Almost 100% of IVRA lower limb blocks are associated with detectable leakage of local anesthetic, compared with 25% of upper limb IVRA procedures.[73] Increased drug leakage following IVRA occurs with fracture manipulation,[74] particularly in the lower limb. In addition, IVRA lower limb blocks require a high dose and volume of local anesthetic to achieve satisfactory analgesia. Lower limb IVRA is also associated with a high incidence of poor-quality block (36.8%).[75]

Many factors apart from the location of the tourniquet may be responsible for leakage of drug past an intact cuff. The occurrence of an interosseous circulation, not amenable to occlusion by a tourniquet, has been demonstrated angiographically,[76] but does not seem to be a major factor in IVRA-related morbidity. Of greater clinical relevance is the association between the rate of fluid injection into the isolated segment and the development of an increased venous pressure within the isolated segment. Venous pressure values greater than 250 mmHg have been recorded 1 minute following bolus injection of 66 mL of saline in volunteers.[77] These data underscore the importance of avoiding rapid injection of drug solutions during IVRA.

The tourniquet pressure required to completely occlude blood flow in a limb is considerably greater than systolic blood pressure as there is considerable attenuation of the applied tourniquet pressure by fat, muscle, and connective tissue within the limb.[78] Tourniquet use is associated with an increase in systolic blood pressure over time[79]; this increase may be excessive, particularly in hypertensive patients.[80] The inflation pressure of the tourniquet must be adjusted appropriately to account for these alterations.

### *Deflation of the Tourniquet*

Symptoms of local anesthetic toxicity (tinnitus and perioral paresthesia) are frequently reported following elective deflation of the tourniquet.[72] These symptoms correlate with the concentration of local anesthetic in the arterial[81–83] rather than venous circulation.[14,84] No safe time interval between local anesthetic drug administration and tourniquet deflation has been established. The current recommendation is to wait 20 minutes from the time the drug has been injected, but this is not based on any scientific evidence. Intermittent deflation rather than a single deflation has been proposed to minimize risk of LA toxicity[81]; however, this does not alter the peak concentration of local anesthetic achieved on tourniquet release but merely prolongs the time for it to be achieved.

### *Tourniquet Pain*

Tourniquet pain is a common complication of IVRA.[72] A double-cuff tourniquet reduces the incidence of tourniquet pain and should be used if the duration of the surgical procedure is anticipated to be longer than 30 minutes. Other less effective treatment options include intravenous sedation/analgesia and temporary deflation, then reinflation, of the cuff. The evidence presented above would suggest that this complication may be reduced by the use of adjuvants such as dexmedetomidine, clonidine, ketorolac, and ketamine or some combinations of these adjuvants to the IVRA.[42,60,64,67] Dexmedetomidine seems to have the best safety profile, but it is also the drug with the least investigation in this role. Tourniquet pain has also been reduced by lidocaine priming with 1 mg/kg given intravenously 5 minutes before IVRA[85] and by using a forearm rescue cuff.[86]

### *Paralysis*

The incidence of neuromuscular dysfunction (a reduction in preoperative motor or sensory function, whether temporary or permanent) following the use of pneumatic tourniquet for a bloodless field is estimated at 1 in 8000.[87] Sporadic case reports exist of damage to ulnar, median, and musculocutaneous nerves associated with IVRA.[88,89] The common etiology of these injuries is direct pressure to the nerves, which exhibit histologic changes of crush injury. Tourniquet time should not exceed 2 hours to avoid capillary and muscle cell damage secondary to tissue acidosis.[87]

### *Compartment Syndrome*

Compartment syndrome[90,91] is an increase in pressure within a muscular compartment to a value greater than perfusion pressure, leading to tissue ischemia. IVRA, particularly when used for reduction of long bone lower limb fractures, is associated with an increased incidence of compartment syndrome.[92] This may well reflect the large volume of drug solution required to provide effective lower limb IVRA and inadequate exsanguination of the limb before IVRA. Compartment syndrome secondary to hypertonic saline instillation, mistakenly used as a diluent for local anesthetic, has been reported.[90,93]

### *Loss of Limb*

Loss of a forearm following IVRA has been reported in a 28-year-old female patient.[94] In the case described, the tourniquet time was 25 minutes, and signs of severe ischemia were apparent on release of the tourniquet. One week after the procedure, the 28-year-old patient had her arm amputated. Histologic examination of the excised limb demonstrated thrombosis of the radial and ulnar arteries. This catastrophic event may have been caused by inadvertent intraarterial drug injection, an idiosyncratic drug reaction, or a drug administration error.

## Reducing Complications

### *Appropriate Drug Selection*

Prilocaine (3–4mg/kg of 0.5%)[95–99] or lidocaine (1.5–3mg/kg)[100–102] are appropriate and safe local anesthetics to administer in IVRA. Levobupivacaine and ropivacaine may become suitable choices in the future, but more studies are required to establish safety. At this time, the evidence is that these drugs are safer than bupivacaine. It remains to be seen if that is safe enough.

### *Reduce the Quantity of Drug Used*

Consider use of a forearm tourniquet technique. This allows use of half as much local anesthetic, thereby reducing the incidence of complications while still providing adequate analgesia.[103–105]

### *Minimize Leakage of Drug Across the Tourniquet*

1. Ensure adequate exsanguination of the limb before tourniquet inflation, a process facilitated by the limb elevation and the application of an Esmarch bandage.[72]
2. Maintain the tourniquet pressure at a level sufficient to prevent venous congestion in the isolated segment of the limb.
3. Do not use excessive volumes of local anesthetic solution. A volume of 0.5mL/kg (40mL total volume) is adequate for upper limb IVRA. In forearm IVRA, a volume of 20mL has been shown to be adequate.[103]
4. Inject the local anesthetic solution over at least 90 seconds.
5. Inject the solution as far distal to the tourniquet as practical.[106]

### *Reduce the Incidence of Tourniquet Pain*

A double-cuff tourniquet is preferable to a single-cuff device.

### *Prevent Ischemia*

1. Ensure that the drug injection cannula is placed in a vein.
2. Do not allow the total tourniquet time to exceed 2 hours.[87,89]

### *Deflate the Tourniquet Appropriately*

An interval of at least 20 minutes between drug administration and tourniquet deflation is suggested.

## Conclusion

IVRA is a safe, simple, and effective regional anesthetic. Repeated evaluations have found success rates in the 95% and above range.[107] Careful attention to detail and a thorough understanding of the limitations and potential complications of the technique are essential to achieve the optimal outcome.

## References


1. Bier A. Uber einen neuen weg lokalanasthesie an den gliedmassen zu erzeugen. Verh Dtsch Ges Chir 1908;37:204–214.
2. Brown EM, McGriff JT, Malinowski RW. Intravenous regional anaesthesia (Bier block): review of 20 years' experience. Can J Anaesth 1989;36(3):307–310.
3. Tucker GT. Pharmacokinetics of local anaesthetics. Br J Anaesth 1986;58:717–731.
4. Bean BP, Cohen CJ, Tsien RW. Lidocaine block of cardiac sodium channels. J Gen Physioly 1983;5:613–642.
5. Reiz S, Nath S. Cardiotoxicity of local anaesthetic agents. Br J Anaesth 1986;58: 736–746.
6. Nath S, Haggmark S, Johansson G, Reiz S. Differential depressant and electrophysiological cardiotoxicity of local anesthetics: an experimental study with special reference to lidocaine and bupivacaine. Anesth Analg 1986;65:1263–1270.
7. Liu P, Covino BM, Giasi R, Covino BG. Acute cardiovascular toxicity of intravenous amide anesthetics in anesthetized ventilated dogs. Anesth Analg 1982;61:317–322.
8. deJong RH, Ronfeld RA, DeRosa RA. Cardiovascular effects of convulsant and supraconvulsant doses of amide local anesthetics. Anesth Analg 1982;61(1):3–9.
9. Enright AC, Smith GG, Wyant GM. Comparison of bupivacaine and lidocaine for intravenous regional analgesia. Can Anaesth Soc J 1980;27(6):553–555.
10. Covino BG. Toxicity of local anesthetics. Acta Anaesthesiol Belg 1988;39:159–164.
11. Ware RJ. Intravenous regional analgesia using bupivacaine. A double blind comparison with lignocaine. Anaesthesia 1979;34(3):231–235.
12. Smith CA, Steinhaus JE, Haynes CD. The safety and effectiveness of intravenous regional anesthesia. South Med J 1968;61:1057–1060.
13. Tucker GT, Boas RA. Pharmacokinetic aspects of intravenous regional anesthesia. Anesthesiology 1971;34:538–549.
14. Kern C, Gamulin Z. Generalised convulsions after intravenous regional anaesthesia with prilocaine. Anaesthesia 1994;49(7):642–643.
15. Bader AM, Concepcion M, Hurley RJ, Arthur GA. Comparison of lidocaine and prilocaine for intravenous regional anesthesia. Anesthesiology 1988;69(3):409–412.
16. Mazze RI, Dunbar RW. Intravenous regional anesthesia – report of 497 cases with toxicity study. Acta Anaesthesiol Scand Suppl 1969;36:27–34.
17. Thorn-Alquist AM. Blood concentrations of local anaesthetics after intravenous regional anaesthesia. Acta Anaesthesiol Scand 1969;13(4):229–240.
18. Clarkson CW, Hondeghem LM. Mechanism for bupivacaine depression of cardiac conduction: fast block of sodium channels during the action potential with slow recovery from block during diastole. Anesthesiology 1985;62(4):396–405.
19. Ware RJ. Intravenous regional analgesia using bupivacaine. Anesthesia 1975;30(6): 817–822.
20. Heath ML. Deaths after intravenous regional anaesthesia from bupivacaine. Br Med J (Clin Res Ed) 1982;285(6346):913–914.
21. Long WB, Rosenblum S, Grady IP. Successful resuscitation of bupivacaine-induced cardiac arrest using cardiopulmonary bypass. Anesth Analg 1989;69(3): 403–406.
22. Reynolds F. Bupivacaine and intravenous regional anaesthesia. Anaesthesia 1984;39(2): 105–107.
23. Atanassoff PG, Aouad R, Hartmannsgruber M, Halaszynski T. Levobupivacaine 0.125% and lidocaine 0.5% for intravenous regional anesthesia in volunteers. Anesthesiology 2002;97:325–328.
24. Huang YF, Pryor ME, Mather LE, Veering BT. Cardiovascular and central nervous system effects of intravenous levobupivacaine in sheep. Anesth Analg 1998;86(4): 797–804.
25. Atanassoff PG, Hartmannsgruber M. Central nervous system side effects are less important after IV regional anesthesia with ropivacaine 0.2% compared to lidocaine 0.5% in volunteers. Can J Anaesth 2002;49(2):169–172.
26. Peng PW, Coleman MM, McCartney CJ, et al. Comparison of anesthetic effect between 0.375% ropivacaine versus 0.5% lidocaine in forearm regional anesthesia. Reg Anesth Pain Med 2002;27(6):595–599.

27. Groban L, Deal DD, Vernon JC, James RL, Butterworth J. Cardiac resuscitation after incremental overdosage with lidocaine, bupivacaine, levobupivacaine and ropivacaine in anesthetized dogs. Anesth Analg 2001;92(1):37–43.
28. Biscoping J, Michaelis G, Hempelmann G. Behavior of plasma concentrations of prilocaine following intravenous regional anesthesia and their relation to methemoglobinemia. Reg Anaesth 1988;11:35–39.
29. Harris WH. Choice of anesthetic agents for intravenous regional anesthesia. Acta Anaesthesiol Scand Suppl 1969;36:47–52.
30. Mazze RI. Methemoglobin concentrations following intravenous regional anesthesia. Anesth Analg 1968;47:122–125.
31. Pitkanen MT, Suzuki N, Rosenberg PH. Intravenous regional anaesthesia with 0.5% prilocaine or 0.5% chloroprocaine. A double-blind comparison in volunteers. Anaesthesia 1992;47:618–619.
32. Schurg R, Biscoping J, Bachmann-M B, Hempelmann G. Intravenous regional anesthesia of the foot using prilocaine. Clinical aspects, pharmacokinetic and pharmacodynamic studies. Reg Anaesth 1990;13:118–121.
33. Bartholomew K, Sloan JP. Prilocaine for Bier's block: how safe is safe? Arch Emerg Med 1990;7:189–195.
34. Arendt-Nielsen L, Oberg B, Bjerring P. Laser-induced pain for quantitative comparison of intravenous regional anesthesia using saline, morphine, lidocaine, or prilocaine. Reg Anesth 1990;15:186–193.
35. Suzuki N, Pitkanen M, Sariola H, Palas T, Rosenberg PH. The effect of plain 0.5% 2-chloroprocaine on venous endothelium after intravenous regional anaesthesia in the rabbit. Acta Anaesthesiol Scand 1994;38:653–656.
36. Palas TA. Don't forget chloroprocaine for IVRA. Reg Anesth 1990;15:271.
37. Pitkanen MT, Suzuki N, Rosenberg PH. Intravenous regional anaesthesia with 0.5% prilocaine or 0.5% chloroprocaine. Anaesthesia 1992;47:618–619.
38. Pitkanen MT, Xu M, Haasio J, Rosenberg PH. Comparison of 0.5% articaine and 0.5% prilocaine in intravenous regional anesthesia of the arm: a cross-over study in volunteers. Reg Anaesth Pain Med 1999;24(2):131–135.
39. Prieto-Alvarez P, Calas-Guerra A, Fuentes-Bellido J, Martinez-Verdera E, Benet-Catala A, Lorenzo-Foz JP. Comparison of mepivacaine and lidocaine for intravenous regional anaesthesia: pharmacokinetic study and clinical correlation. Br J Anaesth 2002;88(4): 516–519.
40. Amiot JF, Bouju P, Palacci JH, Ballinere E. Intravenous regional anaesthesia with ketamine. Anaesthesia 1985;40:899–901.
41. Durrani Z, Winnie AP, Zsigmond EK, Burnett ML. Ketamine for intravenous regional anesthesia [see comments]. Anesth Analg 1989;68:328–332.
42. Gorgias NK, Maidatsi PG, Kyriakidis AM, Karakoulas KA, Alvanos DN, Giala MM. Clonidine versus ketamine to prevent tourniquet pain during intravenous regional anesthesia with lidocaine. Reg Anesth Pain Med 2001;26:512–517.
43. Hannington-Kiff JG. Intravenous regional sympathetic block with guanethidine. Lancet 1974:1019–1020.
44. Blanchard J, Ramamurthy S, Walsh N, Hoffman J, Schoenfeld L. Intravenous regional sympatholysis: a double-blind comparison of guanethidine, reserpine and normal saline. J Pain Symptom Manage 1990;5:357–361.
45. Walker SM, Cousins MJ. Complex regional pain syndromes: including "reflex sympathetic dystrophy" and "causalgia." Anaesth Intensive Care 1997;25:113–125.
46. Hannington-Kiff JG. Rheumatoid arthritis – interventional treatment with regionally applied drugs and the use of sympathetic modulation: discussion paper. J R Soc Med 1990;83:373–376.
47. Kaplan R, Thomas P, Tepper H, Strauch B. The treatment of frostbite with guanethidine. Lancet 1981;2(8252):940–941.
48. Aarts HF. Regional intravascular sympathetic blockade for better results in flap surgery. An experimental study of free flaps, island flaps, and pedicle flaps in the rabbit ear. Plast Reconstr Surg 1980;66:690–698.
49. Jadad AR, Carroll D, Glynn CJ, McQuay HJ. Intravenous regional blockade for pain relief in reflex sympathetic dystrophy: a systematic review and a randomized double-blind crossover study. J Pain Symptom Manage 1995;10:13–20.

50. Coffman JD. Drug therapy: vasodilator drugs in peripheral vascular disease. N Engl J Med 1979;300:713–717.
51. Hannington-Kiff JG. Pharmacological target blocks in hand surgery. J Hand Surg Br 1984;9:29–36.
52. Sharpe E, Milaszkiewicz R, Carli F. A case of prolonged hypotension following intravenous guanethidine block. Anaesthesia 1987;42:1081–1084.
53. Woo R, McQueen J. Apnea and syncope following intravenous guanethidine Bier block in the same patient on two different occasions. Anesthesiology 1987;67:281–282.
54. Kalmanovitch DVA, Hardwick PB. Hypotension after guanethidine block. Anaesthesia 1988;43:256.
55. Choyce A, Peng P. A systematic review of adjuncts for intravenous regional anesthesia for surgical procedures. Can J Anaesth 2002;49(1):32–45.
56. Armstrong P, Power I, Wildsmith JA. Addition of fentanyl to prilocaine for intravenous regional anaesthesia. Anaesthesia 1991;46:278–280.
57. Arthur JM, Heavner JE, Mian T, Rosenberg PH. Fentanyl and lidocaine versus lidocaine for Bier block. Reg Anesth 1992;17:223–227.
58. McGlone R, Heyes F, Harris P. The use of muscle relaxant to supplement local anaesthetics for Bier's blocks. Arch Emerg Med 1988;5:79–85.
59. Elhakim M, Sadek RA. Addition of atracurium to lidocaine for intravenous regional anaesthesia. Acta Anaesthesiol Scand 1994;38:542–544.
60. Reuben SS, Steinberg RB, Kreitzer JM, Duprat KM. Intravenous regional anesthesia using lidocaine and ketorolac. Anesth Analg 1995;81:110–113.
61. Steinberg RB, Reuben SS, Gardner G. The dose-response relationship of ketorolac as a component of intravenous regional anesthesia with lidocaine. Anesth Analg 1998;86: 791–793.
62. Jones NC, Pugh SC. The addition of tenoxicam to prilocaine for intravenous regional anesthesia. Anaesthesia 1996;51:446–448.
63. Corpataux J-B, Van Gissel EF, Donald FA, Forster A, Gamulin Z. Effect on postoperative analgesia of small-dose lysine acetylsalicylate added to prilocaine during intravenous regional anesthesia. Anesth Analg 1997;84:1081–1085.
64. Reuben SS, Steinberg RB, Klatt JL, Klatt ML. Intravenous regional anesthesia using lidocaine and clonidine. Anesthesiology 1999;91:654–658.
65. Gentili M, Bernard J-M, Bonnet F. Adding clonidine to lidocaine for intravenous regional anesthesia prevents tourniquet pain. Anesth Analg 1999;88(6):1327–1330.
66. Kleinschmidt S, Stockl W, Wilhelm W, Larsen R. The addition of clonidine to prilocaine for intravenous regional anaesthesia. Eur J Anaesthesiol 1997;14:40–46.
67. Memis D, Turan A, Karamanhoglu B, Pamukcu Z, Kurt I. Adding dexmedetomidine to lidocaine for intravenous regional anesthesia. Anesth Analg 2004;98:835–840.
68. Turan A, Karamanlyoglu B, Memis D, Kaya G, Pamukcu Z. Intravenous regional anesthesia using prilocaine and neostigmine. Anesth Analg 2002;95:1419–1422.
69. Robinson DA, Shimmings KI. Uncomplicated accidental early tourniquet deflation during intravenous regional anaesthesia with prilocaine. Anaesthesia 1989;44(1): 83–84.
70. Aronson HB, Vatashsky E. Inadvertent tourniquet release five minutes after intravenous regional bupivacaine. Anaesthesia 1980;35:1208–1210.
71. Mazze RI, Dunbar RW. Plasma lidocaine concentrations after caudal, lumbar epidural, axillary block, and intravenous regional anesthesia. Anesthesiology 1966;27(5): 574–679.
72. Dunbar RW, Mazze RI. Intravenous regional anesthesia: experience with 779 cases. Anesth Analg 1967;46(6):806–813.
73. Davies JA, Walford AJ. Intravenous regional anaesthesia for foot surgery. Acta Anaesthesiol Scand 1986;30:145–147.
74. Quinton DN, Hughes J, Mace PF, Aitkenhead AR. Prilocaine leakage during tourniquet inflation in intravenous regional anaesthesia: the influence of fracture manipulation. Injury 1988;19:333–335.
75. Kim DD, Shuman C, Sadr B. Intravenous regional anesthesia for outpatient foot and ankle surgery: a prospective study. Orthopedics 1993;16:1109–1113.
76. Cotev S, Robin GC. Experimental studies on intravenous regional anaesthesia using radioactive lignocaine. Br J Anaesth 1966;38(12):936–940.

77. Lawes EG, Johnson T, Pritchard P, Robbins P. Venous pressures during simulated Bier's block. Anaesthesia 1984;39:147–149.
78. Davies J, Hall I, Wilkey A, et al. Intravenous regional analgesia. The danger of the congested arm and the value of occlusion pressure. Anaesthesia 1984;39:416–421.
79. Valli H, Rosenberg PH, Kytta J, et al. Arterial hypertension associated with the use of a tourniquet with either general or regional anaesthesia. Acta Anaesthesiol Scand 1987; 31:279–283.
80. Ogden PN. Failure of intravenous regional analgesia using a double cuff tourniquet. Anaesthesia 1984;39:456–459.
81. Sukhani R, Garcia CJ, Munhall RJ, et al. Lidocaine disposition following intravenous regional anesthesia with different tourniquet deflation technics. Anesth Analg 1989; 68:633–637.
82. Hargrove RL, Hoyle JR, Boyes RN, et al. Blood levels of local anesthetics following intravenous regional anesthesia. Acta Anaesthesiol Scand Suppl 1969;36: 115–120.
83. Thorn-Alquist AM. Blood concentrations of local anaesthetics after intravenous regional anaesthesia. Acta Anaesthesiol Scand 1969;13:229–240.
84. Hargrove RL, Hoyle JR, Parker JB. Blood lignocaine levels following intravenous regional analgesia. Anaesthesia 1966;21(1):37–41.
85. Estebe J-P, Gentili ME, Langlois G, Mouilleron P, Bernard F, Ecoffey C. Lidocaine priming reduces tourniquet pain during intravenous regional anesthesia: a preliminary study. Reg Anesth Pain Med 2003;28(2):120–123.
86. Perlas A, Peng PW, Plaza MB, Middleton WJ, Chan VW, Sanandaji K. Forearm rescue cuff improves tourniquet tolerance during intravenous regional anesthesia. Reg Anesth Pain Med 2003;28(2):98–102.
87. Love BR. The tourniquet. ANZ J Surg 1978;48(1):66–70.
88. Bolton CF, McFarlane RM. Human pneumatic tourniquet paralysis. Neurology 1978; 28(8):787–793.
89. Larsen UT, Hommelgaard P. Pneumatic tourniquet paralysis following intravenous regional analgesia. Anaesthesia 1987;42(5):526–528.
90. Mabee JR, Bostwick TL, Burke MK. Iatrogenic compartment syndrome from hypertonic saline injection in Bier block. J Emerg Med 1994;12(4):473–476.
91. Quigley JT, Popich GA, Lanz UB. Compartment syndrome of the forearm and hand: a case report. Clin Orthop Relat Res 1981;(161):247–251.
92. Maletis GB, Watson RC, Scott S. Compartment syndrome. A complication of intravenous regional anesthesia in the reduction of lower leg shaft fractures. Orthopedics 1989; 12(6):841–846.
93. Hastings H 2nd, Misamore G. Compartment syndrome resulting from intravenous regional anesthesia. J Hand Surg 1987;12(4):559–562.
94. Luce EA, Mangubat E. Loss of hand and forearm following Bier block: a case report. J Hand Surg [Am] 1983;8(3):280–283.
95. Pitkanen M, Kytta J, Rosenberg PH. Comparison of 2-chloroprocaine and prilocaine for intravenous regional anaesthesia of the arm: a clinical study. Anaesthesia 1993;48(12): 1091–1093.
96. Armstrong P, Brockway M, Wildsmith JA. Alkalinisation of prilocaine for intravenous regional anaesthesia. Anaesthesia 1990;45(1):11–13.
97. Paul DL, Logan MR, Wildsmith JA. The effects of injected solution temperature on intravenous regional anaesthesia. Anaesthesia 1988;43(5):362–364.
98. Prien T, Goeters C. Intravenous regional anesthesia of the arm and foot using 0.5, 0.75 and 1.0 percent prilocaine. Anasth Intensivther Notfallmed 1990;25(1):59–63.
99. Armstrong P, Watters J, Whitfield A. Alkalinisation of prilocaine for intravenous regional anaesthesia. Suitability for clinical use. Anaesthesia 1990;45(11):935–937.
100. Plourde G, Barry PP, Tardif L, et al. Decreasing the toxic potential of intravenous regional anaesthesia. Can J Anaesth 1989;36(5):498–502.
101. Colizza WA, Said E. Intravenous regional anesthesia in the treatment of forearm and wrist fractures and dislocations in children. Can J Surg 1993;36(3):225–228.
102. Turner PL, Batten JB, Hjorth D, et al. Intravenous regional anaesthesia for the treatment of upper limb injuries in childhood. ANZ J Surg 1986;56(2):153–155.
103. Plourde G, Barry P-P, Tardif L, Lepage Y, Hardy J-F. Decreasing the toxic potential of intravenous regional anaesthesia. Can J Anaesth 1989;36(5):498–502.

104. Karalezli N, Karalezli K, Iltar S, Cimen O, Aydogan N. Results of intravenous regional anaesthesia with distal forearm application. Acta Orthop Belg 2004;70: 401–405.
105. Reuben SS, Steinberg RB, Maciolek H, Manikantan P. An evaluation of the analgesic efficacy of intravenous regional anesthesia with lidocaine and ketorolac using a forearm versus upper arm tourniquet. Anesth Analg 2004;95:457–460.
106. El-Hassan KM, Hutton P, Black AM. Venous pressure and arm volume changes during simulated Bier's block. Anaesthesia 1984;39(3):229–235.
107. Brill S, Middleton W, Brill G, Fisher A. Bier's block: 100 years old and still going strong! Acta Anaesthesiol Scand 2004;48(1):117–122.

# 13 The Evidence-Based Safety of Pediatric Regional Anesthesia and Complications

Lynn M. Broadman and Ryan A. Holt

In the first edition of "Complications in Regional Anesthesia," Broadman[1] produced a chapter that essentially reported a synopsis of all of the complications that were available at that time in the English-language literature that were associated with the placement of regional blocks in infants and children, and the limited safety record associated with caudal block placements. The caudal block safety record was based on three moderately sized series, 750–7800 blocks, which had been safely performed by anesthesiologists that are now recognized authorities in the field of pediatric regional anesthesia.[2–4] All of the potential problems or complications associated with the placement of regional anesthesia blocks at the time of the first writing were unfortunately derived from single case reports.

In this chapter, your authors, Broadman and Holt, will focus their attention on the established safety record of pediatric regional anesthesia. This evidenced-based safety record was derived from data contained in the very large French (ADERPEF) study,[5] the most recent ASA Closed Claims Review,[6] the first 2000 adverse events reported in the Australian Incident Monitoring Study,[7] the 2001 Italian literature review on caudal block safety,[8] and a single-center experience with 1132 spinal anesthetics.[9] Finally, we will update the case report section on specific complications by adding new relevant cases that were reported in the peer-reviewed literature after 1997.

## The Evidenced-Based Safety Record of Pediatric Regional Anesthesia

Perhaps the best single article on the overall safety of pediatric regional anesthesia is the 1-year prospective, multicenter (ADARPEF) study.[5] In this study, Giaufré, Dalens, and Gombert collected data on the complications encountered by 164 of the 309 ADARPEF members (French-Language Society of Pediatric Anesthesia) who voluntarily agreed to participate in this 1-year study. The members worked at hospitals in France, Belgium, and Italy, and the study ran from May 1, 1993 to April 30, 1994. Data were collected and evaluated from a total of 85,412 anesthetics, of which 61,003 involved general anesthesia only. These general anesthetics were excluded from further analysis. The remaining 24,409 cases contained some element of regional anesthesia (local infiltration, neuraxial, or peripheral blocks), and the anesthesia records from cases in which a complication or adverse outcome occurred were subjected to a very detailed analysis. Eighty-nine percent of the aforementioned blocks were placed under general anesthesia.

Peripheral blocks and local infiltration techniques were used in 9396 (38%) of the 24,409 regional cases. Local infiltration was the single most common "peripheral block technique" and was safely performed 5306 times. Surprisingly, there were no complications with either the placement of any of the peripheral blocks or the local infiltration cases, and many of these blocks were placed in the youngest patients.

All of the complications in this large series (23/24,409) occurred during the placement of central blocks. A total of 15,013 central blocks were placed, accounting for 61.5% of all regional anesthetic block placements. The caudal block was the most common central block. Twelve thousand one hundred eleven caudal blocks were placed and only 12 adverse incidents were encountered, for an incident rate of 1/1000 blocks. Heretofore, caudal blocks were viewed as the most simple pediatric regional technique and it was assumed that they were virtually free of any untoward outcomes. Based on the evidence contained in the Giaufré study,[5] this may not be the case and the same vigilance that one uses when placing more demanding central neuraxial blocks may be warranted when placing "routine" caudal blocks. There were no complications associated with any of the 372 thoracic epidural blocks. It can only be assumed that all of these blocks were placed by the most skilled pediatric anesthetists. The lumbar epidural block was associated with the highest adverse outcome odds ratio of 5/1000. There were 10 adverse incidents associated with the placement of the 2024 lumbar epidural blocks. Again, all 23 of the adverse events occurred during placement of neuraxial blocks and there were no complications associated with the placement of either peripheral nerve blocks or thoracic epidurals.

Two of the 23 complications recorded by Giaufré et al.[5] occurred in one patient. Dural puncture was the most frequent complication. Of the eight dural punctures, four resulted in total spinals. Two of the eight inadvertent dural punctures caused the patients to have postdural puncture headaches (PDPHs). There were six intravascular injections resulting in two seizures, two cardiac arrhythmias, and two that did not produce any adverse reactions. The seizures and arrhythmias took place despite there being a previous negative test dose in five of the six cases. Two complications were directly related to needle placement and management of a catheter. One rectal puncture and one kinked catheter were also reported. The two sacral postoperative paresthesias were likely the result of positioning because they took place after lumbar epidurals and completely resolved very early in the recovery process. There were three overdoses in the series. Two of these occurred with local anesthetic solutions and one with morphine. There was one "delayed block." Finally, there was one burn-related necrotic lesion over the gluteal region of a child after placement of a caudal catheter. This burn likely occurred secondary to cautery grounding pad placement over an area of skin that had been cleansed with surgical alcohol just before the placement of the caudal catheter. This first-degree burn resolved within 3 days and did not require any form of treatment. Again, it should be noted that two complications occurred in the same patient during their caudal block placement.

Several conclusions can be drawn from the Giaufré study data.[5] It should be noted that the use of improper equipment was blamed for the cause of the adverse event in 11 cases. It is imperative that our readers only use a needle of the correct length, gauge, and bevel for every pediatric block. One could also draw the conclusion that experience could have prevented many of these complications; however, it should be noted that 18 of the complications resulted from blocks placed by experienced practitioners. The majority of thoracic epidurals were performed in infants younger than 6 months of age, and one can only surmise that these blocks were placed by very experienced pediatric anesthesiologists. A similar situation may have existed for peripheral nerve blocks leading to their perfect safety record. Based on the Giaufré data,[5] one should consider a peripheral nerve block whenever possible as opposed to a neuraxial block because they seem to be associated with fewer adverse outcomes.

The American Society of Anesthesiologists' Closed Claims Analysis provides a potential source for defining specific risks of regional anesthesia. In 1999, Cheney et al.[6] reviewed 2651 claims not previously reviewed since 1990, and 445 of these claims were the result of nerve injuries; however, *none of the claims involved pediatric patients.*

The first conclusion that one can deduce from this closed claims update[6] is that there is often no cause and effect relationship between anesthesia/surgery and perioperative nerve injuries. This is especially true with ulnar neuropathies. All of the ulnar neuropathies occurred in older patients and may have been related to positioning during surgery. There were eight patients who had lower-body procedures performed under a neuraxial block who sustained ulnar neuropathies. Therefore, one should be cautious when positioning all patients for surgery, and this should include pediatric patients. Similar injuries also occurred to the long thoracic nerve in adult patients who were awake during epidural anesthesia and in patients receiving brachial plexus or lumbosacral plexus blocks. Perhaps the reason one does not see such injuries in children is that they are more flexible and can tolerate positioning-related nerve stretching without sustaining any injury.

There were only 13 claims in adult patients for brachial plexus injuries, and in only four of the cases was a paresthesia reported at any time during any of these block placements. This should be somewhat reassuring to pediatric anesthesiologists because most pediatric brachial plexus blocks are placed under light general anesthesia, and even if these pediatric brachial plexus blocks were placed in awake or lightly sedated children most of the younger children would be unable to report a paresthesia. This closed claims report would suggest that there is a very low correlation between patients sustaining a paresthesia during block placement and resultant nerve injury. More importantly, virtually all pediatric peripheral blocks are now placed with either a nerve stimulator or ultrasonic guidance and a paresthesia is not needed to ensure block success.

There were 50 adult claims for spinal cord injury during regional anesthesia. The most common etiologies included spinal hematoma, chemical injury, anterior spinal artery syndrome, and meningitis. Thirteen of the claims resulted from block placements in anticoagulated placements. For the most part, children do not receive anticoagulation therapy and those who do are usually undergoing cardiac anesthesia. This may explain why there are no spinal, caudal, or epidural closed claims in children.

Ninety-three percent of the 67 lumbosacral adult nerve root injuries occurred during neuraxial anesthesia. Major risk factors included the elicitation of paresthesias during block placements and multiple attempts at block placement. It should be noted that 13 of the 23 sciatic injuries were associated with patient positioning. When performing lower-extremity nerve blocks in children, one should glean the following messages from the adult closed claims data: accurate needle placements must be obtained with either a nerve stimulator or ultrasonic guidance, and one should have a low threshold to abandon blocks when placement difficulties are encountered.

The Australian Incident Monitoring Study (AIMS) provides another opportunity to evaluate the safety and risks associated with the use of regional anesthesia. Fox et al.[7] took data from the first 2000 incidents that occurred in the AIMS program and scrutinized the cases that were done under regional anesthesia. There were a total of 160 cases in which regional anesthesia was associated with a complication; however, *none of these cases involved pediatric patients.* The cases were then subdivided into six groups according to the type of regional block that was performed. The groups were epidural, spinal, brachial plexus, intravenous regional anesthesia, ocular blocks, and local infiltration. Not surprisingly, circulatory problems were frequently seen in the spinal and epidural groups. These complications included hypotension, bradycardia/tachycardia, and cardiac arrest. One would expect that similar problems would only be rarely encountered in the pediatric patients. Hypotension is not a problem in children younger than 7 or 8 years of age even when they develop a high spinal or epidural block.[9] Unintentional dural puncture was also a common complication in the AIMS study, and it frequently resulted in the development of a PDPH which required treatment with an epidural blood patch. PDPHs are rarely seen in pediatric patients younger than 10 years of age.[10] Pediatric PDPHs will be discussed in detail in a later section of this article.

All of the remaining incidences reported by the AIMS study[7] could potentially occur in pediatric patients with the same frequency as Fox and colleagues found in adults. There were 24 drug errors in AIMS. The small size of pediatric patients would likely make small drug errors that much more clinically significant. In this study, there were three incidences of delayed hypoxia/respiratory depression which occurred after the injection of epidural morphine. Respiratory depression, apnea, bradycardia, and periodic breathing are all major concerns when one anesthetizes former premature infants. In fact, the use of the caudal/epidural agent clonidine has been implicated as the causal agent in a recent postoperative apnea case report.[11]

An interesting conclusion one can draw from the AIMS study[7] is the very low incidence of perioperative mortality which was found in patients who received the benefits associated with having had a regional anesthetic. Unfortunately, only the numerator is known in the AIMS study, so one cannot make sweeping statements about the morbidity and mortality rate associated with regional versus general anesthesia. There was only one death in the 2000 AIMS patients and it was directly attributable to surgical hemorrhage. There were one case of pulmonary edema following hypotensive resuscitation and one case of neuraxial block–induced cardiac arrest. Both of these patients were successfully resuscitated.

Brachial plexus block–related complications were usually the result of local anesthetic toxicity. The AIMS study authors emphasized that the majority of these complications occurred in ASA class I–III patients and most of the incidents were immediately recognized and treated by a vigilant anesthetist. Infants younger than 6 months of age are particularly sensitive to the toxic effects of local anesthetics, and the AIMS study highlights the risks of using excessive doses to place brachial plexus blocks or the failure to recognize intravascular injections.

### *The Safety Profile of Spinal Anesthesia*

Further support for the safety and efficacy of pediatric neuraxial anesthesia can be found in the low incidence of complications recently reported in a rather large series of 1132 spinal anesthetics by Puncuh and colleagues.[9] The children in this study ranged in age from 6 months to 14 years. Older patients were sedated with oral midazolam (0.6 mg/kg) whereas younger children received this drug via the rectal route. The maximum dose of midazolam was 15 mg irrespective of the patient's weight. An intravenous line was then inserted before placing a hyperbaric bupivacaine spinal with a 25-gauge Sprotte needle. The authors reported a success rate of 98%, which was defined as "not having to induce general anesthesia." All blocks took less than 5 minutes to perform, and complications or problems were only rarely encountered during any of the block placements. Seventeen children had intraoperative hypotension (defined as a decrease in systolic blood pressure by 20% or more from baseline). As expected, this phenomenon was rarely noted in children younger than 10 years of age (9/942) or less than 1% of the children in this younger age group. Seven children had transient oxygen desaturation, and this was likely the result of excessive intraoperative sedation with propofol, midazolam, or thiopental. Finally, one child developed bronchospasm for unknown reasons. The incidence of postoperative complications was also very low. Five children developed a PDPH; unfortunately, the ages of these children were not reported, but none of them required an epidural blood patch. Nine of the children reported a transient self-limited backache. There were no neurologic deficits or mortalities in any patient in this study.

## *A Summary of Specific Complications Including Recent Reports*

### Air Loss of Resistance to Locate Epidural Space

Air loss of resistance techniques for caudal or epidural blockade should be avoided in pediatric patients. Reports indicate that children can develop a life-threatening venous air embolism from small quantities of air used during loss of resistance identification of the caudal epidural space.[12] Schwartz and Eisenkraft[13] reported circulatory collapse in a 9-month-old infant who had 3.0mL of air injected into the lumbar epidural space. In fact, children may be at more risk than adults because of their high incidence of probe-patent foramen ovale (up to 50% in children younger than 5 years of age).[14]

Because of the lower extension of the dural sac, the risk of dural puncture theoretically is higher in infants and small children than in adults or older children. However, this complication is technique dependent and easily recognized if gentle aspiration is performed after placement of the needle and before the first injection of drug. If a dural puncture is noted, it would be prudent to abandon attempts at caudal blockade because of the risk of total spinal block.[15]

### Infection and Associated Risks

One of the most feared complications of neuraxial anesthesia is infection, and it has been recently shown by Holt et al.[16] that a significant number of long-term indwelling catheters will ultimately become infected. The Holt study involved adult patients in whom about 1000 long-term indwelling epidural catheters were followed prospectively for a 17-month period of time. These catheters were left in place from 1 to 270 days and 147 catheter tips were sent for culture for various reasons. Seventy-eight of the 147 catheter tips were ultimately shown to be culture positive. Sixty-four of these 78 tips (82%) grew either *staphylococci* or *corynebacteria*; both of these bacteria are common skin flora. However, only 59 of the 78 patients were suspected of having an epidural-related catheter infection at the time the catheter tip was sent for culture. Twenty of these 59 patients had both insertion site– and catheter tip–positive cultures. Twenty-three other catheter tip–positive patients had systemic signs and symptoms of infection which could have been caused by the epidural catheter, such as meningitis, neurologic deficits, epidural abscess, back pain, or fever. Twelve of these 23 patients died during the study period, but it was not reported if the cause of death was the result of the catheter-related infections or the patients' underlying disease. These authors, Holt et al.,[16] demonstrated that the longer one leaves an epidural catheter in place the more likely it becomes that any given patient will ultimately develop a catheter-related infection. Epidural catheter infections are extremely rare if catheters are left in place for 2 days or less, but the incidence increases dramatically over the next 2 weeks. It should be noted that the average duration of catheterization for patients with only local symptoms was 8 days, whereas those with generalized symptoms had their catheters in place for an average of 15 days. Again, 82% of the infections were caused by normal skin flora supporting the conclusion that local spread is the most common route for the development of catheter tip–positive cultures/infections. Moreover, in the majority of central nervous system infections, localized signs and symptoms were present before the development of these more serious infections. This emphasizes the need for all anesthesiologists and pain medicine physicians to promptly remove catheters that appear to be infected. Finally, these authors recommended that cryptic and overt catheter-related infections, including meningitis and epidural abscess, be promptly diagnosed via lumbar puncture and magnetic resonance imaging studies.

More germane to the pediatric population is a recent study by McNeely and colleagues[17] in which they prospectively studied and cultured the lumbar epidural (n = 46) and caudal catheter tips (n = 45) from pediatric patients in whom all 91 catheters had been placed under aseptic conditions in the operating room and then used to provide short-term postoperative analgesia.[16] On discontinuation of the epidural infusion, the skin was decontaminated with 70% alcohol and then cultured. The distal catheter tip and hub were also cultured. Nine of the caudal catheter tips (20%) were colonized, whereas only two of the lumbar epidural tips (4%) grew bacteria ($P < .02$). Staphylococcus was the predominant skin and catheter tip organism in both groups, but only the caudal catheters grew gram-negative organisms (4/9) (42%). The results of this study suggest that the risk of producing a clinically significant epidural infection is quite low when one uses either a lumbar epidural or caudal catheter to provide short-term postoperative analgesia in the pediatric population. However, the incidence of catheter tip colonization significantly increases when the caudal route is used and it is more likely that the tip will be colonized with more pathogenic gram-negative organisms.

A novel approach to reducing or eliminating caudal catheter tip colonization and localized infections has recently been reported by Fujinaka et al.[18] These researchers demonstrated that by subcutaneous tunneling caudal catheters, infections and catheter tip colonizations could be eliminated. They prospectively studied 18 infants and toddlers in whom caudal catheters were left in place for an average of 3.9 days. Surprisingly, there was a zero incidence of either catheter tip colonization or the development of localized infection in any child. However, one must use caution when attempting to apply these data to the management of long-term indwelling chronic pain catheters because the length of catheterization was brief and the number of patients enrolled in this study was very small.

An older study by Strafford and colleagues[19] also substantiates the belief that epidural infections following the administration of protracted epidural analgesia via indwelling catheters is a very rare event in infants and children. These authors retrospectively reviewed the records of 1620 caudal/epidural catheter placements in infants and children over a 6-year period. The catheters were left in place for as long as 14 days, median 2.4 days. Seventy catheters (3.7%) were placed via the caudal approach; however, the majority of these catheters were lumbar epidural catheters (93%). A combination of bupivacaine and fentanyl was the most common perfusate. This study reported a 0% incidence of clinically significant infections in postoperative patients, a rate that is not statistically different from the spontaneous abscess rate of 0.2–1.2 cases per 10,000 hospital admissions.[20] Epidural abscess was not a reported complication in any of the patients in the Strafford study[19] who received postoperative analgesia via a caudal/epidural catheter. However, one terminally ill child with a necrotic epidural tumor did develop *Candida* colonization of her epidural space.

Meunier and colleagues[21] reported two cases in which infants with biliary atresia developed localized skin infections at their lumbar epidural puncture sites. Both children had undergone Kasai procedures and had received epidural analgesia for the first 48 postoperative hours, at which time the catheters were removed. On the fifth postoperative day, each child was noted to have an area of induration and a small pustule at the catheter entry site. In each case, the pus was evacuated and sent for culture. No organisms were isolated in the first case, so antibiotic therapy was not instituted. The second child was noted to have a recurrent collection of fluctuant subcutaneous material in the area of catheter insertion and underwent surgical incision and drainage of his subcutaneous abscess on postoperative days 6 and 12. His *Staphylococcus aureus* infection was also treated with an appropriate course of oxacillin.

However, the most distressing pediatric infection-related case report in the literature is by Larsson and colleagues.[22] These authors document the formation of an epidural abscess in a 1-year-old boy with severe visceral pain secondary to a rare condition, chronic intestinal pseudoobstruction. His pain could not be managed with parenteral narcotics and over a 6-month time span, from when he was 7 months old until he was 1 year of age, he had three lumbar epidural catheters placed for pain control. Each remained in place from 3 to 12 days. The child's third catheter had been deliberately placed more cephalad than previous ones in order to better target the area of nonoperative chronic visceral pain and to minimize bupivacaine infusion requirements. It had been placed through a L1–L2 puncture site and the catheter tip had been threaded cephalad to T11–12. Eleven days after the placement of this third catheter, the concentration of bupivacaine had to be increased from 0.125% to 0.375%. Despite the large dose of bupivacaine being infused (1.1 mg/kg/h), the child's pain could not be adequately controlled and parenteral narcotics were administered. The next day (day 12), tender swelling was noted at the epidural catheter penetration site. The catheter was immediately removed. A bacterial culture from the epidural catheter tip revealed the growth of *Pseudomonas aeruginosa* which was sensitive to tobramycin. A magnetic resonance imaging confirmed the presence of an epidural abscess extending T5 to L5. The abscess was noted to be deforming and dislocating the medulla in this area. Surprisingly, the child had not developed any neurologic symptoms. He was treated nonsurgically with intravenously administered antibiotics. The abscess could not be detected on a follow-up computed axial tomography study 11 days after the institution of antibiotic therapy. He survived this event without sequelae. These authors provide the following invaluable tip. When one notes a sudden and otherwise unexplained decrease in the ability of previously effective epidural catheter to continue to provide adequate pain control, an epidural abscess should be included in the differential problem list.[22]

Larsson and colleagues[22] suggest that their patients' continuous bacteremia from his necrotizing enterocolitis may have led to the seeding of his epidural catheter and the subsequent development of his epidural abscess. Likewise, both children in the Meunier report[21] were known to have congenital biliary atresia and had undergone a recent Kasai procedure; as such, they probably had ascending cholangitis and bacteremia.

It is the opinion of Broadman and Holt that children with known or suspected bacteremia/septicemia are probably not suitable candidates to receive neuraxial anesthesia or analgesia.

It is common practice for many pediatric anesthesiologists and their dental colleagues to induce anesthesia in children with congenital heart disease, start a peripheral intravenous line, and then have the surgeons perform a dental block before having completed the infusion of prophylactic antibiotic therapy (SBE prophylaxis). However, an article by Roberts et al.[23] demonstrated a significant increase in bacteremia after buccal infiltration analgesia (16%), modified intraligamental analgesia (50%), and intraligamental analgesia (97%). All of these blocks are common techniques used by pedodontists to supplement general anesthesia and to provide postoperative analgesia. The Roberts study involved 143 children varying in age from 23 months to 19 years. Fifty consecutive children had blood cultures drawn after the induction of anesthesia but before any dental manipulation (baseline). The remaining 93 children were randomized to receive a dental block via one of three aforementioned techniques and a postblock blood culture was obtained 30 seconds after each injection. Therefore, each child had only one blood culture drawn. There were 4/50 children who had spontaneous or "background" bacteremia (8%); this finding was quite surprising and suggests that children with congenital heart disease may be at ongoing risk for the development of endocarditis from dental-based bacteremia. There was a significant increase in bacteremia from all of the dental blocks ($P < .0001$) when compared with baseline values. This study certainly has implications for the timing of SBE prophylaxis administration and the performance of dental blocks. The authors conclude that the modified technique should be used when possible in children at risk for developing endocarditis. Based on the findings of Roberts et al.,[23] Broadman and Holt believe that SBE prophylaxis should be started in all at-risk children before any dental blocks or manipulations are undertaken.

### The Advantages of Caudal Catheters

Lumbar and thoracic epidural anesthesia poses certain advantages over caudal anesthesia in infants and children undergoing upper abdominal and thoracic procedures. Both of the former techniques allow for the targeting of local anesthetic solutions at the site of surgery and therefore reduce the potential for toxic drug reactions and other morbidities. Although both of these techniques, lumbar and thoracic epidural catheter placements, have been well described in children in the older literature,[24,25] it was the belief that both of these blocks were technically difficult and even hazardous to perform in infants and children. However, a recent report by Giaufré and associates[5] refutes these early opinions and clearly demonstrates that thoracic epidural blocks are quite safe when placed by a skilled pediatric anesthetist. However, caudal catheters are very easy to place and the catheter tips may be threaded cephalad to the desired level, thereby affording one the opportunity to provide thoracoabdominal anesthesia/analgesia without the associated risks of either spinal cord trauma or local anesthetic toxicity.[26,27]

### Problems Encountered During the Cephalad Advancement of Lumbar Epidural Catheters

An article by Blanco and colleagues[28] demonstrated that it is very difficult and sometimes impossible to advance a catheter that has been placed in the lumbar epidural space cephalad to a thoracic level in infants and children older than 1 year of age. The Blanco group studied 39 infants and children who ranged in age from 0 to 96 months. They used an 18-gauge Tuohy needle and air loss of resistance techniques to properly identify the epidural space at the L-4/L-5 interspace in all study patients. Unfortunately, only 7/39 (18%) of the 19-gauge, unstyletted, polyethylene, multiorifice catheters could be advanced cephalad to the T-12 level. Twenty-three of the 39 catheters (59%) simply formed a loop at or about the L-4/L-5 region. Eight of the catheters were difficult to place. The fact that a catheter was easy to place did not positively correlate with the ability to advance the catheter tip cephalad. There were no inadvertent dural punctures and all catheters were removed without difficulty.

Why did the Blanco group[28] encounter so much difficulty passing 19-gauge catheters cephalad, and Bösenburg et al.[26] and Gunter and Eng[27] did not? Perhaps it relates to the fact that Bösenburg et al.[26] placed their catheters in infants younger than 1 year of age, and one would suspect that most of the infants in the Bösenburg study had not yet assumed upright posture. Therefore, they had not developed lumbar lordosis and 19/20 of Bösenburg's catheters easily passed cephalad.

Gunter and Eng[27] circumvented this problem in older infants and children by using wire styletted microcatheters. Broadman, Holt, and their colleague David Rosen have been using a wire styletted, open-end, microcatheter for several years and coiling has not been a problem (Sims 20/24 Micro Catheter System®).

### Postdural Puncture Headache

The incidence of PDPH in children following spinal anesthesia or an inadvertent "wet tap" during placement of an epidural block is quite low, and Wee and Colleagues[10] suggest that the problem rarely occurs in children younger than 10 years of age. However, these authors point out that PDPH is quite common in older pediatric patients and the incidence increases with age. Wee et al.[10] prospectively studied 105 children with malignant disease who ranged from 3 to 18 years of age. All of the children were having a lumbar puncture performed under general anesthesia, and all of the punctures were performed with a 22-gauge spinal needle with a "cutting point."

The parents of each child were given a questionnaire to answer over the 3-day period after the diagnostic/therapeutic lumbar puncture and the questionnaire was targeted to answer the following questions: What was the incidence of PDPH in children and did such headaches spontaneously resolve with time and hydration? Ninety-seven questionnaires were returned (92%). *None of the children younger than 10 years of age developed a PDPH.* Of the children aged 10–12 years, 2 of 17 developed a headache (11.8%). The older children aged 13–18 years had an incidence of 50% (5/10). Adolescent girls in this study had headaches twice as frequently as did boys and this sex-related difference is consistent with the incidence of PDPH reported by Raskin[29] in adults. The reason for the low incidence of PDPH in children younger than 10 years of age is unknown, but it may be related to the lower CSF pressures found in this age group.[30]

A case report by McHale and O'Donovan[31] suggests that there is a role for the use of epidural blood patch techniques in pediatric patients with PDPHs that fail to respond to conservative therapy. McHale and O'Donovan injected 8 mL of blood into the epidural space of a 39-kg boy (0.2 mL/kg) while he was under general anesthesia and his classic PDPH symptoms promptly resolved. The child had had a classic PDPH for 4 days following an inadvertent subarachnoid puncture during a lumbar epidural catheter placement with an 18-gauge Tuohy epidural needle. The volume of blood used in this report is consistent with the amount found in earlier case reports.[32,33] However, the best single reference to help one manage the placement of an epidural blood patch in infants and children is an article by Kumar and colleagues.[34] These authors point out that an epidural blood patch provides effective treatment for PDPH in pediatric patients when the child has not responded to conventional therapy and symptoms persist for more than a week. Sedation and EMLA® cream may be beneficial adjuncts to reduce the pain and emotional trauma of blood patch therapy. Practitioners should consider the child's age and level of maturity when determining whether conscious or deep sedation will be required. The volume of autologous blood recommended varies from 0.5 to 0.75 mL/kg, and should be injected slowly.[34]

### Problems with Test Dosing

There is no effective test dosing method or other technique for the reliable detection of the intravascular injection of local anesthetic solutions during block placements in children simultaneously undergoing general anesthesia with volatile agents. Desparmet and colleagues[35] studied 65 children, ranging in age from 1 month to 11 years of age, and found that children who received an intravenous epinephrine-containing solution without atropine pretreatment did not demonstrate a consistent increase in their heart rates. Furthermore, 94% of children who received atropine premedication followed by intravenous epinephrine had only a brief heart rate increase of greater than 10 bpm, (peaking at 45 seconds and lasting to 60 seconds postinjection).[35] It must be emphasized that the atropine injection in this study was given to patients with a stable end-tidal halothane concentration of 1.0%. Increases in heart rate of 10 bpm or more may be noted after needle placements in children who are not so deeply anesthetized. Perillo and colleagues[36] performed a similar study comparing two intravenous doses of isoproterenol (0.05 μg/kg and 0.075 μg/kg). As in the epinephrine study by Desparmet and colleagues,[35] Perillo et al.[36] were unable to show any consistent or predictable relationship between the infusion of the aforementioned test doses of isoproterenol and increases in heart rate.

As in adults, it is important to administer the local anesthetic solution in small increments and carefully monitor for signs of systemic toxicity rather than to rely completely on a test-dosing technique.

### The Toxicity of Local Anesthetics

Bupivacaine is one of the most frequently used local anesthetic agents for pediatric caudal and epidural blocks. This agent can be used safely if maximum dosage guidelines are followed. However, complications relating to neurologic and cardiac toxicity have been reported.

Whereas the toxic plasma bupivacaine level for adults is estimated to be 4.0 μg/mL,[37] the level in infants and children is not known. Plasma levels that are less than 2.0 μg/mL are thought to be safe in children and have not been associated with neurologic or cardiac toxicity.[38] However, a number of factors indicate that one should use caution when applying adult toxicity data to children. The metabolism of local anesthetics is greatly reduced in the neonate, because of both decreased plasma pseudocholinesterase and decreased hepatic microsomal activity.[39,40] Also, alpha$_1$-acid glycoprotein (AGP) concentrations are quite low in infants younger than 2 months of age and they do not reach adult levels until after the first year of life.[41] Alpha$_1$-AGP is important because it is the primary binding substrate for cationic drugs such as local anesthetics. Albumin and other plasma proteins only have a very minor role in the binding of local anesthetic solutions. Reduced levels of alpha$_1$-AGP allow for more of the local anesthetic solution to remain in the unbound or free form, and it is only the unbound fraction of local anesthetics that can precipitate toxic reactions such as seizure activity and myocardial depression.

Children eliminate drugs faster than newborns and infants but more slowly than adults. This slower rate of elimination requires particular attention to continuous infusions of local anesthetic. The larger cardiac output of pediatric patients is a factor in the relatively rapid increase of local anesthetic blood levels, especially in the vessel-rich organs such as the brain and heart.

Other factors that have been noted to potentially increase susceptibility to bupivacaine toxicity include concomitant administration of volatile agents,[42] acidosis,[43] hypoxia,[44] and hyponatremia and hyperkalemia,[45] as well as rapid increases in plasma bupivacaine levels.[46]

Several studies have evaluated bupivacaine plasma levels following the administration of single bolus doses to pediatric patients. After lumbar epidural administration of 0.25% bupivacaine (3.0 mg/kg), Eyres and colleagues[47] noted that plasma levels peaked at 20 minutes and ranged from about 1.0 to 2.0 μg/mL. Ecoffey et al.[24] studied 10 infants and children who ranged in age from 3 to 36 months. Six of the infants had thoracic epidural catheters and four had lumbar catheters. Peak plasma levels occurred in these infants 20 minutes after the bolus administration of 0.5% bupivacaine (3.75 mg/kg). All of their plasma levels were less than 1.8 μg/mL with the exception of one child who had a plasma level of 2.2 μg/mL.[24] Eyres and coworkers[48] found that plasma bupivacaine concentrations ranged from 1.2 to 1.4 μg/mL after the caudal injection of 0.25% bupivacaine (3 mg/kg) in children. Stow and colleagues[49] also noted that peak plasma bupivacaine concentrations were reached at around 20 minutes after caudal administration to children. In each of the aforementioned studies,[24,47–49] the peak plasma levels of bupivacaine were less than those that are considered to be toxic in adults, and all of the peak plasma levels occurred 20 minutes after administration by caudal, lumbar, and thoracic injections.

Desparmet and colleagues[50] evaluated plasma bupivacaine levels in six children who were given a loading dose of 0.25% bupivacaine (0.5 mL/kg) without epinephrine injected into the lumbar epidural space, followed in 30 minutes by an infusion of the same drug at a rate of 0.08 mL/kg/h. Plasma bupivacaine levels were assayed from specimens obtained at 4-hour intervals between 24 and 48 hours after the start of the infusion, and then every 2 hours until 10 hours had elapsed following termination of all infusions. Plasma levels in these six children were highly variable, ranging from 0.2 to 1.2 μg/mL. No increase was noted in plasma levels between 24 and 48 hours. However, research on adults has shown that continuous epidural infusions of bupivacaine produce constant plasma levels until approximately 50 hours after the start of infusion when a dramatic increase occurs.[51]

McIlvaine et al.[52] evaluated plasma bupivacaine levels in children receiving intrapleural infusions at rates of 0.5–2.5 mg/kg/h. Plasma bupivacaine levels ranged from 1.0 to 7.0 μg/mL. None of these children were noted to experience any signs of toxicity;

however, this may be attributable either to the small number of patients in the series, or to the fact that some of the children received diazepam within the first 24 hours after surgery.

Agarwal and colleagues[53] reported two cases of neurotoxicity related to continuous bupivacaine infusions. Both patients received 0.25% bupivacaine with 1:200,000 of epinephrine. The first case involved a 9.4-kg 3-year-old girl with chronic interstitial lung disease who was scheduled for a right middle lobe lung biopsy. During the procedure, an intrapleural catheter was placed. It should be noted that systemic absorption of local anesthetic agents is far greater in the intrapleural space than in either the intercostal or caudal epidural space. One hour after a bolus dose of 0.66 mg/kg of bupivacaine was administered, an infusion of 0.25 mg/kg/h was begun. Five hours later the infusion was increased to 0.5 mg/kg/h because of complaints of increased discomfort. Twenty-one hours after the start of the infusion, the patient had two tonic-clonic seizures which were treated with intravenous phenobarbital (100 mg). The patient's bupivacaine plasma level was 5.6 μg/mL at the time of her seizures. The second patient to develop seizures from systemic accumulation of bupivacaine was a 26-kg 9-year-old girl with cerebral palsy. She was a former premature infant, but at the time of the report, she was an otherwise healthy child, scheduled for selective dorsal rhizotomy. After a bolus of bupivacaine (1.25 mg/kg) was injected into her caudal epidural catheter, an infusion at the rate of 1.25 mg/kg/h was started. Fifty-six hours after the start of the infusion, the patient had three tonic-clonic seizures that were successfully treated with phenobarbital. The patient's plasma bupivacaine level at the time of the first seizure was 5.4 μg/mL.

Of interest in the report by Agarwal and colleagues[53] is the complete absence in both cases of prodromal warning signs, which might have alerted caregivers of the impending onset of acute bupivacaine neurotoxicity. Both patients were reported to be calm, cooperative, and restful just before the onset of their seizure activity. The only unusual complaint was from the second patient, who reported a "falling" or "tumbling" sensation several hours before the onset of her seizures.[53] Early central nervous system manifestations of toxicity may not be apparent in children because they are less likely to articulate their symptoms. In infants and toddlers who are awake, these symptoms may be misinterpreted as irritability or "fussiness." The first signs of local anesthetic toxicity in a pediatric patient may be dysrhythmias or cardiovascular collapse.[54,55]

McCloskey and colleagues[56] reported three cases in which children experienced toxic side effects from their continuous epidural bupivacaine infusion. Bupivacaine 0.25% with 1:200,000 of epinephrine was used in all three patients. The first case was a 3.89-kg 1-day-old newborn scheduled for direct closure of exstrophy of the bladder. Bupivacaine solution in bolus doses of 2.5, 1.87, and 1.87 mg/kg was administered at hours 0, 1.5, and 3.0, respectively. At hour 4.5, an infusion was begun at the rate of 2.5 mg/kg/h. Ten hours after the start of the infusion, the patient developed bradycardia and hypotension. The infusion was discontinued and the newborn was quickly intubated. Bag and mask ventilation with oxygen was instituted and epinephrine (10 μg/kg) was given intravenously. The sinus bradycardia suddenly changed to ventricular tachycardia, which partially responded to three bolus doses of lidocaine (1.0 mg/kg) and one dose of sodium bicarbonate (1.0 mEq/kg). Normal sinus rhythm was reestablished through the intravenous infusion of phenytoin (5.0 mg/kg). However, 2 hours later, the patient's rhythm reverted once again to ventricular tachycardia and generalized tonic-clonic seizure activity was noted. Both were treated successfully with intravenous diazepam, 0.25 mg/kg and serially administered phenytoin for a total dose of 7.0 mg/kg. The plasma bupivacaine level at the time the infusion was discontinued was 5.6 μg/mL, and 12 hours later it had only decreased to 3.7 μg/mL. The child had no neurologic sequelae as a result of the aforementioned events and enjoyed an uneventful recovery.

The second patient reported by McCloskey and colleagues[56] was a 45-kg 8-year-old child scheduled for bladder augmentation. Bolus doses of bupivacaine 1.40, 0.83, 0.55, and 1.00 mg/kg were given at 0, 1.5, 3.5, and 5.5 hours, respectively, via his epidural catheter. An infusion of 1.67 mg/kg/h was begun at hour 9.5. After another 25 hours, the patient experienced two generalized tonic-clonic seizures which responded to diazepam. The plasma bupivacaine level shortly after the seizure was 6.6 μg/mL. The third patient was a 12-kg 4-year-old girl with bilateral knee trauma resulting from a motor vehicle accident. There were no signs of head trauma. The patient received bupivacaine boluses during surgery of 2.50, 1.67, 1.67, and 1.67 mg/kg at hours 0, 2.0, 4.0, and 5.5, respectively. A bupivacaine infusion was begun 3.0 hours after the last intraoperative dose at the rate of 1.67 mg/kg/h. At hour 26, the patient's level of analgesia decreased from T-10 to L-2. A leak at the catheter insertion site was noted, and the catheter was replaced. A 0.42 mg/kg bolus was given and the infusion was reinstituted at 2.0 mg/kg/h. Eight hours later, the patient experienced a generalized tonic-clonic seizure which resolved with diazepam. The patient's plasma bupivacaine level was 10.2 μg/mL at the time of her seizure. Neurologic examinations of all three patients after seizure activity resolved were normal.

The infusion rates for all three patients in the aforementioned case report were excessively high. This led McCloskey and colleagues[56] to develop infusion guidelines based on extrapolations from linear pharmacokinetic projections for bolus caudal and epidural bupivacaine levels. They suggested 0.4 mg/kg/h for infants younger than 6 months and 0.75 mg/kg/h for older children.[56] However, lower infusion rates, which provide adequate analgesia, yet pose less potential for toxic complications, have been established by Berde.[57] The Berde recommended dosage guidelines for epidural bupivacaine infusions include a loading dose of 2.0–2.5 mg/kg and an infusion rate not in excess of 0.4–0.5 mg/kg/h in older infants, toddlers, and children and less than 0.2–0.25 mg/kg/h in neonates.

The second complication related to bupivacaine toxicity is cardiac dysrhythmia. This is perhaps a more serious complication because it may be refractory to conventional treatment. Maxwell and colleagues[55] have successfully used phenytoin in the treatment of two neonates with bupivacaine-induced cardiac toxicity. The first patient in the Maxwell article[55] is the same 3.89-kg 1-day-old newborn with exstrophy of the bladder presented by McCloskey et al.[56] The second patient was a 4.4-kg full-term infant, also with exstrophy of the bladder, who received three caudal bolus doses of bupivacaine, 2.50, 1.25, and 1.75 mg/kg, at 0, 2.5, and 4.5 hours, respectively. Five minutes after the third dose was administered, the patient developed a wide-complex tachydysrhythmia. All anesthetic agents were discontinued, and 100% oxygen was administered. After bretylium 5.0 mg/kg was administered, the patient's heart rate increased from 120 to 240 bpm and his blood pressure decreased from 90/60 to 65/40 torr. Normal sinus rhythm was reestablished after phenytoin was administered in divided doses for a total dose of 7.0 mg/kg.

Broadman and Holt suggest that if inadequate analgesia persists after the maximum dose of bupivacaine has been administered and incorrect needle placement and other technical problems have been ruled out, it is unwise to administer additional bupivacaine. Either an epidural opioid can be added to the local anesthetic solution or a systemic opioid can be used in conjunction with the epidural infusion. Moreover, it may simply be more prudent in such cases to simply discontinue the epidural catheter/infusion and use systemic opioids or other analgesics.

An older report[55] suggests that a continuous infusion of caudal or epidural lidocaine may be preferable to bupivacaine because of the ability to rapidly and easily monitor plasma concentrations of the former agent in most hospital laboratories. Unfortunately, many hospital laboratories no longer perform in-house lidocaine assays; therefore, there may not be any advantage to using a long-term lidocaine infusion. More importantly, the newer isomer-specific agent ropivacaine has been extensively studied in the pediatric population and it may be the agent of choice for long-term infusion analgesia in infants and children.

### *Levobupivacaine and Ropivacaine Toxicity in Children*

A complete Medline® search was conducted by your authors from 1997 through May 2005. This search was facilitated through the use of Procite®. We can say without reservation that there seems to be zero adverse outcomes or reactions in pediatric patients associated with the use of either levobupivacaine or ropivacaine during the placement of axis or peripheral blocks. However, there are two recent adverse reaction case reports in adult patients that clearly show that toxic reactions can occur with either of these new local anesthetic agents.[58,59]

However, there are several studies involving infants and children in which ropivacaine has been successfully used to provide intraoperative anesthesia and postoperative analgesia without any adverse outcomes or complications.[60–66] There are advantages to using ropivacaine in lieu of bupivacaine. However, the most important advantage of ropivacaine is its well-established reduced cardiotoxicity profile which has been clearly demonstrated in animal models.[67] It has also been shown that when ropivacaine and bupivacaine are used in equipotent doses in pediatric patients, the resultant peak plasma concentrations are much lower in the ropivacaine group.[62] The pharmacokinetics of ropivacaine has been recently studied in the pediatric population. Apparently, the use of ropivacaine in children is associated with a longer elimination half-life and a larger volume of distribution when compared with adults.[63] The pharmacodynamic profile for ropivacaine has also been defined in pediatric patients. Concentrations of 0.2% ropivacaine or less have been shown to produce both excellent intraoperative and postoperative analgesia.[64] In fact, dangerously high peak plasma concentrations were noted when higher concentrations of ropivacaine (0.375%–0.5%) were used with a total dose of 3.5 mg/kg.[65] These relatively high doses were associated with peak plasma levels of 4.33–5.6 μg/mL.[65] Although no toxic side effects were noted in the aforementioned study, it would be prudent to limit total doses of ropivacaine to 3.0 mg/kg or less. If more intense intraoperative motor blockade is needed and higher concentrations of ropivacaine are used, then one can decrease peak plasma ropivacaine levels by using epinephrine (1:200,000).[66] Van Obbergh and colleagues[66] recently showed that the addition of epinephrine reduced peak ropivacaine plasma levels by approximately 33% after caudal injection. However, caution is warranted when applying the above ropivacaine data to neonates and chronically ill pediatric patients because neither of these groups were specifically targeted.

### *Spinal Opioids, Clonidine, and Respiratory Depression*

The use of either epidural opioids or clonidine alone or in concert with local anesthetic agents has gained widespread acceptance with many pediatric anesthetists during the past decade. However, delayed respiratory depression is always possible, whether the opioid is administered via the caudal, epidural, or spinal route, especially in young infants. This is particularly true with concomitant administration of systemic opioids.

Nichols and colleagues[68] studied the disposition and respiratory effects of subarachnoid morphine in 10 infants and children undergoing craniofacial surgery. All of these children required cerebrospinal fluid (CSF) drainage as part of the surgical procedure; this was accomplished by placing a subarachnoid catheter at the L4-L5 interspace. The same catheter was used to administer subarachnoid morphine (2.0 μg/kg) before the conclusion of surgery, and then to sample and measure the CSF concentration of morphine at 6, 12, and 18 hours. Corresponding plasma concentrations of morphine were determined by radioimmunoassay. Subarachnoid morphine produced a reduction in both the slope and the intercept of the ventilatory response curve; this reduction was greatest 6 hours after morphine administration, and the ventilatory response only partially recovered 12 and 18 hours later. This study documents that infants and children may experience respiratory depression for at least 18 hours after subarachnoid morphine administration and that appropriate monitoring and safeguards are essential.

The pharmacokinetic parameters observed after epidural morphine administration in older children have been found to be similar to those previously measured in adults, including a significant decrease in the minute ventilatory response to breathing an end-tidal $CO_2$ pressure of 55 torr. Breathing such a mixture caused a significant shift in the $CO_2$ response curve for more than 22 hours after epidural morphine administration.[69] Krane and colleagues[70] demonstrated that caudal morphine in a dose of 33μg/kg provides excellent analgesia with a lower incidence of the delayed respiratory depression. Such delayed respiratory depression was previously reported by Krane[71] when a larger dose of 100μg/kg was administered to a 2.5-year-old boy. Valley and Bailey[72] reported the use of caudal morphine (70μg/kg diluted with normal saline) in 138 children undergoing major abdominal, thoracic, and orthopedic surgery. Children weighing less than 5kg received 3.0mL of solution, whereas those weighing 5–15kg received 5.0mL and those weighing more than 15kg received 10mL of solution. Of note is the high incidence of respiratory depression that occurred in 11 children in this study.[72] Of these 11 children, 10 were younger than 1 year of age and most had received concomitant systemic opioids along with the extradural opioids. The mean time from the administration of caudal morphine until the onset of respiratory depression in this group was 3.8 hours; *no respiratory depression occurred in any child more than 12 hours after the administration of the last dose of caudal morphine.* All episodes of respiratory depression were successfully managed with naloxone (5–20μg/kg) followed by the infusion of naloxone at the rate of 2–10μg/kg/h.

Bailey and colleagues[73] compared the efficacy of caudal, epidural, and intravenous butorphanol in reducing the incidence of adverse side effects associated with epidural morphine. They found that there was no difference in the incidence of adverse side effects between the children who had received butorphanol and those who had not. However, Lawhorn and Brown[74] found a decreased incidence of opioid-related complications when butorphanol (40μg/kg) was added to epidural morphine (80μg/kg).

The addition of clonidine to epidural morphine seems to provide prolonged analgesia without increasing the incidence of adverse side effects.[75] However, as reported earlier in this chapter, there has been a recent case report in which a former 32-week gestational-age neonate, who was 38 weeks' postconceptional age at the time of his elective inguinal hernia repair, received epidural clonidine and experienced significant periods of apnea and bradycardia.[11] This child essentially served as his own control because he received two separate caudal epidural anesthetics. The caudal blocks served as his total anesthetic during both surgeries. The first hernia repair was conducted with caudal bupivacaine (0.25%) and no periods of apnea were observed. One week later, a second herniorrhaphy was required. This time he received a caudal block that contained both bupivacaine (0.125%) and clonidine (1.8μg/kg). Unfortunately, the infant experienced profound periods of apnea and bradycardia for more than 12 hours after the second anesthetic. Caution is warranted should one elect to administer either caudal or epidural clonidine to pediatric patients at risk for the development of apnea, bradycardia, or periodic breathing.

## Conclusion

At the time of this writing, 2005, the safety and efficacy of pediatric regional anesthesia has been well established. That being said, there are still rare but serious complications that can occur should one elect to use regional anesthesia techniques in infants and children; however, many of these problems can be avoided by using good techniques, selecting the proper materials and patients, and by providing appropriate follow-up care to detect early signs and symptoms of serious complications. The benefits of using regional anesthesia either alone or in conjunction with general anesthesia in pediatric patients are not limited to just obtaining better postoperative pain control,[76] but also to a decreased need for postoperative ventilation[77] and a decreased response to stress.[78] Even in pediatric cardiac surgery where patients may be at an increased risk of developing an epidural hematoma because of total body heparinization during bypass, expert opinion has weighed in favor of using spinal axis anesthesia/analgesia to provide our pediatric patients with profound postoperative pain relief.[79]

*Acknowledgments*

The authors thank Heather Harris, Emily Stewart, Karen Holt, and David Chasey for their assistance in the research and preparation of this chapter.

## References

1. Broadman LM. Complications of pediatric regional anesthesia. In: Finucane BT, ed. Complications of Regional Anesthesia. 2nd ed. Philadelphia: Churchill Livingstone; 1999: 245–256.
2. Dalens B, Hasnouai A. Caudal anesthesia in pediatric surgery: success rate and adverse effects in 750 consecutive patients. Anesth Analg 1989;68:83–89.
3. Broadman LM, Rice LJ. Neural blockade for pediatric surgery. In: Cousins MJ, Bridenbaugh PO, eds. Neural Blockade in Clinical Anesthesia and Pain Management. 3rd ed. Philadelphia: JB Lippincott; 1998:615–636.
4. Veyckemans F, Van Obbergh LJ, Gouverneur JM. Lessons from 1100 pediatric caudal blocks in a teaching hospital. Reg Anesth 1992;17:119–125.
5. Giaufré E, Dalens B, Gombert A. Epidemiology and morbidity of regional anesthesia in children: a one-year prospective survey of the French-Language Society of Pediatric Anesthesiologists. Anesth Analg 1996;83:904–912.
6. Cheney FW, Domino KB, Caplan RA, Posner KL. Nerve injury associated with anesthesia: a closed claims analysis. Anesthesiology 1999;90:1062–1069.
7. Fox MAL, Webb RK, Singleton R, et al. Problems with regional anaesthesia: an analysis of 2000 incident reports. Anaesth Intensive Care 1993;21:646–649.
8. Zadra N, Giusti F. Il Blocco caudale in pediatria. Minerva Anestesiol 2001;67(suppl 1): 126–131.
9. Puncuh F, Lampugnani E, Kokki H. Use of spinal anaesthesia in paediatric patients: a single centre experience with 1132 cases. Pediatr Anesth 2004;14:564–567.
10. Wee LH, Lam F, Cranston AJ. The incidence of post dural puncture headache in children. Anaesthesia 1996;51:1164–1166.
11. Fellmann C, Gerber AC, Weiss M. Apnoea in a former preterm infant after caudal bupivacaine with clonidine for inguinal herniorrhaphy. Pediatr Anaesth 2002;12:637–640.
12. Guinard J-P, Borboen M. Probable venous air embolism during caudal anesthesia in a child. Anesth Analg 1993;76:1134–1135.
13. Schwartz N, Eisenkraft JB. Probable venous embolism during epidural placement in the infant. Anesth Analg 1993;76:1136–1138.
14. Nora JJ. Etiologic aspects of heart disease. In: Adams FH, Emmanouilides CG, eds. Heart Disease in Infants, Children and Adolescents. 3rd ed. Baltimore: Williams & Wilkins; 1983:14.
15. Desparmet J. Total spinal anesthesia after caudal anesthesia in an infant. Anesth Analg 1990;70:665–667.
16. Holt HM, Andersen SS, Andersen O, et al. Infections following epidural catheterization. J Hosp Infect 1995;30:253–260.
17. McNeely JK, Trentadue NC, Rusy LM, Farber NE. Culture of bacteria from lumbar and caudal epidural catheters used for postoperative analgesia in children. Reg Anesth 1997; 22:428–431.
18. Fujinaka W, Hinomoto N, Saeki S, et al. Decreased risk of catheter infection in infants and children using subcutaneous tunneling for continuous caudal anesthesia. Acta Med Okayama 2001;55:283–287.

19. Strafford MA, Wilder RT, Berde CB. The risk of infection from epidural analgesia in children. A review of 1620 cases. Anesth Analg 1995;80:234–238.
20. Baker AS, Ojemann RG, Swartz MN, Richardson EP. Spinal epidural abscess. N Engl J Med 1975;293:463–468.
21. Meunier JF, Norwood P, Dartayet B, et al. Skin abscess with lumbar epidural catheterization in infants. Is it dangerous? Report of two cases. Anesth Analg 1997;84:1248–1249.
22. Larsson BA, Lundberg S, Olsson GL. Epidural abscess in a one-year-old boy after continuous epidural analgesia. Anesth Analg 1997;84:1245–1247.
23. Roberts GJ, Simmons NB, Longhurst P, Hewitt PB. Bacteraemia following local anaesthetic injections in children. Br Dent J 1998;185:295–298.
24. Ecoffey C, Dubousset A-M, Samii K. Lumbar and thoracic epidural anesthesia for urologic and upper abdominal surgery in infants and children. Anesthesiology 1986;65:87–90.
25. Ruston FG. Epidural anaesthesia in infants and children. Can Anaesth Soc J 1954;1: 37–40.
26. Bösenberg AT, Bland BAR, Schulte-Steinberg O, Downing JW. Thoracic epidural anesthesia via caudal route in infants. Anesthesiology 1988;69:265–269.
27. Gunter JB, Eng C. Thoracic epidural anesthesia via the caudal approach in children. Anesthesiology 1992;76:935–938.
28. Blanco D, Llamazares J, Rincón R, et al. Thoracic epidural anesthesia via the lumbar approach in infants and children. Anesthesiology 1996;84:1312–1316.
29. Raskin NH. Lumbar puncture headache: a review. Headache 1990;30:197–200.
30. Tobias JD. Postdural puncture headache in children: etiology and treatment. Clin Pediatr 1990;33:110–113.
31. McHale J, O'Donovan FC. Postdural puncture symptoms in a child. Anaesthesia 1997; 52:688–690.
32. Purtock RV, Buhl JL, Abram SE. Epidural blood patch in a nine-year-old boy. Reg Anesth 1984;9:154–155.
33. Roy L, Vischoff D, Lavoie J. Epidural blood patch in a seven-year-old child. Can J Anaesth 1995;42:621–624.
34. Kumar V, Maves T, Barcellos W. Epidural blood patch for treatment of subarachnoid fistula in children. Anaesthesia 1991;46:117–118.
35. Desparmet J, Mateo J, Ecoffey C, Mazoit X. Efficiency of an epidural test dose in children anesthetized with halothane. Anesthesiology 1990;72:249–251.
36. Perillo M, Sethna NF, Berde CB. Intravenous isoproterenol as a marker for epidural test-dosing in children. Anesth Analg 1993;76:178–181.
37. Tucker GT. Pharmacokinetics of local anaesthetics. Br J Anaesth 1986;58:717–731.
39. Sethna NF, Berde CB. Pediatric regional anesthesia. In: Gregory G, ed. Pediatric Anesthesia. 3rd ed. New York: Churchill Livingstone; 1994:281–317.
39. Morgan D, McQuillan D, Thomas J. Pharmacokinetics and metabolism of the anilide local anesthetics in neonates. Eur J Clin Pharmacol 1978;13:365–371.
40. Mazoit JX, Denson DD, Samii K. Pharmacokinetics of bupivacaine following caudal anesthesia in infants. Anesthesiology 1988;68:387–391.
41. Lerman J, Strong HA, Le Dez KM, et al. Effects of age on serum concentration of alpha$_1$-acid glycoprotein and the binding of lidocaine in pediatric patients. Clin Pharmacol Ther 1989;46:219–245.
42. Eyres RL, Kidd J, Oppenheimer R, Brown TCK. Local anaesthetic plasma levels in children. Anaesth Intensive Care 1978;6:243–247.
43. Rosen MA, Thigpen JW, Shnider S, et al. Bupivacaine-induced cardiotoxicity in hypoxic and acidotic sheep. Anesth Analg 1985;64:1089–1096.
44. Heavner JE, Dryden CF, Sanghani V, et al. Severe hypoxia enhances central nervous system and cardiovascular toxicity of bupivacaine in lightly anesthetized pigs. Anesthesiology 1992;77:142–147.
45. Timour Q, Freysz M, Mazze R, et al. Enhancement by hyponatremia and hyperkalemia of ventricular conduction and rhythm disorders caused by bupivacaine. Anesthesiology 1990;72:1051–1056.
46. Scott DB. Evaluation of clinical tolerance of local anesthetic agents. Br J Anaesth 1975; 47:328–333.
47. Eyres RL, Hastings C, Brown TCK, Oppenheim RC. Plasma bupivacaine concentrations following lumbar epidural anesthesia in children. Anaesth Intensive Care 1986;14: 131–134.

48. Eyres RL, Bishop W, Oppenheim RC, Brown TCK. Plasma bupivacaine concentrations in children during caudal epidural analgesia. Anesth Intensive Care 1983;11:20–26.
49. Stow PJ, Scott A, Phillips A, White JB. Plasma bupivacaine concentrations during caudal analgesia and ilioinguinal-iliohypogastric nerve block in children. Anaesthesia 1988; 43:650–653.
50. Desparmet J, Meistelman C, Barre J, Saint-Maurice C. Continuous epidural infusion of bupivacaine for postoperative pain relief in children. Anesthesiology 1987;67:108–110.
51. Richter O, Klein K, Abel J, et al. The kinetics of bupivacaine plasma concentrations during epidural anesthesia following intraoperative bolus injection and subsequent continuous infusion. Int J Clin Pharmacol Ther Toxicol 1984;22:611–617.
52. McIlvaine WB, Knox RF, Fennessey PV, Goldstein M. Continuous infusion of bupivacaine via intrapleural catheter for analgesia after thoracotomy in children. Anesthesiology 1988; 69:261–264.
53. Agarwal R, Gutlove DP, Lockhart CH. Seizures occurring in pediatric patients receiving continuous infusion of bupivacaine. Anesth Analg 1992;75:284–286.
54. Ved SA, Pinosky M, Nicodemus H. Ventricular tachycardia and brief cardiovascular collapse in two infants after caudal anesthesia using a bupivacaine-epinephrine solution. Anesthesiology 1993;79:1121–1123.
55. Maxwell LG, Martin LD, Yaster M. Bupivacaine-induced cardiac toxicity in neonates: successful treatment with intravenous phenytoin. Anesthesiology 1994;80:682–686.
56. McCloskey JJ, Haun SE, Deshpande JK. Bupivacaine toxicity secondary to continuous caudal infusion in children. Anesth Analg 1992;75:287–290.
57. Berde CB. Convulsions associated with pediatric regional anesthesia. Anesth Analg 1992;75:164–166.
58. Klein SM, Pierce T, Rubin Y, et al. Successful resuscitation after ropivacaine-induced ventricular fibrillation. Anesth Analg 2003;97:901–903.
59. Crews JC, Rothman TE. Seizure after levobupivacaine for interscalene brachial plexus block. Anesth Analg 2003;96:1188–1190.
60. Ivani G, Lampugnani E, De Negri P, Lönnqvist P, Broadman L. Ropivacaine vs bupivacaine in major surgery in infants. Can J Anaesth 1999;46:467–469.
61. Broadman LM, Ivani G. Caudal blocks. Tech Reg Anesth Pain Manage 1999;3:150–156.
62. Ala-Kokko TI, Karinen J, Raiha E, et al. Pharmacokinetics of 0.75% ropivacaine and 0.5% bupivacaine after ilioinguinal-iliohypogastric nerve block in children. Br J Anaesth 2002; 89:438–441.
63. Habre W, Bergesio R, Johnson C, et al. Pharmacokinetics of ropivacaine following caudal analgesia in children. Paediatr Anaesth 2000;10:143–147.
64. Deng XM, Xiao WJ, Tang GZ, et al. The minimum local anesthetic concentration of ropivacaine for caudal analgesia in children. Anesth Analg 2002;94:1465–1468.
65. Paut O, Schreiber E, Lacroix F, et al. High plasma ropivacaine concentrations after fascia iliaca compartment block in children. Br J Anaesth 2004;92:416–418.
66. Van Obbergh LJ, Roelants FA, Veyckemans F, Verbeeck RK. In children, the addition of epinephrine modifies the pharmacokinetics of ropivacaine injected caudally. Can J Anaesth 2003;50:593–598.
67. Morrison SG, Dominguez JJ, Frascarolo P, Reiz S. A comparison of the electrocardiographic cardiotoxic effects of racemic bupivacaine, levobupivacaine, and ropivacaine in anesthetized swine. Anesth Analg 2000;90:1308–1314.
68. Nichols D, Yaster M, Lynn A, et al. Disposition and respiratory effects of intrathecal morphine in children. Anesthesiology 1993;79:733–738.
69. Attia J, Ecoffey C, Sandouk P, et al. Epidural morphine in children. Pharmacokinetics and $CO_2$ sensitivity. Anesthesiology 1986;65:590–594.
70. Krane EJ, Tyler DC, Jacobson LE. The dose response of caudal morphine in children. Anesthesiology 1989;71:48–52.
71. Krane EJ. Delayed respiratory depression in a child after caudal epidural morphine. Anesth Analg 1988;67:79–82.
72. Valley RD, Bailey AG. Caudal morphine for postoperative analgesia in infants and children: a report of 138 cases. Anesth Analg 1991;72:120–124.
73. Bailey AG, Valley RD, Freid EB, Calhoun P. Epidural morphine combined with epidural or intravenous butorphanol for postoperative analgesia in pediatric patients. Anesth Analg 1994;79:340–344.

74. Lawhorn CD, Brown RE. Epidural morphine with butorphanol in pediatric patients. J Clin Anesth 1994;6:91–94.
75. Jamail S, Monin S, Begon C, et al. Clonidine in pediatric caudal anesthesia. Anesth Analg 1994;78:663–666.
76. Callow LB, Rosen DA, Rosen KR, et al. Optimal pain relief following cardiac surgery in children. Circulation 1992;86:I-501.
77. Huang JJ, Hirshberg G. Regional anaesthesia decreases the need for postoperative mechanical ventilation in very low birth weight infants undergoing herniorrhaphy. Paediatr Anaesth 2001;11:705–709.
78. Tuncer S, Yosunkaya A, Reisli R, et al. Effect of caudal block on stress responses in children. Pediatr Int 2004;46:53–57.
79. Rosen D, Rosen KR, Hammer GB. Pro: regional anesthesia is an important component of the anesthetic technique for pediatric patients undergoing cardiac surgical procedures. J Cardiothorac Vasc Anesth 2002;16:374–378.

# 14 Complications of Obstetric Regional Anesthesia

Paul J. O'Connor

The major trend in the provision of anesthesia services to pregnant women over the past 25 years has been the increasing use of regional anesthetic techniques for labor and operative delivery.[1] According to the latest report on Confidential Enquiries into Maternal Deaths in the United Kingdom, at least 80% of cesarean deliveries are now performed under regional block.[2] The report highlights that the likelihood of dying from anesthesia is now 1 per 100,000 cesarean deliveries, more than 30 times less than it was during the 1960s. This reduction in mortality is clearly associated with the increased use of regional anesthesia, to which no deaths were attributed in this triennium.[2] This was not always the case, and it is only 15 years since deaths resulting from regional anesthesia in the United States were evenly divided between local anesthetic toxicity and high spinal/epidural anesthesia.[3] In contrast to regional anesthesia, the safety of general anesthesia remains unchanged since 1982–1984, and the risk of death attributable to general anesthesia is now estimated to be 1 death per 20,000 cesarean deliveries.[2] Death is only the tip of the morbidity iceberg, however, and obstetric regional anesthesia was the source of more than one-third of anesthesia malpractice insurance claims in the United States during the 1980s and 1990s.[4,5] Obstetric anesthetists must be familiar with the differential diagnosis of postpartum injuries to be able to recognize rare but potentially life-threatening complications of regional anesthesia. Such injuries may be intrinsic to labor and delivery or they may result directly or indirectly from obstetric or anesthetic intervention.[6]

## Postdural Puncture Headache

This topic has been addressed in detail in Chapters 9 and 10 but from different perspectives, and when you combine the information gleaned from three different points of view your knowledge of this topic will be more complete.

Accidental dural puncture with an epidural needle is reported to occur in about 0.5%–2% of parturients. Among those who experience this complication, 70%–80% will develop a headache.[7,8] The most identifiable characteristic of the headache is postural dependence, seen in about 80% of patients. It is frequently severe and causes significant limitation of daily activity. The distribution is typically frontal/occipital and it may be accompanied by neck/shoulder stiffness, photophobia, or nausea and vomiting.[9] Intentional dural puncture with a 27- or 29-gauge pencil-point needle as part of a combined spinal-epidural (CSE) technique also leads to postdural puncture headache (PDPH) in about 0.5%–1.5% of cases.[10,11] Dural puncture leads to loss of cerebrospinal fluid (CSF) and lowering of CSF pressure but the actual mechanism producing the headache is not clear. One theory is that decreased CSF pressure causes the brain to sag when the patient assumes the upright position, resulting in traction on pain-sensitive blood vessels in the brain. Another explanation may be that loss of CSF volume produces a compensatory venodilatation causing headache.

The initial management of PDPH is by conservative measures including bedrest, oral analgesics, and gentle rehydration. Cerebral vasoconstrictors such as caffeine and sumatriptan have been found to be effective in relieving dural puncture headache in some cases but are not frequently used.[12] Overall success rates with conservative measures are disappointing, and, in the absence of contraindications (fever, local infection, or coagulopathy), 60%–80% of parturients with PDPH receive an autologous epidural blood patch (EBP).[7,9,13] A recent Cochrane Review concluded that evidence does not support routine use of EBP in the treatment of PDPH.[14] However, this practice has an established role in obstetric regional anesthesia, and, for ethical reasons, it is unlikely that a randomized, controlled trial (RCT) of epidural blood patching will be performed.[15] Indeed, the low frequency of PDPH and the difficulty in blinding treatment would make such a study almost impossible. The best alternative source of evidence is therefore prospective audit. A large prospective survey of 65,000 parturients in the United Kingdom, which returned detailed information on 404 patients with PDPH, revealed that the rate of epidural blood patching was 59%.[9] A similar Australian audit of 12,500 parturients yielded 100 cases of accidental dural puncture, 81 (81%) of whom developed PDPH and 58 (58%) of whom received at least one blood patch.[13] Another (retrospective) review of more than 15,000 obstetric epidurals yielded 72 patients with accidental dural puncture, 55 (76%) of whom developed PDPH and 45 (63%) of whom had a blood patch.[7]

The initial rate of success with epidural blood patching in the study by Banks et al.[13] was 67% (complete success). A further 28% had partial resolution of symptoms (partial success), although 31% of patients experienced a recurrence. In a retrospective audit of more than 5000 maternity epidurals, 48 patients had one or more blood patches resulting in complete and permanent relief of symptoms in only 33%, and partial relief in 50%.[16] Results for complete and partial success from a second blood patch in this study were 50% and 36%, respectively. On average, therefore, only about 60% of patients undergoing EBP obtain complete or partial relief from symptoms. Success rates may improve if treatment is delayed for 48 hours or more, but this figure is still substantially lower than that traditionally quoted. Failure to obtain symptomatic relief with one EBP should prompt a search for an alternative diagnosis. A second EBP may be performed when more sinister causes of the headache such as meningitis, intracranial hemorrhage, or cerebral venous thrombosis have been considered.

It is clear that the incidence and severity of PDPH are related to the size and shape of the hole in the dura.[17] Although specific data confirming this with regard to epidural needles are lacking, common sense suggests that it is better to choose an 18-gauge epidural needle than a 16 or 17 gauge. In the case of spinal needles, a 27-gauge needle with an atraumatic tip may represent the optimum balance between dural puncture headache and the risk of technical failure.[18–20] Maintenance of the supine position after dural tap is not effective in reducing the incidence of PDPH. Prophylactic blood patching through a resited epidural catheter has been advocated following a wet tap but results have been disappointing.[21] Subarachnoid catheterization is another option involving placement of the epidural catheter intrathecally at the time of accidental dural puncture. This avoids the need to resite the epidural (with the attendant risk of a second dural tap) but has not been shown to reduce the incidence of PDPH. One study suggested that the need for epidural blood patching might be reduced with this technique, but there are lingering doubts about spinal catheters and the possibility of failure to distinguish catheters located in the subarachnoid space from epidural catheters is a legitimate concern.[7]

The most common complication of EBP is low back pain, which is usually self-limiting.[22] Significant low back pain during the performance of EBP is usually taken as an indication to discontinue the procedure. In the absence of pain in the back, buttocks, or legs, the ideal volume of blood to be injected is controversial but is probably between 10 and 20 mL. Serious complications of EBP are rarely reported.[23,24]

## Hypotension

Spinal anesthesia has become the method of choice for anesthesia for elective cesarean delivery.[25] It is frequently accompanied by hypotension, which may be defined in absolute terms as a systolic blood pressure of 90 or 100 mm Hg or in relative terms as a percentage (usually less than 80%) of baseline. Hypotension caused by a reduction in systemic vascular resistance is normally compensated by an increase in cardiac output. This is attenuated under spinal anesthesia by an increase in venous capacitance because of venodilatation in the mesenteric bed. The situation is further compounded in pregnancy by aortocaval compression. Thus, instead of a compensatory increase, cardiac output usually decreases.[26] It is the combined effect of reduced cardiac output and decreased systemic vascular resistance that accounts for hypotension after spinal anesthesia.

The placental bed is maximally dilated at term and therefore unable to autoregulate when perfusion pressure is reduced. Uterine blood flow is therefore pressure dependent. As a consequence of this, prolonged maternal hypotension is damaging to the fetus and it is also frequently associated with maternal nausea and vomiting. Treatment has traditionally consisted of uterine displacement, crystalloid preloading, and use of vasopressors. The results of pretreatment with intravenous crystalloids before spinal anesthesia have generally been disappointing. In a recent RCT, the incidence of hypotension in mothers having elective cesarean delivery was 85% despite the administration of 2 L of lactated Ringer's solution as a preload before spinal anesthesia.[27] Studies of this kind have led to a reappraisal of the role of fluid preloading.[28–31] A recent systematic review found that crystalloid was inconsistent in preventing hypotension and that colloid was significantly better.[32] However, disadvantages of colloid include the additional cost and the possibility of anaphylactoid reactions.[33] Interestingly, the same review also concluded that wrapping the legs with elastic bandages consistently and significantly reduced the incidence of hypotension compared with leg elevation.[32]

Ephedrine has been the drug of choice for more than 30 years in the treatment of maternal hypotension in obstetric spinal anesthesia when conservative measures fail. This is largely attributable to a seminal study in 1974, which found that ephedrine preserved uterine blood flow in pregnant sheep much better than alpha-adrenergic agonists such as methoxamine or metaraminol.[34] Ephedrine thus became the "gold standard" for this application and, as recently as 2001, a survey of obstetric anesthetists in the United Kingdom found that more than 95% used ephedrine as the sole vasopressor, with only 0.4% choosing phenylephrine.[35] Interest in phenylephrine was rekindled in 1988 by Ramanathan and Grant[36], who found that it did not cause fetal acidosis when treating maternal hypotension. Numerous studies have confirmed these findings and have almost all reported higher umbilical artery (UA) pH values in neonates born to phenylephrine-treated mothers.[26,37–39] A systematic review in 2002 summarized findings from seven RCTs comparing ephedrine with phenylephrine.[40] In this review, phenylephrine was associated with higher UA pH values than ephedrine although there was no difference in the incidence of fetal acidosis (UA pH $< 7.20$) or in Apgar scores $<7$ at 1 and 5 minutes. What is the significance of these findings? Neonatal acid-base studies and Apgar scores are essentially surrogate outcomes for neonatal well-being. However, we may never have studies with sufficient power to detect clinically significant outcome differences in the neonate. What we can say is that a growing body of evidence supports the use of phenylephrine as a valid alternative to ephedrine. When there is hypotension and bradycardia, ephedrine continues to be the drug of choice.[30] Otherwise, phenylephrine has not been shown to be deleterious to the fetus and it may well be the better agent.

There are limited data comparing ephedrine and phenylephrine with regard to other maternal outcomes of interest including nausea and vomiting and bradycardia. One study found that the incidence of nausea was 66% in ephedrine-treated mothers compared with 17% in the phenylephrine group.[41] The figures for vomiting were 36% and 0%, respectively. A recent study seeking to define the optimum regime for phenylephrine administration compared the effects of titrating the infusion to 80%, 90%, or 100% of baseline blood pressure.[42] The authors found that maintaining the blood pressure at 100% of baseline was associated with the best outcome for the baby (highest UA pH) and the mother (less nausea or vomiting) despite a median total dose of 1.5 mg of phenylephrine given to mothers in the 100% group.

Low-dose spinal anesthesia for cesarean delivery combines a small dose of intrathecal local anesthetic with an opioid in an effort to reduce the incidence of hypotension. When used as part of a CSE technique, the epidural catheter is available for "rescue analgesia." Studies to date suggest that intrathecal anesthesia may be achieved with as little as 5 mg of bupivacaine combined with an opioid, with epidural supplementation in 5%–15% of patients.[43–46] Although the technique is promising, and one might intuitively expect a reduction in the incidence of hypotension and nausea with such low doses, there are insufficient data to support this conclusion.

In summary, a combination of a colloid preload and leg wrapping may be most efficacious for the prevention of hypotension under spinal anesthesia for cesarean delivery. Apart from this, one may choose ephedrine or phenylephrine as a vasopressor. There is an abundance of evidence to suggest that phenylephrine is at least as good as ephedrine and a more liberal use of this drug is probably justified.

## Complications of Combined Spinal-Epidural Blockade

The CSE technique has increased in popularity in the last decade. Advantages include early onset of maternal analgesia and greater maternal satisfaction compared with epidural only, although satisfaction scores with both techniques are high.[47,48] Compared with traditional (but not low-dose) epidurals, there is a reduced incidence of instrumental delivery, probably secondary to a reduction in the dose of local anesthetic used throughout labor.[49] This leads to a reduction in motor block, which may facilitate maternal ambulation and lead to better satisfaction.

Complications that are common to both CSE and epidurals include technical failure, hypotension, pruritus, urinary retention, and backache, as well as rare but serious events such as neuraxial hematoma and meningitis. Pruritus is strongly associated with the use of intrathecal opioids and, although usually mild, it may cause considerable distress in some patients.[50] Treatment usually consists of an antihistamine. Naloxone or nalbuphine are reserved for severe cases, because there is a risk of breakthrough pain. Respiratory depression may occur also and is discussed under the heading of Complications of Neuraxial Opioids.

One might intuitively expect an increase in the incidence of PDPH following intentional dural puncture during CSE.[51] However, the reliability of correctly identifying the epidural space may be enhanced by the observation of CSF return through the spinal needle in addition to loss of resistance per se.[52] This could lead to a reduction in the incidence of accidental dural puncture with the epidural needle. Alternatively, intrathecal opioids may provide prophylaxis against the development of PDPH.[53] Studies have not shown an increased incidence of accidental dural tap or PDPH with CSE, and this has been confirmed by a recent Cochrane review.[10,11,48,54–56]

Fetal heart rate (FHR) abnormalities, especially prolonged bradycardia, may follow the induction of labor analgesia.[57] These abnormalities usually respond to simple measures such as maternal repositioning, supplemental oxygen, treatment of hypotension if present, and, occasionally, tocolysis. There is a lack of agreement in the literature concerning the association between spinal opioids and nonreassuring FHR patterns. Several studies have reported uterine hyperactivity and an increased incidence of nonreassuring FHR following intrathecal sufentanil in doses ranging from 1.5 to 7.5 µg.[58,59] A metaanalysis of published randomized trials in 2002 concluded that intrathecal opioids increase the risk of fetal bradycardia.[60] This is in contrast to a previous literature review in 2000 that concluded that these abnormalities occur with similar frequencies in association with any method of effective labor pain relief.[57] A large trial of more than 1000 nulliparous patients randomly allocated to receive "traditional" epidural, low-dose epidural infusion, or CSE was published in 2001.[49] Patients in the CSE group received 2.5 mg of bupivacaine plus fentanyl 25 µg intrathecally. Although the study did not report FHR abnormalities, the rate of cesarean delivery was the same in all groups. Compared with "traditional" epidural analgesia, neonates born to mothers who received CSE were more likely to have 1-minute Apgar scores ≤7, but this difference was not significant. Apart from this, the incidence of 5-minute Apgar scores ≤7, the rate of admission to neonatal units, and the requirement for resuscitation were identical in the CSE group compared with "traditional." Similar neonatal and obstetric outcome data were found in the studies in which differences in FHR patterns were reported in association with intrathecal sufentanil.[58,59] From these studies, it would seem that any differences in FHR associated with low-dose intrathecal opioids do not translate into a difference in outcome. It has been pointed out that these outcome measures are somewhat crude, however, and there is a possibility that the studies were not powered to detect such a difference if it exists. This question requires further study.

Because it is difficult to test epidural catheters placed as part of a CSE technique, there were concerns that untested catheters might be less reliable for labor analgesia, and in particular when used for obstetric emergencies. This has not been shown to be a problem. One study found a reduced incidence of CSE catheter replacement although a large prospective study of more than 2000 parturients failed to confirm this.[10,11] CSE may also carry an increased risk of a high block because of the possibility of leakage of epidural drug across the dura mater. This is unlikely to be a problem in cases of dural perforation with a 26- or 27-gauge spinal needle.

There is also a possibility of high block because of cephalad shift of subarachnoid local anesthetic secondary to external compression of the dural sac by an epidural bolus. To overcome this mass effect, it may be prudent to use a continuous epidural infusion or to delay the administration of an epidural bolus for at least 15–20 minutes after intrathecal injection.

## Complications of Neuraxial Opioids

The discovery of spinal opioid receptors in the late 1970s led to the widespread use of dilute solutions of local anesthetics and opioids for epidural analgesia in labor and more recently to the use of spinal opioids for cesarean delivery.[61,62] The most troublesome side effects include pruritus, nausea and vomiting, and respiratory depression. A systematic review of RCTs of intrathecal opioids for cesarean delivery in 1999 reported pooled data (for different drugs and doses) from 15 studies including more than 500 patients.[63] The incidence of pruritus was 50%–80% and did not differ between fentanyl, sufentanil, and morphine. However, nausea and vomiting occurred less frequently with the lipophilic drugs such as fentanyl and sufentanil than with morphine. Another metaanalysis compared intrathecal opioids and epidural local anesthetics for labor analgesia.[50] The odds ratio of pruritus for spinal opioids versus epidural local anesthetics was 14. The odds ratio of nausea was 0.95, although the duration of follow-up was not clear and the analysis did not include studies of patients receiving intrathecal meperidine.

Respiratory depression is the most feared side effect of intrathecal opioids. There have been several cases of respiratory arrest following sufentanil and fentanyl for labor analgesia.[64–68] The authors of one report performed a retrospective review of almost 4900 parturients who had received intrathecal sufentanil as part of a CSE technique for labor in their institution and found only one case of respiratory arrest (0.021%), which occurred following 10 μg of sufentanil.[65] Delayed onset respiratory depression is a particular concern with morphine, and may occur 12–24 hours after a single dose. Among the 15 studies included in the previously mentioned systematic review, respiratory depression (respiratory rate < 10 breaths/minute) was reported in only one patient (1/485) following a dose of 0.1 mg of spinal morphine.[63] However, a prospective series of almost 900 patients who were given a relatively high dose of 0.2 mg of intrathecal morphine for cesarean delivery reported eight cases of respiratory depression (1%), defined as a respiratory rate ≤8 and/or $Sao_2$ ≤85%.[69] The true incidence of this complication is unknown, but it may be more likely to occur in obese patients (all eight patients in this study were noted to be markedly obese) and with the coadministration of systemic opioids.[65]

It has also been demonstrated that both epidural and intrathecal morphine are associated with reactivation of herpes simplex labialis in mothers undergoing cesarean delivery.[70,71] A recent study found that the risk of herpes simplex labialis reactivation within 30 days postoperatively in mothers receiving 0.25 mg of spinal morphine was 38%, compared with 17% in those who received systemic morphine for postoperative analgesia.[71] The mechanism involved is unclear and may involve pruritus leading to scratching of the skin in the distribution of the trigeminal nerve.[72]

## Backache

The association of postpartum backache with epidural analgesia in labor has been the subject of controversy since it was first reported in 1990[73] (Chapter 10). A difficulty in studying this question is that ideally it requires ongoing follow-up between 6 weeks and a year after delivery. In two early studies, the incidence of new-onset postpartum backache was 18%–19% among mothers who had epidural analgesia in labor compared with 11%–12% in those who did not.[73,74] The study by MacArthur et al.[73] is by far the largest in the literature and the most controversial. More than 30,000 postal questionnaires were sent out between 1 and 9 years after delivery. The number of questionnaires returned was 11,700, giving a response rate of 38.9%. More than half of the women had changed address, and when this was taken into account the authors quoted an adjusted response rate of 79% (of those still living at the same address who could be presumed to have received the questionnaire). Despite the huge number of responses in absolute terms, two main problems arise. Depending on actual or adjusted response rate, the study may have been subject to significant selection bias (women with postpartum health problems may be more likely to respond). Secondly, the accuracy of distant recall after a period as long as 9 years is questionable. This might lead to underreporting of both antenatal backache (which is strongly correlated with postpartum back pain) as well as new-onset postpartum backache.

Studies since about 1994 have enrolled smaller numbers of mothers but have generally been of a more robust prospective design, have obtained follow-up data within 2 months to 2 years after delivery, and have achieved response rates of 75%–99%.[75–79] These studies have reported a much lower incidence of backache and have failed to demonstrate an association with epidural analgesia. One study from 1995 with a 99% follow-up reported that 14% of women in the epidural group had new onset of low back pain at 6 weeks postpartum compared with only 7% in the nonepidural group, but the difference was not significant and the authors stated in their discussion that this may have been attributable to a lack of power.[76] In a prospective study of more than 600 parturients, with a response rate of 75% 3 months after delivery, Russell et al.[77] identified only 33 cases of new-onset backache. This was markedly different from the results of their earlier retrospective study.[74] Unsurprisingly, given the low incidence, they were unable to detect a difference between mothers who had received an epidural and those who had not. Howell et al.[79] performed a follow-up study of patients who had been randomly allocated to receive epidural (n = 184) versus nonepidural (n = 185) analgesia in labor and found no significant differences in the onset or duration of low back pain. These authors also performed a number of objective measurements of spinal mobility on 241 of these mothers and found no significant differences.

These findings may be attributable in part to changes in obstetric practice since 1978, smaller-gauge epidural needles, and changes in drug/dose combinations (with or without a spinal component), which result in greater preservation of maternal muscle tone. Overall, however, given that the proportion of mothers who receive epidural or CSE analgesia in labor is 70% in many centers, it would be reassuring to have a larger prospective study evaluating this issue using modern neuraxial techniques.

## Systemic Toxicity of Local Anesthetics

Systemic local anesthetic toxicity may occur after the rapid, accidental intravenous injection of large doses of local anesthetic usually intended for delivery into the epidural space. As plasma levels increase, minor symptoms of central nervous system (CNS) toxicity are followed by convulsions, CNS depression, and coma. In the later stages of toxicity, cardiovascular manifestations predominate and include hypotension, bradycardia, and cardiac arrest. Cardiovascular toxicity with bupivacaine develops almost simultaneously with CNS toxicity, however, and this drug was responsible for a cluster of maternal deaths in the United States between 1979 and 1984, when local anesthetic toxicity was one of the leading causes of maternal death during regional anesthesia.[3]

More recent data suggest that the incidence of serious complications related to drug toxicity following epidural blockade in modern obstetric anesthesia is very low. There were no cardiac arrests and only two cases of convulsions reported out of a total of almost 190,000 obstetric epidurals in three large series.[80–82] Data for obstetric spinals are less clearcut, with one case reported by Auroy et al.[81] out of a total 5640 obstetric spinals. Overall, these data suggest that good standards of practice are effective in reducing the incidence of life-threatening complications. With epidural techniques, the risk is minimized by aspirating the catheter, use of a test dose, and, above all, fractionating the dose. A number of recent developments have also contributed to reducing the risk of systemic toxicity. The widespread use of epidural opioids has facilitated a reduction in the concentration of epidural local anesthetics, thereby reducing cumulative drug dosages. Also, the use of CSE techniques avoids the need for a large epidural bolus to establish a block and may further reduce this risk. Finally, newer local anesthetic agents such as levobupivacaine may have an improved cardiovascular safety profile, although large studies are awaited.[83,84]

## Unintended High Block

The injection of large doses of local anesthetic into the subarachnoid space in the belief that the drug is being injected epidurally leads to extensive sensory and motor block. Aspiration for CSF and administration of a test dose containing local anesthetic are designed to prevent this from happening but are not foolproof. In extreme cases, inadvertent intrathecal injection produces a "total" spinal which is characterized by blockade of the cervical segments of the spinal cord and brainstem. This leads to diaphragmatic paralysis and apnea and requires ventilatory support. Severe hypotension requiring fluids and vasopressors may also occur because of extensive sympathetic blockade.

A so-called "epidural" catheter may also lie in the subdural space. This is classically described as a potential space between the dura and arachnoid mater, extending from the second sacral vertebra into the cranial cavity. Although it has also been implicated in block failure, subdural injection of local anesthetic drug usually produces a block that is unexpectedly high with a somewhat slow onset of 20–35 minutes.[85] Unlike subarachnoid block, motor block is variable, hypotension is not usually severe, and sacral dermatomes are frequently spared.[80] Because of the slower onset, a subdural catheter is not detected by a test dose.

The incidence of inadvertent subarachnoid or subdural injection has been reported in several large series.[80,82,86] The largest prospective series was reported by Jenkins[80] in 2005 and involved more than 145,000 maternity epidurals between 1987 and 2003. Using predefined diagnostic criteria (which did not include radiologic confirmation of the position of the catheter), the author reported 51 cases of intrathecal injection (1/2900 epidurals), 35 cases of inadvertent subdural injection (1/4200), and nine cases of high or total spinal (1/16,200). These incidence rates are higher than a previous large prospective series but lack of standardization of diagnostic criteria makes comparison difficult.[86] Fractionation of the dose when administering a bolus is the best way to limit the consequences of injection through a misplaced catheter.

## Neurologic Deficits and Labor Analgesia

Immediate postpartum neurologic complications as a consequence of central neural blockade are uncommon. The largest prospective series of almost 123,000 neuraxial blocks in parturients was reported in 1995 by Scott and Tunstall.[86] There were 46 neuropathies, virtually all involving a single spinal or peripheral nerve, with a rate of 3.5/10,000 epidurals and 5.4/10,000 spinals (overall rate 3.7/10,000). Complete recovery was reported in 1–12 weeks and there were no confirmed cases of permanent disability. Similar data were reported in a recent French study in which the incidence of neurologic injury was 0.6/10,000 with a significantly increased risk after spinal (3.5/10,000) compared with epidural (0/10,000).[81] From these and other prospective studies published since 1995, the incidence ranges from 0 to 3.7 per 10,000 neuraxial blocks (Table 14-1).[81,82,86–89] Possible mechanisms of injury are discussed below.

Table 14-1. Results from Prospective Studies of Neurologic Complications Attributed to Neuraxial Blockade in Parturients

| Author | Year | N | Details | Incidence/10,000 |
|---|---|---|---|---|
| Scott and Tunstall[86] | 1995 | 122,989 | 46 mononeuropathies | 3.7* |
| Holdcroft et al.[87] | 1995 | 13,007 | 1 peripheral neuropathy | 0.8 |
| Paech et al.[82] | 1998 | 10,995 | 1 traumatic mononeuropathy | 0.9 |
| Auroy et al.[81] | 2002 | 35,372† | 2 peripheral neuropathies | 0.6 |
| Dar et al.[88] | 2002 | 2,615 | | 0‡ |
| Wong et al.[89] | 2003 | 6,048 | Radicular pain after spinal | 1.7 |

*No distinction drawn between obstetric palsies and neurologic injuries attributed to neuraxial blockade.

†This represents the subset of 35,372 obstetric patients within a larger study.

‡Six women had sacral numbness of unknown etiology after cesarean delivery under epidural or CSE. Neuraxial blockade may have contributed to these indirectly.

## Direct Trauma

Direct trauma to the spinal cord, conus medullaris, or spinal nerve roots may be secondary to needle/catheter trauma or intraneural injection of local anesthetic. Most of the reported cases concern radiculopathy involving a single nerve root (Table 14-1) and most are reversible.[86] The possibility of damage to the conus medullaris is of far greater consequence to the patient, however. A report in 2001 described seven cases of damage to the conus medullaris following spinal or CSE anesthesia, six of them in obstetric patients.[90] Spinal needle insertion was painful in all cases but only one patient reported pain on injection. Magnetic resonance imaging (MRI) showed a syrinx in the conus in six cases. The patients experienced unilateral sensory loss, pain, foot drop ($n = 6$), and urinary symptoms ($n = 3$). Symptoms persisted up to 18 months in some cases and may have been permanent. MRI studies in adults without spinal deformity have shown that the position of the tip of the conus medullaris follows a normal distribution ranging from the middle third of T12 to the upper third of L3 with a mean conus position corresponding to the lower third of L1.[91] According to this study, the conus extends below L1/2 in approximately 20% of normal adults. Given this intrinsic variability and bearing in mind that identification of lumbar interspaces based on surface anatomy is unreliable in many patients, it is important to reiterate that one should not knowingly insert a spinal needle above the spinous process of L3.[90,92] This recommendation is reinforced by a report in 2004 of a further three spinal cord injuries in obstetric patients leading to permanent neurologic injury following needle trauma (two epidural and one spinal).[93]

## Transient Neurologic Symptoms

The syndrome of short-lived painful sensations in the buttocks and/or legs after spinal anesthesia is known as transient neurologic symptoms (TNS) and was first reported in 1993[94] (Chapter 9). It may appear up to 24 hours after uneventful spinal anesthesia and usually lasts for 1–4 days. The etiology of the condition is unclear. The majority of cases occur after the administration of hyperbaric lidocaine for spinal anesthesia, and a recent review found that it is seven to eight times more likely to occur with lidocaine (or mepivacaine) than with bupivacaine, prilocaine, or procaine.[95] Studies of patients undergoing spinal anesthesia with lidocaine show that the incidence of TNS varies from 0% to 40%.[96] Pregnancy may offer some protection against TNS, but the risk is increased in ambulatory patients and after surgery in the lithotomy position.[97–99] TNS can be distinguished from more serious complications of neuraxial blockade by the fact that it is not associated with any abnormality on neurologic examination, MRI, or electrophysiologic testing.[96] Treatment with nonsteroidal anti-inflammatory drugs is sufficient in most cases. Given the suitability of long-acting local anesthetic agents for spinal anesthesia for cesarean delivery, the increased likelihood of TNS in the setting of ambulatory surgery, especially in the lithotomy position, and the overall sevenfold increased risk of TNS with spinal lidocaine compared with bupivacaine, one may question whether there are appreciable benefits for its routine use in obstetrics.[100]

## Cauda Equina Syndrome

Cauda equina syndrome proper is the triad of paraparesis/paraplegia of leg and buttock muscles, saddle anesthesia with sensory deficits below the groin, and incompetence of bladder and rectal sphincters causing incontinence of urine and feces.[101] Although it has been reported following spinal and epidural anesthesia in the general patient population, it is important to state that there are no reports of cauda equina syndrome following neuraxial blockade in obstetrics.[81,93,102] Anesthetic factors that have been implicated include spinal microcatheters, direct local anesthetic toxicity, and cord compression caused by hematoma formation or EBP.[24,103,104] Reports of the syndrome in the early 1990s after continuous spinal anesthesia led to the withdrawal of spinal microcatheters from the United States.[103] Hyperbaric 5% lidocaine was implicated in six cases that occurred in Sweden, leading to the recommendation that it should be administered in concentrations not greater than 2% up to a maximum dose of 60mg.[104] However, it is not clear that the risks are greater with lidocaine because the recent study by Moen et al.[93] reported eight cases involving hyperbaric lidocaine with a further 11 involving hyperbaric (n = 6) and isobaric (n = 5) bupivacaine 0.5%.

## Anterior Spinal Artery Syndrome

This syndrome may occur spontaneously in the obstetric population or in association with neuraxial blockade with an incidence of less than two per million.[105] Symptoms are attributed to interruption of the blood supply to the anterior two-thirds of the spinal cord via the artery of Adamkiewicz in the thoracolumbar region. The clinical features include paraplegia or quadriplegia, loss of pain and temperature sensation, and bowel and bladder incontinence with relative sparing of proprioception, vibration, and light touch. A recent review summarizing three cases in the obstetric anesthesia literature suggested that hypotension, vasoconstriction (caused by the use of adrenaline-containing local anesthetic solutions), and increased CSF pressure (resulting from injection of large volumes of epidural local anesthetic) might have contributed to spinal cord ischemia.[106]

## Meningitis

When appropriate aseptic precautions are taken, bacterial meningitis following neuraxial anesthesia in obstetric patients is very rare. The risk is somewhat greater with subarachnoid block than epidural because the intact dura mater serves as a barrier to the spread of infection. In a retrospective study that included 1,260,000 spinals and 450,000 epidurals (200,000 for labor analgesia), Moen et al.[93] reported that the incidence of purulent meningitis was 1/53,000 spinals, approximately double the rate for epidural blockade. There is a theoretical risk that CSE may be associated with a small increased risk of bacterial meningitis, although there is no evidence for this. Patients usually present within 24–48 hours of the anesthetic procedure with pyrexia, headache, nausea and vomiting, photophobia, signs of meningism, and occasionally seizures. It is essential for rapid diagnosis that a thorough neurologic examination is performed, followed in most cases by a lumbar puncture and a computed tomography of the brain, before the initiation of broad-spectrum antibiotic therapy pending examination of the CSF and identification of the organism.

Aseptic meningitis may also occur as a possible complication of regional anesthesia and is thought to be the result of chemical irritation of the spinal cord and meninges. The clinical picture is similar to bacterial meningitis except that the CSF is sterile.

## Epidural Abscess

Epidural abscess may occur spontaneously because of hematogenous spread or as a rare but serious complication of obstetric regional anesthesia. It is difficult to be precise in quoting the incidence rate. There was only one case in a retrospective study of more than 500,000 obstetric epidurals and none at all in a prospective study of

108,000 obstetric epidurals by the same group.[86,105] A 1-year prospective Danish study in the general population reported nine cases, giving a much higher incidence of approximately 1 per 2000 epidural catheters used.[107] However, the mean duration of catheterization in patients who developed an epidural abscess in this study was 11 days and there were no cases in patients whose catheters were removed after 2 days.

The most common presenting complaint is backache with localized tenderness accompanied by fever and leukocytosis. This is followed by the development of symptoms of spinal cord compression including radicular pain, loss of lower limb sensory and motor function, and bladder dysfunction. Onset is slower than in the case of bacterial meningitis and the patient may present 4–10 days postpartum.[106] The most common infecting organism is *Staphylococcus aureus* which was isolated in 6 of 9 cases (67%) in the Danish study and 4 of 8 cases (50%) summarized by Loo et al.[106,107] The chances of a good functional recovery depend on early diagnosis (immediate MRI for preference) and aggressive surgical management as an adjunct to antibiotic therapy.

## Spinal Epidural Hematoma

This condition may arise spontaneously in the obstetric patient population, or, rarely, in association with obstetric epidural blockade.[108] Large retrospective studies have each reported a single epidural hematoma from a combined total of more than 700,000 obstetric epidurals, giving an incidence of 0.2–0.5 per 100,000.[93,105] Spinal hematoma after obstetric spinal blockade was also reported in one patient in the Swedish series.[93] A review of 10 cases of spinal hematoma after obstetric epidural blockade found that most cases were associated with an identifiable deficiency in the coagulation system.[109] Vandermeulen et al.[110] identified 61 case of spinal hematoma following central neuraxial blockade in the entire world literature between 1906 and 1994. As in the review by Abramovitz and Beilin,[109] there was evidence of hemostatic abnormality in the majority of cases, the incidence of hematoma appeared to be greater after continuous epidural versus spinal, and approximately half occurred at the time of epidural catheter removal.

Clinical management of parturients with thrombocytopenia or those taking aspirin or low-molecular-weight heparin (LMWH) for thromboprophylaxis requires individual assessment of the specific risks and benefit to each individual. A survey of practice patterns in obstetric anesthesia found that 100% of respondents would place an epidural catheter in an otherwise healthy patient with a platelet count $>100 \times 10^9$ per liter.[111] Only about 60% were prepared to do so with a platelet count between 80 and $99 \times 10^9$ platelets per liter and fewer than 20% with a platelet count below this. The risk of spinal hematoma associated with the use of LMWH has been addressed in guidelines presented by the American Society of Regional Anesthesia.[112] The recommendations are based on placing and removing needles and catheters during periods of low LMWH activity. In the case of patients on prophylactic LMWH, it is suggested that needle placement (and catheter removal) should be delayed for 10–12 hours after the previous dose. After catheter removal, the next dose of LMWH should be deferred for at least 2 hours. Concomitant administration of antiplatelet medication probably carries an additional risk of hemorrhagic complications but this cannot be quantified.

The signs and symptoms of spinal cord hematoma are similar to other causes of spinal cord compression such as epidural abscess. Recognition may be delayed, however, in the presence of a dense block and dilute solutions of local anesthetic and opioid permit more accurate assessment of neurologic status. New onset of back pain, radicular pain, progressive lower extremity numbness or weakness, and bowel/bladder dysfunction require immediate investigation (preferably MRI scan). It has been recommended that neurosurgical intervention within 8 hours of the development of symptoms offers the best chance of a full recovery, but the likelihood of permanent neurologic damage remains high.[93,110]

## Intracranial Subdural Hematoma

This is a rare but potentially life-threatening complication of central neuraxial blockade.[113] It is more frequently reported after accidental dural puncture during epidural anesthesia but it may also occur following subarachnoid block.[113,114] Scott and Hibbard[105] found one case in 505,000 obstetric epidurals whereas a recent Swedish study reported two cases in 200,000 epidurals.[93] The mechanism is thought to be the result of CSF leakage causing traction and eventual rupture of intracranial subdural veins. Loo et al.[106] summarized eight cases, all of which took place after epidural block complicated by inadvertent dural puncture. The most consistent clinical feature was persistent headache, frequently misdiagnosed as PDPH, and the definitive diagnosis was made between 8 and 42 days postpartum. The authors concluded that a persistent or recurrent postspinal headache should alert the anesthesiologist to the possibility of a cranial subdural hematoma. The differential diagnosis of atypical headache in parturients should also include subarachnoid hemorrhage, either as the result of a ruptured intracranial aneurysm or as an extremely rare complication of spinal anesthesia.[115]

## Intrinsic Obstetric Nerve Palsies

It has been estimated that intrinsic obstetric nerve palsies may be 3–4 times as likely to occur as are neurologic sequelae of regional blockade.[116] However, maternal morbidity and mortality have decreased considerably during the past 50 years in the Western world and fewer women now recognize that childbirth carries any risk. As a result, in cases in which an anesthesiologist has inserted a needle in a parturient's back, it is practically axiomatic that almost any postnatal symptom can be attributed to it.[117] Neurologic complications secondary to pregnancy and childbirth may be difficult to distinguish from those attributable to regional anesthesia. Risk factors for nerve injury were identified in a retrospective review of almost 24,000 deliveries by Ong et al.[118] These included primiparity, instrumental delivery, and epidural or general anesthesia. However, patients in this study who received some form of anesthetic also had longer labors and were more likely to have instrumental delivery and the authors concluded that a direct causal relationship with epidural (or general) anesthesia was highly unlikely. A study of more than 6000 parturients by Wong et al.[89] found that laboring women with postpartum nerve injury were more likely to be nulliparous, to have had a prolonged second stage of labor, and assisted vaginal delivery. Nerve injury was also more likely among women who had regional blockade but the difference was not statistically significant. However, the association between epidural analgesia and prolongation of labor (and possibly increased instrumental delivery rates) has been confirmed in several systematic reviews, and neuraxial blockade could therefore contribute indirectly to postpartum nerve injury.[119–121] Furthermore, in the presence of a regional block, parturients may not appreciate symptoms of impending injury, which would ordinarily prompt a change in maternal position.[122]

The relative infrequency of nerve injuries, the overlap of putative risk factors, and the fact that symptoms usually resolve spontaneously make it difficult to establish causality in some cases. It is therefore incumbent upon obstetric anesthetists to be familiar with known intrinsic obstetric palsies, both to facilitate rapid diagnosis of conditions that require immediate treatment and to reduce medicolegal risk. The principal obstetric causes of postpartum nerve injury include nerve compression by the fetal head, midforceps deliveries, and improper positioning during delivery. The injuries are mostly unilateral and last from a few days to a few months.[86,88,89,118] In addition to lumbar nerve roots, injuries often involve the lateral femoral cutaneous nerve, the lumbosacral plexus, the common peroneal nerve, and the femoral nerve. These injuries are briefly described below. The interested reader is referred to a textbook of neurology in pregnancy for a more comprehensive discussion.[116]

### *Meralgia Paresthetica*

This is a sensory mononeuritis involving the lateral femoral cutaneous nerve, which supplies the skin over the anterolateral aspect of the upper thigh. The nerve is prone to injury as it passes beneath (or bisects) the inguinal ligament. Symptoms may arise during the latter half of pregnancy or in association with maternal pushing in the lithotomy position.

### *Lumbosacral Plexus and Common Peroneal Nerve Injuries*

Compression of the lumbosacral trunk (L4-5) by the fetal head against the sacral ala may result in foot drop, the most common obstetric nerve palsy during the last century. Patients present with weakness of ankle dorsiflexion and eversion, and numbness along the lateral aspect of the lower leg and dorsum of the foot. Symptoms are usually unilateral (on the side opposite the fetal occiput) and it is classically associated with midforceps rotation. Foot drop may also occur because of compression of the common peroneal nerve against the head of the fibula when the knees are hyperflexed.

### *Femoral Nerve Palsy*

Injury to the femoral nerve is relatively common after labor and delivery.[88,89] The nerve can be compressed within the pelvis by the fetal head during vaginal delivery or by surgical retractors during cesarean delivery. It can also be compressed more peripherally under the inguinal ligament because of exaggerated hip flexion. Symptoms include limited thigh flexion, quadriceps weakness (especially seen on climbing stairs), absent or reduced knee jerk, and loss of sensation over the anterior thigh and medial calf.

### *Obturator Nerve Palsy*

Damage to the obturator nerve during labor and delivery is relatively uncommon. The nerve can be compressed against the lateral pelvic wall or in the obturator canal resulting in decreased sensation over the medial thigh and weakness of hip adduction and internal rotation.

## Evaluation of Neurologic Deficit in the Parturient

The most important step in evaluating a postanesthetic neurologic deficit is to rule out a rapidly expanding mass lesion such as an epidural abscess or hematoma.[1] If this is suspected, the patient should have urgent MRI followed by decompressive laminectomy within 8 hours. With nonprogressive deficits, it is essential to try and elicit the mechanism whereby the damage has occurred, and it would be wise to involve a neurologist as soon as possible.[122] Electromyography may be helpful in defining both the anatomic location of the injury as well as estimating when it took place.

## Paracervical Block

Paracervical block (PCB) has been used for labor analgesia since the 1940s. It provides a therapeutic alternative for first-stage labor pain when central neuraxial blockade is contraindicated or unavailable.[123] The technique is relatively easy to perform and involves transvaginal injection of local anesthetic into the paracervical tissues. Approximately 75% of women report good or excellent first-stage labor analgesia after PCB.[124] The utility of the technique is limited by its short duration of action and injections may have to be repeated. Increasing uptake of neuraxial techniques and concerns about fetal bradycardia have also contributed to a decrease in popularity of PCB in recent years.

The most common complication of PCB is fetal bradycardia, with an overall incidence of about 15%.[124] FHR changes are usually transient with an onset of approximately 2–10 minutes after PCB. The etiology is unclear and has been attributed to vasoconstriction of the uterine arteries, uterine hypertonicity, direct local anesthetic toxicity, or a combination of factors. A recent study compared hemodynamic effects and efficacy of PCB versus epidural analgesia for labor.[125] The authors reported an increased uterine artery pulsatility index, providing support for the theory that uterine artery vasoconstriction is at least partly responsible for fetal bradycardia with this technique. The study lacked power to detect a difference in analgesic efficacy but there was a trend toward better analgesia after epidural block and 38% of PCB patients required a "rescue" epidural. Neonatal Apgar scores and UA pH values were within normal limits and did not differ between groups. Maternal complications of PCB are rare and include systemic local anesthetic toxicity, paracervical abscess or hematoma formation, and sacral plexus neuropathy.[126]

## Consent for Neuraxial Blocks in Labor

The view that anesthesiologists should obtain separate, written consent for anesthesia has been strongly articulated in a recent review.[127] Although most anesthetic interventions are intended to *facilitate* surgical treatment, neuraxial blockade for labor analgesia represents a special case in which anesthetic intervention *is* the treatment. As such, obstetric anesthesiologists would seem to have a duty to obtain consent of a legal standard similar to that which a surgeon might obtain before an operation.[127] The scope of risk disclosure which is required in law varies between jurisdictions but is increasingly moving toward the "reasonable patient" standard, defined by the Canadian Supreme court in 1980. This held that the adequacy of the consent explanation is to be judged by what a reasonable patient in that particular patient's circumstance would have expected to hear before consenting to or refusing treatment.[128] Specifically, this is increasingly taken to include "when adverse outcome is severe even though its occurrence is rare."[129] The ability of laboring patients to give informed consent has been affirmed in a prospective survey by Jackson et al.[130], who concluded that, in the majority of cases, such ability was unaffected by labor pain, anxiety, or prior opioid administration. Clearly, most women want to have the risks of neuraxial blockade explained to them. Even when this is not the case, anesthesiologists should understand that rare but serious risks are considered material to the consent process and *require* disclosure.[128] Whether one agrees that this should include a signed consent form is debatable but it seems prudent, at the very least, to document the consent process in the patient notes, including details of risks discussed.

## Regional Anesthesia in a Parturient with an Anticipated Difficult Airway

The failure rate of spinal or CSE anesthesia for cesarean delivery can be as high as 2%.[25] Opinions differ about the advisability of choosing a regional technique in a parturient with a known or anticipated difficult airway, because there is a possibility of having to convert to a general anesthetic. For elective cesarean deliveries, however, neuraxial blockade is a reasonable choice provided that one avoids a high block. In this scenario, there is time to formulate a strategy for securing the airway in a controlled manner in the event of block failure. The risk of an excessively high block may be minimized by a CSE technique with a low-dose spinal component with epidural supplementation if required. Converting a neuraxial block to a general anesthetic may carry a risk of hemodynamic instability and this should also be anticipated. The real problem arises in the extreme case of an emergency cesarean delivery in which there is an immediate threat to the life of the mother or the fetus. General anesthesia is still associated with a risk of maternal death because of complications of airway management, and failure to intubate is reported with a frequency of 1/249 (0.4%).[131,132] This is a very difficult clinical scenario in which the time required to perform a regional block must be balanced against the urgency of the delivery and the possibility of failure to intubate. If a general anesthetic is preferred, the chosen airway strategy will clearly depend on the skills and preference of the individual practitioner but should certainly include the availability of a second anesthesiologist where possible.[133]

## Regional Anesthesia and Obstetric Hemorrhage

It has been shown that regional anesthesia is associated with a reduction in blood loss in both obstetric and nonobstetric patients.[134–136] An RCT of 341 parturients for cesarean delivery found that blood loss was significantly greater after general anesthesia compared with spinal or epidural.[134] A prospective cohort study of 2751 elective and nonelective cesarean deliveries reported that general anesthesia was an independent risk factor for intraoperative blood loss >1000 mL and/or blood transfusion.[135]

In mothers known to be at increased risk of hemorrhage, regional anesthesia for cesarean delivery is controversial, however, and there are concerns that neuraxial blockade may exacerbate hypotension by obtunding the sympathetic response to hypovolemia. Massive hemorrhage associated with placenta previa is a recognized cause of morbidity and mortality.[3] Recent trends suggest that anesthesiologists are increasingly prepared to use regional anesthesia for cesarean delivery in patients with placenta previa in the absence of significant (volume >500 mL of blood) ante partum hemorrhage and provided that the placenta is not underlying the surgical incision.[137,138] Evidence in support of this practice is provided by one small RCT and two retrospective reviews.[139–141] Hong et al.[139] randomly allocated 25 mothers undergoing cesarean delivery for grade 4 placenta previa to receive general anesthesia or epidural and found that patients undergoing general anesthesia were more likely to require a blood transfusion. Frederiksen et al.[140] reviewed 93,000 deliveries at a single institution in the United States from 1976 to 1997 and reported 514 cesarean deliveries for placenta previa. They concluded that general anesthesia was an independent predictor of the need for blood transfusion. A subsequent study in the United Kingdom by Parekh et al.[141] confirmed this finding. These data clearly demonstrate that regional anesthesia is not contraindicated for cesarean delivery for placenta previa. However, one should be cautious in applying these findings to any one individual patient, particularly in the presence of active bleeding or when the position of the placenta is unfavorable.

## Conclusion

Tremendous strides have been made in obstetric anesthesia in the past 40 years, thanks to pioneers such as Hingson, Bonica, and Bromage, who went to great lengths to firmly establish continuous epidural anesthesia as the gold standard for pain relief in labor. Not too long ago, anesthesia was listed as one of the major causes of maternal death. The practice change from general to regional anesthesia for obstetric surgical intervention has saved many lives in recent years. The introduction of the intrathecal and epidural opioids has added a new dimension to obstetric anesthesia care but has also added some new side effects and complications to deal with. The use of the CSE technique has given the obstetric anesthesiologist some additional options when dealing with obstetric patients. The problems of headache, backache, and the occasional nerve injury continue to be reported, but these complications are not always anesthesia related and we should be aware of that. There is no doubt that obstetric anesthesia care has improved greatly in recent years.

## References


1. Wlody D. Complications of regional anesthesia in obstetrics. Clin Obstet Gynecol 2003; 46:667–678.
2. Confidential Enquiry into Maternal and Child Health. Why Mothers Die 2000–2002: The Sixth Report of the Confidential Enquiry into Maternal Death in the United Kingdom. London: RCOG Press; 2004.
3. Hawkins JL, Koonin LM, Palmer SK, et al. Anesthesia-related deaths during obstetric delivery in the United States, 1979–1990. Anesthesiology 1997;86:277–284.
4. Clyburn PA. Early thoughts on 'Why Mothers Die 2000–2002.' Anaesthesia 2004;59:1157–1159.
5. Lee LA, Posner KL, Domino KB, et al. Injuries associated with regional anesthesia in the 1980s and 1990s: a closed claims analysis. Anesthesiology 2004;101:143–152.
6. Wong CA. Neurologic deficits and labor analgesia. Reg Anesth Pain Med 2004;29: 341–351.
7. Rutter SV, Shields F, Broadbent CR, et al. Management of accidental dural puncture in labour with intrathecal catheters: an analysis of 10 years' experience. Int J Obstet Anesth 2001;10:177–181.
8. Paech M, Banks S, Gurrin L. An audit of accidental dural puncture during epidural insertion of a Tuohy needle in obstetric patients. Int J Obstet Anesth 2001;10:162–167.
9. Chan TM, Ahmed E, Yentis SM, et al. Postpartum headaches: summary report of the National Obstetric Anaesthetic Database (NOAD) 1999. Int J Obstet Anesth 2003; 12:107–112.
10. Van de Velde M, Teunkens A, Hanssens M, et al. Post dural puncture headache following combined spinal epidural or epidural anaesthesia in obstetric patients. Anaesth Intensive Care 2001;29:595–599.
11. Norris MC, Fogel ST, Conway-Long C. Combined spinal-epidural versus epidural labor analgesia. Anesthesiology 2001;95:913–920.
12. Berger CW, Crosby ET, Grodecki W. North American survey of the management of dural puncture occurring during labour epidural analgesia. Can J Anaesth 1998;45:110–114.
13. Banks S, Paech M, Gurrin L. An audit of epidural blood patch after accidental dural puncture with a Tuohy needle in obstetric patients. Int J Obstet Anesth 2001;10:172–176.
14. Sudlow C, Warlow C. Epidural blood patching for preventing and treating post-dural puncture headache. Cochrane Database Syst Rev 2002;(2):CD001791.
15. Horlocker TT, Brown DR. Evidence-based medicine: haute couture or the emperor's new clothes? Anesth Analg 2005;100:1807–1810.
16. Williams EJ, Beaulieu P, Fawcett WJ, et al. Efficacy of epidural blood patch in the obstetric population. Int J Obstet Anesth 1999;8:105–109.
17. Smedstad KG. Dealing with post-dural puncture headache – is it different in obstetrics? Can J Anaesth 1998;45:6–9.
18. Turnbull DK, Shepherd DB. Post-dural puncture headache: pathogenesis, prevention and treatment. Br J Anaesth 2003;91:718–729.
19. Vallejo MC, Mandell GL, Sabo DP, et al. Postdural puncture headache: a randomized comparison of five spinal needles in obstetric patients. Anesth Analg 2000;91:916–920.
20. Choi PT, Galinski SE, Takeuchi L, et al. PDPH is a common complication of neuraxial blockade in parturients: a meta-analysis of obstetrical studies. Can J Anaesth 2003;50: 460–469.
21. Scavone BM, Wong CA, Sullivan JT, et al. Efficacy of a prophylactic epidural blood patch in preventing post dural puncture headache in parturients after inadvertent dural puncture. Anesthesiology 2004;101:1422–1427.

22. Abouleish E, Vega S, Blendinger I, et al. Long-term follow-up of epidural blood patch. Anesth Analg 1975;54:459–463.
23. Safa-Tisseront V, Thormann F, Malassine P, et al. Effectiveness of epidural blood patch in the management of post-dural puncture headache. Anesthesiology 2001;95:334–339.
24. Diaz JH. Permanent paraparesis and cauda equina syndrome after epidural blood patch for postdural puncture headache. Anesthesiology 2002;96:1515–1517.
25. Shibli KU, Russell IF. A survey of anaesthetic techniques used for caesarean section in the UK in 1997. Int J Obstet Anesth 2000;9:160–167.
26. Thomas DG, Robson SC, Redfern N, et al. Randomized trial of bolus phenylephrine or ephedrine for maintenance of arterial pressure during spinal anaesthesia for Caesarean section. Br J Anaesth 1996;76:61–65.
27. Riley ET, Cohen SE, Rubenstein AJ, et al. Prevention of hypotension after spinal anesthesia for cesarean section: six percent hetastarch versus lactated Ringer's solution. Anesth Analg 1995;81:838–842.
28. McKinlay J, Lyons G. Obstetric neuraxial anaesthesia: which pressor agents should we be using? Int J Obstet Anesth 2002;11:117–121.
29. Rout C, Rocke DA. Spinal hypotension associated with Cesarean section: will preload ever work? Anesthesiology 1999;91:1565–1567.
30. Vallejo MC, Ramanathan S. Should alpha-agonists be used as first line management of spinal hypotension? Int J Obstet Anesth 2003;12:243–245.
31. Riley ET. Spinal anaesthesia for Caesarean delivery: keep the pressure up and don't spare the vasoconstrictors. Br J Anaesth 2004;92:459–461.
32. Morgan PJ, Halpern SH, Tarshis J. The effects of an increase of central blood volume before spinal anesthesia for cesarean delivery: a qualitative systematic review. Anesth Analg 2001;92:997–1005.
33. Weeks S. Reflections on hypotension during Cesarean section under spinal anesthesia: do we need to use colloid? Can J Anaesth 2000;47:607–610.
34. Ralston DH, Shnider SM, DeLorimier AA. Effects of equipotent ephedrine, metaraminol, mephentermine, and methoxamine on uterine blood flow in the pregnant ewe. Anesthesiology 1974;40:354–370.
35. Burns SM, Cowan CM, Wilkes RG. Prevention and management of hypotension during spinal anaesthesia for elective Caesarean section: a survey of practice. Anaesthesia 2001;56:794–798.
36. Ramanathan S, Grant GJ. Vasopressor therapy for hypotension due to epidural anesthesia for cesarean section. Acta Anaesthesiol Scand 1988;32:559–565.
37. Moran DH, Perillo M, LaPorta RF, et al. Phenylephrine in the prevention of hypotension following spinal anesthesia for cesarean delivery. J Clin Anesth 1991;3:301–305.
38. Hall PA, Bennett A, Wilkes MP, et al. Spinal anaesthesia for caesarean section: comparison of infusions of phenylephrine and ephedrine. Br J Anaesth 1994;73:471–474.
39. LaPorta RF, Arthur GR, Datta S. Phenylephrine in treating maternal hypotension due to spinal anaesthesia for caesarean delivery: effects on neonatal catecholamine concentrations, acid base status and Apgar scores. Acta Anaesthesiol Scand 1995;39:901–905.
40. Lee A, Ngan KW, Gin T. A quantitative, systematic review of randomized controlled trials of ephedrine versus phenylephrine for the management of hypotension during spinal anesthesia for cesarean delivery. Anesth Analg 2002;94:920–926.
41. Cooper DW, Carpenter M, Mowbray P, et al. Fetal and maternal effects of phenylephrine and ephedrine during spinal anesthesia for cesarean delivery. Anesthesiology 2002;97:1582–1590.
42. Ngan Kee KW, Khaw KS, Ng FF. Comparison of phenylephrine infusion regimens for maintaining maternal blood pressure during spinal anaesthesia for Caesarean section. Br J Anaesth 2004;92:469–474.
43. Fan SZ, Susetio L, Wang YP, Cheng YJ, et al. Low dose of intrathecal hyperbaric bupivacaine combined with epidural lidocaine for cesarean section – a balance block technique. Anesth Analg 1994;78:474–477.
44. Vercauteren MP, Coppejans HC, Hoffmann VL, et al. Small-dose hyperbaric versus plain bupivacaine during spinal anesthesia for cesarean section. Anesth Analg 1998;86:989–993.
45. Vercauteren MP, Coppejans HC, Hoffmann VH, et al. Prevention of hypotension by a single 5-mg dose of ephedrine during small-dose spinal anesthesia in prehydrated cesarean delivery patients. Anesth Analg 2000;90:324–327.

46. Ben-David B, Miller G, Gavriel R, et al. Low-dose bupivacaine-fentanyl spinal anesthesia for cesarean delivery. Reg Anesth Pain Med 2000;25:235–239.
47. Hepner DL, Gaiser RR, Cheek TG, et al. Comparison of combined spinal-epidural and low dose epidural for labour analgesia. Can J Anaesth 2000;47:232–236.
48. Wilson MJ, Cooper G, MacArthur C, et al. Randomized controlled trial comparing traditional with two "mobile" epidural techniques: anesthetic and analgesic efficacy. Anesthesiology 2002;97:1567–1575.
49. Comparative Obstetric Mobile Epidural Trial (COMET) Study Group. Effect of low-dose mobile versus traditional epidural techniques on mode of delivery: a randomised controlled trial. Lancet 2001;358:19–23.
50. Bucklin BA, Chestnut DH, Hawkins JL. Intrathecal opioids versus epidural local anesthetics for labor analgesia: a meta-analysis. Reg Anesth Pain Med 2002;27:23–30.
51. Dunn SM, Connelly NR, Parker RK. Postdural puncture headache (PDPH) and combined spinal-epidural (CSE). Anesth Analg 2000;90:1249–1250.
52. Balestrieri PJ. The incidence of postdural puncture headache and combined spinal-epidural: some thoughts. Int J Obstet Anesth 2003;12:305–306.
53. Brownridge P. Spinal anaesthesia in obstetrics. Br J Anaesth 1991;67:663.
54. Norris MC, Grieco WM, Borkowski M, et al. Complications of labor analgesia: epidural versus combined spinal epidural techniques. Anesth Analg 1994;79:529–537.
55. Albright GA, Forster RM. The safety and efficacy of combined spinal and epidural analgesia/anesthesia (6,002 blocks) in a community hospital. Reg Anesth Pain Med 1999;24:117–125.
56. Hughes D, Simmons SW, Brown J, Cyna AM. Combined spinal-epidural versus epidural analgesia in labour. Cochrane Database Syst Rev 2003;(4):CD003401.
57. Norris MC. Intrathecal opioids and fetal bradycardia: is there a link? Int J Obstet Anesth 2000;9:264–269.
58. Van de Velde M, Vercauteren M, Vandermeersch E. Fetal heart rate abnormalities after regional analgesia for labor pain: the effect of intrathecal opioids. Reg Anesth Pain Med 2001;26:257–262.
59. Van de Velde M, Teunkens A, Hanssens M, et al. Intrathecal sufentanil and fetal heart rate abnormalities: a double-blind, double placebo-controlled trial comparing two forms of combined spinal epidural analgesia with epidural analgesia in labor. Anesth Analg 2004;98:1153–1159.
60. Mardirosoff C, Dumont L, Boulvain M, et al. Fetal bradycardia due to intrathecal opioids for labour analgesia: a systematic review. BJOG 2002;109:274–281.
61. Chestnut DH, Laszewski LJ, Pollack KL, et al. Continuous epidural infusion of 0.0625% bupivacaine-0.0002% fentanyl during the second stage of labor. Anesthesiology 1990; 72:613–618.
62. Vertommen JD, Vandermeulen E, Van Aken H, et al. The effects of the addition of sufentanil to 0.125% bupivacaine on the quality of analgesia during labor and on the incidence of instrumental deliveries. Anesthesiology 1991;74:809–814.
63. Dahl JB, Jeppesen IS, Jorgensen H, et al. Intraoperative and postoperative analgesic efficacy and adverse effects of intrathecal opioids in patients undergoing cesarean section with spinal anesthesia: a qualitative and quantitative systematic review of randomized controlled trials. Anesthesiology 1999;91:1919–1927.
64. Greenhalgh CA. Respiratory arrest in a parturient following intrathecal injection of sufentanil and bupivacaine. Anaesthesia 1996;51:173–175.
65. Ferouz F, Norris MC, Leighton BL. Risk of respiratory arrest after intrathecal sufentanil. Anesth Analg 1997;85:1088–1090.
66. Katsiris S, Williams S, Leighton BL, et al. Respiratory arrest following intrathecal injection of sufentanil and bupivacaine in a parturient. Can J Anaesth 1998;45:880–883.
67. Kehl F, Erfkamp S, Roewer N. Respiratory arrest during caesarean section after intrathecal administration of sufentanil in combination with 0.1% bupivacaine 10ml. Anaesth Intensive Care 2002;30:698–699.
68. Kuczkowski KM. Respiratory arrest in a parturient following intrathecal administration of fentanyl and bupivacaine as part of a combined spinal-epidural analgesia for labour. Anaesthesia 2002;57:939–940.
69. Abouleish E, Rawal N, Rashad MN. The addition of 0.2mg subarachnoid morphine to hyperbaric bupivacaine for cesarean delivery: a prospective study of 856 cases. Reg Anesth 1991;16:137–140.

70. Boyle RK. Herpes simplex labialis after epidural or parenteral morphine: a randomized prospective trial in an Australian obstetric population. Anaesth Intensive Care 1995; 23:433–437.
71. Davies PW, Vallejo MC, Shannon KT, et al. Oral herpes simplex reactivation after intrathecal morphine: a prospective randomized trial in an obstetric population. Anesth Analg 2005;100:1472–1476.
72. Gieraerts R, Navalgund A, Vaes L, et al. Increased incidence of itching and herpes simplex in patients given epidural morphine after cesarean section. Anesth Analg 1987; 66:1321–1324.
73. MacArthur C, Lewis M, Knox EG, et al. Epidural anaesthesia and long term backache after childbirth. BMJ 1990;301:9–12.
74. Russell R, Groves P, Taub N, et al. Assessing long term backache after childbirth. BMJ 1993;306:1299–1303.
75. Breen TW, Ransil BJ, Groves PA, et al. Factors associated with back pain after childbirth. Anesthesiology 1994;81:29–34.
76. Macarthur A, MacArthur C, Weeks S. Epidural anaesthesia and low back pain after delivery: a prospective cohort study. BMJ 1995;311:1336–1339.
77. Russell R, Dundas R, Reynolds F. Long term backache after childbirth: prospective search for causative factors. BMJ 1996;312:1384–1388.
78. Macarthur AJ, MacArthur C, Weeks SK. Is epidural anesthesia in labor associated with chronic low back pain? A prospective cohort study. Anesth Analg 1997;85:1066–1070.
79. Howell CJ, Dean T, Lucking L, et al. Randomised study of long term outcome after epidural versus non-epidural analgesia during labour. BMJ 2002;325:357.
80. Jenkins JG. Some immediate serious complications of obstetric epidural analgesia and anaesthesia: a prospective study of 145,550 epidurals. Int J Obstet Anesth 2005;14: 37–42.
81. Auroy Y, Benhamou D, Bargues L, et al. Major complications of regional anesthesia in France: The SOS Regional Anesthesia Hotline Service. Anesthesiology 2002;1274–1280.
82. Paech MJ, Godkin R, Webster S. Complications of obstetric epidural analgesia and anaesthesia: a prospective analysis of 10,995 cases. Int J Obstet Anesth 1998;7:5–11.
83. Kopacz DJ, Allen HW. Accidental intravenous levobupivacaine. Anesth Analg 1999; 89:1027–1029.
84. Breslin DS, Martin G, Macleod DB, et al. Central nervous system toxicity following the administration of levobupivacaine for lumbar plexus block: a report of two cases. Reg Anesth Pain Med 2003;28:144–147.
85. Collier CB. Accidental subdural injection during attempted lumbar epidural block may present as a failed or inadequate block: radiographic evidence. Reg Anesth Pain Med 2004;29:45–51.
86. Scott DB, Tunstall ME. Serious complications associated with epidural/spinal blockade in obstetrics: a two-year prospective study. Int J Obstet Anesth 1995;133–139.
87. Holdcroft A, Gibberd FB, Hargrove RL, et al. Neurological complications associated with pregnancy. Br J Anaesth 1995;75:522–526.
88. Dar AQ, Robinson AP, Lyons G. Postpartum neurological symptoms following regional blockade: a prospective study with case controls. Int J Obstet Anesth 2002;11:85–90.
89. Wong CA, Scavone BM, Dugan S, et al. Incidence of postpartum lumbosacral spine and lower extremity nerve injuries. Obstet Gynecol 2003;101:279–288.
90. Reynolds F. Damage to the conus medullaris following spinal anaesthesia. Anaesthesia 2001;56:238–247.
91. Saifuddin A, Burnett SJ, White J. The variation of position of the conus medullaris in an adult population. A magnetic resonance imaging study. Spine 1998;23:1452–1456.
92. Van Gessel EF, Forster A, Gamulin Z. Continuous spinal anesthesia: where do spinal catheters go? Anesth Analg 1993;76:1004–1007.
92. Moen V, Dahlgren N, Irestedt L. Severe neurological complications after central neuraxial blockades in Sweden 1990–1999. Anesthesiology 2004;101:950–959.
94. Schneider M, Ettlin T, Kaufmann M, et al. Transient neurologic toxicity after hyperbaric subarachnoid anesthesia with 5% lidocaine. Anesth Analg 1993;76:1154–1157.
95. Zaric D, Christiansen C, Pace NL, et al. Transient neurologic symptoms after spinal anesthesia with lidocaine versus other local anesthetics: a systematic review of randomized, controlled trials. Anesth Analg 2005;100:1811–1816.

96. Pollock JE. Transient neurologic symptoms: etiology, risk factors, and management. Reg Anesth Pain Med 2002;27:581–586.
97. Aouad MT, Siddik SS, Jalbout MI, et al. Does pregnancy protect against intrathecal lidocaine-induced transient neurologic symptoms? Anesth Analg 2001;92:401–404.
98. Wong CA, Slavenas P. The incidence of transient radicular irritation after spinal anesthesia in obstetric patients. Reg Anesth Pain Med 1999;24:55–58.
99. Freedman JM, Li DK, Drasner K, et al. Transient neurologic symptoms after spinal anesthesia: an epidemiologic study of 1,863 patients. Anesthesiology 1998;89:633–641.
100. Schneider MC, Birnbach DJ. Lidocaine neurotoxicity in the obstetric patient: is the water safe? Anesth Analg 2001;92:287–290.
101. De Jong RH. The spinal inquisition: heresy of neurotaxonomy. Anesthesiology 1999;90: 318–319.
102. Auroy Y, Narchi P, Messiah A, et al. Serious complications related to regional anesthesia: results of a prospective survey in France. Anesthesiology 1997;87:479–486.
103. Rigler ML, Drasner K, Krejcie TC, et al. Cauda equina syndrome after continuous spinal anesthesia. Anesth Analg 1991;72:275–281.
104. Loo CC, Irestedt L. Cauda equina syndrome after spinal anaesthesia with hyperbaric 5% lignocaine: a review of six cases of cauda equina syndrome reported to the Swedish Pharmaceutical Insurance 1993–1997. Acta Anaesthesiol Scand 1999;43:371–379.
105. Scott DB, Hibbard BM. Serious non-fatal complications associated with extradural block in obstetric practice. Br J Anaesth 1990;64:537–541.
106. Loo CC, Dahlgren G, Irestedt L. Neurological complications in obstetric regional anaesthesia. Int J Obstet Anesth 2000;9:99–124.
107. Wang LP, Hauerberg J, Schmidt JF. Incidence of spinal epidural abscess after epidural analgesia: a national 1-year survey. Anesthesiology 1999;91:1928–1936.
108. Szkup P, Stoneham G. Case report: spontaneous spinal epidural haematoma during pregnancy: case report and review of the literature. Br J Radiol 2004;77:881–884.
109. Abramovitz S, Beilin Y. Thrombocytopenia, low molecular weight heparin, and obstetric anesthesia. Anesthesiol Clin North Am 2003;21:99–109.
110. Vandermeulen EP, Van Aken H, Vermylen J. Anticoagulants and spinal-epidural anesthesia. Anesth Analg 1994;79:1165–1177.
111. Beilin Y, Bodian CA, Haddad EM, et al. Practice patterns of anesthesiologists regarding situations in obstetric anesthesia where clinical management is controversial. Anesth Analg 1996;83:735–741.
112. Horlocker TT, Wedel DJ, Benzon H, et al. Regional anesthesia in the anticoagulated patient: defining the risks. Reg Anesth Pain Med 2004;29:1–16.
113. Yildirim GB, Colakoglu S, Atakan TY, et al. Intracranial subdural hematoma after spinal anesthesia. Int J Obstet Anesth 2005;14:159–162.
114. Ayorinde BT, Mushambi MC. Extradural haematoma in a patient following manual removal of the placenta under spinal anaesthesia: was the spinal to blame? Int J Obstet Anesth 2002;11:216–218.
115. Eggert SM, Eggers KA. Subarachnoid haemorrhage following spinal anaesthesia in an obstetric patient. Br J Anaesth 2001;86:442–444.
116. Donaldson JO. Neurology of Pregnancy. 2nd ed. Philadelphia: WB Saunders; 1989.
117. Reynolds F. Maternal sequelae of childbirth. Br J Anaesth 1995;75:515–517.
118. Ong BY, Cohen MM, Esmail A, et al. Paresthesias and motor dysfunction after labour and delivery. Anesth Analg 1987;66:18–22.
119. Liu EH, Sia AT. Rates of caesarean section and instrumental vaginal delivery in nulliparous women after low concentration epidural infusions or opioid analgesia: systematic review. BMJ 2004;328:1410.
120. Leighton BL, Halpern SH. The effects of epidural analgesia on labor, maternal, and neonatal outcomes: a systematic review. Am J Obstet Gynecol 2002;186:S69–S77.
121. Zhang J, Klebanoff MA, DerSimonian R. Epidural analgesia in association with duration of labor and mode of delivery: a quantitative review. Am J Obstet Gynecol 1999;180: 970–977.
122. Holloway J, Seed PT, O'Sullivan G, et al. Paraesthesiae and nerve damage following combined spinal epidural and spinal anaesthesia: a pilot survey. Int J Obstet Anesth 2000;9:151–155.
123. Littleford J. Effects on the fetus and newborn of maternal analgesia and anesthesia: a review. Can J Anaesth 2004;51:586–609.

124. Rosen MA. Paracervical block for labor analgesia: a brief historic review. Am J Obstet Gynecol 2002;186:S127–S130.
125. Manninen T, Aantaa R, Salonen M, et al. A comparison of the hemodynamic effects of paracervical block and epidural anesthesia for labor analgesia. Acta Anaesthesiol Scand 2000;44:441–445.
126. Chestnut DH. Alternative regional anesthetic techniques: paracervical block, lumbar sympathetic block, pudendal nerve block and perineal infiltration. In: Chestnut DH, ed. Obstetric Anesthesia. Philadelphia: Mosby; 2004:387–396.
127. White SM, Baldwin TJ. Consent for anaesthesia. Anaesthesia 2003;58:760–774.
128. Smedstad KG, Beilby W. Informed consent for epidural analgesia in labour. Can J Anaesth 2000;47:1055–1059.
129. Jenkins K, Baker AB. Consent and anaesthetic risk. Anaesthesia 2003;58:962–984.
130. Jackson A, Henry R, Avery N, et al. Informed consent for labouring epidurals: what labouring women want to know. Can J Anaesth 2000;47:1068–1073.
131. Hawkins, JL. Maternal morbidity and mortality: anesthetic causes. Can J Anaesth 2002; 49(6):R6.
132. Barnardo PD, Jenkins JG. Failed tracheal intubation in obstetrics: a 6-year review in a UK region. Anaesthesia 2000;55:685–694.
133. Practice guidelines for management of the difficult airway: an updated report by the American Society of Anesthesiologists Task Force on Management of the Difficult Airway. Anesthesiology 2003;98:1269–1277.
134. Lertakyamanee J, Chinachoti T, Tritrakarn T, et al. Comparison of general and regional anesthesia for cesarean section: success rate, blood loss and satisfaction from a randomized trial. J Med Assoc Thai 1999;82:672–680.
135. Hager RM, Daltveit AK, Hofoss D, et al. Complications of cesarean deliveries: rates and risk factors. Am J Obstet Gynecol 2004;190:428–434.
136. Rodgers A, Walker N, Schug S, et al. Reduction of postoperative mortality and morbidity with epidural or spinal anaesthesia: results from overview of randomised trials. BMJ 2000;321:1493.
137. Peel WJ. A survey of the anaesthetic management of patients presenting for caesarean section with 'high-risk' obstetric conditions. Int J Obstet Anesth 1996;5:219–220.
138. Bonner SM, Haynes SR, Ryall D. The anaesthetic management of Caesarean section for placenta praevia: a questionnaire survey. Anaesthesia 1995;50:992–994.
139. Hong JY, Jee YS, Yoon HJ, et al. Comparison of general and epidural anesthesia in elective cesarean section for placenta previa totalis: maternal hemodynamics, blood loss and neonatal outcome. Int J Obstet Anesth 2003;12:12–16.
140. Frederiksen MC, Glassenberg R, Stika CS. Placenta previa: a 22-year analysis. Am J Obstet Gynecol 1999;180:1432–1437.
141. Parekh N, Husaini SW, Russell IF. Caesarean section for placenta praevia: a retrospective study of anaesthetic management. Br J Anaesth 2000;84:725–730.

# 15 Complications of Catheter Techniques

Per H. Rosenberg

## Catheter Materials and Characteristics

Catheters for prolongation of nerve blocks were first used in the 1940s, when ureteral lacquered silk catheters were applied in continuous caudal (sacral) analgesia,[1,2] continuous subarachnoid block,[3] and continuous lumbar epidural block.[4] Thereafter, there has been a steady development in plastic material technology and polyethylene and polyvinyl catheters have been followed by presently used nylon (polyamide), polyurethane, and Teflon (tetrafluoroethylene) catheters. Still today, there seems to be no universally ideal catheter material, and the material, design, and diameter of regional anesthesia and analgesia catheters are chosen according to the specific requirements associated with the various blocks. Overall, the catheter material is such that in a case of resistance or obstruction, the catheter must not break.[5] For example, an epidural catheter should advance into and through the needle rather than flex excessively when resistance is encountered, and yet still bend and deflect off tissue.[6] The deflection property has been solved in some of the epidural catheters by a "soft" and flexible steel coil extension of the tip (e.g., Arrow Flextip®). An intrathecal catheter should be soft, relatively thin, and resistant to kinking. However, a brachial plexus catheter has to be relatively stiff and blunt. In addition to acceptable tissue compatibility, the catheter must also withstand the destructive (solubilizing) action of the neurolytic drug solutions administered through the catheters, such as 6%–10% phenol or 100% ethanol.

Although not as critical as the design of the distal tip of a catheter, the problems of developing suitable and safe adapters for syringes and pumps have not yet been completely solved. Despite special adapter designs that resist high pressures and prevent the catheter tip from collapsing, untight locking is still a practical problem.[7]

## Epidural Catheters

### *Trauma and Malposition of Catheter*

Typical trauma caused by the introduction of epidural catheters is rupture of epidural veins. Bloody taps are, in fact, quite common, in particular in obstetric patients, when the epidural veins are extended. Inadvertent cannulation of an epidural vein has been reported in 1.3%–15.7% of parturients[8,9], and this seems to occur more often when the patient is in the sitting position.[9] An inadvertent cannulation may result in systemic toxicity of local anaesthetics,[10] inadequate pain relief,[11] or epidural hematoma with neurologic complications.[12] It seems possible to reduce the risk of epidural vein cannulation by the catheter by injecting fluid (e.g., saline) before and during the catheterization,[13,14] or by using a catheter with a flexible tip.[15]

Epidural catheter tips have three different basic designs. One has an open tip (i.e., a single orifice), another a bullet-formed tip with several (usually three) orifices near the tip, and a third having an open tip behind a protruding flexible wire coil. The risks related to the use of the multiorifice epidural catheter have received considerable attention in the light of reports of local anesthetic toxicity caused by malpositioning of the catheter in a blood vessel.[10,16,17] The different orifices may be in different anatomic spaces at the same time. For example, a subdural or subarachnoid catheterization may have occurred, leaving a proximal orifice outside, i.e., in the epidural space. Similarly, the distal orifice may be in an epidural vein and the two proximal ones in the epidural space.[18] The study by Beck and coworkers[18] revealed that, in many instances, all available tests for exclusion of an intravascular catheter were insufficient; the aspiration test for blood and injecting a test dose of local anesthetic solution containing epinephrine, therefore, do not seem to be reliable when multiorifice catheters are used. The abandonment of multiorifice epidural catheters from clinical use has been advocated[18,19] because their advantages have not been demonstrated, but potential, as well as real, dangers have been shown.

The catheter with the flexible protrusion at the tip (Arrow Flextip®) has proven useful for safe placement of the catheter, but problems have been encountered at the removal of the catheter. Uncoiling of the reinforced wire has occasionally been encountered, and a few of these cases have been reported.[20,21] Fortunately, the uncoiled wires have not broken. With this particular catheter (fine stainless-steel wire reinforcement lining the polyvinyl chloride tubing), it is possible to confirm the catheter tip location (placement) with low current electrical stimulation relatively simply via an attached electrocardiogram adapter at the connector of the catheter.[22] By observing the motor response (e.g., truncal or limb movement) and varying the stimulation current, it may be possible to detect both subarachnoid placement and intravascular placement of the epidural catheter.[23] However, the sensitivity and specificity of this electrical stimulation test (so-called Tsui test) for the detection of a malpositioned epidural catheter has not been evaluated.

There are reports of so-called secondary vessel migration[24–27] or dural perforation.[28–30] Epidural catheters have been shown to move 1–2cm inward or outward during the period of epidural therapy independent of whether the catheter had been tunneled or fixed to the skin by suture.[31]

In any case, to reduce the risk of inadvertent subarachnoid or intravascular injection through an epidural catheter, a test dose should be injected before starting the epidural anesthetic or analgesic therapy. To detect an inadvertent subarachnoid injection, the dose of the local anesthetic should be such that it rapidly produces demonstrable sensory and motor block. The detection of an intravascular injection has relied on the presence of a small amount (5–15μg) of epinephrine in the local anesthetic solution.[32,33] Recommended epidural test dose drugs include lidocaine (60–100mg), mepivacaine (60–100mg), and bupivacaine (10–15mg).[32] However, the validity of epinephrine in the test dose during labor epidural analgesia has been questioned because aspiration alone detects almost all inadvertent intravascular catheters.[34] If an epinephrine-containing epidural test dose is used in labor analgesia, excellent specificity and good sensitivity of the test could be achieved by recording beat-to-beat maternal heart rate by cardiotocography.[35] Despite a negative result of the initial epidural test dose, each additional epidural dosing (top-up), usually without epinephrine, should be considered a test dose, i.e., the patient needs to be observed and examined for symptoms of local anesthetic toxicity or unexpectedly rapid reestablishment of the motor block.

Other possible malpositions of epidural catheters do not usually result in life-threatening or other serious complications. Such positions include transforaminal escape,[36] curling of the catheter to the lateral and anterior side of the dural "tube,"[36,37] and interligament or intramuscular placement. These malpositions may lead to inadequate analgesia or none, and in the first two instances even to unilateral analgesia. The catheter may, in rare instances, enter the subdural space unnoticed.[38–40] Although the space between the dura and the arachnoid mater membranes is a potential space, injection of local anesthetic into this space may spread unpredictably; for example, in the study by Boys and Norman,[41] 40 mg of bupivacaine (8 mL of bupivacaine 5 mg/mL) injected subdurally resulted in an analgesic dermatomal spread from L2 to C7.

Most of the malpositions of the epidural catheter can be avoided by a careful technique, which includes accurate identification of the epidural space before threading the catheter and advancing the catheter, with no forceful movement, not more than 3–4 cm into the epidural space.

## *Knotting and Breaking of Catheters*

Catheters may be deflected by connective tissue bands, blood vessels or nerve roots that lie in the path, curling up or doubling back after passing only a short distance. In the study by Blanco and coworkers,[42] 48% of easily advanced catheters intended to be inserted from the lumbar to the thoracic level remained at the L4-5 level (circles, figure-of-eight, wavy-line form; Figure 15-1). Approaching the epidural space at an angle of 120–135 degrees may facilitate entry and ascent[43]; however, this approach may present a greater risk of vascular puncture[36] and a risk that the needle may not follow the aimed route between the skin and the epidural space.[44] There are a few cases in the literature of catheter knots occurring on caudally placed catheters[45,46] and on lumbar epidurally placed catheters.[47–49] A knotted catheter can usually be removed by applying a firm, steady pull.[47,48] The knot presumably becomes tighter and smaller,

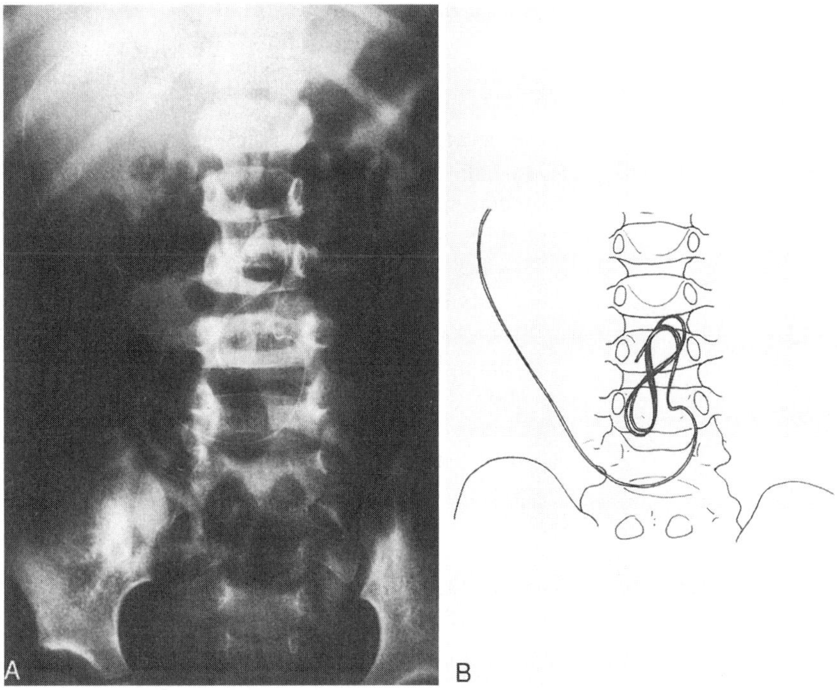


**FIGURE 15-1.** Radiograph **(A)** and corresponding drawing **(B)** of an epidural catheter (19-gauge multiorifice catheter) introduced at L4-5 level with the intention of advancing it to the thoracic level. The catheter has formed a figure-of-eight. (From Blanco et al.[42] Reprinted with permission from Lippincott Williams & Wilkins.)

approaching the size of the normal catheter. It may be advisable to test the tensile strength of an unused catheter before pulling a knotted catheter out and to let the anesthetic effect wear off before removal attempt, so that nerve root involvement in the knot can be detected.[47] Surgical removal of the catheter may occasionally be indicated, such as when the catheter makes a sling and a knot.[50]

Shearing of the catheter near the needle tip may occur when the catheter is withdrawn with the needle still in place. In a retrospective series of 26,490 lumbar epidural analgesic blocks via catheter, 12 cases of broken or sheared off catheter were found (4.5 per 10,000 cases).[51] This risk has been reduced by manufacturing Tuohy needles with a blunt upper edge of the orifice. In case of a break of the catheter just below the skin, a small incision is made under local anesthetic infiltration, and the distal piece is grasped (e.g., with a hemostat) and is pulled out. Deep breaks within the spinal canal should as a rule be left where they are. A catheter piece will be walled off by fibrous tissue after a few weeks, remaining immured and innocuous within the epidural space.[36] Very rarely, persistent symptoms, or other reasons may lead to search for the foreign body by computed tomography scan and roentgenograms, and exploratory laminectomy.[52]

It is unlikely that normally positioned epidural catheters would break during removal. It has been shown that catheters removed with the patient in the sitting position requires a force more than 2.5 times greater than that required in the lateral position.[53] Even in the sitting position, the margin of safety with respect to catheter breakage during removal seems to be quite high.[53] Gripping an epidural catheter with a hemostat during removal might result in accidental breakage of the catheter.[54] Also, the reinforced Arrow catheter may break and it has been shown that the fracture may occur at the traction site rather than at the fixed site.[55]

### *Epidural Hematoma*

Epidural needles or catheters can cause trauma to epidural veins, but in the presence of normal hemostatic mechanisms, the bleeding stops spontaneously. The incidence of bloody tap from epidural needle or catheter puncture is 1%–10%[36,56] and as high as 18% in pregnant patients.[13] In their review of 46 cases of spinal hematoma after epidural techniques, Vandermeulen and coworkers[57] note that in 32 cases a catheter had been used. Interestingly, in 15 of the 32 epidural catheter cases, spinal bleeding occurred immediately after the removal of the catheter, with therapeutic plasma levels of heparin still in place. The majority of the patients (62%) underwent decompression laminectomies with evacuation of the hematoma. In the patients who made good or partial recovery of neurologic function, surgery was performed within 8 hours of the development of paraplegia. If surgery is delayed, complete paralysis may ensue.[58,59]

Patients fully anticoagulated with a continuous heparin infusion should have the infusion discontinued 2–4 hours before catheter removal.[60] Heparinization should not be initiated for at least an hour after catheter placement.[61] Patients receiving antiplatelet medication who will undergo subsequent heparinization seem to be at risk for spinal hematoma and should be followed closely.[62] The timing of epidural catheter removal in an anticoagulated patient is also important. The present rule is to remove an indwelling catheter in a patient receiving intravenous or subcutaneous (low-molecular-weight) heparin under the same conditions in which the placement is considered safe. It is therefore performed 10–12 hours after the last dose of heparin, and anticoagulation should not be reinstituted for at least 2 hours after catheter removal.[60] Epidural anesthesia can be safely performed in a patient receiving antiplatelet therapy with acetylsalicylic acid (aspirin)[60] and with the modern antiplatelet drugs (e.g., clopidogrel, ximelagatran); precautions regarding timing should be taken according to the pharmacokinetics of each individual drug.

### *Epidural Abscess and Infection*

Epidural abscess is a rare complication that can result in permanent neurologic deficit. It has been reported after epidural anesthesia[36,63] and during the use of indwelling epidural catheters for chronic pain treatment.[64] The review by Kee and coworkers[63] describes 16 cases of epidural catheter-related abscesses published between 1974 and 1991. A disproportionate number of cases had involved thoracic catheters. The causative organism had been isolated in 11 cases; *Staphylococcus aureus* was identified in nine and *S. epidermidis* in two. Despite positive bacterial culture (*S. aureus* and *S. epidermidis*) from four catheter tips after 5 days of postoperative epidural treatment in 200 patients, none of the patients had signs and symptoms of skin or epidural infection.[65] The positive bacterial cultures probably resulted from skin contamination on removal of the catheters. A few cases of fistula formation after epidural catheterization for postoperative pain treatment in surgical patients have been reported.[66,67]

In patients with infectious skin wounds or abscesses, or septicemia, epidural catheterization has been considered relatively contraindicated.[68] This concept has been questioned based on results from epidural catheterization in 69 patients with localized skin infections.[69] In this series, a single case of spondylitis was the only serious complication, but this seemed not to be related to the epidural technique. On 12 occasions, the catheter was removed because of local infection in the skin at the puncture site. These beneficial results from one particular hospital should not be regarded as a signal allowing less vigilance in the maintenance of epidural catheters.[70] The risk of epidural infections is still there, which is indicated by several published case reports during the past few years.[71–73] The incidence of catheter-related epidural abscess is difficult to assess accurately. Not all epidural abscesses are caused by needle punctures or catheter contamination. Interestingly, epidural abscesses unrelated to anesthesia or analgesia have been reported with an incidence as high as 0.2–1.2 per 10,000 hospital admissions.[74]

Signs and symptoms of epidural abscess may be similar to those of epidural hematoma, except that the patient is febrile. Diagnosis is best made by magnetic resonance imaging, although computed tomography would be necessary if the patient has an implanted metal (other than titanium) port.[75]

The continuous successful use of anesthesia or analgesia via the epidural route requires constant alertness for sterile technique during puncture and catheter insertion, use of bacterial filters, aseptic maintenance of catheter and adapter, and regular observation of possible infectious symptoms. If a catheter is to be kept longer than 5–7 days, tunneling under the skin is a preventive measure against catheter contamination and infections. Intraluminal spread of bacterial infection may also be prevented by filling the catheter with, for example, bupivacaine 5 mg/mL, which has antimicrobial action.[76] The antimicrobial effect has been found much weaker with ropivacaine.[77] This protective action is more apparent than real and, therefore, omission of a bacterial filter in the epidural catheter cannot be recommended.

### *Headache and Backache*

Postdural puncture headache (PDPH) may result from accidental dural puncture by the needle or by the catheter (see also the section Trauma and Malposition of Catheter, above). As shown from the anesthesia records of 9000 obstetric patients receiving epidural analgesia,[78] 19 epidural catheter punctures (migrations) of dura mater occurred, resulting in PDPH in six of these patients (31.6%). In the same survey, it was observed that 99 epidural needle punctures of dura mater caused 48 cases of PDPH (48.5%). In contrast, when an epidural catheter (20 gauge) has been used for continuous spinal anesthesia, the incidence of PDPH has been surprisingly low, in the range of 1%.[79,80]

In a series of 26,490 lumbar epidural analgesic catheters in obstetrics, only two of the six patients with identified inadvertent catheter-induced dural puncture developed PDPH.[51] Because the subarachnoid administration is not always evident or identified after the initial epidural test dose or therapeutic bolus dose, an epidural test dose (either with local anesthetic with epinephrine, or local anesthetic alone) should be given before the subsequent top-up.[81] From a practical point of view, the amount of local anesthetic in an epidural top-up dose for labor analgesia could be similar to that in an adequate test dose.[82]

Some anesthesiologists perform a prophylactic epidural blood patch when the epidural needle or catheter has punctured dura mater,[75,83] despite the fact that this is associated with a certain degree of morbidity (backache nerve root irritation).[84,85] A recent study showed no effect on the incidence of PDPH of the prophylactic epidural blood patch in obstetric patients.[86]

The incidence of backache after a successful and atraumatic epidural block (with or without catheter) does not seem to be higher than that in a normal surgical population receiving general anesthesia.[36] However, in parturients, the incidence of backache is higher, regardless of whether they received anesthesia or not.[68]

### *Neurologic Injury*

Most of the rare neurologic complications developing at placement or during the use of epidural analgesia are caused by traumatic puncture, bleeding, or infection.

The risk of neurologic damage related to lumbar epidural catheter placement or infusion seems to be very low,[87,88] as it is when the catheter is placed under general anesthesia.[89] However, several case reports describe neural injury when thoracic epidural catheters have been placed under general anesthesia.[90–92] This has created a vivid, and even emotional, discussion among regional anesthesiologists but, overall, most authorities recommend that thoracic epidural puncture and catheterization in adults must not be performed while the patient is under heavy sedation or general anesthesia.[93–95]

Rare cases of either cutaneous cerebrospinal fluid (CSF)-leaking fistula after dural perforation by the epidural catheter[96] and a cutaneous epidural fistula (probably related to infection)[67] have been reported.

### *Wrong Solution*

Accidental injection of the wrong drug into epidural catheters may occur. There are surprisingly numerous cases of epidural injections of potassium chloride (KCl).[36,97,98] Typically, injection of KCl results in severe pain in the lower part of the body, and can be relieved by the administration of an epidural steroid.[98]

The intravenous thiopental solution has a high pH (pH 10–11) and is irritating to tissues. It has also been erroneously injected into an epidural catheter and treated as above, with epidural administration of methylprednisolone.[99]

A questionnaire survey in the United Kingdom among obstetric anesthesiologists revealed that drugs that erroneously have been administered into the epidural catheter include, e.g., meperidine instead of alfentanil or fentanyl, metronidazole instead of saline, water instead of saline, ephedrine instead of bupivacaine.[100] Among the neuromuscular blocking agents, succinylcholine and vecuronium[101] and pancuronium[102] have been accidentally administered epidurally.

The list of anecdotal reports of erroneous epidural drug administrations includes in addition bicarbonate, Ringer's solution, midazolam, nicardipine, pentazocine, and mixtures of atropine and neostigmine. As long as the drug solutions do not irritate the tissues and the incident is immediately detected, no permanent harm usually develops. These patients need close observation and proper monitoring. It is obvious that greater vigilance and better labeling of drug vials and syringes as well as of the various infusion lines are needed to avoid this kind of accident.

### *Combined Spinal and Epidural Anesthesia*

In combined spinal-epidural (CSE) anesthesia, the epidural catheter and the spinal needle are placed either through separate vertebral interspaces, or in the same interspace by using the epidural needle as an introducer for the spinal needle

("needle-through-needle").[103] In the former double-segment technique, the epidural catheter is usually placed first, whereas in the latter single-segment technique, the intrathecal injection is performed before the epidural catheterization. In a modified single-segment technique, the spinal needle and the epidural needle are introduced next to each other; the epidural catheter is placed first followed by removal of the spinal needle stylet and the intrathecal injection for the spinal block.[104]

The risk of epidural catheter migration through the dural hole made by the spinal needle has been a matter of much discussion. In the 1980s, when regular Tuohy needles were used as part of the CSE technique, the risk of dural penetration through the spinal needle path in the dura was considered not to be greater than that in regular epidural catheterization, at least when the tip of the Tuohy needle was turned 180° before the epidural catheter was introduced.[105] However, in the study by Carter and coworkers,[106] when the Tuohy needle was not turned 180° before catheterization, inadvertent puncture of the dura with the catheter was found to occur in 3% of the cases.

Modern CSE sets include Tuohy-type epidural needles with an extra aperture in the curved tip of the needle ("back eye") for passing of the spinal needle. Thereby the risk of epidural catheter penetration through the dural hole made by the spinal needle is further diminished, and is practically eliminated. Another technical improvement for the general success of the "needle-through-needle" CSE technique is the built-in reliable locking devices to keep the spinal needle from moving during manipulation and injection.

The complications of the use of the epidural catheter in the CSE technique are essentially the same as in regular epidural anesthesia and analgesia. The only notable exception is the risk of unnoticed neural injury at the time of epidural catheter introduction in cases in which the spinal block has been introduced first by using a normal block dose. Because of the rapid development of the spinal block, the patient may not respond with a paresthesia reaction. In the techniques in which the epidural catheter has been introduced first, the incidence of paresthesias during epidural catheter introduction has been 10% in the "needle-through-needle" technique[107] and 6.5 % in the single-segment "side-by-side" needle technique.[104]

## Subarachnoid Catheters

### *Technical Problems and Complications*

Continuous spinal anesthesia was repopularized in the 1980s, with the development of microcatheters (29 and 32 gauge).[108] From the very beginning, and still today, the problems encountered with microcatheters have centered around technical difficulties in passing the thin catheter through a small needle. Coiling and kinking of the catheters, catheter breakage, and failure to aspirate were noted already in the initial trials. Built-in and removable stylets have been applied for the prevention of kinking and breakage.[109,110] The considerable failure rate for inserting the thin 32-gauge microcatheter experienced in our own department, 25%,[111,112] have been similar to those in other studies.[113] Literature on continuous spinal anesthesia using large-caliber equipment (epidural catheters) rarely makes any mention of unsuccessful lumbar puncture or catheter insertion. However, in three studies on continuous spinal anesthesia with 20-gauge catheters, unsuccessful catheterization occurred in 4.3%,[114] 3.2%,[79] and 1% of cases.[115]

A practical problem encountered with the 32-gauge polyurethane catheter with removable stylet, and occasionally with the 28-gauge nylon catheter, has been stretching during attempts to remove the catheter.[112,116] Catheter breakage during removal may occur.[108,112,116] If the break point is outside the skin or immediately below the surface, the distal part of the catheter may be retrieved after first repositioning the patient in a "curved back" position and carefully pulling the catheter hand or hemostat. As with sheared-off epidural catheter pieces, if the remnant is deeper below the skin, it is recommended to leave it as it is.

### *Hemorrhage*

The subarachnoid puncture with a needle and the insertion of a plastic catheter can cause damage to blood vessels and the nervous tissue. No serious bleeding complications (e.g., spinal hematoma) from continuous intrathecal catheters have been reported in the literature. However, a considerable number of erythrocytes were observed in the CSF of several patients who were given continuous spinal (intrathecal) anesthesia via a 22-gauge epidural catheter.[117] The erythrocyte count in this small patient population seemed to be independent of whether or not the patients had received low-molecular-weight heparin for thromboprophylaxis preoperatively (hip or knee arthroplasties), or intravenous heparin intraoperatively (vascular surgery). The amounts of erythrocytes (maximally $20 \times 10^9$/L), which result in macroscopically blood-tinged CSF, can easily be handled by arachnoid villi and, therefore, from a neuropathologic point of view the hemorrhage can be considered insignificant. No neurologic complications ensued in that particular patient population.[117] The finding of no significant complications attributable to the presence of erythrocytes in the CSF during continuous spinal anesthesia is substantiated by the results of a prospective study in which minor hemorrhage was observed in the puncture needle of the spinal catheter in 18 of 46 cases.[118] This particular study also indicates that preoperative antiplatelet nonsteroidal antiinflammatory drug therapy does not increase the risk of spinal hematoma associated with spinal or epidural anesthesia.

### *Infectious Complications*

Serious infectious complications associated with continuous spinal anesthesia have not been reported. In a study of 66 surgical patients in our own department, in which CSF was sampled at intervals of 24 hours, an excess of leukocytes was observed in the 24-hour sample of one patient.[117] The bacterial culture showed *S. epidermidis*. The patient was symptom free with no leukocytosis in the blood and was treated with intravenous antibiotics. The fact remains that the excess of leukocytes in the CSF would not have been detected in the symptom-free phase had repeat CSF sampling not been performed as scheduled. Standl and coworkers[119] reported one contaminated catheter tip (*S. epidermidis*) in 100 spinal catheters used for postoperative analgesia and removed after 24 hours.

Both of these cases probably represent contamination from normal skin bacterial flora; *S. epidermidis*, for example, is readily adherent to plastic material indwelling in the body. The presence of bupivacaine (3.75–5 mg/mL) inside the catheter may prevent microorganism growth to some extent.[76,77] Furthermore, a bacterial filter (diameter 0.22 µg) must always be used on the catheters.

### *Headache and Neurologic Complications*

The primary factor that has limited the use of continuous spinal anesthesia is the belief that the relatively large size of the puncture needle, as well as the use of epidural catheters as intrathecal catheters, requiring insertion through still larger needles, will result in a high incidence of PDPH. This contention is controversial, however (Table 15-1). In the particular study that clearly renewed interest in the use of the continuous spinal technique, there was only one case of PDPH among 117 surgical patients who received a 20-gauge intrathecal catheter through an 18-gauge needle.[79] The reason for this low incidence of PDPH was postulated to be an inflammatory reaction in the dura mater and the arachnoid surrounding the puncture site, which, as a result of edema and fibrinous exudate, would seal the hole in the dura after catheter removal. With

TABLE 15-1. Number of Subarachnoid Catheterization Failures and PDPHs in Various Study Materials During 1991–1996

| Patients (no.) | Age (y) | Catheter size (gauge) | Difficult insertion | PDPHs (no.) | Reference |
|---|---|---|---|---|---|
| 45 | >75 | 20 | NA* | 0 | 120 |
| 20 | 16–43 | 32 | 5 | 0 | 121 |
| 226 | 19–94 | 20–21 | NA* | 0 | 122 |
| 20 | 55–78 | 24 | 1 | 1 | 107 |
| 20 | 61–80 | 32 | 6 | 0 | 97 |
| 20 | 66–86 | 22 | 1 | 0 | 86 |
| 30 | 5178 | 28 | 2 | 1 | 123 |
| 10 | <5 | 28 | NA* | 0† | 98 |
| 100 | 22–86 | 28 | 0 | 1 | 96 |
| 30 | >70 | 20 | NA* | 0 | 124 |

*Not reported.
†Leakage of CSF along the catheter in three children.

the use of the 32-gauge microcatheter, the incidence of PDPH in the first report was 4%.[108] In elderly patients, the incidence of PDPH associated with the 32-gauge spinal catheter has been zero.[111,112] Microcatheters for continuous spinal anesthesia have also been used in children.[125] Extravasation was noticed when the 28-gauge catheter was left in situ for 24 hours in some of the pediatric patients. Catheters smaller than 27 gauge are no longer approved by the regulatory agencies of various countries (others have released warnings), which seems to be the logical reason why continuous spinal techniques are rarely used in children nowadays. The reason for withdrawal of microcatheters (smaller than 27 gauge) for spinal anesthesia from the North American market was the report of at least 14 cases of cauda equina syndrome after continuous spinal anesthesia to the Food and Drug Administration (FDA) in the beginning of 1990s. An official Safety Alert was issued by the FDA in May 1992. However, in most European countries, 28-gauge, but not 32-gauge, catheters are in routine use today. The occurrence of the above-mentioned cauda equina syndromes is not, obviously, caused by the catheter per se, but indirectly so that the thin catheter easily turns into the caudal direction[126] and an injected hyperbaric local anesthetic solution becomes pooled in the vicinity of the roots of the cauda equina, producing direct local anesthetic tissue toxicity.[127,128] Therefore, when small-bore catheters are used for continuous spinal anesthesia, the catheters should not be advanced more than 3–4 cm into the subarachnoid space, and hyperbaric local anesthetic solution should be considered contraindicated.

Better and predictable positioning of the tip of the intrathecal catheter can be achieved by using directional puncture needles (Tuohy, Sprotte).[129]

The problem of predicting the positioning of the catheter tip in the intrathecal space, and in order to eliminate leakage of CSF through the puncture hole in the dura, around the inserted catheter, the spinal catheter (22 or 24 gauge) may be introduced over the spinal needle (27 or 29 gauge).[129] Despite the relatively ingenious technical approach, this catheter set has turned out to be technically rather difficult to handle.[130]

## Brachial Plexus Catheters

### *Technical Complications*

Difficulty in insertion of a brachial plexus catheter is typically associated with multiple puncture attempts, which may lead to tissue trauma, bleeding, and infection. Even in the perivascular block techniques, accidental puncture of a blood vessel by the needle is not uncommon, but accidental intravascular catheter insertion seems to be rare. We, however, encountered such a complication during insertion of an interscalene brachial plexus catheter (outer diameter 0.85 mm). The misplacement of the catheter into the vertebral artery was verified radiographically (Figure 15-2).[131]

Blood vessel puncture is a common risk in all the various techniques, but otherwise, each of the various approaches (more than 20) of the brachial plexus block has its own more or less specific risks of puncture complications.[132] Typically, the supraclavicular approaches carry the risk of pleural puncture. In recent years, ultrasound guidance of the block performance has become popular in some centers[133,134] and the experts claim that the needles can be directed with great accuracy. Whereas ultrasound guidance has not been found helpful in directing the insertion of the catheter, the closeness of the tip of a peripheral nerve catheter to the plexus can be verified by introducing a metal wire into the catheter for nerve stimulation.[135]

Technical failures during the continuous block therapy may occur. Thus, leakage of the local anesthetic solution to the skin occurs relatively often, in particular in the interscalene approaches in which the distance from the tip to skin is narrow, and the hole made by the introducer cannula is large. Catheters may become dislodged (slide out) because of insufficient fixation and patient mobilization activities.[136]

A case report describes knotting of an axillary brachial plexus catheter which was revealed at removal 3 days after insertion.[137]

### *Neurologic Complications*

Diaphragmatic paralysis caused by phrenic nerve block occurs always in association with a successful interscalene brachial plexus block,[138,139] and often associated with other supraclavicular approaches to the brachial plexus.[132,140] In continuous interscalene brachial plexus analgesia blocks, the diaphragmatic motility is depressed as long as the local anesthetic infusion is continuous.[141] Despite the fact that deterioration in spirometric parameters can be shown (Table 15-2), the patient rarely experiences any subjective symptoms of respiratory insufficiency. Obviously, bilateral interscalene

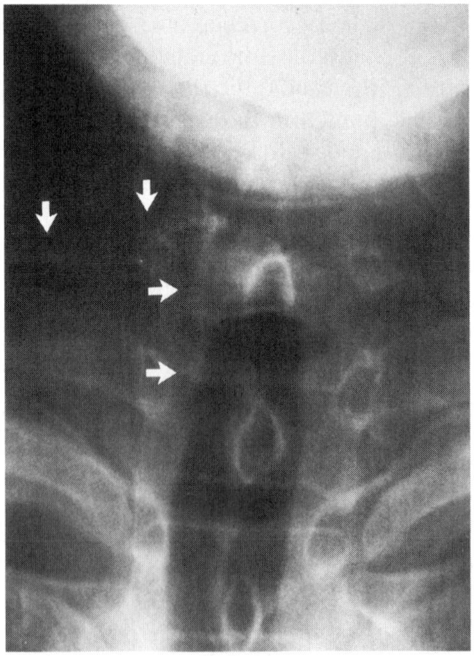

**FIGURE 15-2.** Radiograph of an interscalene brachial plexus catheter (outer diameter 0.85 mm) inadvertently placed in the vertebral artery. The white arrows indicate the position of the catheter filled with contrast medium. A 90-degree bend of the catheter has occurred. (From Tuominen et al.[131] Reprinted with permission from Lippincott Williams & Wilkins.)

TABLE 15-2. Changes in Ipsilateral Diaphragmatic Motion*

| | Interval | |
|---|---|---|
| | 3h | 24h |
| Diaphragmatic motion (%) | 12 ± 8 | 48 ± 30 |
| FVC (%) | 58 ± 23 | 74 ± 29 |
| $FEV_1$ (%) | 59 ± 22 | 76 ± 30 |

*Source:* Modified from Pere et al.[139]
Data are mean ± SD.
*As measured from a double-exposure chest radiograph (percentage from the preoperative value), and in forced vital capacity (FVC) and forced expiratory volume in one second ($FEV_1$) (percentage of predicted normal value) after continuous interscalene brachial plexus block with bupivacaine.

blocks are not recommended. In addition to a 100% incidence of phrenic block, stellate ganglion block (approximately 17%) and hoarseness (recurrent laryngeal nerve block, approximately 35%) have been observed at the end of 24-hour interscalene infusion of bupivacaine 2.5 mg/mL.[136]

Deterioration of hearing on the ipsilateral side has also been shown in some patients during continuous interscalene infusions of bupivacaine.[142] Reversible hearing impairment was recorded in four of 20 surgical patients who received an initial interscalene brachial plexus block for surgery with bupivacaine 7.5 mg/mL, followed by a continuous infusion of bupivacaine 2.5 mg/mL for 24 hours. Although this side effect was not accompanied by signs of Horner's syndrome, it was assumed that hearing impairment was related to the sympathetic block at the ear region.

Rare neurologic complications also include accidental catheterization of the epidural space during attempt to perform an interscalene brachial plexus block,[143] and the development of acute transient neurologic symptoms[120] or persistent neurologic deficit of the upper extremity after the placement of an interscalene brachial plexus catheter for postoperative pain relief.[121]

### *Infectious Complications*

Infectious problems during continuous brachial plexus analgesia are rare, probably because the duration of the treatment usually does not last more than a few days. Furthermore, as long as bupivacaine is used for the infusions, some protection against bacterial growth is provided by this particular local anesthetic.[76,77] In a series of continuous axillary brachial plexus block, of the 11 catheter tips cultured, there were three positive cultures with *S. aureus*, coagulase-negative staphylococcus, *Pseudomonas maltophilia*, and group B streptococcus.[122] The duration of the indwelling catheters was 3.6 days for negative cultures and 8.6 days for positive cultures, on average. No specific antibiotic treatment was given because evidence of local or systemic infection was absent.

Localized infection (*S. aureus*) terminated a 118-day implanted axillary brachial plexus block catheterization and self-administration of local anesthetic in a patient with sympathetically maintained pain of the upper extremity.[123]

## Intercostal, Paravertebral, and Interpleural Catheters

Continuous techniques for intercostal and paravertebral block are used relatively rarely because in most cases where such continuous technique might be used, the analgesic technique of choice is epidural analgesia. One of the first described continuous intercostal techniques consisted of insertion of six plastic cannulas in separate intercostal spaces with the patient under light general anesthesia.[124] There was one case of pneumothorax among 140 patients, which seems to be in accord with the incidence of pneumothorax from the needle puncture in intercostal block (i.e., pneumothorax/intercostal puncture).[144,145] In the most proximal part of the intercostal space, the local anesthetic solution can easily spread over to the next 1–2 interspaces[146,147] and, therefore, it may suffice to place only one catheter even when several adjacent ribs are fractured and painful. For practical reasons, a standard (multiple sideholes) may be placed via a Tuohy needle. The technique is not problem-free, because in the volunteer study by Crossley and Hosie[147] three of the 10 catheterizations failed and one subject developed temporary neuritis within the nerve distribution of the intercostal nerve.

The correct positioning of percutaneously placed intercostal catheters may be difficult to predict.[148] The measurement of intercostal space pressure via the catheter may be helpful in confirming the position of the catheter tip in the intercostal space, at least when compared with the negative pressure in the interpleural space.[149] Most accurate positioning of the intercostal catheter can be achieved by placing the catheter either along the intercostal nerves posteriorly[150] or extrapleurally in the paravertebral space[151] under visual control, before the thoracotomy wound is closed. There is a report of breakage of such a catheter during its removal, probably as the result of an unintentionally tight suture.[150]

Pneumothorax is a possible complication of cannulation and catheterization of the paravertebral space. Cannulation pneumothoraces have been reported in 0.26%[152] and 0.5%.[153] Two recent studies on the use of continuous thoracic paravertebral analgesia[154,155] reported no pleural punctures, and excellent postoperative analgesia. Cannulation of a vein in the paravertebral space by the epidural catheter has been reported,[156] and recannulation in the same paravertebral space seems to be successful.

The interpleural regional analgesia technique became popular in the late 1980s and was used for pain relief after surgery and trauma in the thoracic region.[157] Pneumothorax was reported in various studies, at a frequency of about 2%, on average. The study by Symreng and coworkers[158] deserves special attention because it points out the frequently occurring damage to the lung tissue by the puncture and the catheter insertion. In their study, an interpleural catheter was placed in 21 anesthetized patients immediately before thoracotomy. When the thorax was opened, three of the catheter tips were found to be outside the pleura, and seven of the tips were within the lung tissue. Eight of the patients had a hole in the lung tissue and three had pneumothorax, two of which were under tension. This study is an important reminder of the fact that such catheters must not be placed just preoperatively in a patient receiving general anesthesia with positive-pressure ventilation.

A few cases of pleural effusion[157,159] have been reported. There is one case of interpleural catheter breakage during the attempt to remove the intraoperatively placed catheter.[160] The sequestered piece of the catheter was left in place in this patient who had undergone thoracotomy for inoperable lung cancer. Phrenic nerve paresis may occur in rare instances.[161] The concurrent sympathetic block sometimes produces Horner's syndrome, particularly when the patient is positioned with a head-down tilt.[162] This cranial sympathetic blockade may be beneficial in the attenuation of chronic neuropathic pain of the upper extremities.[163]

In recent years, the popularity of the interpleural technique has diminished at the expense of the thoracic epidural technique. Some new development still occurs and the interpleural technique has been used for postoperative pain after thoracotomy, applying an "epidural-like" analgesic mixture (bupivacaine plus fentanyl).[164]

## Lower Extremity Nerve Block Catheters

Continuous peripheral nerve block catheters have been used in all major technique such as three-in-one block, lumbar plexus block, psoas compartment block, sciatic nerve block (all approaches), and femoral nerve block.

After the first case reports on insertion of a plastic catheter (18-gauge Teflon intravenous cannula) in the fascial sheath of the femoral nerve,[165] the technique has developed to include advancing either an epidural catheter or a specially designed catheter 15–20 cm upward along the femoral nerve, close to the lumbar spine.[166] In the published literature, only a few technical complication have been reported. An acute compression syndrome of the femoral nerve was developed 30 hours after catheter insertion, with the 20-gauge Teflon catheter still in place.[167] A case of femoral nerve injury has been reported after continuous psoas compartment block, possibly attributable to direct needle trauma to the spinal nerve roots rather than to damage by the catheter.[168]

As in other continuous catheter techniques, catheter misplacements may occur and, e.g., intrathecal placement of posterior lumbar plexus block catheters[169] and intrathecal[170] or epidural placement[171] of psoas compartment catheters have been reported.

Infectious complications are rare; one case of a thigh abscess was reported after continuous popliteal sciatic nerve block.[172] Recent case reports on bleeding after removal of peripheral nerve block catheters in patients receiving LMWH[173] have activated the discussion on whether guidelines are needed also for peripheral nerve block catheters associated with anticoagulant use.

## References


1. Manalan SA. Caudal block anesthesia in obstetrics. J Indiana Med Assoc 1942;45:564–565.
2. Adams RC, Lundy JS, Seldon TH. Continuous caudal anesthesia or analgesia: a consideration of the technic, various uses and some possible dangers. JAMA 1943;25:152–158.
3. Tuohy EB. Continuous spinal anesthesia: a new method of utilising a ureteral catheter. Surg Clin North Am 1945;25:834–840.
4. Curbelo MM. Continuous peridural segmental anesthesia by means of ureteral catheter. Anesth Analg Curr Res 1949;28:13–22.
5. Edell TA, Ramamurthy S. Catheters for neural blockade: materials and design. Tech Reg Anesth Pain Manage 1998;2:103–110.
6. Eckmann DM. Variations in epidural catheter manufacture: implications for bending and stiffness. Reg Anesth Pain Med 2003;28:37–42.
7. Niemi L, Pitkänen M, Tuominen M, Rosenberg PH. Technical problems and side effects associated with continuous intrathecal or epidural postoperative analgesia in patients undergoing hip arthroplasty. Eur J Anaesthesiol 1994;11:469–474.
8. Bahar M, Chanimov M, Cohen ML, et al. The lateral recumbent head-down position decreases the incidence of epidural veinous puncture during catheter insertion in obese patients. Can J Anaesth 2004;51:577–580.
9. Harney D, Moran CA, Whitty R, Harte S, Geary M, Gardiner J. Influence of posture on the incidence of vein cannulation during epidural catheter placement. Eur J Anaesthesiol 2005;22:103–106.
10. Ryan DW. Accidental intravenous injection of bupivacaine: a complication of obstetric epidural anaesthesia. Br J Anaesth 1973;45:907–908.
11. Hylton RR, Eger EI II, Rovno SH. Intravascular placement of epidural catheters. Anesth Analg Curr Res 1964;43:379–382.
12. Usubiaga JE. Neurological complications following epidural anesthesia. Int Anesthesiol Clin 1975;13:1–153.
13. McNeill MJ, Thorburn J. Cannulation of the epidural space. A comparison of 18- and 16-gauge needles. Anaesthesia 1988;43:154–155.
14. Mannion D, Walker R, Clayton K. Extradural vein puncture – an avoidable complication. Anaesthesia 1991;46:585–587.
15. Banwell BR, Morley-Forster P, Krause R. Decrease incidence of complications with the Arrow (FlexTip Plus) epidural catheter. Can J Anaesth 1998;45:370–372.
16. Hartley M. A strange case of inadvertent spinal. Br J Anaesth 1975;47:420.

17. Ward CF, Osborne R, Benumof JL, Saidman LJ. A hazard of double-orifice epidural catheters. Anesthesiology 1978;48:362–364.
18. Beck H, Brassow F, Doehn M, Bause H, Dziadzka A, Schulte am Esch J. Epidural catheters of multi-orifice type: dangers and complications. Acta Anaesthesiol Scand 1986;30:549–555.
19. Morrison LM, Buchan AS. Comparison of complications associated with single-holed and multi-holed extradural catheters. Br J Anaesth 1990;64:183–185.
20. Woehlck HJ, Bolla B. Uncoiling of wire in Arrow Flextip epidural catheter on removal. Anesthesiology 2000;92:907–909.
21. Bastien JL, McCarroll MG. Uncoiling of Arrow Flextip Plus epidural catheter reinforcing wire during catheter removal: an unusual complication. Anesth Analg 2004;98:554–555.
22. Tsui BC, Gupta S, Finucane B. Confirmation of epidural catheter placement using nerve stimulation. Can J Anaesth 1998;45:640–644.
23. Tsui BC, Gupta S, Finucane B. Detection of subarachnoid and intravascular epidural catheter placement. Can J Anaesth 1999;46:675–678.
24. De Vore JS, Asrani R. Bupivacaine-induced seizure in obstetrics. Anesthesiology 1978; 48:386–387.
25. Ravindran R, Albrecht W, McKay M. Apparent intravascular migration of an epidural catheter. Anesth Analg 1979;58:252–253.
26. Zebrowski ME, Gutsche BB. More on intravascular migration of an epidural catheter. Anesth Analg 1979;58:531.
27. Dickson MA, Doyle E. The intravascular migration of an epidural catheter. Paediatr Anaesth 1999;9:273–275.
28. Robson JA, Brodsky JB. Latent dural puncture after lumbar epidural block. Anesth Analg 1977;56:725–726.
29. Skowronski GA, Rigg JRA. Total spinal block complicating epidural analgesia in labour. Anaesth Intensive Care 1981;9:274–276.
30. Sasakawa T, Nagashima M, Hamada I, et al. Delayed subarachnoid migration of an epidural catheter: a case report [Japanese]. Masui 2004;53:284–286.
31. Chadwick VL, Jones M, Poulton B, Fleming BG. Epidural catheter migration: a comparison of tunnelling against a new technique of catheter fixation. Anaesth Intensive Care 2003;31:518–522.
32. Blomberg RA, Löfström JB. The test dose in regional anaesthesia. Acta Anaesthesiol Scand 1991;35:465–468.
33. Gaiser RR. The epidural test dose in obstetric anesthesia: it is not obsolete. J Clin Anesth 2003;15:474–477.
34. Norris MC, Ferrenbach D, Dalman H, et al. Does epinephrine improve the diagnostic accuracy of aspiration during labor epidural analgesia? Anesth Analg 1999;88:1073–1076.
35. Gieraerts R, Van Zundert A, De Wolf A, Vaes L. Ten ml bupivacaine 0.125% with 12.5 micrograms epinephrine is a reliable epidural test dose to detect inadvertent intravascular injection in obstetric patients. A double-blind study. Acta Anaesthesiol Scand 1992;36: 656–659.
36. Bromage PR. Epidural Analgesia. Philadelphia: WB Saunders; 1978.
37. Usubiaga JE, Reis AD, Usubiaga LE. Epidural misplacement of catheters and mechanisms of unilateral blockade. Anesthesiology 1970;32:158–161.
38. Hartrick CT, Pither CE, Pai U, Raj PP, Tomsick TA. Subdural migration of an epidural catheter. Anesth Analg 1985;64:175–178.
39. Orbegozo M, Sheikh T, Slogoff S. Subdural cannulation and local anesthetic injection as a complication of an intended epidural anesthetic. J Clin Anesth 1999;11:129–131.
40. Collier CB. Accidental subdural injection during attempted lumbar epidural block may present as a failed or inadequate block: radiographic evidence. Reg Anesth Pain Med 2004;29:7–8.
41. Boys JE, Norman PF. Accidental subdural analgesia. Br J Anaesth 1975;47:1111–1113.
42. Blanco D, Llmazares J, Rincón R, Ortiz M, Vidal F. Thoracic epidural anesthesia via the lumbar approach in infants and children. Anesthesiology 1996;84:1312–1316.
43. Blomberg RG. Technical advantages of the paramedian approach for lumbar epidural puncture and catheter introduction. Anaesthesia 1988;43:837–843.
44. Gallart JL, Blanco D, Samsó E, Vidal F. Clinical and radiological evidence of the epidural plica mediana dorsalis. Anesth Analg 1990;71:689–701.

45. Nicholson MJ. Complication associated with the use of extradural catheter in obstetric anesthesia. Anesth Analg 1965;44:245–247.
46. Chun L, Karp M. Unusual complications from placement of catheters in caudal canal in obstetrical anesthesia. Anesthesiology 1966;27:96–97.
47. Browne RA, Politi VL. Knotting of an epidural catheter: a case report. Can Anaesth Soc J 1979;26:142–144.
48. Gozal D, Gozal Y, Beilin B. Removal of knotted epidural catheters. Case reports. Reg Anesth 1996;21:71–73.
49. Hsin ST, Chang FC, Tsou MY, et al. Inadvertent knotting of a thoracic epidural catheter. Acta Anaesthesiol Scand 2001;45:255–257.
50. Riegler R, Pernetzky A. Unremovable epidural catheter due to a sling and a knot. A rare complication of epidural anesthesia in obstetrics [German]. Reg Anaesth 1983;6:19–21.
51. Crawford JS. Some maternal complications of epidural analgesia for labour. Anaesthesia 1985;40:1219–1225.
52. Tanaka S, Sanuki M, Kinoshita H. Accidental severance of epidural catheter used in a patient with postoperative delirium [Japanese]. Masui 2004;53:559–561.
53. Boey SK, Carrie LE. Withdrawal forces during removal of lumbar extradural catheters. Br J Anaesth 1994;73:833–835.
54. Nishio I, Sekiguchi M, Aoyama Y, Asano S, Ono A. Decreased tensile strength of an epidural catheter during its removal by grasping with a hemostat. Anesth Analg 2001;93:210–212.
55. Tsui BC, Finucane B. Tensile strength of 19- and 20-gauge Arrow epidural catheters. Anesth Analg 2003;97:1524–1526.
56. Moir DD, Thorburn J. Obstetric anaesthesia and analgesia. 3rd ed. London: Bailliere Tindall; 1986.
57. Vandermeulen EP, Van Aken H, Vermylen J. Anticoagulants and spinal-epidural anesthesia. Anesth Analg 1994;79:1165–1177.
58. Schmidt A, Nolte H. Subdural and epidural hematomas following epidural anesthesia. A literature review [German]. 1992;41:276–284.
59. Brockmeier V, Moen H, Karlsson BR, Fjeld NB, Reiestad F, Steen PA. Interpleural or thoracic epidural analgesia for pain after thoracotomy. A double blind study. Acta Anaesthesiol Scand 1993;38:317–321.
60. Horlocker TT, Wedel DJ, Benzon H, et al. Regional anesthesia in the anticoagulated patient: defining the risks (the second ASRA Consensus Conference on Neuraxial Anesthesia and Anticoagulation). Reg Anesth Pain Med 2003;28(3):172–197.
61. Rao TLK, El-Etr AA. Anticoagulation following placement of epidural and subarachnoid catheters: an evaluation of neurologic sequelae. Anesthesiology 1981;55:618–620.
62. Ruff RL, Dougherty JH. Complications of lumbar puncture followed by anticoagulation. Stroke 1982;12:879–882.
63. Kee WD, Jones P, Worth RJ. Extradural abscess complicating extradural anaesthesia for caesarean section. Br J Anaesth 1992;69:647–652.
64. Du Pen SL, Petersen DG, Williams A, Bogosian AJ. Infection during chronic epidural catheterization: diagnosis and treatment. Anesthesiology 1990;73:905–909.
65. Nickels JH, Poulos JG, Chaoki K. Risks of infection from short-term epidural catheter use. Reg Anesth 1989;14:88–89.
66. Wanscher M, Riishede L, Krogh B. Fistula formation following epidural catheter. A case report. Acta Anaesthesiol Scand 1985;29:552–553.
67. Schregel W, Hartmann K, Schmitz C, Baumgartner D, Cunitz G. An infected fistula following a peridural catheter [German]. Anaesthesist 1992;41:346–347.
68. Bromage PR. Neurologic complications of regional anesthesia in obstetrics. In: Shnider SM, Levinson G, eds. Anesthesia for Obstetrics. 3rd ed. London: Williams & Wilkins; 1993:433–453.
69. Jakobsen KB, Christensen M-K, Carlsson P. Extradural anaesthesia for repeated surgical treatment in the presence of infection. Br J Anaesth 1995;75:536–540.
70. Carson D, Wildsmith JAW. The risk of extradural abscess [editorial]. Br J Anaesth 1995;75:520–521.
71. Heller AR, Ragaller M, Koch T. Epidural abscess after epidural catheter for pain release during pancreatitis. Acta Anaesthesiol Scand 2000;44:1024–1027.
72. Ansari A, Davies DW, Lohn JW, Culpan P, Etherington G. Extensive epidural abscess associated with an unremarkable recovery. Anaesth Intensive Care 2004;32:825–829.

73. Volk T, Hebecker R, Ruecker G, Perka C, Haas N, Spies C. Subdural empyema combined with paraspinal abscess after epidural catheter insertion. Anesth Analg 2005;100:1222–1223.
74. Baker AS, Ojemann RG, Schwartz MN, Richardson EP Jr. Spinal epidural abscess. N Engl J Med 1975;293:463–468.
75. Stevens RA. Neuraxial blocks. In: Brown DL, ed. Regional Anesthesia and Analgesia. Philadelphia: WB Saunders; 1996.
76. Rosenberg PH, Renkonen OV. Antibacterial activity of bupivacaine and morphine. Anesthesiology 1985;62:178–179.
77. Pere P, Lindgren L, Vaara M. Poor antibacterial effect of ropivacaine: comparison with bupivacaine. Anesthesiology 1999;91:884–886.
78. Kalas DB, Hehre FW. Continuous lumbar peridural anesthesia in obstetrics. VIII. Further observations on inadvertent lumbar puncture. Anesth Analg 1972;51:192–195.
79. Denny N, Masters R, Pearson D, Read J, Sihota M, Selander D. Postdural puncture headache after continuous spinal anesthesia. Anesth Analg 1987;66:791–794.
80. Pitkänen M. Continuous spinal anaesthesia. Curr Opin Anaesthesiol 1992;5:676–680.
81. Moore DC, Batra MS. The components of an effective dose prior to epidural block. Anesthesiology 1981;55:693–696.
82. Van Zundert A, Vaes L, Soetens M, et al. Every dose given in epidural analgesia for vaginal delivery can be a test dose. Anesthesiology 1987;67:436–440.
83. Cheek TG, Banner R, Sasuter J, Gutsche BB. Prophylactic extradural blood patch is effective. A preliminary communication. Br J Anaesth 1988;61:340–342.
84. Ostheimer GW, Palahniuk RJ, Shnider SM. Epidural blood patch for post-lumbar puncture headache. Anesthesiology 1974;41:307–308.
85. Walpole JB. Blood patch for spinal headache. A recurrence and a complication. Anaesthesia 1975;30:783–785.
86. Scavone BM, Wong CA, Sullivan JT, Yaghmour E, Sherwani SS, McCarthy RJ. Efficacy of a prophylactic epidural blood patch in preventing post dural puncture headache in parturients after inadvertent dural puncture. Anesthesiology 2004;101:1422–1427.
87. Auroy Y, Narchi P, Messiah A, Litt L, Rouvier B, Samii K. Serious complications related to regional anesthesia: results of a prospective survey in France. Anesthesiology 1997;87:479–486.
88. Auroy Y, Benhamou D, Bargues L, et al. Major complications of regional anesthesia in France. The SOS Regional Anesthesia Hotline Service. Anesthesiology 2002;97:1274–1280.
89. Horlocker TT, Abel MD, Messick JM Jr, Schroeder DR. Small risk of serious neurologic complications related to lumbar epidural catheter placement in anesthetized patients. Anesth Analg 2003;96:1547–1552.
90. Bromage PR, Benumof JL. Paraplegia following intracord injection during attempted epidural anesthesia under general anesthesia. Reg Anesth Pain Med 1998;23:104–107.
91. Wilkinson PA, Valentine A, Gibbs JM. Intrinsic spinal cord lesion complicating epidural anaesthesia and analgesia: report of three cases. J Neurol Neurosurg Psychiatry 2002;72:537–539.
92. Kao MC, Tsai SK, Tsou MY, Lee HK, Guo WY, Hu JS. Paraplegia after delayed detection of inadvertent spinal cord injury during thoracic epidural catheterization in an anesthetized elderly patient. Anesth Analg 2004;99:580–583.
93. Bromage PR, Benumof JL. Safety of epidurals: further comment and response [letter]. Reg Anesth Pain Med 1999;24:274–275.
94. Rosenquist RW, Birnbach DJ. Epidural insertion in anesthetized adults: will your patient thank you? Anesth Analg 2003;96:1545–1546.
95. Drasner K. Thoracic epidural anesthesia: asleep at the wheel? [editorial] Anesth Analg 2004;99:578–579.
96. Motsch J, Hutschenreuter K. Cutaneous cerebrospinal fluid fistula associated with secondary puncture of the dura caused by a peridural catheter [German]. Reg Anaesth 1984;7:74–76.
97. Lin D, Becker K, Shapiro HM. Neurologic changes following epidural injection of potassium chloride and diazepam. A case report with laboratory correlations. Anesthesiology 1986;65:210–212.
98. Liu K, Chia Y-Y. Inadvertent epidural injection of potassium chloride. Report of two cases. Acta Anaesthesiol Scand 1995;39:1134–1137.

99. Forestner JE, Raj PP. Inadvertent epidural injection of thiopental: a case report. Anesth Analg 1975;54:406–407.
100. Yentis SM, Randall K. Drug errors in obstetric anaesthesia: a national survey. Int J Obstet Anesth 2003;12:246–249.
101. Kasaba T, Uehara K, Katsuki H, Ono Y, Takasaki M. Analysis of inadvertent epidural injection of drugs [Japanese]. Masui 2000;49:1391–1394.
102. Krataijan J, Laeni N. Accidental epidural injection of pancuronium. Anesth Analg 2005;100:1546–1547.
103. Rawal N, Van Zundert A, Holmström B, Crowhurst JA. Combined spinal-epidural technique. Reg Anesth 1997;22:406–423.
104. Cook TM. 201 combined spinal-epidurals for anaesthesia using a separate needle technique. Eur J Anaesthesiol 2004;21:679–683.
105. Rawal N, Schollin J, Wesström G. Epidural versus combined spinal epidural block for cesarean section. Acta Anaesthesiol Scand 1988;32:61–66.
106. Carter LC, Popat MT, Wallace DH. Epidural needle rotation and inadvertent dural puncture with catheter. Anaesthesia 1992;47:447–448.
107. Puolakka R, Pitkänen MT, Rosenberg PH. Comparison of technical and block characteristics of different combined spinal-epidural anesthesia techniques. Reg Anesth Pain Med 2001;26:17–23.
108. Hurley RJ, Lambert DH. Continuous spinal anesthesia with a microcatheter technique: preliminary experience. Anesth Analg 1990;70:97–102.
109. Hurley RJ. Continuous spinal anesthesia: a historical perspective. Reg Anesth 1993;18:390–393.
110. Rosenberg PH. Novel technology: needles, microcatheters, and combined techniques. Reg Anesth 1998;23:363–369.
111. Silvanto M, Pitkänen M, Tuominen M, Rosenberg PH. Technical problems associated with the use of 32-gauge and 22-gauge spinal catheters. Acta Anaesthesiol Scand 1992;36:295–299.
112. Pitkänen M, Tuominen M, Rosenberg P, Wahlström T. Technical and light microscopic comparison of four different small-diameter catheters used for continuous spinal anesthesia. Reg Anesth 1992;17:288–291.
113. Guinard J-P, Chiolero R, Mavrocordatos P, Carpenter RL. Prolonged intrathecal fentanyl analgesia via 32-gauge catheters after thoracotomy. Anesth Analg 1993;77:936–941.
114. Jöhr M. Continuous spinal anesthesia using bupivacaine. Report of experience [German]. Reg Anaesth 1988;11:71–73.
115. Van Gessel E, Forster A, Gamulin Z. A prospective study of feasibility in a university hospital. Anesth Analg 1995;80:880–885.
116. De Vera HV, Ries M. Complication of continuous spinal microcatheters: should we seek their removal if sheared? Anesthesiology 1991;74:794.
117. Lindgren L, Silvanto M, Scheinin B, Kauste A, Rosenberg PH. Erythrocyte counts in the cerebrospinal fluid associated with continuous spinal anaesthesia. Acta Anaesthesiol Scand 1995;39:396–400.
118. Horlocker TT, Wedel DJ, Schroeder DR, et al. Preoperative antiplatelet therapy does not increase the risk of spinal hematoma associated with regional anesthesia. Anesth Analg 1995;80:303–309.
119. Standl T, Eckert S, Schulte am Esch J. Microcatheter continuous spinal anaesthesia in the postoperative period: a prospective study of its effectiveness and complications. Eur J Anaesthesiol 1995;12:273–279.
120. Borgeat A, Ekatodramis G, Kalberer F, Benz C. Acute and nonacute complications with interscalene block and shoulder surgery: a prospective study. Anesthesiology 2001;95:875–880.
121. Dullenkopf A, Zingg P, Curt A, Borgeat A. Persistent neurological deficit of the upper extremity after a shoulder operation under general anesthesia combined with a preoperatively placed interscalene catheter [German]. Anaesthesist 2002;51:547–551.
122. Gaumann DM, Lennon RL, Wedel DJ. Continuous axillary block for postoperative pain management. Reg Anesth 1988;13:77–82.
123. Aguilar JL, Domingo V, Samper D, Roca G, Vidal F. Long-term brachial plexus anesthesia using a subcutaneous implantable injection system. Reg Anesth 1995;20:242–245.

124. Ablondi MA, Ryan JF, O'Connell CT, Haley RW. Continuous intercostal nerve blocks for postoperative pain relief. Anesth Analg 1966;45:185–190.
125. Payne KA, Moore SW. Subarachnoid microcatheter anesthesia in children. Reg Anesth 1994;19:237–242.
126. Standl T, Beck H. Radiological examination of the intrathecal position of microcatheters in continuous spinal anaesthesia. Br J Anaesth 1993;71:803–806.
127. Lambert RJ, Hurley RJ. Cauda equina syndrome and continuous spinal anesthesia. Anesth Analg 1991;72:817–819.
128. Lambert LA, Lambert DH, Strichartz GR. Irreversible conduction block in isolated nerve by high concentration of local anesthetics. Anesthesiology 1994;80:1082–1093.
129. Pitkänen M. Continuous spinal anesthesia and analgesia. Tech Reg Anesth Pain Manage 1998;2:96–102.
130. Puolakka R, Pitkänen MT, Rosenberg PH. Comparison of three catheter sets for continuous spinal anesthesia in patients undergoing total hip or knee arthroplasty. Reg Anesth Pain Med 2000;25:584–590.
131. Tuominen M, Pere P, Rosenberg PH. Unintentional arterial catheterization and bupivacaine toxicity associated with continuous interscalene brachial plexus block. Anesthesiology 1991;75:356–358.
132. Winnie AP. Plexus Anesthesia. Vol 1. Fribourg: Mediglobe SA; 1990.
133. Kapral S, Krafft P, Eisenberger K, Fitzgerald R, Gosch M, Weinstabl C. Ultrasound-guided supraclavicular approach for regional anesthesia of the brachial plexus. Anesth Analg 1994;78:507–513.
134. Chan VW. Applying ultrasound imaging to interscalene brachial plexus block. Reg Anesth Pain Med 2003;28:340–343.
135. Boezaart AP, De Beer JF, Nell ML. Early experience with continuous cervical paravertebral block using a stimulating catheter. Reg Anesth Pain Med 2003;28:406–413.
136. Tuominen M, Haasio J, Hekali R, Rosenberg PH. Continuous interscalene brachial plexus block: clinical efficacy, technical problems and bupivacaine plasma concentrations. Acta Anaesthesiol Scand 1989;33:84–88.
137. Hubner T, Gerber H. Knotting of a catheter in the plexus brachialis. A rare complication [German]. Anaesthesist 2003;52:606–607.
138. Urmey WF, Talts KH, Sharrock NE. One hundred percent incidence of hemidiaphragm paresis with interscalene brachial plexus anesthesia as diagnosed by ultrasonography. Anesth Analg 1991;72:498–503.
139. Pere PJ, Pitkänen MT, Rosenberg PH, et al. Effect of continuous interscalene brachial plexus block on diaphragmatic motion and on ventilatory function. Acta Anaesthesiol Scand 1992;36:53–57.
140. Farrar MD, Scheybani M, Nolte H. Upper extremity block effectiveness and complications. Reg Anesth 1981;6:133–134.
141. Pere P. The effect of continuous interscalene brachial plexus block with 0.125% bupivacaine plus fentanyl on diaphragmatic motility and ventilatory function. Reg Anesth 1993; 18:93–97.
142. Rosenberg PH, Lamberg TS, Tarkkila P, Marttila T, Björkenheim J-M, Tuominen M. Auditory disturbances associated with interscalene brachial plexus block. Br J Anaesth 1995;74:89–91.
143. Mahoudeau G, Gaertner E, Launoy A, Ocquidant P, Loewenthal A. Interscalenic block: accidental catheterization of the epidural space [French]. Ann Fr Anesth Reanim 1995;14:438–441.
144. Moore DC, Bridenbaugh LD. Pneumothorax, its incidence following intercostal nerve block. JAMA 1962;182:135–138.
145. Shanti CM, Carlin AM, Tyburski JG. Incidence of pneumothorax from intercostal nerve block for analgesia in rib fractures. J Trauma 2001;51:536–539.
146. O'Kelly E, Garry B. Continuous pain relief for multiple fractured ribs. Br J Anaesth 1981;53:989–991.
147. Crossley AWA, Hosie HE. Radiographic study of intercostal nerve block in healthy volunteers. Br J Anaesth 1987;59:149–154.
148. Mowbray A, Wong KKS, Murray JM. Intercostal catheterization. An alternative to the paravertebral space. Anaesthesia 1987;42:958–961.
149. Kawamata M, Omote K, Namiki A, Miyabe M. Measurement of intercostal and pleural pressures by epidural catheter. Anaesthesia 1994;49:208–210.

150. Olivert RT, Nauss LA, Payne S. A technique for continuous intercostal nerve block analgesia following thoracotomy. J Thorac Cardiovasc Surg 1980;80:308–311.
151. Sabanathan S, Smith PJ, Pradhan GN, Hashimi H, Eng JB, Mearns AJ. Continuous intercostal nerve block for pain relief after thoracotomy. Ann Thorac Surg 1988;46: 425–426.
152. Tenicela R, Pollan SB. Paravertebral-peridural block technique: a unilateral thoracic block. Clin J Pain 1990;6:227–234.
153. Naja Z, Lönnqvist PA. Somatic paravertebral nerve blockade. Incidence of failed block and complications. Anaesthesia 2001;56:1184–1188.
154. Dhole S, Mehta Y, Saxene H, Juneja R, Trehan N. Comparison of continuous thoracic epidural and paravertebral blocks for postoperative analgesia after minimally invasive direct coronary artery bypass surgery. J Cardiothorac Vasc Anesth 2001;15:288–292.
155. Marret E, Bazelly B, Taylor G, et al. Paravertebral block with ropivacaine 0.5% versus systemic analgesia for pain relief after thoracotomy. Ann Thorac Surg 2005;79:2109–2114.
156. Eason MJ, Wyatt R. Paravertebral thoracic block – a reappraisal. Anaesthesia 1979;34: 638–642.
157. Strømskag KE, Minor B, Steen PA. Side effects and complications related to interpleural analgesia: an update. Acta Anaesthesiol Scand 1990;34:473–477.
158. Symreng T, Gomez MN, Johnson B, Rossi NP, Chiang CK. Intrapleural bupivacaine technical considerations and intraoperative use. J Cardiothorac Anesth 1989;3:139–143.
159. Murrell G. A new complication of the intrapleural catheter method for postoperative analgesia. Anaesth Intensive Care 1988;16:499–500.
160. Rosenberg PH, Scheinin BM, Lepäntalo MJ, Lindfors O. Continuous interpleural infusion of bupivacaine for analgesia after thoracotomy. Anesthesiology 1987;67:811–813.
161. Lauder GR. Interpleural analgesia and phrenic nerve paralysis. Anaesthesia 1993;48: 315–316.
162. Parkinson SK, Mueller JB, Rich TJ, Little WL. Unilateral Horner's syndrome associated with interpleural catheter injection of local anesthetic. Anesth Analg 1989;68:61–62.
163. Reiestad F, McIlvane WB, Kvalheim L, Stokke T, Pettersen B. Interpleural analgesia in treatment of upper extremity reflex sympathetic dystrophy. Anesth Analg 1989;69:671–673.
164. Karakaya D, Baris S, Özkan F, et al. Analgesic effect of interpleural bupivacaine with fentanyl for post-thoracotomy pain. J Cardiothorac Vasc Anesth 2004;18:461–465.
165. Rosenblatt RM. Continuous femoral anesthesia for lower extremity surgery. Anesth Analg 1980;59:631–632.
166. Postel J, März P. Continuous blockade of the lumbar plexus ("3-in-1 block") in perioperative pain therapy [German]. Reg Anaesth 1984;7:140–143.
167. Jöhr M. A complication of continuous blockade of the femoral nerve [German]. Reg Anaesth 1987;10:37–38.
168. Al-Nasser B, Palacios JL. Femoral nerve injury complicating psoas compartment block. Reg Anaesth Pain Med 2004;29:361–363.
169. Pousman RM, Mansoor Z, Sciard D. Total spinal anesthetic after continuous posterior lumbar plexus block. Anesthesiology 2003;98:1281–1282.
170. Litz RJ, Vicent O, Wiessner D, Heller AR. Misplacement of a psoas compartment catheter in the subarachnoid space. Reg Anesth Pain Med 2004;29:60–64.
171. Rotzinger M, Neuburger M, Kaiser H. Inadvertent epidural placement of a psoas compartment catheter. Case report of a rare complication [German]. Anaesthesist 2004;53: 1069–1072.
172. Compere V, Cornet C, Fourdrinier V, et al. Thigh abscess as a complication of continuous popliteal sciatic nerve block. Br J Anaesth 2005;95(2):255–256.
173. Bickler P, Brandes J, Lee M, Bozic K, Chesbro B, Claassen J. Bleeding complications from femoral and sciatic nerve catheters in patients receiving low molecular weight heparin. Anesth Analg 2006;103:1036–1037.

# 16 Regional Anesthesia Complications Related to Acute Pain Management

Narinder Rawal

There is a large variety of available routes for administration of analgesic drugs to manage postoperative pain; these include: enteral (oral, sublingual, buccal, transmucosal), rectal, parenteral [subcutaneous, intramuscular (i.m.), intravenous (i.v.)], surface (topical, transdermal), cavity (intranasal, inhalational, intra-articular), and neural (neuraxial and peripheral) routes. Table 16-1 shows the regional techniques available to manage postoperative pain. The problems associated with regional techniques generally are covered elsewhere in this book; these include technique-related issues, infection, nerve injury, systemic local anesthetic (LA) toxicity, etc. Also, it is clear that "epidural analgesia" is not a generic term. Its effects on outcome and complications may differ depending on whether epidural injections consist of opioids, LAs, or both. In addition, the insertion site for the epidural catheter (lumbar, low thoracic, or high thoracic) will significantly alter physiologic effects when LAs are used.

This chapter will outline the complications associated with the use of regional techniques for the management of pain in the postoperative period in inpatients and those undergoing day surgery.

## Neuraxial Blocks and Risks of Severe Neurologic Complications

Severe complications caused by central neuraxial blocks (CNBs) are believed to be extremely rare, but the incidence is probably underestimated. In a recent Swedish retrospective study of complications during 1990–1999 after CNB (1,260,000 spinal blocks and 450,000 epidural blocks), 127 severe neurologic complications were reported.[1] These included spinal hematoma (n = 33), cauda equina syndrome (n = 32), meningitis (n = 29), epidural abscess (n = 13), and miscellaneous (n = 20). Permanent neurologic damage was observed in 85 patients. The incidence of complications after spinal blockade was within 1:20,000–30,000 in all patient groups. The incidence after obstetric epidural blockade was 1:25,000; in the remaining patients it was 1:3600 ($P < .0001$). In this study, a 55 times greater risk of spinal hematoma was noted after epidural block in female patients undergoing knee arthroplasty (1:3600) as compared with patients receiving epidural block for obstetric indications (1:200,000) ($P < .0001$).

TABLE 16-1. Regional techniques for postoperative analgesia

- Central blocks (epidural, spinal, combined spinal–epidural)
- Peripheral blocks
  Proximal and distal nerves
  Perineural – during surgery (amputation)
  Intercostal, paravertebral
- Incisional (subcutaneous, subfascial)
- Intraarticular, intrabursal
- Intraperitoneal
- Supraperiosteal

This study is the most comprehensive retrospective study performed to detect serious neurologic complications after CNB. The authors concluded that more complications than expected were found. Complications occur significantly more often following epidural than spinal blockade, and these complications are different. Obstetric patients carry a significantly lower incidence of complications. Osteoporosis was proposed as a previously neglected risk factor. One-third of all spinal hematomas were seen in patients receiving thromboprophylaxis in association with neuraxial block in accordance with the current guidelines and in the absence of any previously known risk factors. Consequently, adherence to guidelines regarding low-molecular-weight heparin may reduce but not completely abolish the risk of spinal hematoma after neuraxial block on the surgical wards. Close surveillance after central neuraxial blockade is mandatory for safe practice. More females than males experience osteoporotic hip fractures and more females need knee or hip arthroplasty. Osteoporosis not only causes a higher number of hip fractures – the spine is also affected with vertebral deformities and fractures. Moreover, the osteoporotic vertebra is enlarged, causing narrowing of the spinal canal. A large number of female patients with pathologically altered spines are therefore subject to CNB.

In this study, only 13 cases of epidural abscess were found, indicating an incidence significantly lower than previously reported.[2,3] The incidence of epidural abscess may be underestimated because these complications may appear late after the patient has left the surgical ward. Risk factors for infection were present in 75% of the patients.

## Organizational Issues – Role of Acute Pain Services

Providing effective analgesia for patients undergoing major surgery is challenging for most anesthesiologists. Continuous thoracic epidural analgesia using a low-dose LA–opioid combination has the potential to provide effective dynamic pain relief, early mobilization, and rehabilitation for patients undergoing major upper abdominal or thoracic procedures. However, in a busy surgical ward, it is not uncommon for epidurals to be ineffective in providing dynamic pain relief. Rarely and catastrophically, major complications occur.[4]

Regional techniques can result in a number of complications, some of which are of major concern because of their potential to cause permanent neurologic damage. These problems can be related to the presence of the catheters in the epidural, subarachnoid, or perineural space, or to drugs infused or drug errors. The availability of acute pain services (APSs) can help in early recognition of these rare complications and to prevent serious harm.

Implementation of invasive analgesic techniques such as epidural anesthesia may lead to increased treatment-related morbidity which will depend on the drugs and adjuvants administered in the epidural catheter and on the monitoring routines. This may range from pruritus to serious complications such as epidural hematoma. Provision of safe analgesia is one of the main objectives of an APS; however, there is very little literature on the role of APSs in preventing or reducing these complications.[5–7] Werner et al.[5] reviewed the literature on APSs, the 44 audits and four clinical trials containing outcome data included 84,097 postoperative patients. The overall incidence of complications (total = 43,576; epidural analgesia = 12,212) was 0.5%–1.2%, comprising in most cases opioid-related respiratory depression.[8,9] The incidence of serious neurologic complications related to the epidural analgesia was reported in six audits (n = 12,940) and in one review. Several authors have emphasized that epidural analgesia, with continuous infusion of LAs on the wards, requires visits including gross neurologic examination by an APS at least once a day.[10]

### *Neurologic Complications on Surgical Wards*

Neurologic injuries caused by neuraxial blockade are in two categories: those that relate to performing the block and those related to an inadequate organization of the postoperative surveillance at the postanesthesia care unit (PACU), the high-dependency unit, or the ward. The review by Werner et al.[5] showed that serious catheter-related epidural complications reported included one case of cauda equina syndrome with persisting urinary incontinence (n = 5602),[11] two cases of meningitis (n = 2287),[12] three cases of intravascular migration of the epidural catheters (n = 1062),[13] and five cases of intradural migration of the catheter (n = 4958).[8,13,14]

### *Technical Incidents*

In a study by Chen et al.,[15] 53 incidents were reported during 1 year in 1275 patients managed by an APS. Twenty-eight incidents were related to malfunctioning infusion devices and 15 incidents to erroneous drug dosing. Thirty-eight of the incidents were detected by the APS and the anesthesiologist. In a safety-assessment study, potentially severe complications were discovered in 0.5% of the patients (16 of 3016), without sequelae.[8]

### *Urinary Retention*

Surgery, anesthesia, and postoperative analgesia are factors that contribute to postoperative urinary retention, which may lead to urinary tract infections. Treatment by an indwelling catheter for a prolonged period, however, increases the incidence of urinary tract infections, septicemia, and mortality.[5]

### *Hypotension*

The reported incidence of clinically significant hypotension requiring APS intervention after epidural analgesia ranges from 0.7%[16–18] to 7.4%.[19] The use of epidural LA drugs is associated with hypotension because of blockade of the sympathetic chain. If the block height reaches the cardiac innervation (between T1 and T5), there may be a marked hypotensive and bradycardic response, particularly in the presence of hypovolemia. Wheatley et al.[4] combined the results of three studies involving nearly 9000 patients and showed that the incidence of hypotension during epidural infusion of LA was 0.7%–3% depending on the concentration used (0.0625%–0.25% bupivacaine) and the criteria for hypotension.[17,20,21] Use of patient-controlled epidural analgesia (PCEA) resulted in a 6.8% incidence of hypotension.[4]

### *Complications Caused by Excessive Motor Blockade*

Excessive lower limb motor blockade is uncommon with low doses of local anesthesia solutions. Scott et al.[22] reported an incidence of 3% with bupivacaine–fentanyl combination. Excessive motor block may result in the development of pressure areas on the heels[23–25] and deep venous thrombosis.[9] Persistent motor blockade of one or both lower limbs in a patient receiving a low-dose combination LA–opioid thoracic epidural should always be treated with suspicion. Stopping the epidural infusion normally results in neurologic improvement within 2 hours. If this does not occur, consideration should be given to excluding a spinal hematoma or abscess. Ropivacaine may produce less motor blockade compared with an equianalgesic dose of bupivacaine, especially if used in low concentrations (0.1%) with fentanyl ($2\,\mu g\,mL^{-1}$).[26]

The literature review by Werner et al. showed that the incidence of clinically significant motor blockade (Bromage grade >0), impeding normal ambulation, was significantly increased with lumbar versus thoracic catheters (7%–50% and 1%–4%, respectively).[11,14,18] An unusually prolonged, unilateral motor block in two patients, lasting 4–10 days, was reported in one audit.[9] Subjective motor weakness was reported in up to 16%–21% of patients (the level of the epidural catheter placement was not reported).[17]

### *Catheter-Incision Congruent Analgesia*

The importance of the site of epidural catheter cannot be overemphasized; the use of "catheter-incision congruent analgesia" involves the placement of epidural catheter corresponding to the dermatomes of the surgical incision. For patients with coronary artery disease who are undergoing upper abdominal or thoracic surgery, the use of thoracic epidural analgesia may provide several physiologic advantages by increasing coronary flow to ischemic areas and attenuating sympathetically mediated coronary vasoconstriction.[27–29] The use of lumbar epidural analgesia in these patients may result in increased sympathetic activity in upper thoracic segments and may increase myocardial oxygen consumption.[27,30] A metaanalysis showed a significant decrease in the incidence of postoperative myocardial infarction with the use of thoracic (congruent) but not lumbar (incongruent) epidural analgesia.[31] A review of the literature comparing epidural analgesia with systemic opioids to assess return of postoperative bowel function showed that all nine trials incorporating "catheter-incision congruent" epidural analgesia noted earlier return of gastrointestinal function, whereas only one of seven trials with "catheter-incision incongruent" epidural analgesia noted earlier return of gastrointestinal function.[32]

### *Catheter Migration*

The tip of the epidural catheter can migrate intrathecally (i.t.) or intravascularly. This must be considered before any bolus dose is administered in the epidural catheter by careful aspiration; a test dose of LA containing epinephrine can also provide evidence of i.v. migration by producing a transient tachycardia. These techniques, and the use of low-dose LA–opioid infusions, can prevent dramatic complications, such as total spinal anesthesia and seizures.[33,34] Unintentional subdural catheter placement or migration can also lead to a high block, requiring intubation.[35] The incidence of i.t. and i.v. migration has been reported as 0.15%–0.18%.[4,36,37]

### *Knotting of Epidural Catheter*

The estimated incidence of knotting of the epidural catheter is 0.0015%. There are 14 case reports in the literature since 1965.[38] The length of the catheter introduced in the epidural space and the design and material of the epidural catheter have been proposed as possible causes. It is generally recommended that the length of catheters in the epidural space should be less than 5 cm.[38]

## Adverse Events Related to Epidural Drug Administration

### *Drug Errors*

The most common drugs involved in errors are LAs and opioids; adjuvants such as clonidine and epinephrine are also involved in errors. All these drugs carry the potential for serious adverse effects. Drug errors can also occur when a wrong drug is administered via the epidural catheter. The incidence remains unclear – glucose,[39] antibiotics,[40] thiopentone,[41,42] potassium chloride[43–45] (resulting in paraplegia), and total parenteral nutrition[46] have all been inadvertently injected. The use of pharmacy-prepared or commercially prepared solutions, extreme care with labeling of epidural catheters and drugs, checking procedures, and the use of dedicated pumps should help avoid these problems.

### *Central Nervous System Toxicity*

The incidence of convulsions, as a result of high plasma concentrations of free LAs, was reported to be 0.01%–0.12% for bupivacaine when 16,870[47] and 40,010[48] epidural blocks were assessed.[4]

## Respiratory Depression – Are Lipophilic Drugs Safer?

The adverse effect of most concern with epidural opioids is respiratory depression. Nearly all available opioids have been used epidurally in the management of postoperative pain. Data from large studies and from several reviews suggest that morphine is by far the most extensively studied opioid worldwide.[49–52] A 17-nation European survey showed that 12 different opioids were used routinely to manage postoperative pain. Morphine and fentanyl are the most frequently used opioids in Europe.[53] Highly lipid-soluble drugs such as fentanyl and sufentanil have a more rapid onset and shorter duration of effect than hydrophilic drugs such as morphine. The long duration of analgesia of epidural morphine allows it to be used as an intermittent bolus dose twice a day, whereas opioids such as fentanyl and sufentanil are better suited for continuous infusion because of their short duration of analgesia.

On the basis of pharmacologic models proposed for spinal opioid transport, the risk of late-onset respiratory depression is high with hydrophilic morphine. In contrast, lipophilic opioids such as fentanyl and sufentanil are considered safe because of segmental localization; minimal drug is available for rostral migration in cerebrospinal fluid (CSF) to reach medullary respiratory centers by diffusion and bulk flow. This has led to the widespread use of fentanyl as a safe opioid for epidural administration. However, the earlier belief that continuous infusions of epidural fentanyl do not cause late-onset respiratory depression has been shown to be incorrect.[54–59] The use of continuous epidural fentanyl infusions has been associated with three deaths caused by respiratory arrest. Two of the patients had sleep apnea syndrome.[60] Similarly, respiratory depression was reported in several patients on postoperative days 2, 3, and 4 in patients receiving epidural sufentanil–bupivacaine infusion for analgesia after major surgery.[61]

In an editorial, Eisenach[62] has stated that the belief that highly lipid-soluble drugs stay fixed at their site of location and do not move in CSF is a myth. Several case reports have demonstrated acute and life-threatening respiratory depression following i.t. fentanyl, sufentanil, and meperidine. Lipid-soluble drugs, be they opioids or LAs, do move rapidly and extensively in CSF and can produce patient harm.[62] There is a widespread misconception that any opioid administered epidurally or i.t. will produce analgesia by a selective spinal mechanism. Recent data suggest that increasing lipid solubility decreases the spinal cord bioavailability of spinally administered opioids. These data help to explain many clinical studies that have demonstrated that the analgesic effect of spinally administered lipid-soluble opioids is partly, if not exclusively, attributable to plasma uptake and distribution to brainstem opioid receptors.[63] The method of lipophilic opioid administration may also be important. It has been demonstrated that epidural fentanyl infusion produces analgesia by uptake into plasma and redistribution to brain and peripheral opioid receptors, whereas fentanyl bolus produces analgesia by a selective spinal mechanism.[64]

The choice of opioid may also depend on hospital or state nursing regulations regarding administration of opioids in epidural or i.t. catheters. This may be one reason why intermittent administration of morphine in epidural catheters is common in countries where nurses are allowed to inject drugs. Conversely, epidural infusion techniques are popular in some countries where nurses are not allowed to inject drugs in epidural or i.t. catheters.

### *Problems with Intraspinal Opioids and LA Combinations*

Epidural LA drugs have many advantages, such as blockade of sympathetic and hormonal responses to surgery and pain and lack of inhibition of bowel function. However, motor block may prevent postoperative mobilization and sympathetic block can result in hypotension. Adjuvants such as opioids, clonidine, and epinephrine have been added to improve analgesia, reduce morbidity, and reduce LA dose and side effects.

It is generally agreed that epidural analgesia using LA and opioid combinations is highly effective in reducing movement-associated pain. However, the optimum combination that has an opioid-sparing synergistic effect, without delaying mobilization, is yet to be established. A variety of factors influence the rate of epidural analgesia infusion that is necessary for effective analgesia. These include the site and type of surgery, type of pain (labor versus postsurgery), choice of opioid and its loading dose, the volume of injectate, the concentration of LA, and patient characteristics that influence epidural pharmacokinetics and pharmacodynamics of the given opioid. Sitting of the catheter tip in the epidural space is also important, thus, bupivacaine 0.1% with fentanyl given through a lumbar catheter was associated with a high incidence of lower limb weakness[65] whereas motor weakness was insignificant when LA (0.1%–0.2% bupivacaine) was administered at the thoracic level.[66,67]

In general there is no agreement about the most suitable drug combinations and dosages. A recent questionnaire survey of United Kingdom epidural practice showed that 103 LA–opioid solutions were used at the 74 centers that responded. In one center, seven different solutions were used.[68] Clearly, there is a need for rationalizing this practice because it has implications for safety, nursing workload, economic costs, and audit data collection.

### *Patient-Controlled Epidural Analgesia*

PCEA may improve analgesia, patient satisfaction, and safety compared with epidural technique using bolus administration or infusion. It has been suggested that epidural PCA with opioids results in a more rapid recovery and shorter hospitalization than i.v. PCA or i.m. opioids.[69] Patients have increased satisfaction partly because of a sense of control and the flexibility to increase analgesic demand to match pain during movement.

Potential benefits of PCA have to be balanced against potential risks. Excessive self-administration of opioid may result in respiratory depression, and of LA in a high incidence of hypotension or motor block. Self-administration of opioids and LAs could exacerbate the effects of displaced epidural catheter into the intravascular or i.t. space resulting in high spinal block, systemic toxicity, or respiratory depression.[58,70]

A report based on experience with 1030 surgical patients using PCEA with bupivacaine and fentanyl showed that PCEA provided effective postoperative analgesia for rest and movement-related pain. The study included abdominal, thoracic, gynecologic, urologic, vascular, orthopedic, and plastic surgical procedures. Although the incidence of side effects was quite low, hypotension (6.8%) and respiratory depression (0.3%) did occur.[58] In a survey of 1057 patients (3858 treatment days), PCEA with bupivacaine–fentanyl was associated with 0.19% severe respiratory depression and one patient was unrousable.[59] Appropriate surveillance is therefore necessary for patients receiving PCEA.

In general, there is a lack of randomized studies to identify the best lipophilic opioid. The ideal combination of LA and opioid for PCEA is unknown. Further studies are needed to determine optimal analgesic solution, background infusion rates, and lockout intervals. Studies are also necessary to evaluate the cost–benefit ratio of this technique.

## Safety of Epidural Versus Intrathecal Opioids

The efficacy, optimal dose, duration of analgesia, and adverse effect profile of epidural opioids have been extensively documented; however, there is a paucity of similar information for i.t. opioids. The i.t. route is a direct one because there is no dura to be penetrated and the drug is deposited close to its site of action – the opioid receptors. Intrathecal administration of opioids immediately produces a high CSF concentration of the drug that is dose dependent. Vascular reabsorption of opioids after i.t. administration does occur to some degree, but is clinically irrelevant. Compared with the i.t. route, epidural administration is complicated by pharmacokinetics of dural penetration, epidural fat deposition, and systemic opioid absorption. Intrathecal administration of opioids has the advantages of simplicity, reliability, and low-dose requirements. To compensate for the effects of systemic uptake and fat sequestration, the epidural dose of morphine is approximately 10- to 20-fold greater than that required for i.t. injection.[71]

Recently it is has been demonstrated that doses as low as 0.1–0.5 mg may provide adequate analgesia after abdominal, orthopedic, and thoracic surgery.[72–77] There is now convincing evidence that doses less than 0.2–0.3 mg provide excellent postoperative analgesia. A systematic review of 15 randomized, controlled trials of i.t. opioids in patients undergoing cesarean section with spinal anesthesia showed that only morphine produced clinically relevant reductions in postoperative pain and analgesic consumption; fentanyl and sufentanil had a minor effect only. The incidence of pruritus was high (43%) but similar to morphine, fentanyl, and sufentanil. However, nausea and vomiting were less frequent with the lipophilic opioids than with morphine. The authors recommend morphine 0.1 mg as the drug and dose of choice.[72]

## Adverse Effects of Intraspinal Opioids

### *Pruritus*

Although systemic administration of opioids is known to cause pruritus, it is most frequent after spinal administration of opioids. It may be generalized but is more likely to be localized to the face, neck, or upper thorax. Pruritus usually occurs within a few hours of injection, may be higher when the i.t. route is used, and is lower following subsequent doses. Pruritus has been associated with almost all opioids. Pregnant patients seem more at risk irrespective of the opioid administered; this may be attributable to interaction of estrogen with opioid receptors. The reported incidence of itching following intraspinal opioids is quite variable. Figures ranging from 0% to 100% have been published in the literature. The probable reason is that if not asked specifically, the majority of patients do not complain about this complication because of its mild nature.

A systematic review of 22 randomized trials of pharmacologic control of opioid-induced pruritus showed an average of 60% of patients had some itching. With epidural and i.t. morphine, there was no evidence that the dose made any difference. Other opioids represented the same range of risk although the data were limited. The authors concluded that pruritus caused by opioid analgesia happens frequently, independent of the opioid used, the route of administration, or the dose. They also concluded that naloxone, naltrexone, nalbuphine, and droperidol were efficacious for opioid-induced pruritus; however, minimal effective doses were unclear. There was little data on the efficacy of interventions for the treatment of established pruritus. None of the other tested drugs, nalmefene, epinephrine, propofol, clonidine, hydroxyzine, or prednisolone, showed any worthwhile benefit.[78]

The systematic review demonstrated that there is "a lack of valid data on the efficacy of interventions for the treatment of established pruritus."[78] This conclusion agrees with an excellent review of the literature by Waxler et al.[79]

### *Urinary Retention*

Bladder overdistention induced by retention is associated with stretching, which may lead to dysfunction of the detrusor muscle. Urinary retention induced by i.t. and epidural opioids is likely related to interaction with opioid receptors located in the sacral spinal cord. This interaction promotes inhibition of sacral parasympathetic nervous system outflow, which causes detrusor muscle relaxation and an increase in maximal bladder capacity leading to urinary retention.[80] The reported incidence of urinary retention following epidural or i.t. opioids varies considerably.[80,81] It is difficult to establish the incidence of urinary retention because the majority of patients who receive epidural or i.t. opioids are high-risk patients undergoing major surgery who are usually catheterized. The incidence is not related to the dose of opioid administered. Urinary retention following i.t. and epidural opioids is much more common than after i.v. or i.m. administration of equivalent doses of opioid.[49,80–84]

Lipophilic opioids may have a more favorable profile. Studies with i.t. fentanyl in volunteers[85] and in patients undergoing knee surgery[86] did not show any significant increase in time to urination. Intrathecal sufentanil alone for extracorporeal shock wave lithotripsy was associated with shorter time to voluntary micturition as compared with spinal lidocaine.[87] It should be noted that i.t. epinephrine increases the time to voluntary micturition.[88] Thus, i.t. lipophilic opioids may be the preferred spinal anesthetic adjuvants for outpatient procedures.[89] If patients are unable to void 6 hours after surgery and naloxone is ineffective, a single in-and-out catheterization is indicated to prevent myogenic bladder damage because of prolonged overdistension.

### *Nausea and Vomiting*

The incidence of nausea and vomiting following i.t. and epidural opioids is approximately 30%.[90] Although nausea and vomiting are generally considered a side effect of opioid administration, intraspinal opioids may actually protect against intraoperative nausea and vomiting (IONV).[91] In patients undergoing caesarean section under regional anesthesia, IONV is quite frequent, especially during uterus exteriorization and peritoneal closure. Several recent studies have shown that the risk of IONV can be reduced when i.t. fentanyl is added to spinal LA for caesarean delivery.[91–94] Indeed, i.t. fentanyl has been shown to be superior to i.v. ondansetron in preventing nausea and vomiting during caesarean delivery.[95]

### *Incidence of Respiratory Depression Following Intraspinal Opioids*

This is the adverse effect of most concern and therefore most widely studied. The true incidence of clinically significant respiratory depression is not known. Because of the rarity of late-onset respiratory depression, small sample sizes and invasive respiratory measurement techniques, the majority of prospective studies of epidural morphine have not detected clinically significant respiratory depression.[96]

It is interesting to note that after more than 25 years of clinical use and hundreds of papers, there is no clear definition of the most serious effect of spinal opioid administration. A review of the literature, which included 209 studies, showed that the term "respiratory depression" has not been clearly defined for the use of i.t. morphine for postoperative analgesia. Although defining bradypnea is better than having no definition, this is inadequate.[97] Several anecdotal reports of late-onset respiratory depression and "near misses" have been published. The results from large surveys involving thousands of patients suggest that the risk of late-onset respiratory depression following epidural morphine is less than 1%; this can be reduced further if certain risk factors are avoided. The risk of respiratory depression following other opioids may or may not be less; current data are inconclusive.

The quoted incidence of respiratory depression when epidural analgesia is supervised by an APS is no higher than the incidence of respiratory depression seen with other forms of opioid analgesia.[53] Regular monitoring of respiratory rate and, more importantly, the level of consciousness seems to be adequate to detect respiratory depression, and is indicated for up to 12 hours after a bolus injection of morphine and for the entire duration of a continuous infusion containing any opioid. The literature review by Werner et al.[5] showed that the incidence of serious postoperative opioid-induced respiratory depression requiring the administration of naloxone depended on the analgesic modality and was 0%–1.7% during fixed-rate morphine infusion (two studies), 0.1%–2.2% during PCA (11 studies), 0.1%–1.0% with spinal infusions of opioids (seven studies), and 0%–0.5% with a mixture of LAs and opioids (three studies).

Available data would suggest that the overall risk of severe respiratory depression from therapeutic doses of opioids is similar (<1%) regardless of the route of administration[53,98–105] (Tables 16-2 and 16-3); therefore, all postoperative patients receiving opioid analgesia, irrespective of route, merit diligent observation for respiratory depression.

TABLE 16-2. Incidence of Respiratory Depression Following Epidural Opioids

| Total no. of patients | Respiratory depression (no. of patients) | Risk of respiratory depression (%) | Reference |
|---|---|---|---|
| 6,000–9,000* | 23 | 0.25–0.4 | 100 |
| 1,085* | 10 | 0.9 | 101 |
| 14,000* | 13 | 0.09 | 102 |
| 4,880* | 12 | 0.25 | 103 |
| 1,106* | 2 | 0.2 | 104 |
| 2,378 | 19 | 0.13 | 105 |
| 49,183† | 45 | 0.09 | 53 |

*Morphine.
†Morphine (n = 33), fentanyl (n = 4), oxycodone (n = 4), diamorphine (n = 4).

TABLE 16-3. Incidence of respiratory depression on surgical wards after epidural LA–opioid combination for postoperative analgesia*

| Study no. | Total no. of patients | Respiratory depression (no. of patients) | Risk of respiratory depression (%) | Opioid | Reference |
|---|---|---|---|---|---|
| 1 | 4,227 | 3 | 0.07 | Morphine | 20 |
| 2 | 1,014 | 4 | 0.4 | Fentanyl | 22 |
| 3 | 614 | 3 | 0.49 | Sufentanil | 61 |
| 4 | 2,000 | 3 | 0.15 | Morphine | 21 |
| 5 | 1,062 | 4 | 0.32 | Fentanyl | 13 |
| 6 | 1,030† | ? | 0.2 | Fentanyl | 58 |
| 7 | 5,602† | 0 | 0 | Sufentanil | 11 |
| 8 | 1,057† | 2 | 0.19‡ | Fentanyl | 59 |

*LA in all studies was bupivacaine. Brodner et al. (study 7) also used ropivacaine.
†PCEA technique.
‡Additionally, one patient was unarousable.

## Intraspinal Opioids and Monitoring Routines

It is clear that respiratory depression following intraspinal opioids is unpredictable and may be associated with any opioid (Tables 16-2 and 16-3). It should be emphasized that respiratory rate alone is inadequate to establish the presence or lack of respiratory depression.[106] Monitoring of level of consciousness is important because increasing sedation is associated with advancing respiratory depression.[52] Data from more than 20,000 patients from the Swedish surveys and from other large studies show that respiratory depression, if it occurs, will manifest itself within 12 hours after injection of morphine.[50,102,107] At our institution, the 12-hour observation routine has been used since 1980 for thousands of patients without any major problems. For lipophilic opioids, the observation period can be reduced, to perhaps 4–6 hours after fentanyl and sufentanil.

Current evidence suggests that most patients can be safely monitored on regular wards if (a) personnel are trained and preprinted guidelines for potential emergencies are provided, (b) patient selection and opioid dosing is appropriate, and (c) respiratory rate and level of sedation are checked every hour. Since 1992, these guidelines have been accepted by the Swedish Society of Anesthesiology and Intensive Care (SFAI). European Society of Regional Anaesthesia (ESRA)[108] has recommended similar guidelines. It should be noted that monitoring routines vary among countries and also among institutions in the same country.[105,109] The efficacy and safety of spinal opioids on surgical wards is best assured when these analgesic techniques are used under the supervision of organized APSs.[6,11]

## Complications of Regional Techniques for Pain Management after Ambulatory Surgery

With the advance of catheter and disposable pump technologies, it is now possible not only to provide superior analgesia with continuous peripheral nerve blocks but also to send patients home with an ambulatory perineural block anesthetic infusion. Patients have been sent home with perineural, intraarticular, surgical wounds, and periosseous (e.g., supraperiosteal and subalveolar) LA infusions.[110] There are now studies showing the efficacy and safety of ambulatory continuous interscalene blocks,[111,112] infraclavicular blocks,[113] axillary blocks,[114] sciatic nerve blocks,[115–117] femoral nerve blocks,[118] psoas compartment blocks,[119] and paravertebral blocks.[120]

Continuing regional anesthesia in the home environment has been demonstrated to reduce analgesic consumption and reduce sleep disturbance. Disposable pumps are now available that use continuous infusions at a variety of preset rates, with or without patient-controlled boluses. Catheter removal may be successfully performed by the patients, by another healthcare provider, or by the patient caregiver with telephone supervision.

However, perineural techniques have a potential for significant complications such as nerve injury,[121] catheter migration leading to local anesthetic toxicity,[122] and unintentional spread of blockade epidurally or i.t.[123] Although this author was the first to report the use of perineural (and incisional and intraarticular) catheter analgesia at home,[110,114] and the perineural catheter technique is still used at our institution, our preference is for incisional and intraarticular catheter techniques because of their simplicity and safety, which are the two most important prerequisites for such techniques at home. Another reason for restrictive use of ambulatory perineural catheters is that in Sweden (and in most countries outside the United States) extensive joint surgery, which is one of the most important indications for perineural catheter techniques, is not an ambulatory procedure at present. Different infiltration techniques have been shown to be pain reducing and opioid sparing after cholecystectomy,[124] inguinal hernia repair,[125] breast surgery,[126] gynecologic laparotomies,[127] orthopedic,[128] anorectal,[129] and cardiac surgery.[130]

The use of incisional and intraarticular LA drugs to treat postoperative pain is an attractive technique because of its simplicity, safety, and low cost. Administration of LA in the wound or joint has several advantages over perineural techniques for postoperative analgesia.[131] Continuous wound infiltration with a disposable infusion pump, with or without a patient-controlled bolus, may provide several days of analgesia. Although these techniques may not be as potent as continuous peripheral nerve blocks, they are credited with being safe and very simple to use. They can be easily combined with a single-injection peripheral nerve block.[131]

## Discharge and Follow-up – Safety Considerations

The discharge and follow-up routines will depend on the type of block for surgery (CNB or peripheral nerve block) and also on whether a simple injection technique or a catheter technique is used. In most centers, the single injection technique is routine; however, catheter technique is being increasingly used to provide superior pain relief after surgical procedures that are associated with moderate to severe pain.

### *Discharge of the Patient with Blocked Extremity*

Many anesthesiologists still consider discharge of patients with insensate extremities controversial. Theoretically, these patients with blocked extremities would be more predisposed to limb injury because of lack of protective pain reflexes and reduced proprioception. Patients undergoing upper limb surgery should be instructed to wear a sling at all times to protect the anesthetized limb, and not to drive.

### *LA Toxicity*

LA toxicity is a potential complication when continuous perineural infusions are used. Although the majority of cases occur when large-volume boluses of local anesthetics are used during block placement, toxicity is still possible with continuous infusion at home. To minimize the risk of toxicity in the ambulatory and home settings, a long-acting local anesthetic with a good safety profile should be used. Low concentrations can provide motor-sensory differential blockade allowing patients to actively participate in their postoperative rehabilitation. Currently, ropivacaine seems to be the best choice. Careful catheter testing should be performed to avoid inadvertent vascular placement and consequent local anesthetic toxicity.[132]

### *Catheter Insertion Site Infection*

The risk of infection is always possible with any percutaneous technique (see Chapter 19). Cuvillon and coworkers[133] demonstrated that the risk of infection of femoral nerve catheters is small, although bacterial colonization is common. They also demonstrated that 57% of 208 femoral catheters were most frequently colonized by *Staphylococcus epidermidis* (71%), *Enterococcus* (10%), and *Klebsiella* (4%). None of the patients demonstrated any clinical evidence of infection or abscess formation. Similarly, catheter tips colonized by bacteria were reported for intraarticular catheters without any signs of clinical infection.[134] Vintar et al.[135] isolated *S. epidermidis* on the tips of 3 of 38 intraarticular catheters; there were no signs of local inflammation, but one patient needed antibiotics to treat increased body temperature. The incidence of infection after arthroscopic surgery is generally very low: 0%–0.2%. Rosseland et al.[136] reported no infection in more than 150 patients treated with an intraarticular catheter. We have not seen any infection after subacromial catheters during the last 8 years.[110,114] Park et al.[137] did not report any infection in their study of intrabursal catheter technique for shoulder surgery. However, intraarticular catheter infection requiring antibiotic treatment has been reported in two patients.[138,139]

All continuous peripheral nerve catheters are at risk for infection. However, with careful attention to aseptic technique during catheter placement, this problem is infrequent in clinical practice. Patients should also be aware of signs and symptoms of infection and contact healthcare professionals immediately in this case.

### *Catheter Dislodgment*

Although catheter dislodgment is a major concern, especially outside the hospital environment, this complication is very uncommon. Several techniques to secure perineural catheters have been reported including suturing, cutaneous sutures, retrograde subcutaneous tunneling, medical adhesive solutions, and 2-octyl cyanoacrylate glue. In addition, some sites are easier to secure catheters (e.g., infraclavicular), decreasing the probability of dislodgment.[132]

### *Catheter Migration*

Migration of perineural catheters is also a potential problem that can lead to serious complications, such as LA toxicity from intravascular migration,[122] interpleural migration of interscalene catheter,[140] centroneuraxial spread from i.t. or epidural migration of lumbar plexus and interscalene catheters.[141,142]

### *Infusion Pump Problems*

To determine the optimal device for safe delivery of LA at home, factors that need to be considered are flow-rate accuracy, infusion flexibility, and total LA volume requirement. In general, there are two types of pumps: single-use elastomeric and multiple-use electronic pumps. Although the nonelectronic elastomeric pumps are not as accurate or as flexible as electronic pumps, studies show that patients prefer simple devices that avoid the need for reprogramming or the problems caused by frequent alarms.[143] There is extensive experience with nonelectronic pumps providing safe and effective postoperative analgesia at home. Simplicity and safety are not mutually exclusive and the physician should ensure that the selected device provides the prescribed dose of LA within reasonable limits.

### *Organizational Issues of Catheter Techniques at Home*

Patient education should begin during the preoperative visit. Audiovisual material and information brochures allow patients to be psychologically prepared for surgery under regional anesthesia and for pain and its management at home. All authors who

Table 16-4. Patient Instructions for Postoperative Patient-controlled Regional Analgesia at Home

| |
|---|
| Inform the patient about the technique and how the "balloon pump" works (oral and written information). Information should also include the following: |
| • Instructions for removal of catheter at the end of treatment |
| • Importance of good hygiene near the wound area |
| • Information about signs of LA toxicity or infection |
| • There should be 24-hour access to anesthesia services. |
| Provide the name and telephone (and beeper) number(s) of the physician to be contacted in case of LA toxicity symptoms or other problems. |
| • Ask the patient to return follow-up data about technique, satisfaction/dissatisfaction in a self-addressed envelope. |
| • Telephone follow-up on the day after surgery by a nurse or physician |

have used ambulatory perineural and incisional catheters emphasize the importance of good organization as a prerequisite for the safe delivery of such analgesic techniques at home. However, there is no consensus on the requirements for such an organization. Some practitioners have patients remove their catheters at home at the conclusion of their infusion, whereas others prefer removing the catheters themselves. Some discharge patients with written instructions regarding catheter removal, and others give verbal instructions over the phone during removal. Some investigators have provided twice-daily home nursing visits, whereas others have relied on daily telephone contact.[144] Studies from the United States show that the organization for perineural catheters is quite elaborate and includes: physician availability at all times, twice-daily home nursing visits in addition to telephone calls, catheter removal by healthcare provider or by the patient's caretaker with instructions on the phone by the anesthesiologist.[145–147] Our organization with the use of incisional and intraarticular catheter techniques is quite simple and consists of verbal and written predischarge information about pump function and use of PCRA rescue analgesic medication, symptoms of LA toxicity, local hygiene, catheter removal, return of completed patient diary, and contact numbers in case of problems (Table 16-4). A nurse from our PACU calls the patient the day after surgery to confirm the proper functioning of the technique. Patient selection is important and before discharge the patients are expected to demonstrate that they have understood the technique by using the pump in the presence of a PACU nurse. Our relatively simple approach is supported by the findings of a recent United States study, which surveyed the use of ambulatory catheter techniques at home. The follow-up survey of patients who had undergone ambulatory perineural infusion showed that 98% of respondents reported feeling "safe" with infusion and felt comfortable removing their catheter at home.[144]

## Conclusion

Sending patients home with perineural, incisional, and intraarticular catheters is a new and evolving area of postoperative pain management. Although no large-scale study of possible problems has been published, the experiences of several centers that routinely use these techniques have not revealed any major complications. Current evidence suggests that these techniques are effective, feasible, and safe in the home environment if appropriate patient selection routines and organization for follow-up are in place. Understandably, follow-up routines are more elaborate for perineural techniques. Further studies are necessary to establish indications for incisional and intraarticular techniques as part of balanced analgesia concept and save the potentially more risky perineural techniques for the remaining patients. Outcome and risk studies are also necessary.

*Acknowledgment*

The author acknowledges the excellent secretarial assistance of Marianne Welamsson.

## References

1. Moen V, Dahlgren N, Irestedt L. Severe neurological complications after central neuraxial blockades in Sweden 1990–1999. Anesthesiology 2004;101:950–959.
2. Hasserius R, Johnell O, Nilsson BE, et al. Hip fracture patients have more vertebral deformities than subjects in population-based studies. Bone 2003;32:180–184.
3. Wang LP, Hauerberg J, Schmidt JF. Incidence of spinal epidural abscess after epidural analgesia: a national 1-year survey. Anesthesiology 1999;91:1928–1940.
4. Wheatley RG, Schug SA, Watson D. Safety and efficacy of postoperative analgesia. Br J Anaesth 2001;87:47–61.
5. Werner MU, Søholm L, Rotbøll-Nielsen P. Does an acute pain service improve postoperative outcome? Anesth Analg 2002;95:1361–1372.
6. Rawal N. Acute pain services revisited: good from far, far from good? Reg Anesth Pain Med 2002;27:117–121.
7. Rawal N. Organization, function, and implementation of acute pain service. Anesthesiol Clin North Am 2005;23:211–225.
8. Shug SA, Torrie JJ. Safety assessment of postoperative pain management by an acute pain service. Pain 1993;55:6–21.
9. Wheatley RG, Madej TH, Jackson IJ, Hunter D. The first year's experience of an acute pain service. Br J Anaesth 1991;67:353–359.
10. Maier C, Kibbel K, Mercker S, Wulf H. Postoperative pain therapy at general nursing stations: an analysis of eight years' experience at an anesthesiological acute pain service. Anaesthesist 1994;43:385–397.
11. Brodner G, Mertes N, Buerkle H, et al. Acute pain management: analysis, implications and consequences after prospective experience with 6349 surgical patients. Eur J Anaesthesiol 2000;17:566–575.
12. Breivik H. Benefit, risks and economics of postoperative pain management programmes. In: Breivik H, ed. Baillière's Clinical Anaesthesiology. Vol 9. London: Baillière Tindall; 1995:403–460.
13. Burstal R, Wegener F, Hayes C, Lantry G. Epidural analgesia: prospective audit of 1062 patients. Anaesth Intensive Care 1998;26:165–172.
14. Breivik H, Högström H, Niemi G, et al. Safe and effective postoperative pain relief: introduction and continuous quality-improvement of comprehensive postoperative pain management programmes. In: Breivik H, ed. Baillière's Clinical Anaesthesiology. London: Baillière Tindall; 1995:423–460.
15. Chen PP, Ma M, Chan S, Oh TE. Incident reporting in acute pain management. Anaesthesia 1998;53:730–735.
16. Blanco J, Blanco E, Rodriguez G, et al. One year's experience with an acute pain service in a Spanish University Clinic hospital. Eur J Anaesthesiol 1994;11:417–421.
17. Tsui SL, Irwin MG, Wong CM, et al. An audit of the safety of an acute pain service. Anaesthesia 1997;52:1042–1047.
18. Bredahl C, Dahl BL, Toft P. Acute pain service: organization and results. Ugeskr Laeger 1998;160:6070–6074.
19. Sartain JB, Barry JJ. The impact of an acute pain service on postoperative pain management. Anaesth Intensive Care 1999;27:375–380.
20. De Leon-Casasola OA, Parker B, Lema MJ, et al. Postoperative epidural bupivacaine-morphine therapy. Experience with 4227 surgical cancer patients. Anesthesiology 1994;81:368–375.
21. Rygnestad T, Borchgrevink PC, Eide E. Postoperative epidural infusion of morphine and bupivacaine is safe on surgical wards. Organisation of the treatment, effects and side-effects in 2000 consecutive patients. Acta Anaesthesiol Scand 1997;41:868–876.
22. Scott DA, Beilby DS, McClymont C. Postoperative analgesia using epidural infusions of fentanyl with bupivacaine. A prospective analysis of 1014 patients. Anesthesiology 1995; 83:727–737.

23. Cohen S, Amar D, Pantuck CB, et al. Adverse effects of epidural 0.03% bupivacaine during analgesia after cesarean section. Anesth Analg 1992;75:753–756.
24. Punt CD, van Neer PA, de Lange S. Pressure sores as a possible complication of epidural analgesia. Anesth Analg 1991;73:657–659.
25. Smet IG, Vercauteren MP, De Jongh RF, et al. Pressure sores as a complication of patient-controlled epidural analgesia after cesarean delivery. Case report. Reg Anesth 1996;21: 338–341.
26. Liu SS, Moore JM, Luo AM, et al. Comparison of three solutions of ropivacaine/fentanyl for postoperative patient-controlled epidural analgesia. Anesthesiology 1999;90:727–733.
27. Wu CL, Thomsen RW. Effect of postoperative epidural analgesia on patient outcomes. Tech Reg Anesth Pain Manage 2003;7:140–147.
28. Davis RF, DeBoer LW, Maroko PR. Thoracic epidural anesthesia reduces myocardial infarct size after coronary artery occlusion in dogs. Anesth Analg 1986;65:711–717.
29. Kock M, Blomberg S, Emanuelsson H, et al. Thoracic epidural anesthesia improves global and regional left ventricular function during stress-induced myocardial ischemia in patients with coronary artery disease. Anesth Analg 1990;71:625–630.
30. Veering BT, Cousins MJ. Cardiovascular and pulmonary effects of epidural anaesthesia. Anaesth Intensive Care 2000;28:620–635.
31. Beattie WS, Badner NH, Choi P. Epidural analgesia reduces postoperative myocardial infarction: a meta-analysis. Anesth Analg 2001;93:853–858.
32. Hodgson PS, Liu SS. Thoracic epidural anaesthesia and analgesia for abdominal surgery: effects on gastrointestinal function and perfusion. Balliere's Clin Anaesthesiol 1999; 13:9–22.
33. Miguel R, Barlow I, Morrell M, et al. A prospective, randomized, double-blind comparison of epidural and intravenous sufentanil infusions. Anesthesiology 1994;81:346–352.
34. Seeling W, Heinrich H. Unexpected intravenous penetration of an epidural catheter. Reg Anaesth 1984;7:137–139.
35. Chauhan S, Gaur A, Tripathi M, Kaushik S. Unintentional combined epidural and subdural block. Case report. Reg Anesth 1995;20:249–251.
36. Ready LB, Loper KA, Nessly M, Wild L. Postoperative epidural morphine is safe on surgical wards. Anesthesiology 1991;75:452–456.
37. Schug SA, Torrie JJ. Safety assessment of postoperative pain management by an acute pain service. Pain 1993;55:387–391.
38. Bizat Z, Boztug N, Onder G, Ertok E. A rare complication of epidural catheter. Acta Anaesthesiol Scand 2005;49:589–590.
39. Whiteley MH, Laurito CE. Neurologic symptoms after accidental administration of epidural glucose. Anesth Analg 1997;84:216–217.
40. Kopacz DJ, Slover RB. Accidental epidural cephazolin injection: safeguards for patient-controlled analgesia. Anesthesiology 1990;72:994–997.
41. Cay DL. Accidental epidural thiopentone. Anaesth Intensive Care 1984;12:61–63.
42. Forestner JE, Raj PP. Inadvertent epidural injection of thiopental: a case report. Anesth Analg 1975;54:406–407.
43. Kulka PJ, Stratesteffen I, Grunewald R, Wiebalck A. Inadvertent potassium chloride infusion in an epidural catheter. Anaesthesist 1999;48:896–899.
44. Lin D, Becker K, Shapiro HM. Neurologic changes following epidural injection of potassium chloride and diazepam: a case report with laboratory correlations. Anesthesiology 1986;65:210–212.
45. Shanker KB, Palkar NV, Nishkala R. Paraplegia following epidural potassium chloride. Anaesthesia 1985;40:45–47.
46. Patel PC, Sharif AM, Farnando PU. Accidental infusion of total parenteral nutrition solution through an epidural catheter. Anaesthesia 1984;39:383–384.
47. Brown DL, Ransom DM, Hall JA, et al. Regional anesthesia and local anesthetic-induced systemic toxicity: seizure frequency and accompanying cardiovascular changes. Anesth Analg 1995;81:321–328.
48. Tanaka K, Watanabe R, Harada T, Dan K. Extensive application of epidural anesthesia and analgesia in a university hospital: incidence of complications related to technique. Reg Anesth 1993;18:34–38.
49. Cousins MJ, Mather LE. Intrathecal and epidural administration of opioids. Anesthesiology 1984;61:276–310.

50. Morgan M. The rational use of intrathecal and extradural opioids. Br J Anaesth 1989;63: 165–188.
51. Rawal N. Spinal opioids. In: Raj PP, ed. Practical Management of Pain. St. Louis: Mosby Year Book; 1992:829–851.
52. Vercauteren MP. The role of perispinal route for postsurgical pain relief. Balliere's Clin Anaesth 1993;7:769–792.
53. Rawal N, Allvin R, EuroPain Study Group on Acute Pain. Epidural and intrathecal opioids for postoperative pain management in Europe – a 17-nation questionnaire study of selected hospitals. Acta Anaesthesiol Scand 1996;40:1119–1126.
54. Brockway MS, Noble DW, Sharwood-Smith GH, McClure JH. Profound respiratory depression after extradural fentanyl. Br J Anaesth 1990;64:243–245.
55. Weightman WM. Respiratory arrest during fentanyl infusion of bupivacaine and fentanyl. Anaesth Intensive Care 1991;19:282–284.
56. Scott DA, Beilby DSN, McClymont C. Postoperative analgesia using epidural infusions of fentanyl with bupivacaine. Anesthesiology 1995;83:727–737.
57. Burstal R, Wegener F, Hayes C, Lantry G. Epidural analgesia: prospective audit of 1062 patients. Anaesth Intensive Care 1998;26:165–172.
58. Liu SS, Allen HW, Olsson GL. Patient-controlled epidural analgesia with bupivacaine and fentanyl on hospital wards: prospective experience with 1030 surgical patients. Anesthesiology 1998;88:688–695.
59. Wigfull J, Welchew E. Survey of 1057 patients receiving postoperative patient-controlled epidural analgesia. Anaesthesia 2001;56:47–81.
60. Ostermeier AM, Roizen MF, Hautkappe M, et al. Three sudden postoperative respiratory arrests associated with epidural opioids in patients with sleep apnea. Anesth Analg 1997;85:452–460.
61. Broekema AA, Gielen MJM, Hennis PJ. Postoperative analgesia with continuous epidural sufentanil and bupivacaine: a prospective study in 614 patients. Anesth Analg 1996; 82:754–779.
62. Eisenach JC. Lipid soluble opioids do move in cerebrospinal fluid. Reg Anesth Pain Med 2001;26:296–297.
63. Bernards CM. Recent insights into the pharmacokinetics of spinal opioids and the relevance to opioid selection. Curr Opin Anaesthesiol 2004;17:441–447.
64. Ginosar Y, Riley ET, Angst MS. The site of action of epidural fentanyl in humans: the difference between infusion and bolus administration. Anesth Analg 2003;97:1428–1438.
65. Parker RK, White PF. Epidural patient-controlled analgesia: an alternative to intravenous patient-controlled analgesia for pain relief after caesarean delivery. Anesth Analg 1992; 75:245–251.
66. Torda TA, Hann P, Mills G, et al. Comparison of extra-dural fentanyl, bupivacaine and two fentanyl-bupivacaine mixtures for pain relief after abdominal surgery. Br J Anaesth 1995;74:35–40.
67. Grass JA. Sufentanil: clinical use as postoperative analgesic – epidural-intrathecal route. J Pain Symptom Manage 1992;7:271–286.
68. Bannon L, Alexander-Williams M, Lutman D. A national survey of epidural practice. Anaesthesia 2001;56(10):1021.
69. Gaffud MP, Bansal P, Lawton C, et al. Surgical analgesia for caesarean delivery with epidural bupivacaine and fentanyl. Anesthesiology 1986;65:331–334.
70. Bush DJ, Kramer DP. Intravascular migration of an epidural catheter during patient-controlled epidural analgesia. Anesth Analg 1993;76:1150–1151.
71. Stoelting RK. Intrathecal morphine: an underused combination for postoperative pain management. Anesth Analg 1989;68:707–709.
72. Dahl JB, Jeppesen IS, Jørgensen H, et al. Intraoperative and postoperative analgesic efficacy and adverse effects of intrathecal opioids in patients undergoing caesarean section with spinal anesthesia. A qualitative and quantitative systematic review of randomized controlled trials. Anesthesiology 1999;91:1919–1927.
73. Mason N, Gondret R, Junca A, Bonnet F. Intrathecal sufentanil and morphine for post-thoracotomy pain relief. Br J Anaesth 2001;86:236–240.
74. Campbell DC, Riben CM, Rooney ME, et al. Intrathecal morphine for postpartum tubal ligation postoperative analgesia. Anesth Analg 2001;93:1006–1011.
75. Gall O, Aubineau JV, Bernière J, et al. Analgesic effect of low-dose intrathecal morphine after spinal fusion in children. Anesthesiology 2001;94:447–452.

76. O'Neill P, Knickenberg C, Bogahalanda S, Booth AE. Use of intrathecal morphine for postoperative pain relief following lumbar spine surgery. J Neurosurg 1985;63:413–416.
77. Holmström B, Laugaland K, Rawal N, Hallberg S. Combined spinal epidural block versus spinal and epidural block for orthopedic surgery. Can J Anaesth 1993;40: 601–606.
78. Kjellberg F, Tramèr MR. Pharmacological control of opioid-induced pruritus: a quantitative systematic review of randomized trials. Eur J Anaesth 2001;18:346–357.
79. Waxler B, Dadabhoy ZP, Stojiljkovic L. Primer of postoperative pruritus for anesthesiologists. Anesthesiology 2005;103:168–178.
80. Rawal N, Möllefors K, Axelsson K, et al. An experimental study of urodynamic effects of epidural morphine and of naloxone reversal. Anesth Analg 1983;62:641–647.
81. Bailey PL, Rhondeau S, Schafer PG, et al. Dose-response pharmacology of intrathecal morphine in human volunteers. Anesthesiology 1993;79:49–59.
82. Martin R, Salbaing J, Blaise G, et al. Epidural morphine for postoperative pain relief: a dose-response curve. Anesthesiology 1982;56:423–426.
83. Stenseth R, Sellevold O, Breivik H. Epidural morphine for postoperative pain: experience with 1085 patients. Acta Anaesthesiol Scand 1985;29:148–156.
84. Peterson TK, Husted SE, Rybro L, et al. Urinary retention during i.m. and extradural morphine analgesia. Br J Anaesth 1982;54:1175–1178.
85. Liu S, Chiu AA, Carpenter RL, et al. Fentanyl prolongs lidocaine spinal anesthesia without prolonging recovery. Anesth Analg 1995;80:730–734.
86. Ben-David B, Solomon E, Levin H, et al. Intrathecal fentanyl with small dose dilute bupivacaine: better anesthesia without prolonging recovery. Anesth Analg 1997;85:560–565.
87. Lau WC, Green CR, Faerber GJ, et al. Intrathecal sufentanil for extracorporeal shock wave lithotripsy provides earlier discharge of the outpatient than intrathecal lidocaine. Anesth Analg 1997;84:1227–1231.
88. Chiu AA, Liu S, Carpenter RL, et al. The effects of epinephrine on lidocaine spinal anesthesia: a cross-over study. Anesth Analg 1995;80:735–739.
89. Hamber EA, Viscomi CM. Intrathecal lipophilic opioids as adjuncts to surgical spinal anesthesia. Reg Anesth Pain Med 1999;24:255–263.
90. Chaney MA. Side effects of intrathecal and epidural opioids. Can J Anaesth 1995;42: 891–903.
91. Pan MH, Wei TT, Shieh BS. Comparative analgesic enhancement of alfentanil, fentanyl, and sufentanil to spinal tetracaine anesthesia for caesarean delivery. Acta Anaesthesiol Sin 1994;32:171–176.
92. Dahlgren G, Hultstrand C, Jakobsson J, et al. Intrathecal sufentanil, fentanyl, or placebo added to bupivacaine for cesarean section. Anesth Analg 1997;85:1288–1293.
93. Palmer CM, Voulgaropoulos D, Alves D. Subarachnoid fentanyl augments lidocaine spinal anesthesia for cesarean delivery. Reg Anesth 1995;20:389–394.
94. Cooper D, Lindsay S, Ryall D, et al. Does intrathecal fentanyl produce acute cross-tolerance to IV morphine? Br J Anaesth 1997;78:311–313.
95. Manullang TR, Viscomi CM, Pace NL. Intrathecal fentanyl is superior to intravenous ondansetron for the prevention of perioperative nausea during caesarean delivery with spinal anesthesia. Anesth Analg 2000;90:1162–1166.
96. Etches RC, Sandler AN, Daley MD. Respiratory depression and spinal opioids. Can J Anaesth 1989;36:165–185.
97. Ko S, Goldstein DH, Van Den Kerkhof EG. Definitions of "respiratory depression" with intrathecal morphine postoperative analgesia: a review of literature. Can J Anaesth 2003;50:679–688.
98. Curry PD, Pacsoo C, Heao DG. Patient-controlled epidural analgesia in obstetric anaesthetic practice. Pain 1994;57:125–128.
99. Etches RC. Respiratory depression associated with patient-controlled analgesia: a review of eight cases. Can J Anaesth 1994;41:125–132.
100. Gustafsson LL, Schildt B, Jacobsen K. Adverse effects of extradural and intrathecal opiates: report of a nation-wide survey in Sweden. Br J Anaesth 1982;54:479–486.
101. Stenseth R, Sellevold O, Breivik H. Epidural morphine for postoperative pain relief: experience with 1085 patients. Acta Anaesthesiol Scand 1985;29:148–156.
102. Rawal N, Arnér S, Gustafsson LL, et al. Present state of epidural and intrathecal opiate analgesia: a nation-wide follow-up survey in Sweden. Br J Anaesth 1987;59:791–799.

103. Fuller JG, McMorland GH, Douglas MJ, Palmer L. Epidural morphine for analgesia after caesarean section: a report of 4880 patients. Can J Anaesth 1990;37:608–612.
104. Ready LB, Loper KA, Nessly M, Wild L. Postoperative epidural morphine is safe on surgical wards. Anesthesiology 1991;75:452–456.
105. Zimmermann DL, Steward J. Postoperative pain management and acute pain service activity in Canada. Can J Anaesth 1993;40:568–575.
106. Rawal N, Wattwil M. Respiratory depression following epidural morphine: an experimental and clinical study. Anesth Analg 1984;63:8–14.
107. Breen TW, Janzen JA. Epidural fentanyl and caesarean section: when should fentanyl be given? Can J Anaesth 1992;39:317–322.
108. Aguilar JL, Benhamou D, Bonnet F, et al. ESRA guide-lines for the use of epidural opioids. Int Monit Reg Anaesth 1997;9:3–8.
109. Romer HC, Russell GN. A survey of the practice of thoracic epidural analgesia in the United Kingdom. Anaesthesia 1998;53:1016–1022.
110. Rawal N, Axelsson K, Hylander J, et al. Postoperative patient-controlled local anesthetic administration at home. Anesth Analg 1998;86:86–89.
111. Klein SM, Grant SA, Greengrass RA, et al. Interscalene brachial plexus block with a continuous catheter insertion system and a disposable infusion pump. Anesth Analg 2000;91:1473–1478.
112. Ilfeld BM, Morey TE, Wright TW, et al. Continuous interscalene brachial plexus block for postoperative pain control at home: a randomized, double-blinded, placebo-controlled study. Anesth Analg 2003;96:1089–1095.
113. Ilfeld BM, Morey TE, Enneking FK. Continuous infraclavicular brachial plexus block for postoperative pain control at home. Anesthesiology 2002;96:1297–1304.
114. Rawal N, Allvin R, Axelsson K, et al. Patient-controlled regional analgesia (PCRA) at home. Anesthesiology 2002;96:1290–1296.
115. Ilfeld BM, Morey TE, Wang RD, Ennekin FK. Continuous popliteal sciatic nerve block for postoperative pain control at home. Anesthesiology 2002;97:959–965.
116. Klein SM, Greengrass RA, Grant SA, et al. Ambulatory surgery for multi-ligament knee reconstruction with continuous dual catheter peripheral nerve blockade. Can J Anaesth 2001;48:375–378.
117. Zaric D, Boysen K, Christiansen J, Haastrup U, Kofoel H, Rawal N. Continuous sciatic nerve block: a new method of analgesia at home after foot surgery – a randomised controlled trial. Acta Anaesthesiol Scand 2004;48:337–341.
118. Chelley JE, Gebhard R, Coupe K, et al. Local anesthetic delivered via a femoral catheter by patient-controlled analgesia pump for pain relief after an anterior cruciate ligament outpatient procedure. Am J Anesthesiol 2001;28:192–194.
119. Ilfeld BM, Morey TE, Enneking FK. Outpatient use of patient-controlled local anesthetic administration via a psoas compartment catheter to improve pain control and patient satisfaction after ACL reconstruction. Anesthesiology 2001;95:A38.
120. Buckenmaier CC II, Kamal A, Rubin Y, et al. Paravertebral block with catheter for breast carcinoma surgery and continuous paravertebral infusion at home. Reg Anesth Pain Med 2002;27:A47.
121. Borgeat A, Ekatodramis G, Kalberer F, Benz C. Acute and non acute complications associated with interscalene block and shoulder surgery: a prospective study. Anesthesiology 2001;95:875–880.
122. Tuominen MK, Pere P, Rosenburg PH. Unintentional arterial catheterization and bupivacaine toxicity associated with continuous interscalene brachial plexus block. Anesthesiology 1991;75:356–358.
123. Cook LB. Unsuspected extradural catheterization in an interscalene block. Br J Anaesth 1991;67:473–475.
124. Moss G, Regal ME, Lichtig L. Reducing postoperative pain, narcotics, and length of hospitalization. Surgery 1986;99:206–210.
125. McLoughlin J, Kelley CJ. Study of the effectiveness of bupivacaine infiltration of the ilioinguinal nerve at the time of hernia repair for postoperative pain relief. Br J Clin Pract 1989;8:281–283.
126. Owen H, Galloway DJ, Mitchell KG. Analgesia by wound infiltration after surgical excision of benign breast lumps. Ann R Coll Surg Engl 1985;67:114–115.
127. Patridge BL, Stabile BE. The effects of incisional bupivacaine on postoperative narcotic requirement, oxygen saturation and length of stay in the postoperative unit. Acta Anaesthesiol Scand 1990;34:486–491.

128. Bourne MH, Johnson KA. Postoperative pain relief using local anesthetic instillation. Foot Ankle 1989;44:964–966.
129. Pryn SJ, Cross MM, Murison SC, et al. Postoperative analgesia for haemorrhoidectomy. Anaesthesia 1989;44:964–966.
130. White PF, Rawal S, Latham P, et al. Use of a continuous local anesthetic infusion for pain management after median sternotomy. Anesthesiology 2003;99:918–923.
131. Rawal N. Ambulatory wound and intra-articular infusions. In: Steele S, Nielsen KC, Klein SM, eds. Ambulatory Anesthesia and Perioperative Analgesia. New York: McGraw-Hill; 2005:503–517.
132. Nielsen KC, Steele S. Ambulatory evaluation and safety considerations. Tech Reg Anesth Pain Manage 2004;8:99–103.
133. Cuvillon P, Ripart J, Lalourcey L. The continuous femoral nerve bock catheter for postoperative analgesia: bacterial colonization, infectious rate and adverse effects. Anesth Analg 2001;93:1045–1049.
134. Axelsson K, Nordensson U, Johanzon E, et al. Patient-controlled regional analgesia (PCRA) with ropivacaine after arthroscopic subacromial decompression. Acta Anaesthesiol Scand 2003;47:993–1000.
135. Vintar N, Rawal N, Veselko M. Intraarticular patient-controlled regional anesthesia after arthroscopy assisted anterior cruciate ligament reconstruction: ropivacaine/morphine/ketorolac versus ropivacaine/morphine. Anesth Analg 2005;101:573–578.
136. Rosseland LA, Stubhaug A, Grevbo F, et al. Effective pain relief from intra-articular saline with or without morphine 2 mg in patients with moderate-to-severe pain after knee arthroscopy: a randomized, double-blind controlled clinical study. Acta Anaesthesiol Scand 2003;47:732–738.
137. Park J-Y, Lee G-W, Kim Y, et al. The efficacy of continuous intra-bursal infusion with morphine and bupivacaine for postoperative analgesia after subacromial arthroscopy. Reg Anesth Pain Med 2002;27:145–149.
138. DeWess FT, Akbari Z, Carline E. Pain control after knee arthroplasty: intraarticular versus epidural anesthesia. Clin Orthop Relat Res 2001;392:226–231.
139. Rasmussen S, Kramh MU, Sperling KP, Pedersen JHL. Increased flexion and reduced hospital stay with a continuous intraarticular morphine and ropivacaine after primary total knee replacement: open intervention study of efficacy and safety of 154 patients. Acta Orthop Scand 2004;75:606–609.
140. Souron V, Reiland Y, De Traverse A. Interpleural migration of an interscalene catheter. Anesth Analg 2003;97:1200–1201.
141. Cook LB. Unsuspected extradural catheterization in an interscalene block. Br J Anaesth 1991;67:473–475.
142. Mathoudeau G, Gaertner E, Launoy A. Interscalenic block: accidental catheterization of the epidural space. Ann Fr Anesth Reanim 1995;14:438–441.
143. Xapdevila X, Macaire P, Aknin P, et al. Patient-controlled perineural analgesia after ambulatory orthopedic surgery: a comparison of electronic versus elastomeric pumps. Anesth Analg 2003;96(2):414–417.
144. Ilfeld B, Morey T, Kayser Enneking F. Portable infusion pumps used for continuous regional analgesia: delivery rate accuracy and consistency. Reg Anesth Pain Med 2003(5);28:424–432.
145. Klein SM, Grant SA, Greengrass RA, et al. Interscalene brachial plexus block infusion pump. Anesth Analg 2000;91:1473–1478.
146. Klein SM, Nielsen KC, Greengrass RA, Aarner DS, Martin A, Steele S. Ambulatory discharge after long-acting peripheral nerve blockade: 2382 blocks with ropivacaine. Anesth Analg 2002;94:65–90.
147. Shah S, Vloka JD, Hadzic A. The future of ambulatory surgery and regional anesthesia. In: Steele S, Nielsen KC, Klein SM, eds. Ambulatory Anesthesia and Perioperative Analgesia. New York: McGraw-Hill; 2005:553–559.

# 17 Complications of Regional Anesthesia in Chronic Pain Therapy

Philip W.H. Peng and Vincent W.S. Chan

Interest in interventional pain management is on the rise, as indicated by an increased enrollment into the anesthesiology pain fellowship programs in North America.[1] The prevalence of treatment-related complications has also increased, as suggested in a recent Closed Claims study.[2] In this chapter, we discuss sympathetic, visceral, and somatic blocks frequently used in the management of chronic pain. To understand how complications arise, it is necessary to review the anatomy and techniques of the blocks, which can be used for diagnostic or therapeutic purposes. It is also important to understand some of the unique drugs used in this setting (e.g., neurolytic agents and corticosteroids). In general, procedure-related damage can result from needle insertion, misplacement or unanticipated spread of the drug, drug toxicity, injection of the wrong substance, or from an idiosyncratic reaction. Postblock physiologic changes may also add to complications.

## Sympathetic Blocks

Sympathetic blockade techniques are frequently used in the diagnosis and treatment of sympathetically mediated pain syndromes, limb ischemia or hypoperfusion, and visceral pain from cancer or nonmalignant conditions.[3] Diagnostic blocks with local anesthetic alone are often performed as a precursor to either a series of blocks or neurolytic block using phenol or ethanol.

### *Stellate Ganglion Block*

The stellate ganglion is formed by the fusion of the inferior cervical and first thoracic sympathetic ganglia lying on the longus colli muscle, anterior to the seventh cervical transverse process and neck of the first rib. The most common approach to the stellate ganglion is an anterior paratracheal approach at the level of the cricoid cartilage (C6). The needle is directed to the prominent anterior tubercle of C6 (Chassaignac's tubercle) followed by a large-volume local anesthetic injection (up to 20 mL). The sympathetic outflow to the head and neck region (cervical trunk) can be blocked independently of the fibers to the upper limb.[4] Thus, development of Horner's syndrome does not guarantee successful sympathetic blockade of the upper limb.

Also described are an anterior C7 paratracheal approach and a posterior T2 paravertebral approach.[5] The posterior approach aims to interrupt sympathetic outflow to the upper extremity with less chance of Horner's syndrome. Thus, it may be indicated for neurolytic blockade when long-term side effects are undesirable.

### Needle Trauma

Structures that lie close to the path of needle insertion are at theoretical, if not actual, risk of injury. Moore[6] documented puncture of pharynx, trachea, and esophagus. Pneumothorax is another recognized risk, especially with the anterior C7 approach, as the dome of the pleura may extend 2.5 cm above the level of the first rib, especially on the right side. The risk of pneumothorax is increased further in tall, thin persons. The incidence of pneumothorax is up to 4% with the posterior approach, which shares many of the risks of the thoracic paravertebral sympathetic block.

### Intravascular Injection

The vessel most at risk for intravascular injection during stellate ganglion block is the vertebral artery. At the level of C7, the vertebral artery lies anterior to the stellate ganglion, before it swings posterior to enter the foramen transversarium of the sixth cervical transverse process. Thus, the anterior C7 paratracheal approach has a greater risk of vertebral artery puncture. Kozody et al.[7] have shown that as little as 2.5 mg of bupivacaine (a test dose) can cause major central nervous system (CNS) effects when accidentally injected into the vertebral artery. A smaller 1-mL test dose is recommended. Intravertebral artery local anesthetic injection may produce dizziness, nausea, light-headedness, and hypotension with low dose and can result in coma, convulsion, and respiratory depression in high dose.[8] These are attributed to the direct effects of local anesthetic on medullary and pontine centers. The duration and nature of the toxic effects depend on the dose injected and global and regional cerebral blood flow, as well as the precise neurovascular anatomy. Local anesthetic-induced neurologic symptoms, which appear after a low-dose injection, are often short-lived (minutes).

Accidental injection of air into the vertebral artery, with subsequent cerebral air embolism was reported by Adelman.[9] This complication represents two errors, not just one. Other vascular structures at risk are the carotid and jugular vessels, which lie lateral to the needle path, but there are no recent reports of puncture.

### Intraspinal Injection

Nerve roots of the brachial plexus exiting from intervertebral foramen may have an accompanying dural cuff. The vertebral canal and its contents lie posteromedial to the stellate ganglion. Thus, dural puncture may occur,[10] either as a result of needle placement too medial or injection into a lateral extension of the perineural dural cuff of the cervical somatic nerve root. Intrathecal injection of local anesthetic will produce a high spinal block, characterized by loss of consciousness, high motor block, hypotension, and apnea. This serious complication necessitates ventilatory and hemodynamic support until it wears off. Subdural injection has also been reported.[11]

Wulf and Maier,[12] in a survey of approximately 45,000 stellate ganglion blocks performed in Germany, reported six subarachnoid blocks and three high epidural injections. Most important of all, care should be taken to avoid inadvertent injection of neurolytic agents into the epidural, subdural, or subarachnoid spaces, because this may lead to long-term neurologic deficit.

### Anomalous Spread of Drug

Even when the drug is injected into the correct anatomic plane, anomalous spread may cause complications. Both bilateral recurrent laryngeal nerve palsy and contralateral Horner's syndrome have been reported.[13] Bilateral block causes unopposed vocal cord adduction and airway obstruction. Local anesthetic spread posteriorly and anterolaterally can produce brachial plexus blockade and phrenic nerve block, respectively. Because of the possibility of somatic spread, it is necessary to check for normal sensory and motor function in the blocked limb when evaluating the success of the sympathetic block.

### Drug Effects

Extensive blockade of the cardiac sympathetic nerves has been reported following a properly performed stellate ganglion block. This resulted in bradycardia, secondary to unopposed vagal tone.[14] Schlack et al.[15] demonstrated in a canine model that left stellate ganglion blockade caused impairment of left ventricular function. The mechanism was asymmetric cardiac contraction and asynchrony, caused by loss of sympathetic tone in the anteroapical segment of the left ventricle, supplied by the left sympathetic chain. Although it is difficult to extrapolate these animal data to humans, who may have different patterns of myocardial innervation, the authors suggest that it may remain a risk in patients with already compromised cardiac function. Data to confirm this are lacking.

One case of migraine has been reported following a stellate ganglion block, presumably caused by an idiosyncratic reaction and a loss of unilateral sympathetic tone in the cerebral vasculature.[16] Absorption of correctly injected local anesthetics to toxic levels is unlikely in stellate ganglion blockade, because the mass of drug used is usually within the therapeutic range.[17] There have been no recent reports of injection of the wrong drug, but it remains a theoretical possibility.

## *Thoracic and Lumbar Sympathetic Blockade*

The sympathetic chain lies in the paravertebral region, receiving fibers from somatic nerve roots via the rami communicantes. In the thoracic region, it lies adjacent to the neck of the ribs, relatively close to the somatic nerve roots and the parietal pleura. Pneumothorax is definitely a possible complication. For this reason, the transcutaneous approach to the thoracic sympathetic chain without radiologic imaging support is not frequently performed. Long-lasting thoracic sympathectomy is usually achieved by surgical ablation, either by thoracotomy or, more recently, thoracoscopy.

In the lumbar region, the sympathetic chain and its ganglia lie on the anterolateral border of the vertebral bodies, separated from the somatic nerve roots by the psoas muscle and fascia. The ganglia are found in variable locations but most consistently found at the L3 level.[18] The classical paramedian technique requires the insertion of a needle 5–6 cm from the posterior midline with the patient in the prone position. The needle passes through the paravertebral muscles, "walks off" the transverse process of L2, L3, or L4, and passes through the psoas muscle and fascia to reach the lumbar sympathetic chain in the anterolateral aspect of the vertebra.

The other approach is more lateral, using fluoroscopy to determine the needle insertion point so that it will pass lateral to the transverse process en route to the anterolateral border of the L2, L3, or L4 vertebrae. The volume of local anesthetic injection also varies, from high volume (e.g., 20 mL) at a single level to low volume at multiple levels. Although no study to date has demonstrated superiority of one approach over the other, the single-level, high-volume technique seems to be most popular.[19]

### Intraspinal and Intravascular Injection

The vertebral column and the spinal canal lie posteromedial to the sympathetic chain. Injection of local anesthetic in the spinal canal is rare, but theoretically possible. Intraspinal injection (intrathecal, epidural, or subdural) and postdural puncture headache (PDPH) can follow puncture of either an extended dural cuff or the intraspinal dura.[20,21] Intravascular injection is a possible complication, because both the aorta and inferior vena cava lie anterior to the sympathetic chain. Puncture of these structures is rarely reported, but it occurs in clinical setting. The vertebral venous plexus is another vascular structure at risk, because it is close to the path of the needle. The risk of intravascular injection into either a perivertebral vein or a major vessel should be minimized by appropriate use of fluoroscopy and contrast medium before the injection of local anesthetic or neurolytic agents.

#### Needle Trauma

Confirmation of needle position with fluoroscopy is necessary when performing neurolytic blocks of the lumbar sympathetic ganglia. The risks of "blind" technique are needle trauma to the kidney, ureter, and bowel. In a cadaver study, three of 80 "blind" needle attempts resulted in needle impalement in grossly osteoporotic vertebral bodies or the hilum of the kidney.[22] These incidents would have been prevented by the use of fluoroscopy.

#### Drug Effects

Complications can occur from the drug used in the sympatholysis, from either local anesthetics or neurolytic agents. Significant sympathetic blockade and postural hypotension may occur, as part of physiologic response to a drug. Another possible undesirable effect is sexual dysfunction in male patients, although this may also be caused by vascular insufficiency, an indication for lumbar sympathetic block in the first place. There remains a possibility that sympathetic blockade of a limb where there is critical fixed stenosis of the arterial supply to one region may vasodilate only the normal vasculature. This will give rise to a "steal" syndrome – deterioration of perfusion to the ischemic area, if there is a fixed inflow.

The most frequent complication associated with lumbar chemical sympathectomy is genitofemoral neuralgia.[23] The genitofemoral nerve arises from the lumbar plexus at the first lumbar segmental level and passes on the ventral surface of the psoas muscle. It emerges from the anterior aspect to supply the groin and upper thigh. The incidence varies between 4% and 15% and most cases are transient, lasting less than 6 weeks.[24]

Ureteric injury is uncommon but can happen following chemical sympathectomy.[25] Whether injury is related to needle trauma or ureterolysis from the neurolytic agents is unclear. Most case reports claimed fluoroscopic confirmation of needle location and delayed presentation of urologic symptoms, suggesting that injury is more likely related to the neurolytic agent. This highlights the importance of limiting the amount of neurolytic agents applied.

### *Intravenous Regional Sympathetic Block*

The technique of intravenous sympathetic blockade has become widespread for treatment of sympathetically mediated pain in the upper limb. The technique is essentially one of perfusion of the isolated limb with a sympatholytic solution. After an interval of 20–30 minutes, when the drug can be assumed to have become fixed to the tissues, the tourniquet is deflated. The block is repeated, usually weekly for three to six times (see Chapter 13).

Sympatholytic agents used for intravenous regional sympathetic block are guanethidine (not available for this use in the United States), bretylium, reserpine, phentolamine, and ketanserin. Guanethidine is one group of drugs that block reuptake of noradrenaline in sympathetic nerve endings for up to 3 days, thus depleting the stores. It should not be used in patients on monoamine oxidase inhibitors for this reason, because there is an initial release of amine from the stores. Guanethidine is usually used in a dose of 10–20mg in up to 40mL of saline or dilute local anesthetic for upper limb. The dose and the volume are usually higher for the lower limb. A recent review on the use of this block in patients with peripheral neuropathic pain and complex regional pain syndromes suggests this block is not an effective analgesic compared with control (normal saline).[26]

**Drug Effects**

Despite the relative simplicity of the technique, there is a risk of unwanted systemic absorption if the drug bypasses the inflated tourniquet or after it is released. Transient decrease in blood pressure on tourniquet release is common,[27] although Sharpe et al.[28] reported prolonged hypotension (80 mm Hg for 1 week) after repeated blocks. Autonomic denervation caused by drug accumulation may be responsible.

Other adverse events following cuff deflation were transient apnea and syncope during intravenous regional anesthesia using guanethidine and lidocaine.[29] Whether this neurologic event was attributable to hypotension or toxic drug reaction is unclear.

### *Celiac Plexus Block*

The celiac plexus innervates the upper abdominal viscera, including pancreas, diaphragm, liver, spleen, stomach, small bowel, ascending and proximal transverse colon, adrenal glands, kidneys, abdominal aorta, and mesentery. It contains preganglionic splanchnic afferent, postganglionic sympathetic fibers, and parasympathetic fibers. Celiac plexus blockade may therefore be indicated in chronic or cancer pain involving these organs – pancreas and stomach being most common.

The greater (T5-10), lesser (T10-11), and least (T12) splanchnic nerves form the preganglionic sympathetic supply for the celiac ganglia. These nerves lie on the thoracic paravertebral border, pierce the diaphragmatic crura, and form the plexus lying on the anterior and lateral aspects of the abdominal aorta, between the origins of the celiac arterial axis and the renal arteries. The celiac ganglia number between one and five and may be up to 4.5 cm in diameter.

Four techniques of blocking the splanchnic nerve and celiac plexus are frequently used. The first is the retrocrural splanchnic nerve block technique. The needles, one on each side, are placed posteriorly and paravertebrally below the twelfth rib and advanced mediad to make contact with the L1 vertebral body. With this approach, the aim is to position the needle tip close to the splanchnic nerves behind the aorta and the diaphragm. A modification of this classical retrocrural technique is to direct the needle more cephalad at the level of the anterolateral margin of T12 vertebra. The theoretical advantage of this modification is to block the visceral sympathetic pathway more effectively with a smaller amount of neurolytic solution.

The second approach is the transcrural technique[30] to block the celiac plexus proper by positioning the needles (one on each side) farther anterior and through the diaphragmatic crura. Under radiologic guidance, the drug is deposited anterior and caudal to the crura and posterior to the aorta. A smaller volume of drug is needed, thus minimizing the risk of somatic block. The third approach is the transaortic approach developed by Ischia[31] using a single needle from the left side of the back. The advantages of this technique are a single needle insertion and a smaller dose requirement of local anesthetic or neurolytic agent, and so a lower risk of retrocrural somatic spread. However, there is a slightly higher risk of hematoma formation.

The fourth approach is a percutaneous anterior approach. Fine needles guided by ultrasound may be used.[32] Visceral or vascular perforation can occur, but the sequelae of perforation may be minimized by antibiotic coverage and avoidance of the technique in "coagulopathic" patients. Celiac plexus block can also be performed under direct vision at the end of laparotomy. Alternatively, endoscopic ultrasound–guided injection is a safe and cost-effective approach.[33] With an ultrasound transducer mounted in front of the viewing lens of the endoscope, the aorta and celiac artery can be easily identified as reference landmarks before injection.

### Hypotension

Because of the sympathetic blockade of splanchnic vasculature, the most common complication of celiac plexus blockade is hypotension. Without adequate prehydration or vasopressor drugs, this may occur in 30%–60% of patients. In a metaanalysis of neurolytic celiac plexus blocks, Eisenberg et al.[34] reported 10 studies covering 571 patients, of whom 217 (38%) had hypotension. Splanchnic vasodilatation and visceral blood pooling contribute to orthostatic hypotension. For this reason, it is recommended that blood pressure and the electrocardiogram be monitored for 2 hours after a block. After block, the patients should remain supine or in the lateral position for at least 1 hour, or until they can stand unaided. A degree of postural hypotension may last up to 2 days.

### Diarrhea

Unopposed parasympathetic activity following celiac plexus block can lead to gastrointestinal hypermotility.[35] Additionally, after a successful celiac plexus block, the patient will need smaller doses of opiate analgesics. The incidence of transient diarrhea may be up to 44%,[34] lasting a few days, but rarely persisting longer. When diarrhea occurs in the presence of preexisting dehydration and pooling of blood in the splanchnic circulation, life-threatening hypovolemia may appear if massive intestinal fluid loss is not replaced. Somatostatin has been suggested as therapy in this situation, and octreotide may have a role in treatment of persistent diarrhea.

### Needle Trauma

Needle puncture and drug injection into the aorta, vena cava, renal vessels, and various viscera have been reported.[36] The anatomy may be distorted by tumor or other mass in the retroperitoneum or abdomen. One expects the risk of hematoma formation to be highest with Ischia's transaortic approach. Aortic puncture is more likely with needle placement on the left side than on the right side. A large retroperitoneal hematoma after vascular puncture may cause hypovolemia and must be differentiated from hypotension caused by splanchnic vasodilatation. Limiting the size of needle and ensuring normal patient coagulation status will reduce the risk of bleeding.

Aortic dissection after formation of an infected pseudoaneurysm has been reported after celiac plexus block,[37] possibly related to the effect of neurolytic agent on the aortic wall. Kaplan et al.[38] reported fatal aortic dissection, which extended to the superior mesenteric and hepatic artery, resulting in extensive liver and bowel infarction.

Unintentional injection between vertebrae producing an incidental discogram was reported by Wilson.[39] Pneumothorax is another theoretical complication, even though the point of needle insertion is below the twelfth rib. Chylothorax has been reported in association with tumor and after puncture of the cisterna chyli during celiac plexus block.[40] The cisterna chyli classically lies anterior to the first two lumbar vertebrae to the right of the aorta, but this is variable. The transdiaphragmatic movement of the retroperitoneal lymph collection is via the lymphatics. Retroperitoneal fibrosis after multiple blocks has been reported.[41]

### Infection

Because of the proximity of the needle path to the bowel, especially with the anterior and endoscopic ultrasound approach, infection is a concern. Retroperitoneal abscess has been reported.[42,43]

### Neurologic and Neurovascular Sequelae

The most serious complications of celiac plexus block are neurologic.[44] There are several mechanisms. Drug misplacement and anomalous or excessive retrocrural spread can affect epidural and lumbar somatic nerve roots. Direct accidental intrathecal injection can also occur. Unintended intrathecal injection of neurolytic agents will lead to permanent paraplegia. Permanent and extensive autonomic blockade may cause male sexual dysfunction.

The arterial supply to the spinal cord may be damaged during celiac plexus block. The anatomy of the blood supply is variable, and the major radicular artery of Adamkiewicz may arise from T7 to L4. In 80% of cases it lies on the left. It enters via a single intervertebral foramen to supply the anterior spinal artery of the lower two-thirds of the cord. Damage to this artery (either mechanical by a needle or chemical by neurolytic drug) may lead to paraplegia. Although radiologically guided techniques minimize the incidence of direct intravascular injection, neurolytic drugs deposited perivascularly may alter arterial reactivity and cause vasospasm. This has been demonstrated in isolated canine lumbar arteries in vitro.[45]

There are several reports of paraplegia following neurolytic celiac plexus block using phenol[46] or alcohol.[47] Injury to artery of Adamkiewicz caused by compression, spasm, or both can lead to anterior spinal artery syndrome.[48] There is a possibility that using only a right-sided approach might lessen the incidence, but it might also diminish the effectiveness. A few reports of transient and reversible paraplegia have also been reported after alcohol celiac plexus block.[49]

The incidence of paraplegia is difficult to estimate, because the total number of blocks performed is not known. It may lie between 0.1% and 0.5%, based on a metaanalysis by Eisenberg et al.[34] Davies[50] surveyed complications of all blocks done in a 5-year period (1986–1990) in England and found four patients with paraplegia among 2730 blocks. Alcohol (50%–99%) was injected under fluoroscopic control in all four patients. This gives a major neurologic complication rate of 1 in 683 (0.15%). In a review by Fugere and Lewis,[51] the overall incidence of all complications (as detailed above plus pain) was approximately 1.8% in 20 series covering 30 years.

In addition to arterial complications, superior mesenteric venous thrombosis has also been reported.[52]

## Drug Effects

Phenol-induced cardiotoxicity may account for a report of cardiac arrest in a patient undergoing intraoperative splanchnic nerve block during laparotomy.[53] Ventricular fibrillation occurred 3 minutes after injection of 30 mL of 6.66% phenol, after negative aspiration under direct vision. The authors cite other reports of cardiac toxicity of phenol, mostly arising from transdermal absorption in dermatologic and plastic surgical practice, where much higher doses are used.

Systemic effects have been reported as a result of absorption of a large volume of alcohol administered for retrocrural celiac plexus block. Measured serum ethanol concentration was up to 39 mg/dL after an injection of 25 mL of 50% ethanol bilaterally[54] and 29 mg/dL after 15 mL of 99.5% ethanol.[55] Although this will not cause any serious impairment, and is below the legally defined limit for intoxication, the authors noted that all patients reported a feeling of mild euphoria. However, toxic alcohol levels may appear in patients who have a genetic deficiency of aldehyde dehydrogenase, which is relatively common in the Japanese population. There is also a possibility of interaction with drugs such as disulfiram or metronidazole, although this has not so far been reported.

In summary, the retrocrural technique has the lowest risk of visceral or vascular puncture, but a higher risk of somatic nerve block because of a larger volume of drug. Transcrural injection requires smaller volumes but has a slightly increased risk of perforation of vital visceral structures. Transaortic celiac plexus block, a single-needle technique, uses the least amount of drug but most likely causes vascular damage and hematoma formation even with a fine needle.

### *Other Visceral Nerve Blocks*

The superior hypogastric nerve and the ganglion impar are two other sites amenable to blockade for chronic or cancer pain of the lower abdominal or pelvic organs.[56] The superior hypogastric plexus is found on the anterior aspect of the sacrum, in the midline. Approach to the superior hypogastric plexus is percutaneous, from a point between the sacral ala and the interspace between the L4 and L5. The needle passes anteromedially and caudad, lateral to the sacral nerve roots and medial to the iliac vessels. The ganglion impar lies on the concavity of the sacrum, and is blocked percutaneously using a specially bent needle inserted toward the sacrococcygeal junction. There are no recent reports of complications from block of this nerve.

### *Facet Joint Block*

The lumbar facet (zygapophyseal) joint has long been considered by some to be a significant source of low back pain[57] whereas cervical facet joint disease is linked to chronic neck pain. The facet or zygapophyseal joints are true synovial joints with considerable sensory innervation and overlap. The medial branch of the posterior ramus supplies the lower pole of one facet joint and the upper pole of the adjoining facet joint.

A diagnostic facet joint injection or a medial branch block may be considered for patients with back pain. Both blocks are believed to have equal diagnostic sensitivity.[58] Real-time fluoroscopic guidance is recommended to ensure accurate needle placement because being off target by a few millimeters can result in aberrant drug spread to intervertebral neural foramen and the epidural space, yielding false-positive results of pain relief.[59] Injection of contrast material (0.5 mL) can enhance accuracy, and local anesthetic injection of 1–1.5 mL (small volume) will decrease the risk of spread to the epidural space or somatic nerves. In the neck, the vertebral artery lies just lateral to the facet joint; thus intravascular injection or damage is a theoretical risk, but so far it has not been reported.

Medial branch block is an easier procedure to perform, also under X-ray control, and is indicated in patients with severe arthritis and narrowed or obliterated joint space. In the neck, the medial branch is farther from the vertebral artery than the facet joint itself.

#### **Increased Pain**

Transient increased pain is the most common side effect (2%–20%) which may last from 6 weeks to 8 months.[60]

#### **Intraspinal Injection**

Spinal anesthesia following attempted lumbar facet block has been reported.[61] These cases may be attributable to erroneous needle placement, possibly through a nerve root dura cuff.

Thomson et al.[62] reported chemical meningism after attempted facet joint block with local anesthetic and steroids, and this was presumably caused by inadvertent intrathecal injection, because there are very few reports of meningism associated with epidural injection of steroids.

#### **Other Complications**

Paraspinal abscess formation and septic joint arthritis have been reported following facet joint injection.[63,64] Excessive local anesthetic injection and spread to the somatic roots can cause ipsilateral weakness, although we have found no recent reports of this obvious complication. This may be caused by excessive anterior needle placement, or excess volume causing joint rupture. It should be remembered that the maximum volume of the facet joint is 1.5 mL.

## Radiofrequency Techniques

Radiofrequency neurotomy interrupts nociceptive pathways by applying heat (60°–75°C) from the tip of an electrode to denervate nerves. This technique is used for treatment of trigeminal neuralgia, dorsal rhizotomy, and dorsal root entry zone interruption for deafferentation syndromes.[65] Radiofrequency procedures can also be used for facet joint denervation in the lumbar and cervical regions. The complications are essentially those caused by needle trauma, needle misplacement, and the low-level heat injury to the nerve. Postblock pain is common in the first 2 weeks after radiofrequency treatment. Cutaneous numbness and dysesthesia is also common but usually resolves in 3 weeks.[65]

## Epidural Blockade

The epidural space may be approached in the cervical, thoracic, lumbar, or sacral regions (via sacral hiatus). The most frequently injected agents are steroids and dilute local anesthetics, although opioid has been used in some circumstances.[19,66] The main indication for epidural steroid injection is relief of radicular pain.[67,68] The transforaminal approach to the epidural space has become popular in recent years because it has proven clinical efficacy over conventional techniques.[69] In the lumbar spine, the needle is aimed at the superior and ventral quadrant of the neural foramen and in cervical spine, the posterior half of the foramen abutting the anterior surface of superior articular process.[70] The major advantage of this approach is drug delivery directly to the site of nerve root impingement, as opposed to only a fraction of the injected dose reaching target with the conventional interlaminar approach.[71]

### *Complications of Epidural Steroid Administration*

Although epidural steroid injection is considered to be safe, life-threatening complications have occurred. This is a major cause of malpractice claims related to chronic pain management in North America.[2,72] Complications specific to steroid injection relate to local or systemic drug effects. Mechanical and traumatic complications can also occur and they are the same as with any epidural injection and are discussed elsewhere (Chapter 10). Specific complications that are discussed include drug neurotoxicity, arachnoiditis, infection, systemic effects of steroids and opioids, and serious neurologic complications related to the transforaminal approach.

#### Arachnoiditis

Arachnoiditis following intentional subarachnoid injection of methylprednisolone acetate can happen. This is documented in a comprehensive review by Abram and O'Connor[73] covering 65 published series and 18 case reports in 6947 patients who received one or more epidural steroid injections and 368 patients who received one or more subarachnoid steroid injections. There were *no* reports of arachnoiditis after epidural injection of steroids when intrathecal injection was excluded. One of the components of the vehicle, polyethylene glycol, has been implicated as the cause of neurotoxicity. Benzon et al.[74] found that nerve conduction was affected by polyethylene glycol at concentrations much higher (seven times) than clinical relevant concentrations. Even at higher concentrations, the conduction defects were reversible. It should be noted that in clinical practice, the solution is always diluted further with either saline or local anesthetic.

#### Infectious Sequelae

The risks of neuraxial infection are present when faulty aseptic technique or bacteremia is present, as for any spinal injection (see Chapter 7). In theory, the immunosuppressive effects of steroids may increase this risk. Epidural abscess following epidural steroid injection have been reported.[75,76] The patients affected were usually diabetic and the most common bacteria cultured was *Staphylococcus aureus*, a likely skin contaminant. However, a recent report described an intradural abscess resulting from epidural steroid injections in a young immunocompetent patient.[77] The culture grew *Aspergillus fumigatus*. Dougherty and Fraser[78] reported bacterial meningitis in two patients. These two cases seem to have been caused by dural puncture and not transdural bacterial spread. Cooper and Sharpe[79] reported a case of *S. aureus* meningitis after repeated epidural steroid injections at weekly intervals.

It would seem that, despite the theoretical increased risk of infection, clinical reports do not indicate that there is any greater incidence associated with epidural steroids than with local anesthetic agents alone, provided the same precautions and contraindications are noted. Even allowing for underreporting, the incidence just from published series and reports appears to be less than 0.01%. Diabetes seems to predispose patients to this complication.

### Systemic Side Effects of Steroid

Suppression of adrenal cortical response has been reported after oral, nasal, inhaled, and parenteral as well as epidural steroid administration. Cushingoid side effects, including fluid retention, electrolyte imbalance, and fat redistribution, have been reported after epidural steroid injections. Stambough et al.[80] reported a case of hypercorticism after two injections a week apart totaling 160mg of methylprednisolone acetate, whereas Tuel et al.[81] reported one case following a single cervical epidural administration of 60mg methylprednisolone acetate. In both cases, return of normal clinical and biochemical functions took weeks to months. Knight and Burnell[82] had reported three occurrences of clinical symptoms consistent with Cushing's syndrome after multiple epidural injections when methylprednisolone acetate, 200mg, was exceeded, in a series of injections over less than 2 weeks. There was no laboratory confirmation.

Iatrogenically induced steroid myopathy (proximal limb) was reported by Boonen et al.[83] after epidural triamcinolone diacetate 60mg. Biochemical adrenal suppression lasted 12 weeks. This case probably represents one tail of a distribution of susceptibility to systemic effect against dosage of steroid given. Maillefert et al.[84] demonstrated biochemical adrenal suppression in a group of nine patients for up to 21 days after a single epidural injection of dexamethasone acetate, 15mg. Clinical signs and symptoms were absent. Kay et al.[85] investigated the effect on the hypothalamic-pituitary-adrenal axis of a series of three epidural injections of methylprednisolone acetate 80mg, at weekly intervals. They also investigated the suppressive effects of concomitant sedation with midazolam, an imidazo-benzodiazepine, a class of drugs known to cause adrenal suppression. Of their 14 patients, five had a subnormal plasma cortisol response to injections of synthetic adrenocorticotropic hormone 1 month after the final epidural injection, but all returned to normal by 3 months. The adrenal suppressive effect of midazolam lasted less than 15 minutes. Significant adrenal suppression was detected in the weeks between the injections although there was no clinical abnormality in any patient. Jacobs et al.[86] suggested that exogenous steroid replacement should be considered for patients having surgery who have had epidural steroids between 1 and 3 months earlier, although the authors were unable to specify predictive factors associated with occurrence or duration of adrenal suppression.

Animal work by Gorski et al.[87] demonstrated failure of adrenal response after experimental hypoglycemia in beagle dogs. The study group of 12 dogs received bupivacaine plus triamcinolone, 2mg/kg epidurally, and showed no increase in plasma cortisol in response to insulin-induced hypoglycemic stress for 4 weeks. The control group all showed the expected increase.

Although there is no consensus for the frequency or dose of steroid administration to prevent systemic side effects, it is prudent not to repeat injections within a 4-week interval and to limit to a maximum of three epidural steroid injections in 6 months based on human and animal data. A recent survey showed that the above clinical guideline was being followed.[19]

### Systemic Side Effects of Epidural Opioid

The addition of epidural morphine to steroid may further relieve low back pain[88] but the associated benefits vary.[89,90] Most of these early studies added 8mg of epidural morphine to the steroid. However, life-threatening ventilatory depression was noted in 3 of 14 patients who received an admixture of steroid and morphine (8mg).[91] Although lower-dose epidural opioid (e.g., morphine 5mg) has been used, the effect produces analgesia for up to 24 hours.[92] The common side effects are pruritus (57%–90%), nausea and vomiting (40%–64%), and urinary retention (20%–43%).[89–92]

Recent surveys show that 2%–10% of anesthesiologists in North America add opioid to epidural steroids.[19,66] It is important to realize that epidural opioids not only have no proven long-term benefits, but death or brain death has been cited in a recent Closed Claims study when injected with epidural steroid.[2] Although the cause–effect relationship cannot be established, clinicians must carefully weigh the limited benefit of epidural opioid against potential serious risks.

### Severe Neurologic Complication Associated with Transforaminal Injections

Although no major complications were reported in two large case series of more than 1000 transforaminal steroid injections,[93,94] severe neurologic complications appeared in subsequent reports.[95] Following cervical transforaminal injections, a fatal anterior spinal artery syndrome,[96] massive cerebellar infarct,[97] and bilateral complete cortical blindness[98] have been reported. Transforaminal injections at lumbar or sacral nerve roots have also resulted in severe paraparesis or paraplegia in four patients.[99,100] Most worrisome is that most of these incidents happened despite fluoroscopic or computed tomography (CT) scan guidance and a presumed "uneventful" injection.

Vascular injury has been implicated as magnetic resonance imaging (MRI) showed spinal cord infarct in these cases. The blood supply to the spinal cord comes from a single anterior spinal artery and two posterior spinal arteries. At each vertebral level, radicular arteries from the aorta travel along with the segmental nerve roots into the neural foramen and supply the corresponding nerve roots. Some of these radicular branches contribute to the perfusion of the anterior spinal cord by joining the anterior spinal artery. The most important radicular artery supplying the lumbar region is the artery of Adamkiewicz (anatomic location discussed earlier in this chapter). In the cervical level, the important contributing radicular artery originates between C3 and C8. Needle trauma to one of the radicular arteries is the likely mechanism of spinal cord injury. Alternatively, the anterior spinal cord circulation can be compromised by a steroid embolus when the preparation is injected intravascularly by accident.[101] Tiso et al.[97] found that both triamcinolone acetonide (Kenalog-40; Bristol-Myers Squibb, Princeton, NJ) and methylprednisolone acetate (Depo-medrol; Pharmacia & Upjohn, Kalamazoo, MI) preparations contain large particles capable of occluding metarterioles and arterioles.

The rate of unintentional intravascular injection using the transforaminal approach is estimated to be 11%.[94] Measures taken to prevent intravascular injection include real-time fluoroscopic guidance and avoidance of needle movement before and during injection. It is important to note that the sensitivity of a positive blood aspirate in detecting intravascular injections is only 45%.

TABLE 17-1. Complications and side effects of epidural steroid injection (interlaminar and caudal approach): aggregate data from published series

| Injection type | No. reported | Complications or side effects | No. (%) |
|---|---|---|---|
| Cervical epidural injections | 1,788* | Neck stiffness,[102] pain[103] | 40 (2.2) |
| | | Facial flushing[102,103] | 24 (1.3) |
| | | Headache[103] | 16 (0.9) |
| | | Nausea/vomiting[102] | 10 (0.6) |
| | | Hypotension (including vagal)[103,104] | 9 (0.5) |
| | | Dural tap[102–104] | 7 (0.4) |
| | | Other (fever, insomnia[103]) | 7 (0.4) |
| Cervical subtotal | | | 123 (6.9) |
| Lumbar, thoracic, and caudal epidural injections | 13,233* | Headache[105–107] | 45 (0.34) |
| | | Dural tap[108,109] | 35 (0.26) |
| | | Hypotension (including vagal)[107,110] | 17 (0.13) |
| | | Systemic steroid effects[111,112] | 6 (0.05) |
| | | Facial flushing[107] | 6 (0.05) |
| | | Other (fever,[113] nausea, bloody tap,[111] DVT,[106] insomnia,[107] increased back/leg pain[107]) | 26 (0.20) |
| Lumbar, thoracic, and caudal subtotal | | | 125 (0.94) |
| Total | 15,021* | All of the above | 248 (1.65) |

*The total number referred to the number of injections in the case series reported in references 73 (review), 102–111, and 114. A number of case series reported no side effects or complications and the references would not be shown in the table.

### Other reactions

Various minor complications have been reported in different case series (Table 17-1).[102–114] Other complications reported in case reports are delayed allergic reaction to an epidural injection of triamcinolone and lidocaine,[115] persistent hiccup presumably caused by systemic effect of steroid,[116] vision loss secondary to retinal hemorrhage,[117] cervical epidural and subdural hematoma,[118,119] and direct spinal cord injury from needle trauma.[120]

In summary, epidural steroid injection is a safe procedure. However, severe and life-threatening complications have been one of the major causes of Closed Claims in North America because of the frequent use of this procedure. Physicians should be cognizant of the systemic effect of the steroid and limit the amount of steroid used and the number of injections per year. Transforaminal injections are gaining popularity but serious neurologic complications can occur. To avoid inadvertent intravascular injection, real-time fluoroscopy is recommended.

## Neural Ablative Procedures

Nerve destruction is reserved mainly as a last resort for patients with debilitating pain related to cancer[121] and occasionally, noncancer conditions (e.g., postherpetic neuralgia[122] and bone graft donor site[123]) that is refractory to conventional treatments. Neurolysis of peripheral nerves (e.g., sciatic, obturator nerves) has also been applied to relieve muscle spasticity following hemiplegic stroke.[124] Because neural ablative procedures are seldom practiced, few clinical studies have documented their relative clinical effectiveness, leaving the practice of these procedures rather empirical. Neurolysis can be achieved in a number of ways: chemically by neurolytic agents such as alcohol and phenol, by radiofrequency coagulation, cryoprobe, and surgery. For the purpose of this discussion, we will focus on complications associated with chemical neurolysis performed by regional anesthetic procedures.

Neurologic complications of chemical neurolysis are drug related and vary according to the site of injection – peripherally on a peripheral nerve and centrally in the epidural or subarachnoid space. Rarely, nonneurologic complications, e.g., bronchospasm secondary to accidental intrabronchial or intrapulmonary injection of phenol during an intercostal nerve block, occur.[125] Because neurologic complications are potentially devastating, it is important to select patients appropriately and include only those with limited life expectancy (no more than 6–12 months). The patient and family must have a clear understanding and realistic expectations before neurolytic procedures. Herein, we will highlight the use of peripheral and central neurolysis to treat malignant somatic pain. Neurolytic blocks for visceral and sympathetically mediated pain have been discussed earlier.

### *Neuropathic Effects of Neurolytic Agents*

Neurolytic agents are applied to section a nerve and disrupt its transmission chemically rather than surgically. Agents frequently used are phenol, alcohol, and glycerol. Less frequently used ones are ammonium sulfate, hypertonic saline, chlorocresol, and butyl aminobenzoate (Butamben). Phenol is usually prepared as an aqueous 5%–7% solution or as a concentrated 10%–12% solution in glycerin. Alcohol is used most often as a 95% solution. Because of the nature of the vehicle solution, phenol in glycerin is hyperbaric whereas alcohol is hypobaric; this is an important consideration when performing central neurolysis.

The neuropathic effect of alcohol and phenol is nonselective. When applied to neural tissues, phenol coagulates proteins and injures perineural blood vessels, causing neural ischemia; ethyl alcohol extracts from neural membrane cholesterol, phospholipid, and cerebroside and causes precipitation of lipoproteins and mucoproteins. There is no proof that small unmyelinated C fibers transmitting nociception are more vulnerable to neurolytic destruction than larger A beta sensory fibers for thermal and mechanical sensation.

### *Neurologic Complications*

Neurolytic agents destroy sensory, sympathetic, and motor nerve fibers indiscriminately, especially when used in high concentrations and large volumes. To lower the risk of neurologic deficit, needle placement must be accurate, aided by nerve stimulator or radiologic guidance. It is wise to first perform a prognostic local anesthetic block in the same target area before neurolysis. This prognostic block allows the patient and physician to assess the resultant pain relief and the extent of potential damage. Neurolytic agents also destroy extraneural structures. Before needle withdrawal, flushing of the needle with saline or air is recommended to avoid skin slough and muscle necrosis.

### *Motor Paresis*

Before a neurolytic agent is applied to peripheral mixed nerves supplying the upper or lower limb, patients must clearly understand that destruction of motor fibers can cause or increase limb weakness. For this reason, neurolysis is ideally reserved for patients with some degree of limb weakness. To preserve residual function, a dilute 3% phenol solution has been used successfully in neurolytic brachial plexus block to alleviate arm pain from lung malignancy.[126] However, analgesia is short-lived with this approach. Another way to limit harm is lesioning more selectively and peripherally at the target site. For example, Kaplan et al.[127] performed a selective paravertebral C5-6 nerve root block, and Patt and Millard[128] performed suprascapular block to treat malignant upper arm pain. The same risk-limiting measures apply when neurolytic block is performed in the lumbosacral plexus for lower extremity pain. On the contrary, although intercostal neurolysis to treat thoracic and abdominal wall pain can impair intercostal muscle function, the damage usually is of little physiologic consequence. However, proximal epidural spread has resulted in paraplegia following phenol intercostal neurolysis.[129]

Central neurolysis performed in the epidural or subarachnoid space can also result in postblock motor paresis.[130] Well-executed, central neurolysis produces neural ablation more selectively, because of greater separation of motor and sensory nerve roots at the spinal cord site of origin. The goal, therefore, is to execute a chemical dorsal rhizotomy (sensory) without ventral rhizotomy (motor).[121] If poorly executed, a cervical and lumbosacral central neurolysis can result in upper and lower limb paresis, respectively. Although rare, quadriplegia caused by anterior spinal artery syndrome has been reported following cervical intrathecal phenol injection.[131]

Subarachnoid phenol injection can cause motor paresis, in addition to sensory, bowel, and bladder dysfunction, as a result of posterior spinal artery thrombosis and spinal cord infarction.[132] Phenol, 8%–12%, and ethanol, 3%–6%, were shown to induce sustained contraction in isolated canine lumbar segmental arteries.[45] Both anterior and posterior spinal syndromes can occur, presumably secondary to vasospasm and/or thrombosis.

Again, one must limit risk by following some important principles. Strict selection criteria should apply to limit central neurolysis to patients with limited life expectancy and whose pain is localized to 2 or 3 dermatomes. First, one must appropriately pick the target of lesioning. For example, malignant pain of soft tissue is treated by targeting specific dermatomes (Figure 17-1), but bony pain in the same area must be treated

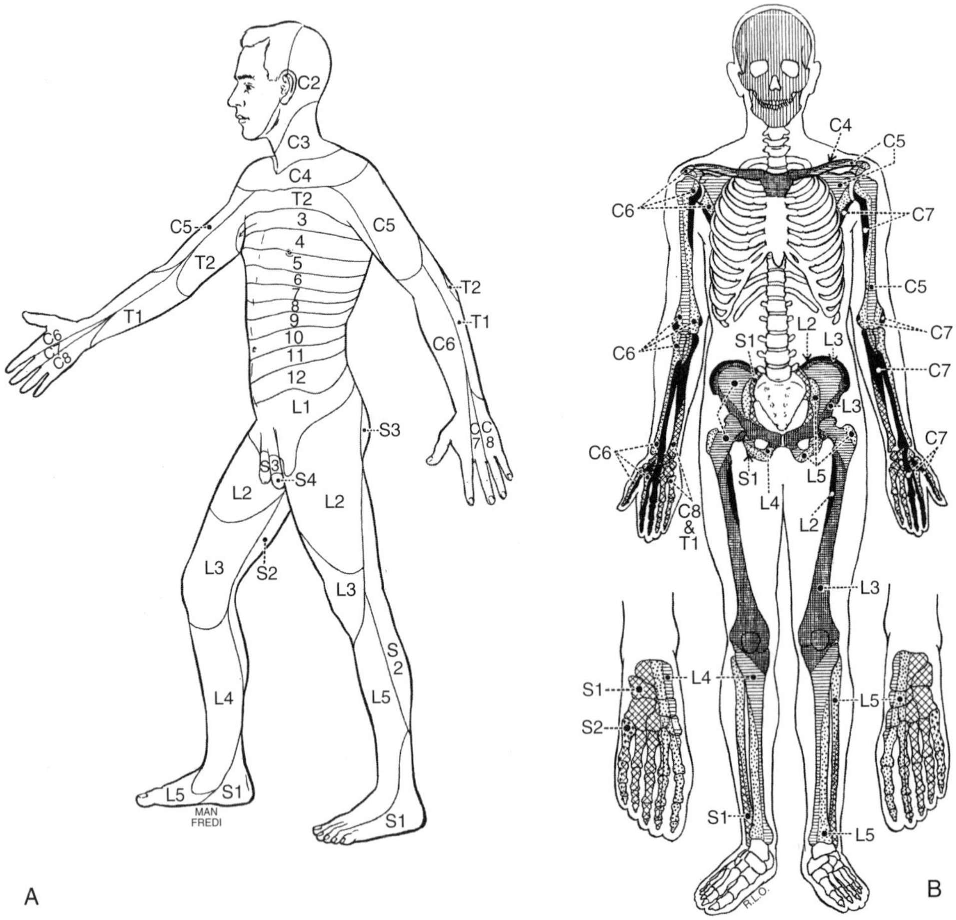


**FIGURE 17-1.** A side view of the dermatomes **(A)** and an anterior view of the sclerotomes indicated by the different styles of shading **(B)**. (Reprinted from Haymaker W, Woodhall B. Peripheral Nerve Injuries. Philadelphia: WB Saunders; 1945:20, 41, with permission from Elsevier.)

**FIGURE 17-2.** The alignment of spinal segments with vertebrae. The bodies and spinous processes of the vertebrae are indicated by Roman numerals, the spinal segments and their respective nerves by Arabic. Note the location where the spinal nerves exit through intervertebral foramina in relationship to their respective vertebral bodies. (Reprinted from Haymaker W, Woodhall B. Peripheral Nerve Injuries. Philadelphia: WB Saunders; 1945:24, with permission from Elsevier.)

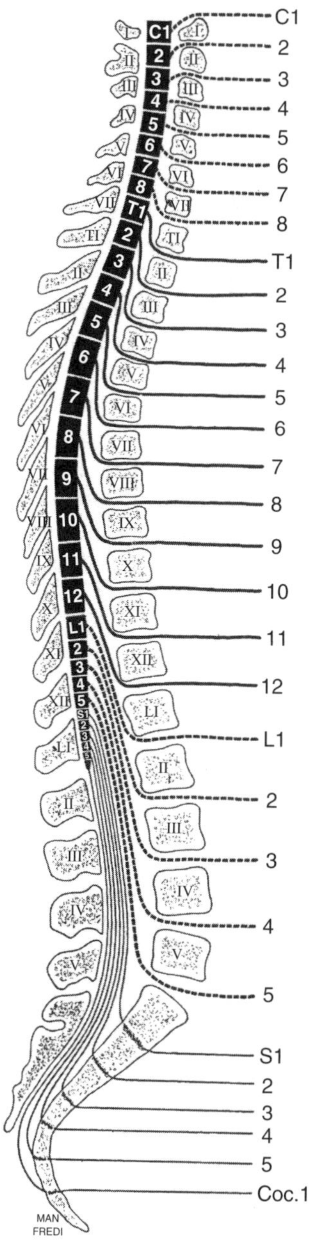


differently, by targeting the responsible sclerotomes, not dermatomes. Second, one must place the neurolytic agent as close to the targeted dorsal root as possible. It is important to recognize that the level at which a particular nerve root leaves the spinal cord is generally higher than the corresponding vertebral body. For example, L3 nerve root leaves the spinal cord at the level of T11-12 vertebral body. Thus, when doing a neurolysis of the L3 root, injection should be made at the T11-12 interspace and *not* L3 (Figure 17-2).

When performing subarachnoid neurolysis, patient positioning is crucial in order to limit inadvertent drug diffusion to the ventral root. Positioning varies according to the choice of neurolytic agent. If hypobaric alcohol is used, the pain site should be positioned uppermost; the opposite is the case when hyperbaric phenol in glycerin is used.[133] Furthermore, to target the dorsal root specifically, the patient should be positioned at a 45-degree angle anteriorly when using hypobaric solution but should be angled posteriorly when a hyperbaric solution is used. Also, the patient should remain in this position for at least 30–45 minutes after injection, to limit spread elsewhere.

Similar to peripheral neurolysis, it is always advisable to first perform a local anesthetic prognostic block to determine adequacy of analgesia, the extent of motor blockade, and paresthesia. One should remember that local anesthetic is not as hypobaric as alcohol, so the resultant block area may be somewhat different. During injection, dose fractionation using 0.1-mL aliquots of alcohol should be used to improve accuracy. If several dermatomal levels are to be blocked, separate subarachnoid injections should be made at each level. One must remember that alcohol does not diffuse well in cerebrospinal fluid (CSF), and injecting a large volume of alcohol at a single spinal level does not reliably block neighboring levels but increases the risk of motor paresis.

When epidural neurolysis is performed, complications can be minimized if an indwelling catheter is used, so that repeated injections can be given in small increments over several days. Before neurolysis, catheter position should be checked with local anesthetic (not more than 5 mL) to document correct spread of drug and correct catheter tip position in relation to dermatomal pain site. Dosing of neurolytic should be slow. For example, no more than 0.2 mL of alcohol is injected as a bolus and 3–5 mL is injected slowly over 20–30 minutes. Also, one must look for reports of tingling and numbness in nontarget areas (e.g., when doing a midthoracic neurolysis, paresthesia in the fifth finger or anterior thigh is indicative that spreading has gone to nontargeted T2 and L2-3 dermatomes. Neurolytic injection must be stopped right away.)[134]

### *Loss of Bladder and Bowel Control*

Destruction of the S2-4 parasympathetic fibers supplying the bladder, rectum, and colon can lead to urinary and fecal incontinence, respectively. Central neurolytic block performed in the lumbosacral region poses the greatest risk, although deficit following thoracic injection has also been reported.[135] Voiding is less likely to be affected after peripheral neurolysis even when performed in the sacral nerves.[136] So far, there is only one report of bladder atony after an S3 S4 alcohol block.[137] To limit risk, it is advisable to do preneurolysis local anesthetic prognostic blocks followed by urodynamic study, perform block under radiologic guidance, and limit injection volume (e.g., 1-mL aliquots at each sacral foramen).

### *Postblock Pain*

Reactive neuritis, neuroma formation, and deafferentation pain are causes of postneurolytic block pain in the denervated area after an initial period of pain relief. Painful paresthesia and neuritis develop in 2%–28% of patients after peripheral neurolysis with phenol or alcohol.[138] Raj[139] suggested that this may be the result of incomplete lesioning and pointed out that when phenol intercostal nerve block was executed with precision under direct vision, neither neuritis pain nor deafferentation pain occurred.[140] Many believed that alcohol is more likely to cause neuritis than phenol, but this is unproven.

Pain, in the form of mechanical hypersensitivity, can occur after peripheral neurolysis. This can be attributable to spontaneous firing of neuromas that were formed by sprouting of injured axons. Deafferentation pain can also appear as a new form of neuropathic pain. Dysesthesia and hyperalgesia may appear in an area of anesthesia, resembling the anesthesia dolorosa seen in gasserian ganglion neurolysis for trigeminal neuralgia. Thus, neurolysis should be limited to patients with short life expectancy.

## Implantable Catheters and Drug Delivery System

Implantable catheters are placed in the epidural[141,142] or subarachnoid (intrathecal)[143] space for long-term delivery of analgesics for treatment of debilitating pain from malignancy[144–146] and nonmalignant[147–149] conditions. Intrathecal analgesia may be preferred over the epidural route because of lower analgesic consumption, fewer drug refills, and fewer mechanical problems.[142,150] Additionally, subarachnoid infusion of baclofen[151] is sometimes used to treat lower limb spasticity from multiple sclerosis or quadriplegia.

There are three types of intraspinal drug delivery systems.[152] Implantable catheters can be connected to: 1) an internalized subcutaneous programmable pump (e.g., Synchromed Infusion Pump, Medtronic Inc.),[153] 2) a subcutaneous port (e.g., the Port-a-Cath port system, Pharmacia-Deltec, Inc.), or 3) an externalized delivery system (e.g., Algoline catheter, Medtronic Inc.). The indwelling end of the catheter in the neuraxial space is sutured in place before it is tunneled subcutaneously from the back to the front. Complications of implantable catheter and drug delivery systems are either mechanical or drug related.[154–156] The safety of the externalized delivery system has notably improved in recent years through a change from bolus administration to continuous infusions and modification of line-insertion techniques.[157] Data from literature surveys are summarized in Tables 17-2 and 17-3 giving the incidence of various complications.[158–179]

### *Infection*

Postimplantation infection is mostly localized but can become systemic. The risk of infection is higher in immunocompromised patients who have had radiation, chemotherapy, or chronic systemic (human immunodeficiency virus) or cutaneous infection. In patients with stomas (e.g., gastrostomy, enterostomy, or nephrostomy), it is important to direct the path of catheter away from these stoma sites, to avoid potential infection. Frequent change of bacterial filters can result in a higher incidence of catheter hub colonization.[180]

Localized infection such as an abscess can be formed anywhere along the implanted catheter. It can be superficial at the catheter exit site or deep in the subcutaneous pocket housing the access port and internalized pump, along the catheter tract, and in the epidural space. Superficial infection often produces purulent exudate at the catheter entry site or localized skin inflammation. A wound or pocket infection often presents as inflammatory skin changes overlying the infected area. Fever and leukocytosis may not appear in immunocompromised patients. Needle aspirate from local seroma or wound hematoma showing white blood cells and positive Gram stain confirms the diagnosis.

Epidural or intrathecal space infection and abscess encapsulation[181] are often manifested in the following manner: pain during injection (not previously present), retrograde flow of infusate and pooling of infused fluid in the paravertebral region, and decreased analgesia despite increased dose of analgesics. Spinal epidural abscess can also manifest as back pain, radicular signs, and spinal cord compression.[171] Common pathogens are skin flora contaminants *S. aureus* and *S. epidermidis*; less common ones are *Escherichia coli*, *Pseudomonas*, *Candida albicans*, and *Mycobacterium* organisms. A localized infection can track along the catheter until it reaches the epidural space. Otherwise, the epidural space is infected through hematogenous spread or through contamination of the analgesic injectate. Diagnosis is confirmed by getting an epidural/subarachnoid aspirate sample for Gram stain and culture as well as a MRI or CT scan to look for abscess. Once detected, both infectious disease and neurosurgery consultants must be involved in patient care.

In the case of an exteriorized catheter, exit site infection can be prevented by regular site cleaning with hydrogen peroxide and chlorhexidine. The catheter and exit site should be protected (e.g., by a minibag) when showering. Bathing in a hot tub is to be avoided. The catheter must always be handled by aseptic technique, and patient and patient's family are instructed to look for signs of inflammation. If an infection occurs, treatments are daily cleaning with chlorhexidine and topical or oral antibiotics. Complete resolution is expected without catheter removal.

Table 17-2. Long-term chronic epidural catheters and related complications

| Investigators | Catheter type (total no.) | Occlusion % (no.) | Minor/major infection % (no.) | Pain on injection % (no.) | Dislodgment/leakage % (no.) | Others % (no.) |
|---|---|---|---|---|---|---|
| Findler et al.,[158] 1982 | Internalized port (6) | 0 | 0/0 | 0 | 0/2 | |
| Malone et al.,[159] 1985 | Tunneled (15) | 0 | 0/0 | 1 | 0/0 | |
| Zenz et al.,[160] 1985 | Externalized nontunneled (139) | 7 (10) | 7 (10)/1 (2) | 0 | 20 (28)/0 | |
| Du Pen,[155,161,162] 1987, 1990, 1999 | Externalized tunneled (350) | 0 | 11 (38)/4 (15) | 0.6 (2) | 0/0 | |
| Downing et al.,[163] 1988 | Externalized nontunneled (23) | 0 | 4 (1)/0 | 0 | 0/0 | |
| Boersma et al.,[164] 1989 | Internalized port (15) | 7 (1) | 0/0 | 0 | 0/7 (1) | |
| Driessen et al.,[165] 1989 | Externalized nontunneled (32) | 22 (7) | NR/NR | NR | 22 (7)/47 (15) | Epidural hematoma (2) |
| | Internalized port (8) | | 13 (1)/NR | | NR/38 (3) | Spinal cord compression caused by epidural fibrosis (2) |
| Hogan et al.,[166] 1991 | Externalized tunneled and nontunneled (36) | 0 | 8 (3)/0 | 11 (4) | 28 (10)/3 (1) | |
| Plummer et al.,[167] 1991 | Internalized port (313) | 11 (31) | 7 (22)/0.8 (1) | 12 (34) | 0/2 (6) | |
| Erdine and Aldemir,[168] 1991 | Externalized nontunneled (175) | 4 (8) | 4 (9)/0 | 0 | 7 (16)/2 (5) | |
| | Internalized port (50) | | | | | |
| Crul and Delhaas,[169] 1991 | Externalized nontunneled (95) | 45 (43) | 4 (4)/0 | 36 (34) | 24 (23)/18 (17) | |
| | tunneled (15) | 27 (4) | 7 (1)/0 | 0 | 0/13 (2) | |
| Smitt et al.,[170] 1998 | Externalized percutaneous short-distance tunneled (72) | 14 (13) | 43 (39)/13 (12), epidural abscess 12 (11) | 9 (8) | 11 (10)/23 (21) | Weakness 6 (5) |
| Sillevis et al.,[171] 1999 | Internalized port (19) | | | | | Sensory deficit 2 (2) Replacement 44 (40) |

TABLE 17-3. Chronic subarachnoid catheters and related complications

| Investigators | Catheter type (total no.) | Duration of use (days) | Occlusion % (no.) | Local/major infection % (no.) | Pain on injection % (no.) | Dislodgment/ leakage | Inflammatory mass/spinal cord compression | Others % (no.) |
|---|---|---|---|---|---|---|---|---|
| Schoeffler et al.,[172] 1986 | Internalized port (37) | NR | NR | NR/meningitis 16 (6) | NR | NR/NR | | NR |
| Crul and Delhaas,[169] 1991 | Externalized tunneled (30) | 10–366 | NR | 7 (2)/NR | NR | 7 (2)/NR | | CSF leak 27 (8)<br>PDPH 10 (3) |
| Plummer et al.,[167] 1991 | Internalized port (17) | Mean 147 | 6 (1) | 6 (1)/NR | NR | NR/NR | | NR |
| Nitescu et al.,[173] 1991 | Externalized tunneled (142) | Median 57 | 0.6 | NR/meningitis 0.7 (1) | NR | 7/NR | | PDPH 10 |
| Nitescu et al.,[174] 1995 | Externalized tunneled (200) | Median 33 | 1 | 0.5/meningitis 0.5 | 4.5 with intermittent injections | 1.5/1.5 | | PDPH 15.5<br>CSF hygroma 1.5 |
| Gilmer-Hill et al.,[175] 1999 | Internalized pump (9) | Mean 137 | NR | NR/NR | NR | NR | NR | Transient urinary retention with intrathecal morphine 67 (6) |
| Anderson and Burchiel,[176] 1999 | Internalized pump (40) | Mean 730 in 20 patients | 2 (1) | NR | NR | 5 (2)/NR | NR | CSF seroma 5 (2) |
| Follett and Naumann,[154] 2000 | Internalized pump (209) | Mean >270 | 2 (5) | Pump pocket infection 5 (11)<br>Wound infection 1 (2)/ meningitis 1 (2) | NR | 1 (2)/1 (3) | NR | CSF leak/hygroma 2 (4) |
| Krames et al.,[177] 2000 | Internalized pump (212) | Mean >460 | 2 (5) | 1 (3)/NR | NR | 5 (10)/NR | NR | CSF/hygroma 1 (3) |
| Coffey and Burchiel,[178] 2002 | Internalized pump (unknown) | Median 735 | NR | NR/NR | NR | NR | ? (41) | Surgical spinal cord/cauda equine decompression (30) |
| Rauck et al.,[143] 2003 | Internalized patient-activated pump (119) | NR | 1 (1) | Occurs but % unknown/ % unknown | NR | 1 (1)/1 (1) | NR | Pump failure (3)<br>CSF leak and seroma occur but % unknown |
| McMillan et al.,[179] 2003 | Internalized pump (7) | Mean 600 | NR | NR/NR | NR | NR | 43 (3)/symptomatic 14 (1) | |
| Thimineur et al.,[148] 2004 | Internalized pump (38) | 1095 | 3 (1) | Pocket 5 (2)/NR | NR | NR | NR | Transverse myelitis 3 (1) |
| Baker et al.,[150] 2004 | Externalized tunneled (100, 81 intrathecal in 76 patients) | Median 24 | NR | 1 (1)/nonfatal meningitis 1 (1)<br>Fatal meningitis 1 (1) | NR | 17/13 | 2 (2) | |

NR, not reported.

However, deep track and epidural/subarachnoid space infections must be treated vigorously by removing the catheter and providing parenteral antibiotic therapy. If the catheter is not removed, deep catheter track infection will recur despite antibiotic treatment. Infection may be prevented with intravenous broad-spectrum antibiotics given 1 hour preoperatively and two doses given after the procedure every 8 hours. Other prophylactic measures include wound irrigation with solution containing antibiotic and using the same fluid to bathe implanted hardware before subcutaneous insertion. Epidural/subarachnoid catheters may be replaced once infection is cleared.[161] Meningitis can occur but is uncommon.

Infection is less likely to occur with the internalized injection port system when implantable catheters are used over the long term. In De Jong's series of 250 epidural catheters, he found that the infection rate for patients with an internalized injection port was half that for the patients with percutaneous catheters (tunneled or nontunneled) – 2.86 infections versus 5.97 per 1000 catheter-days, respectively.[182] Patients in the injection port group did not have infection during the first 70 days of use but those with percutaneous catheters did. In this study, catheter tunneling did not offer any protection from infection, most likely because the tunnel was too short (no more than 30 cm). Interestingly, a large prospective multicenter study showed only a small number of superficial infections with implantable intrathecal catheters.[183]

## *Drug-Related Complications*

Implantable catheters are usually infused with opioids and local anesthetic, less often with $\alpha_2$-agonists (e.g., clonidine), ziconotide,[184] and baclofen.[151] In general, drug-related complications arise when drugs are used in high concentrations and large doses leading to systemic and neurologic toxic sequelae. A summary of literature data is found in Table 17-4.[185–187]

Long-term spinal opioid administration can cause constipation, urinary retention (especially in men with prostate enlargement), nausea, vomiting, nightmares, and pruritus, in descending frequency.[188,189] These side effects are often transient in patients who are tolerant to opioids. Endocrine side effects associated with chronic administration include decreased libido and impotence in men and amenorrhea in premenopausal women because of subnormal levels of sexual hormones.[190] Respiratory depression is rare, but extremely large doses of spinal opioid can cause CNS hyperexcitability manifested as muscle twitching, myoclonus, and eventually seizure.

When switching a patient from systemic opioid to spinal opioid, it is important to remember slow tapering of the systemic opioid dose, to avoid opioid withdrawal syndrome. When side effects of one opioid persist because of large doses, switching to another opioid type is helpful (e.g., from morphine to fentanyl or sufentanil). Another recommendation is to lower the opioid dose by adding a local anesthetic to maintain analgesic efficacy.[191] Other less common side effects are allodynia, paranoia, Meniere-like symptoms, nystagmus, endocrine suppression, and polyarthralgia.[156]

Potential complications of long-term high-dose local anesthetic administration are exaggerated sympathetic blockade, intolerable sensory loss, persistent motor block, CNS toxicity, and loss of bowel and bladder function (Table 17-4). Postural hypotension occurs in as many as 10% of patients during the first 24 hours but usually disappears.[191] This can be corrected easily with intravenous fluid therapy. In the final days of life, many terminally ill patients become dehydrated, and the local anesthetic dose should be reduced at this time. Local anesthetic switching is recommended should intrathecal tachyphylaxis developed.[192]

Intolerable paresthesia and motor paresis affecting ambulation are complications secondary to chronic epidural or intrathecal infusion of local anesthetic. They are dose-related neurologic events that must be balanced against analgesia. Du Pen et al.[191] noted that 50% of the patients receiving epidural bupivacaine, 0.25%, developed profound sensory anesthesia lasting more than 4 days; the figure reached 82% when

TABLE 17-4. Opioid and bupivacaine (B) and related complications

| Investigators | Route of administration (total patients) | Drugs and duration of use (days) | Intolerable paresthesia % (no.) | Motor paresis % (no.) | Postural hypotension % (no.) | Bowel/bladder dysfunction % (no.) | Other % (no.) |
|---|---|---|---|---|---|---|---|
| Driessen et al.,[165] 1989 | Epidural (40) | Morphine (mean 81) | NR | ? Spinal cord compression 5 (2) | NR | Impaired micturition 5 (2)<br>Constipation 10 (4) | NR |
| Hogan et al.,[166] 1991 | Epidural (16) | Morphine alone (6)<br>Opioid and B (10) (median 32) | Hyperesthesia and allodynia during epidural morphine 6 (1) | 31 (5) | NR | NR | NR |
| Erdine and Aldemir,[168] 1991 | Epidural (225) | Morphine (mean 47) | NR | NR | Hypotension 0.8 (2) | Urinary retention 4 (8) | NR |
| Du Pen et al.,[185] 1992 | Epidural (68) | Opioid and B (mean 60–120) | 50 when B >0.25%<br>82 when >0.3% | 0 when B <0.15%<br>15 when B is between 0.15% and 0.25%<br>60 when B >0.35%<br>85 when >0.4% | 9 (6) | Constipation 7 (16)<br>0 when B <0.15% | NR |
| Sjoberg et al.,[186] 1994 | Intrathecal (53 but 27 with normal neurologic function) | Morphine and B (mean 29) | Paresthesia, no allodynia 41 (11/27) | Paresis 33 (9/27) | 2 (1) | Late urinary retention 33 (9/27) | NR |
| Nitescu et al.,[187] 1995 | Intrathecal (200) | Opioid and B (mean 33) | NR | 4 (7) | NR | NR | 0 |
| Baker et al.,[150] 2004 | Intrathecal (81) | Diamorphine and B (median 24) | Persistent 1 (1) | Persistent 9 (7) | Symptomatic 17 (14) | Retention 12 (10)/ incontinence 10 (8) | Respiratory arrest 4 (3) |

NR, not reported.

0.3% bupivacaine was used. Similarly, persistent motor blockade is dose related; it occurred in 60% of patients who received 0.35% bupivacaine and in 85% of the patients when 0.4% bupivacaine was used. Interestingly, all patients could ambulate freely and had no difficulty voiding when the infused bupivacaine solution was weaker than 0.15%. Alternatively, motor impairment can be lessened by the technique of patient-controlled bolus administration on demand.[193] Breakthrough pain is relieved, without reliance on high doses, when infused hourly.

Local anesthetic–induced CNS toxicity is rare, even with long-term epidural infusion. Many patients develop decreasing bupivacaine clearance during infusion.[194] It is not unusual to see increasing plasma bupivacaine concentrations in the last days of life. Plasma levels may reach as high as 10.8μg/mL (total, toxic level is 4μg/mL) and 1.01μg/mL (free, toxic level 0.24μg/mL), but most patients are asymptomatic, without toxic symptoms. Du Pen[155] noted generalized tremors in 12 of 68 patients in the terminal stage, but this was not related to high bupivacaine plasma level. None of the patients showed signs of myoclonic activity, seizure, or cardiotoxicity.

### *Mechanical Complications*

In a recent study,[151] technical incidents were noted in 37% of patient who had implanted indwelling catheters. Catheters can dislodge, dislocate, rupture, kink, leak, occlude, thrombose, or migrate. When this happens, failure of spinal drug delivery will result in an acute loss of analgesia despite drug escalation. Leakage can present as a subcutaneous swelling at the insertion site or in the paravertebral region because drug is being infused subcutaneously. If not recognized, an opioid abstinence syndrome[196] (fever, vomiting, anorexia, hallucinations) can occur that requires systemic opioid rescue. Percutaneous catheters are more likely to dislodge. de Jong and Kansen[197] noted that 21% of catheters became dislodged in the percutaneous group but none in the injection port group. Suspicion of catheter misplacement can be confirmed by a radiocontrast study (e.g., an epidurogram). Catheter obstruction may be a result of filter failure or, less frequently, vertebral compression, tumor, fibrosis, or epidural infection. Occlusion occurs significantly more often in catheters connected to the injection port than in others.[197]

Pain on injection is another mechanical problem. Chronic drug administration leads to tissue reaction around the epidural catheter and epidural fibrosis. Several remedies are useful: injection of opioid in smaller volume, injection of a small dose of local anesthetic before the opioid bolus, and intermittent steroid injections to relieve ongoing inflammation. If all these measures fail and symptoms persist, catheter replacement or change to a subarachnoid catheter is necessary.

Internalized access ports and permanent pumps are housed subcutaneously. If the subcutaneous pocket is too superficial, the device can impinge on ribs, iliac crest, or other bones. This produces discomfort, impairs skin healing of the wound, and increases the risk of skin erosion, especially in cachectic patients. However, if the created pocket is too deep, access and reservoir refilling will be difficult. Malfunction of today's highly sophisticated implanted pump is unusual. More likely, drug under- or overdose is the result of human error in pump programming.

### *Inflammatory Mass*

One of the growing concerns with the implanted intrathecal delivery system is development of an inflammatory mass around the catheter tip.[179,198–200] Not only can the mass block effective drug delivery to the target neural site, but spinal cord compression has been reported. The incidence of inflammatory mass formation is estimated to be 0.04% after 1 year of therapy but up to 1.15% after 6 years.[199] Recent animal studies demonstrate that inflammatory reaction and granuloma formation at the catheter tip is triggered by high morphine concentration in the infusate (12mg/day equivalent to 36mg/day in humans).[201,202] Although hydromorphone has also been implicated, a recent animal study fails to show such an association.[203] When clonidine (0.25–1 mg/day) is added to low-dose morphine (1.5 mg/day), clonidine was found to reduce granuloma formation in a dose-dependent manner.[204] Although this finding is intriguing, clonidine protective effect on larger doses of intrathecal morphine or on other opioids is largely unknown.

Given the current state of knowledge, it is recommended to keep the concentration and total daily dose of intrathecal opioid as low as possible. When a large dose of morphine is required for pain relief, a more potent drug such as hydromorphone should be considered as a substitute. Physicians should be vigilant in monitoring for early symptoms and signs of granuloma formation (e.g., loss of analgesic efficacy, unexplained thoracic or lumbar radicular pain, and recent change in bowel and bladder function). Imaging studies such as contrast-enhanced T1-weighted MRI or CT myelography should be performed to rule out any suspicious lesion.[200]

### *Miscellaneous*

Surgical bleeding associated with implantation is rare but catheter-induced epidural hematoma has been reported.[166,168] Caution must be exercised when the platelet count is below 60,000 or there is suspicion of tumor invasion into the epidural space. Catheter passage in this situation can provoke epidural bleeding.

With a subarachnoid catheter, the incidence of CSF leak and PDPH may be 10%–15%. Those who develop PDPH usually become asymptomatic in 2–4 days; epidural blood patch is seldom required. Persistent CSF leakage externally can present as a CSF hygroma, a subcutaneous fluid collection under the back wound. A big hygroma can cause skin breakdown and lead to development of a CSF cutaneous fistula and increased risk of infection.[205]

Finally, indwelling epidural catheters can migrate intravenously, subdurally,[206] or intrathecally.[207] Reported cases of epidural catheter migration are limited to those used postoperatively. Drug toxicity caused by catheter migration during long-term administration has not been reported.

## Spinal Cord Stimulation

Spinal cord stimulation (SCS) is indicated for intractable pain from failed back surgery syndrome, complex regional pain syndrome, and vascular insufficiency (peripheral vascular disease or refractory angina). A few randomized, controlled studies[208,209] show a modest degree of pain relief but no significant improvement in physical function, activities of daily living, or work capacity.

Before a permanent SCS implantation, patient screening, psychologic assessment, and a trial stimulation are required. The electrode can be inserted percutaneously or by laminotomy (paddle electrode). An external power source is required, either in the form of an implantable pulse generator with a built-in battery or an implantable device powered by an external power supply utilizing radiofrequency-coupling with an antenna taped to the skin over the receiver.

### *Complications of SCS*

In general, two categories of complications are noted – implantable procedure related and stimulator related. Potential risks related to the implantable procedure are similar to those associated with intraspinal catheter implantation. These include bleeding, infection (superficial or deep), inadvertent dural puncture, CSF hygroma, nerve injury, and malposition of the subcutaneous generator. Technical problems seen with SCS are related to electromechanical failures. Failure to overlap stimulator-induced paresthesia with patient's pain distribution can result in a loss of pain relief with time because of physical migration or malposition of the electrodes. This happens more often with the single channel leads. Lead and wire breakage, fibrosis around implanted electrodes, fatigue fracture of conductors, insulation, and radiofrequency receiver failure are other technical problems. Variation of stimulator-induced paresthesia and pain relief with body posture has also been reported.

According to a recent systematic review,[210] the weighted average of the complication rate is 34%. Reported complications are local infection at the receiver/stimulator site or at the connector between the lead and electrode (4.5%), pain at the electrode connector or receiver/stimulator (6%), stimulator revision other than battery replacement (23%), temporary/permanent removal of stimulator (6%), and biologic complication such as dural puncture (2.5%). Surgical removal of the infected stimulator component is usually required.

North et al.[211] also reported serious infection at the receiver site requiring removal (1/33) and electrode migration or malposition requiring hardware revision (3/33). However, there is no reported morbidity, e.g., spinal cord compression, bacterial meningitis, or life-threatening infection in more than 20 years of practice. Surgical wound infection was found in 5% (16/320) of the patients, but all were superficial. A second implantation was possible after treatment with antibiotic and removal of the original hardware. Outright hardware failures, e.g., electronic malfunction of the implanted receiver, lead fatigue fracture, insulation failure, and electrode migration were infrequent complications with new equipment and techniques.

Allergic reactions to SCS are rare[114] but can happen as a result of reaction to the components of stimulator. Similar to a pacemaker, SCS is composed of titanium (generator casing), platinum and iridium (electrodes), and polyurethane (lead covering); all can trigger an allergic reaction. Generalized swelling and hives are generally transient but stimulator removal may be required in severe cases.

In summary, the complications rate of spinal cord stimulator is high, mainly in the form of migration or malposition of the electrode. However, major life-threatening complications are rare.

## References


1. Lema M. What's the name of the game? ASA Newslett 2002;66:1.
2. Fitzgibbon DR, Posner KL, Domino KB, Caplan RA, Lee LA, Cheney FW. Chronic pain management: American Society of Anesthesiologists Closed Claims Project. Anesthesiology 2004;100:98–105.
3. Breivik H. Sympathetic blocks. In: Breivik H, Campbell W, Eccleston C, eds. Clinical Pain Management: Practical Applications and Procedures. 1st ed. London: Arnold; 2003:233–246.
4. Hogan QH, Abram SE. Diagnostic and prognostic neural blockade. In: Cousins MJ, Bridenbaugh PO, eds. Neural Blockade in Clinical Anesthesia and Management of Pain. 3rd ed. Philadelphia: Lippincott-Raven; 1998:837–878.
5. Raj PR. Stellate ganglion block. In: Waldman SD, Winnie AP, eds. Interventional Pain Management. 1st ed. Philadelphia: WB Saunders; 1996:267–274.
6. Moore DC. Puncture of organs and blood vessels. In: Complications of Regional Anaesthesia. Springfield, IL: Charles C. Thomas; 1955.
7. Kozody R, Ready LB, Barsa JE, Murphy TM. Dose requirement of local anaesthetic to produce grand mal seizure during stellate ganglion block. Can Anaesth Soc J 1982;29: 489–491.
8. Ellis JS Jr, Ramamurthy S. Seizure following stellate ganglion block after negative aspiration and test dose. Anesthesiology 1986;64:533–534.
9. Adelman MH. Cerebral air embolism complicating stellate ganglion block. J Mt Sinai Hosp 1948;15:28.
10. Stannard CF, Glynn CJ, Smith SP. Dural puncture during attempted stellate ganglion block. Anaesthesia 1990;45:952–954.
11. Bruyns T, Devulder J, Vermeulen H, De Colvenaer L, Rolly G. Possible inadvertent subdural block following attempted stellate ganglion blockade. Anaesthesia 1991;46: 747–749.

12. Wulf H, Maier C. Complications and side effects of stellate ganglion blockade. Results of a questionnaire survey [German]. Anaesthesist 1992;41:146–151.
13. Allen G, Samson B. Contralateral Horner's syndrome following stellate ganglion block. Can Anaesth Soc J 1986;33:112–113.
14. Tochinai H, Wakusawa R, Segawa Y, Iwabuchi T, Goto T. Case of severe arrhythmia after stellate ganglion block [Japanese]. Masui 1974;23:548–552.
15. Schlack W, Schafer S, Thamer V. Left stellate ganglion block impairs left ventricular function. Anesth Analg 1994;79:1082–1088.
16. Lehmann LJ, Warfield CA, Bajwa ZH. Migraine headache following stellate ganglion block for reflex sympathetic dystrophy. Headache 1996;36:335–337.
17. Romanoff ME, Ellis JS Jr. Bupivacaine toxicity after stellate ganglion block. Anesth Analg 1991;73:505–506.
18. Rocco AG, Palombi D, Raeke D. Anatomy of the lumbar sympathetic chain. Reg Anesth 1995;20:13–19.
19. Peng PW, Castano ED. Survey of chronic pain practice by anesthesiologists in Canada. Can J Anaesth 2005;52:383–389.
20. Artusio JD, Stevens RA, Lineberry PJ. Postdural puncture headache after lumbar sympathetic block: a report of two cases. Reg Anesth 1991;16:288.
21. Waldman SD. Horner's syndrome resulting from a lumbar sympathetic block. Anesthesiology 1989;70:882.
22. Cherry DA, Rao DM. Lumbar sympathetic and coeliac plexus blocks. An anatomical study in cadavers. Br J Anaesth 1982;54:1037–1039.
23. Furlan AD, Lui PW, Mailis A. Chemical sympathectomy for neuropathic pain: does it work? Case report and systematic literature review. Clin J Pain 2001;17:327–336.
24. Reid W, Watt JK, Gray TG. Phenol injection of the sympathetic chain. Br J Surg 1970;57:45–50.
25. Antao B, Rowlands TE, Singh NP, McCleary AJ. Pelviureteric junction disruption as a complication of chemical lumbar sympathectomy. Cardiovasc Surg 2003;11:42–44.
26. Kingery WS. A critical review of controlled clinical trials for peripheral neuropathic pain and complex regional pain syndromes. Pain 1997;73:123–139.
27. Kalmanovitch DV, Hardwick PB. Hypotension after guanethidine block. Anaesthesia 1988;43:256.
28. Sharpe E, Milaszkiewicz R, Carli F. A case of prolonged hypotension following intravenous guanethidine block. Anaesthesia 1987;42:1081–1084.
29. Woo R, McQueen J. Apnea and syncope following intravenous guanethidine Bier block in the same patient on two different occasions. Anesthesiology 1987;67:281–282.
30. Singler RC. An improved technique for alcohol neurolysis of the celiac plexus. Anesthesiology 1982;56:137–141.
31. Ischia S, Luzzani A, Ischia A, Faggion S. A new approach to the neurolytic block of the coeliac plexus: the transaortic technique. Pain 1983;16:333–341.
32. Montero MA, Vidal LF, Aguilar Sanchez JL, Donoso BL. Percutaneous anterior approach to the coeliac plexus using ultrasound. Br J Anaesth 1989;62:637–640.
33. Klapman JB, Chang KJ. Endoscopic ultrasound-guided fine-needle injection. Gastrointest Endosc Clin North Am 2005;15:169–177.
34. Eisenberg E, Carr DB, Chalmers TC. Neurolytic celiac plexus block for treatment of cancer pain: a meta-analysis. Anesth Analg 1995;80:290–295.
35. Chan VW. Chronic diarrhea: an uncommon side effect of celiac plexus block. Anesth Analg 1996;82:205–207.
36. Takahashi M, Yoshida A, Ohara T, et al. Silent gastric perforation in a pancreatic cancer patient treated with neurolytic celiac plexus block. J Anesth 2003;17:196–198.
37. Sett SS, Taylor DC. Aortic pseudoaneurysm secondary to celiac plexus block. Ann Vasc Surg 1991;5:88–91.
38. Kaplan R, Schiff-Keren B, Alt E. Aortic dissection as a complication of celiac plexus block. Anesthesiology 1995;83:632–635.
39. Wilson PR. Incidental discography during celiac plexus block. Anesthesiology 1992; 76:314–316.
40. Fine PG, Bubela C. Chylothorax following celiac plexus block. Anesthesiology 1985;63: 454–456.
41. Pateman J, Williams MP, Filshie J. Retroperitoneal fibrosis after multiple coeliac plexus blocks. Anaesthesia 1990;45:309–310.

42. Navarro-Martinez J, Montes A, Comps O, Sitges-Serra A. Retroperitoneal abscess after neurolytic celiac plexus block from the anterior approach. Reg Anesth Pain Med 2003; 28:528–530.
43. Gress F, Schmitt C, Sherman S, Ciaccia D, Ikenberry S, Lehman G. Endoscopic ultrasound-guided celiac plexus block for managing abdominal pain associated with chronic pancreatitis: a prospective single center experience. Am J Gastroenterol 2001;96:409–416.
44. De Conno F, Caraceni A, Aldrighetti L, et al. Paraplegia following coeliac plexus block. Pain 1993;55:383–385.
45. Brown DL, Rorie DK. Altered reactivity of isolated segmental lumbar arteries of dogs following exposure to ethanol and phenol. Pain 1994;56:139–143.
46. Galizia EJ, Lahiri SK. Paraplegia following coeliac plexus block with phenol. Case report. Br J Anaesth 1974;46:539–540.
47. Cherry DA, Lamberty J. Paraplegia following coeliac plexus block. Anaesth Intensive Care 1984;12:59–61.
48. Takeda J, Namai H, Fukushima K. Anterior spinal artery syndrome after left celiac plexus block. Anesth Analg 1996;83:178–179.
49. Wong GY, Brown DL. Transient paraplegia following alcohol celiac plexus block. Reg Anesth 1995;20:352–355.
50. Davies DD. Incidence of major complications of neurolytic coeliac plexus block. J R Soc Med 1993;86:264–266.
51. Fugere F, Lewis G. Coeliac plexus block for chronic pain syndromes. Can J Anaesth 1993;40:954–963.
52. Fitzgibbon DR, Schmiedl UP, Sinanan MN. Computed tomography-guided neurolytic celiac plexus block with alcohol complicated by superior mesenteric venous thrombosis. Pain 2001;92:307–310.
53. Gaudy JH, Tricot C, Sezeur A. Serious heart rate disorders following perioperative splanchnic nerve phenol nerve block [French]. Can J Anaesth 1993;40:357–359.
54. Jain S, Hirsch R, Shah N, Bedford R. Blood levels of ethanol following celiac plexus block. Anesth Analg 1989;68(suppl):S135.
55. Noda J, Umeda S, Mori K, Fukunaga T, Mizoi Y. Acetaldehyde syndrome after celiac plexus alcohol block. Anesth Analg 1986;65:1300–1302.
56. Plancarte R, Amescua C, Patt RB, Aldrete JA. Superior hypogastric plexus block for pelvic cancer pain. Anesthesiology 1990;73:236–239.
57. Frymoyer JW. Back pain and sciatica. N Engl J Med 1988;318:291–300.
58. Dreyfuss PH, Dreyer SJ. Lumbar zygapophysial (facet) joint injections. Spine J 2003; 3:50S–59S.
59. Dreyfuss P, Schwarzer AC, Lau P, Bogduk N. Specificity of lumbar medial branch and L5 dorsal ramus blocks. A computed tomography study. Spine 1997;22:895–902.
60. Marks RC, Houston T, Thulbourne T. Facet joint injection and facet nerve block: a randomised comparison in 86 patients with chronic low back pain. Pain 1992;49:325–328.
61. Marks R, Semple AJ. Spinal anaesthesia after facet joint injection. Anaesthesia 1988;43: 65–66.
62. Thomson SJ, Lomax DM, Collett BJ. Chemical meningism after lumbar facet joint block with local anaesthetic and steroids. Anaesthesia 1991;46:563–564.
63. Cook NJ, Hanrahan P, Song S. Paraspinal abscess following facet joint injection. Clin Rheumatol 1999;18:52–53.
64. Orpen NM, Birch NC. Delayed presentation of septic arthritis of a lumbar facet joint after diagnostic facet joint injection. J Spinal Disord Tech 2003;16:285–287.
65. Lord SM, Bogduk N. Radiofrequency procedures in chronic pain. Best Pract Res Clin Anaesthesiol 2002;16:597–617.
66. Cluff R, Mehio AK, Cohen SP, Chang Y, Sang CN, Stojanovic MP. The technical aspects of epidural steroid injections: a national survey. Anesth Analg 2002;95:403–408.
67. Abram SE. Treatment of lumbosacral radiculopathy with epidural steroids. Anesthesiology 1999;91:1937–1941.
68. Waldman SD. Cervical epidural nerve block. In: Waldman SD, Winnie AP, eds. Interventional Pain Management. Philadelphia: WB Saunders; 1996:275.
69. Gajraj NM. Selective nerve root blocks for low back pain and radiculopathy. Reg Anesth Pain Med 2004;29:243–256.

70. Rathmell JP, Aprill C, Bogduk N. Cervical transforaminal injection of steroids. Anesthesiology 2004;100:1595–1600.
71. Stojanovic MP, Vu TN, Caneris O, Slezak J, Cohen SP, Sang CN. The role of fluoroscopy in cervical epidural steroid injections: an analysis of contrast dispersal patterns. Spine 2002;27:509–514.
72. Peng PW, Smedstad KG. Litigation in Canada against anesthesiologists practicing regional anesthesia. A review of closed claims. Can J Anaesth 2000;47:105–112.
73. Abram SE, O'Connor TC. Complications associated with epidural steroid injections. Reg Anesth 1996;21:149–162.
74. Benzon HT, Gissen AJ, Strichartz GR, Avram MJ, Covino BG. The effect of polyethylene glycol on mammalian nerve impulses. Anesth Analg 1987;66:553–559.
75. Knight JW, Cordingley JJ, Palazzo MG. Epidural abscess following epidural steroid and local anaesthetic injection. Anaesthesia 1997;52:576–578.
76. Huang RC, Shapiro GS, Lim M, Sandhu HS, Lutz GE, Herzog RJ. Cervical epidural abscess after epidural steroid injection. Spine 2004;29:E7–E9.
77. Saigal G, Donovan Post MJ, Kozic D. Thoracic intradural *Aspergillus* abscess formation following epidural steroid injection. AJNR Am J Neuroradiol 2004;25:642–644.
78. Dougherty JH Jr, Fraser RA. Complications following intraspinal injections of steroids. Report of two cases. J Neurosurg 1978;48:1023–1025.
79. Cooper AB, Sharpe MD. Bacterial meningitis and cauda equina syndrome after epidural steroid injections. Can J Anaesth 1996;43:471–474.
80. Stambough JL, Booth RE Jr, Rothman RH. Transient hypercorticism after epidural steroid injection. A case report. J.Bone Joint Surg Am 1984;66:1115–1116.
81. Tuel SM, Meythaler JM, Cross LL. Cushing's syndrome from epidural methylprednisolone. Pain 1990;40:81–84.
82. Knight CL, Burnell JC. Systemic side-effects of extradural steroids. Anaesthesia 1980; 35:593–594.
83. Boonen S, Van Distel G, Westhovens R, Dequeker J. Steroid myopathy induced by epidural triamcinolone injection. Br J Rheumatol 1995;34:385–386.
84. Maillefert JF, Aho S, Huguenin MC, et al. Systemic effects of epidural dexamethasone injections. Rev Rhum Engl Ed 1995;62:429–432.
85. Kay J, Findling JW, Raff H. Epidural triamcinolone suppresses the pituitary-adrenal axis in human subjects. Anesth Analg 1994;79:501–505.
86. Jacobs S, Pullan PT, Potter JM, Shenfield GM. Adrenal suppression following extradural steroids. Anaesthesia 1983;38:953–956.
87. Gorski DW, Rao TL, Glisson SN, Chinthagada M, El-Etr AA. Epidural triamcinolone and adrenal response to hypoglycemic stress in dogs. Anesthesiology 1982;57:364–366.
88. Cohn ML, Huntington CT, Byrd SE, Machado AF, Cohn M. Epidural morphine and methylprednisolone. New therapy for recurrent low-back pain. Spine 1986;11:960–963.
89. Dallas TL, Lin RL, Wu WH, Wolskee P. Epidural morphine and methylprednisolone for low-back pain. Anesthesiology 1987;67:408–411.
90. Brechner VL. Epidural morphine and methylprednisolone: new therapy for recurrent low-back pain. Spine 1987;12:827.
91. Rocco AG, Frank E, Kaul AF, Lipson SJ, Gallo JP. Epidural steroids, epidural morphine and epidural steroids combined with morphine in the treatment of post-laminectomy syndrome. Pain 1989;36:297–303.
92. Glynn C, Dawson D, Sanders R. A double-blind comparison between epidural morphine and epidural clonidine in patients with chronic non-cancer pain. Pain 1988;34:123–128.
93. Botwin KP, Gruber RD, Bouchlas CG, Torres-Ramos FM, Freeman TL, Slaten WK. Complications of fluoroscopically guided transforaminal lumbar epidural injections. Arch Phys Med Rehabil 2000;81:1045–1050.
94. Furman MB, O'Brien EM, Zgleszewski TM. Incidence of intravascular penetration in transforaminal lumbosacral epidural steroid injections. Spine 2000;25:2628–2632.
95. Rathmell JP, Benzon HT. Transforaminal injection of steroids: should we continue? Reg Anesth Pain Med 2004;29:397–399.
96. Brouwers PJ, Kottink EJ, Simon MA, Prevo RL. A cervical anterior spinal artery syndrome after diagnostic blockade of the right C6-nerve root. Pain 2001;91:397–399.
97. Tiso RL, Cutler T, Catania JA, Whalen K. Adverse central nervous system sequelae after selective transforaminal block: the role of corticosteroids. Spine J 2004;4:468–474.

98. McMillan MR, Crumpton C. Cortical blindness and neurologic injury complicating cervical transforaminal injection for cervical radiculopathy. Anesthesiology 2003;99: 509–511.
99. Houten JK, Errico TJ. Paraplegia after lumbosacral nerve root block: report of three cases. Spine J 2002;2:70–75.
100. Huntoon MA, Martin DP. Paralysis after transforaminal epidural injection and previous spinal surgery. Reg Anesth Pain Med 2004;29:494–495.
101. Baker R, Dreyfuss P, Mercer S, Bogduk N. Cervical transforaminal injection of corticosteroids into a radicular artery: a possible mechanism for spinal cord injury. Pain 2003;103:211–215.
102. Cicala RS, Westbrook L, Angel JJ. Side effects and complications of cervical epidural steroid injections. J Pain Symptom Manage 1989;4:64–66.
103. Botwin KP, Castellanos R, Rao S, et al. Complications of fluoroscopically guided interlaminar cervical epidural injections. Arch Phys Med Rehabil 2003;84:627–633.
104. Waldman SD. Complications of cervical epidural nerve blocks with steroids: a prospective study of 790 consecutive blocks. Reg Anesth 1989;14:149–151.
105. Goebert HW Jr, Jallo SJ, Gardner WJ, Wasmuth CE. Painful radiculopathy treated with epidural injections of procaine and hydrocortisone acetate: results in 113 patients. Anesth Analg 1961;40:130–134.
106. Harley C. Extradural corticosteroid infiltration. A follow-up study of 50 cases. Ann Phys Med 1967;9:22–28.
107. Botwin KP, Gruber RD, Bouchlas CG, et al. Complications of fluoroscopically guided caudal epidural injections. Am J Phys Med Rehabil 2001;80:416–424.
108. Ridley MG, Kingsley GH, Gibson T, Grahame R. Outpatient lumbar epidural corticosteroid injection in the management of sciatica. Br J Rheumatol 1988;27:295–299.
109. Wagner AL. CT fluoroscopy-guided epidural injections: technique and results. AJNR Am J Neuroradiol 2004;25:1821–1823.
110. Johnson BA, Schellhas KP, Pollei SR. Epidurography and therapeutic epidural injections: technical considerations and experience with 5334 cases. AJNR Am J Neuroradiol 1999;20:697–705.
111. Forrest JB. The response to epidural steroid injections in chronic dorsal root pain. Can Anaesth Soc J 1980;27:40–46.
112. Wallace G, Solove GJ. Epidural steroid therapy for low back pain. Postgrad Med 1985;78:213–215, 218.
113. Abram SE. Subarachnoid corticosteroid injection following inadequate response to epidural steroids for sciatica. Anesth Analg 1978;57:313–315.
114. Ochani TD, Almirante J, Siddiqui A, Kaplan R. Allergic reaction to spinal cord stimulator. Clin J Pain 2000;16:178–180.
115. Simon DL, Kunz RD, German JD, Zivkovich V. Allergic or pseudoallergic reaction following epidural steroid deposition and skin testing. Reg Anesth 1989;14:253–255.
116. McAllister RK, McDavid AJ, Meyer TA, Bittenbinder TM. Recurrent persistent hiccups after epidural steroid injection and analgesia with bupivacaine. Anesth Analg 2005; 100:1834–1836.
117. Young WF. Transient blindness after lumbar epidural steroid injection: a case report and literature review. Spine 2002;27:E476–E477.
118. Reitman CA, Watters W III. Subdural hematoma after cervical epidural steroid injection. Spine 2002;27:E174–E176.
119. Williams KN, Jackowski A, Evans PJ. Epidural haematoma requiring surgical decompression following repeated cervical epidural steroid injections for chronic pain. Pain 1990;42:197–199.
120. Hodges SD, Castleberg RL, Miller T, Ward R, Thornburg C. Cervical epidural steroid injection with intrinsic spinal cord damage. Two case reports. Spine 1998;23:2137–2142.
121. Candido K, Stevens RA. Intrathecal neurolytic blocks for the relief of cancer pain. Best Pract Res Clin Anaesthesiol 2003;17:407–428.
122. Lauretti GR, Trevelin WR, Frade LC, Lima IC. Spinal alcohol neurolysis for intractable thoracic postherpetic neuralgia after test bupivacaine spinal analgesia. Anesthesiology 2004;101:244–247.
123. Mahli A, Coskun D, Altun NS, Simsek A, Ocal E, Kostekci M. Alcohol neurolysis for persistent pain caused by superior cluneal nerves injury after iliac crest bone graft

harvesting in orthopedic surgery: report of four cases and review of the literature. Spine 2002;27:E478–E481.
124. Jang SH, Ahn SH, Park SM, Kim SH, Lee KH, Lee ZI. Alcohol neurolysis of tibial nerve motor branches to the gastrocnemius muscle to treat ankle spasticity in patients with hemiplegic stroke. Arch Phys Med Rehabil 2004;85:506–508.
125. Atkinson GL, Shupak RC. Acute bronchospasm complicating intercostal nerve block with phenol. Anesth Analg 1989;68:400–401.
126. Mullin V. Brachial plexus block with phenol for painful arm associated with Pancoast's syndrome. Anesthesiology 1980;53:431–433.
127. Kaplan R, Aurellano Z, Pfisterer W. Phenol brachial plexus block for upper extremity cancer pain. Reg Anesth 1988;13:58.
128. Patt RB, Millard R. A role for peripheral neurolysis in the management of intractable cancer pain. Pain 1990;5(suppl):S358.
129. Kowalewski R, Schurch B, Hodler J, Borgeat A. Persistent paraplegia after an aqueous 7.5% phenol solution to the anterior motor root for intercostal neurolysis: a case report. Arch Phys Med Rehabil 2002;83:283–285.
130. McGarvey ML, Ferrante FM, Patel RS, Maljian JA, Stecker M. Irreversible spinal cord injury as a complication of subarachnoid ethanol neurolysis. Neurology 2000;54:1522–1524.
131. Totoki T, Kato T, Nomoto Y, Kurakazu M, Kanaseki T. Anterior spinal artery syndrome – a complication of cervical intrathecal phenol injection. Pain 1979;6:99–104.
132. Hughes JT. Thrombosis of the posterior spinal arteries. A complication of an intrathecal injection of phenol. Neurology 1970;20:659–664.
133. Slatkin NE, Rhiner M. Phenol saddle blocks for intractable pain at end of life: report of four cases and literature review. Am J Hosp Palliat Care 2003;20:62–66.
134. Korevaar WC. Transcatheter thoracic epidural neurolysis using ethyl alcohol. Anesthesiology 1988;69:989–993.
135. Swerdlow M. Intrathecal and extradural block. In: Relief of Intractable Pain. 2nd ed. Amsterdam: Excerpta Medica; 1978.
136. Robertson DH. Transsacral neurolytic nerve block. An alternative approach to intractable perineal pain. Br J Anaesth 1983;55:873–875.
137. Goffen BS. Transsacral block. Anesth Analg 1982;61:623–624.
138. Wood KM. The use of phenol as a neurolytic agent: a review. Pain 1978;5:205–229.
139. Raj PP. Peripheral neurolysis in the management of pain. In: Waldman SD, Winnie AP, eds. Interventional Pain Management. Philadelphia: WB Saunders; 1996:392.
140. Roviaro GC, Varoli F, Fascianella A, et al. Intrathoracic intercostal nerve block with phenol in open chest surgery. A randomized study with statistical evaluation of respiratory parameters. Chest 1986;90:64–67.
141. DuPen SL. Epidural techniques for cancer pain management: when, why, and how? Curr Rev Pain 1999;3:183–189.
142. Mercadante S. Epidural treatment in advanced cancer patients. Anesth Analg 2004;98: 1503–1504.
143. Rauck RL, Cherry D, Boyer MF, Kosek P, Dunn J, Alo K. Long-term intrathecal opioid therapy with a patient-activated, implanted delivery system for the treatment of refractory cancer pain. J Pain 2003;4:441–447.
144. Kedlaya D, Reynolds L, Waldman S. Epidural and intrathecal analgesia for cancer pain. Best Pract Res Clin Anaesthesiol 2002;16:651–665.
145. Ferrante FM. Neuraxial infusion in the management of cancer pain. Oncology (Williston Park) 1999;13:30–36.
146. Smith TJ, Staats PS, Deer T, et al. Randomized clinical trial of an implantable drug delivery system compared with comprehensive medical management for refractory cancer pain: impact on pain, drug-related toxicity, and survival. J Clin Oncol 2002;20:4040–4049.
147. Prager JP. Neuraxial medication delivery: the development and maturity of a concept for treating chronic pain of spinal origin. Spine 2002;27:2593–2605.
148. Thimineur MA, Kravitz E, Vodapally MS. Intrathecal opioid treatment for chronic nonmalignant pain: a 3-year prospective study. Pain 2004;109:242–249.
149. Cherry DA, Gourlay GK, Eldredge KA. Management of chronic intractable angina – spinal opioids offer an alternative therapy. Pain 2003;102:163–166.

150. Baker L, Lee M, Regnard C, Crack L, Callin S. Evolving spinal analgesia practice in palliative care. Palliat Med 2004;18:507–515.
151. Plassat R, Perrouin VB, Menei P, Menegalli D, Mathe JF, Richard I. Treatment of spasticity with intrathecal baclofen administration: long-term follow-up, review of 40 patients. Spinal Cord 2004;42:686–693.
152. Prager JP. Neuraxial medication delivery: the development and maturity of a concept for treating chronic pain of spinal origin. Spine 2002;27:2593–2605.
153. Ripamonti C, Brunelli C. Randomized clinical trial of an implantable drug delivery system compared with comprehensive medical management for refractory cancer pain: impact on pain, drug-related toxicity, and survival. J Clin Oncol 2003;21:2801–2802.
154. Follett KA, Naumann CP. A prospective study of catheter-related complications of intrathecal drug delivery systems. J Pain Symptom Manage 2000;19:209–215.
155. Du Pen S. Complications of neuraxial infusion in cancer patients. Oncology (Williston Park) 1999;13:45–51.
156. Wallace M, Yaksh TL. Long-term spinal analgesic delivery: a review of the preclinical and clinical literature. Reg Anesth Pain Med 2000;25:117–157.
157. Dickson D. Risks and benefits of long-term intrathecal analgesia. Anaesthesia 2004;59:633–635.
158. Findler G, Olshwang D, Hadani M. Continuous epidural morphine treatment for intractable pain in terminal cancer patients. Pain 1982;14:311–315.
159. Malone BT, Beye R, Walker J. Management of pain in the terminally ill by administration of epidural narcotics. Cancer 1985;55:438–440.
160. Zenz M, Piepenbrock S, Tryba M. Epidural opiates: long-term experiences in cancer pain. Klin Wochenschr 1985;63:225–229.
161. Du Pen SL, Peterson DG, Williams A, Bogosian AJ. Infection during chronic epidural catheterization: diagnosis and treatment. Anesthesiology 1990;73:905–909.
162. DuPen SL, Peterson DG, Bogosian AC, Ramsey DH, Larson C, Omoto M. A new permanent exteriorized epidural catheter for narcotic self-administration to control cancer pain. Cancer 1987;59:986–993.
163. Downing JE, Busch EH, Stedman PM. Epidural morphine delivered by a percutaneous epidural catheter for outpatient treatment of cancer pain. Anesth Analg 1988;67:1159–1161.
164. Boersma FP, Noorduin H, Vanden Bussche G. Epidural sufentanil for cancer pain control in outpatients. Reg Anesth 1989;14:293–297.
165. Driessen JJ, de Mulder PH, Claessen JJ, van Diejen D, Wobbes T. Epidural administration of morphine for control of cancer pain: long-term efficacy and complications. Clin J Pain 1989;5:217–222.
166. Hogan Q, Haddox JD, Abram S, Weissman D, Taylor ML, Janjan N. Epidural opiates and local anesthetics for the management of cancer pain. Pain 1991;46:271–279.
167. Plummer JL, Cherry DA, Cousins MJ, Gourlay GK, Onley MM, Evans KH. Long-term spinal administration of morphine in cancer and non-cancer pain: a retrospective study. Pain 1991;44:215–220.
168. Erdine S, Aldemir T. Long-term results of peridural morphine in 225 patients. Pain 1991;45:155–159.
169. Crul BJ, Delhaas EM. Technical complications during long-term subarachnoid or epidural administration of morphine in terminally ill cancer patients: a review of 140 cases. Reg Anesth 1991;16:209–213.
170. Smitt PS, Tsafka A, Teng-van de Zande F, et al. Outcome and complications of epidural analgesia in patients with chronic cancer pain. Cancer 1998;83:2015–2022.
171. Sillevis SP, Tsafka A, van den BM, et al. Spinal epidural abscess complicating chronic epidural analgesia in 11 cancer patients: clinical findings and magnetic resonance imaging. J Neurol 1999;246:815–820.
172. Schoeffler P, Pichard E, Ramboatiana R, Joyon D, Haberer JP. Bacterial meningitis due to infection of a lumbar drug release system in patients with cancer pain. Pain 1986;25:75–77.
173. Nitescu P, Appelgren L, Hultman E, Linder LE, Sjoberg M, Curelaru I. Long-term, open catheterization of the spinal subarachnoid space for continuous infusion of narcotic and bupivacaine in patients with "refractory" cancer pain. A technique of catheterization and its problems and complications. Clin J Pain 1991;7:143–161.

174. Nitescu P, Sjoberg M, Appelgren L, Curelaru I. Complications of intrathecal opioids and bupivacaine in the treatment of "refractory" cancer pain. Clin J Pain 1995;11:45–62.
175. Gilmer-Hill HS, Boggan JE, Smith KA, Wagner FC Jr. Intrathecal morphine delivered via subcutaneous pump for intractable cancer pain: a review of the literature. Surg Neurol 1999;51:12–15.
176. Anderson VC, Burchiel KJ. A prospective study of long-term intrathecal morphine in the management of chronic nonmalignant pain. Neurosurgery 1999;44:289–300.
177. Krames ES, Chapple I, The 8703 W. Catheter Study Group. Reliability and clinical utility of an implanted intraspinal catheter used in the treatment of spasticity and pain. Neuromodulation 2000;3:7–14.
178. Coffey RJ, Burchiel K. Inflammatory mass lesions associated with intrathecal drug infusion catheters: report and observations on 41 patients. Neurosurgery 2002;50:78–86.
179. McMillan MR, Doud T, Nugent W. Catheter-associated masses in patients receiving intrathecal analgesic therapy. Anesth Analg 2003;96:186–190.
180. De Cicco M, Matovic M, Castellani GT, et al. Time-dependent efficacy of bacterial filters and infection risk in long-term epidural catheterization. Anesthesiology 1995;82:765–771.
181. Gaertner J, Sabatowski R, Elsner F, Radbruch L. Encapsulation of an intrathecal catheter. Pain 2003;103:217–220.
182. de Jong PC, Kansen PJ. A comparison of epidural catheters with or without subcutaneous injection ports for treatment of cancer pain. Anesth Analg 1994;78:94–100.
183. Krames ES, Chapple I, The 8703 W. Catheter Study Group. Reliability and clinical utility of an implanted intraspinal catheter used in the treatment of spasticity and pain. Neuromodulation 2000;3:7–14.
184. Staats PS, Yearwood T, Charapata SG, et al. Intrathecal ziconotide in the treatment of refractory pain in patients with cancer or AIDS: a randomized controlled trial. JAMA 2004;291:63–70.
185. Du Pen SL, Kharasch ED, Williams A, et al. Chronic epidural bupivacaine-opioid infusion in intractable cancer pain. Pain 1992;49:293–300.
186. Sjoberg M, Nitescu P, Appelgren L, Curelaru I. Long-term intrathecal morphine and bupivacaine in patients with refractory cancer pain. Results from a morphine:bupivacaine dose regimen of 0.5:4.75 mg/ml. Anesthesiology 1994;80:284–297.
187. Nitescu P, Sjoberg M, Appelgren L, Curelaru I. Complications of intrathecal opioids and bupivacaine in the treatment of "refractory" cancer pain. Clin J Pain 1995;11:45–62.
188. Winkelmuller M, Winkelmuller W. Long-term effects of continuous intrathecal opioid treatment in chronic pain of nonmalignant etiology. J Neurosurg 1996;85:458–467.
189. Naumann C, Erdine S, Koulousakis A, Van Buyten JP, Schuchard M. Drug adverse events and system complications of intrathecal opioid delivery for pain: origins, detection, manifestations, and management. Neuromodulation 1999;2:92–107.
190. Abs R, Verhelst J, Maeyaert J, et al. Endocrine consequences of long-term intrathecal administration of opioids. J Clin Endocrinol Metab 2000;85:2215–2222.
191. Du Pen SL, Kharasch ED, Williams A, et al. Chronic epidural bupivacaine-opioid infusion in intractable cancer pain. Pain 1992;49:293–300.
192. Yang CP, Yeh CC, Wong CS, Wu CT. Local anesthetic switching for intrathecal tachyphylaxis in cancer patients with pain. Anesth Analg 2004;98:557–558.
193. Buchser E, Durrer A, Chedel D, Mustaki JP. Efficacy of intrathecal bupivacaine: how important is the flow rate? Pain Med 2004;5:248–252.
194. Sjoberg M, Nitescu P, Appelgren L, Curelaru I. Long-term intrathecal morphine and bupivacaine in patients with refractory cancer pain. Results from a morphine:bupivacaine dose regimen of 0.5:4.75 mg/ml. Anesthesiology 1994;80:284–297.
195. de Jong PC, Kansen PJ. A comparison of epidural catheters with or without subcutaneous injection ports for treatment of cancer pain. Anesth Analg 1994;78:94–100.
196. Taha J, Favre J, Janszen M, Galarza M, Taha A. Correlation between withdrawal symptoms and medication pump residual volume in patients with implantable SynchroMed pumps. Neurosurgery 2004;55:390–393.
197. de Jong PC, Kansen PJ. A comparison of epidural catheters with or without subcutaneous injection ports for treatment of cancer pain. Anesth Analg 1994;78:94–100.
198. Perren F, Buchser E, Chedel D, Hirt L, Maeder P, Vingerhoets F. Spinal cord lesion after long-term intrathecal clonidine and bupivacaine treatment for the management of intractable pain. Pain 2004;109:189–194.

199. Yaksh TL, Hassenbusch S, Burchiel K, Hildebrand KR, Page LM, Coffey RJ. Inflammatory masses associated with intrathecal drug infusion: a review of preclinical evidence and human data. Pain Med 2002;3:300–312.
200. Peng P, Massicotte EM. Spinal cord compression from intrathecal catheter-tip inflammatory mass: case report and a review of etiology. Reg Anesth Pain Med 2004;29:237–242.
201. Gradert TL, Baze WB, Satterfield WC, Hildebrand KR, Johansen MJ, Hassenbusch SJ. Safety of chronic intrathecal morphine infusion in a sheep model. Anesthesiology 2003;99:188–198.
202. Yaksh TL, Horais KA, Tozier NA, et al. Chronically infused intrathecal morphine in dogs. Anesthesiology 2003;99:174–187.
203. Johansen MJ, Satterfield WC, Baze WB, Hildebrand KR, Gradert TL, Hassenbusch SJ. Continuous intrathecal infusion of hydromorphone: safety in the sheep model and clinical implications. Pain Med 2004;5:14–25.
204. Yaksh TL, Horais KA, Tozier NA, et al. Chronically infused intrathecal morphine in dogs. Anesthesiology 2003;99:174–187.
205. Nitescu P, Sjoberg M, Appelgren L, Curelaru I. Complications of intrathecal opioids and bupivacaine in the treatment of "refractory" cancer pain. Clin J Pain 1995;11:45–62.
206. Hartrick CT, Pither CE, Pai U, Raj PP, Tomsick TA. Subdural migration of an epidural catheter. Anesth Analg 1985;64:175–178.
207. Barnes RK. Delayed subarachnoid migration of an epidural catheter. Anaesth Intensive Care 1990;18:564–566.
208. Kemler MA, De Vet HC, Barendse GA, Van Den Wildenberg FA, van Kleef M. The effect of spinal cord stimulation in patients with chronic reflex sympathetic dystrophy: two years' follow-up of the randomized controlled trial. Ann Neurol 2004;55:13–18.
209. North RB, Kidd DH, Farrokhi F, Piantadosi SA. Spinal cord stimulation versus repeated lumbosacral spine surgery for chronic pain: a randomized, controlled trial. Neurosurgery 2005;56:98–106.
210. Turner JA, Loeser JD, Deyo RA, Sanders SB. Spinal cord stimulation for patients with failed back surgery syndrome or complex regional pain syndrome: a systematic review of effectiveness and complications. Pain 2004;108:137–147.
211. North RB, Kidd DH, Farrokhi F, Piantadosi SA. Spinal cord stimulation versus repeated lumbosacral spine surgery for chronic pain: a randomized, controlled trial. Neurosurgery 2005;56:98–106.

# 18 Major Neurologic Injury Following Central Neural Blockade

David J. Sage and Steven J. Fowler

This chapter discusses major injuries such as paraplegia caused by epidural, caudal, and spinal anesthetic techniques.

For an individual patient, choice of technique will be based at least in part on the evidence for outcome benefit presented in Chapter 3, and on the potential for serious side effects presented here. A distinction can be drawn between the separate "background" risks of techniques of general anesthesia, sedation, and regional anesthesia, and "superimposed" patient risk factors for technique-related injury. Readers will share the authors' frustration at the lack of precise background incidence data and our inability to accurately quantify superimposed risk for these severe injuries. Furthermore, as the benefits of regional anesthesia become better understood, two trends have emerged from the literature published over the last 50 years that make individual patient assessment even more difficult. First, it is apparent that the very low complication rates for epidural and spinal anesthesia in obstetric patients cannot be extrapolated to the broad surgical population. Second, general anesthetic techniques have gradually become safer and less disruptive of normal physiology whereas the invasiveness of regional techniques has altered little. This includes the grave risks introduced for central neural blockade (CNB) by the presence of sepsis or coagulopathy, which are negligible additional risks for the safety of general anesthesia.

As with all anesthetic procedures, complication rates also reflect the psychomotor skills of the operator, judgment, and the possibility of system error in addition to individual human error. The devastating effects of contaminated local anesthetic described in the Woolley and Roe cases more than 50 years ago in the United Kingdom[1,2] and the "epidemic" of spinal hematomas created by a change in deep venous thrombosis prophylaxis more recently in the United States[3,4] both serve as stark reminders that the basic causes of injury described in this chapter remain unchanged.

## Causes

Spinal cord compression from bleeding or abscess, and the less common causes of serious neurologic injury attributable to neuraxial blockade, are listed in Table 18-1. Considering the everyday use of epidural and spinal anesthesia in developed countries and the extreme rarity of acute spinal cord pathology from all causes, careful

Table 18-1. Causes of Spinal Cord and Nerve Root Injury Associated with Neuraxial Blockade

1. Cord compression
    - Hematoma
        - Needle or catheter trauma
        - Tumor, vascular anomaly
        - Coagulopathy
        - Idiopathic
    - Abscess
        - Exogenous infection via needle/catheter
        - Hematogenous
        - Local spread (e.g., paravertebral)
2. Cord ischemia
    - Anterior spinal artery syndrome
3. Cord trauma
    - Needle/catheter damage
    - Toxic injectate
4. Arachnoiditis
    - Wrong drug
    - Infection
    - Local anesthetic neurotoxicity

investigation including consideration of noniatrogenic causes (Table 18-2) is mandatory. This evaluation is described in Chapter 21.

Intercurrent disease may precipitate catastrophe (such as preexisting spinal cord meningioma)[5], and other coincidental pathology such as spinal stenosis or space-occupying cord lesion can lead to cord compression when triggered by the additional volume of local anesthetic injection. It is well known that temporary obstetric palsies occur with and without neuraxial blockade.[6] Surgical damage[7] or patient positioning[8,9] may actually be more common causes of permanent nerve injury than regional anesthesia. However, proving that the regional technique was not responsible may still be impossible even with advanced diagnostic techniques. Thus, there is significant potential for misclassification of these injuries.

## Incidence

Because of the perceived benefits, neuraxial techniques are being performed more often in increasingly complex cases. Improvements in diagnosis and follow-up surveillance, along with changes in technique, equipment, drugs, and protocols, have made

Table 18-2. Coincidental Conditions Mimicking Neurologic Injury from Caudal, Epidural, or Spinal Anesthesia

- Spinal tumors
- Spinal vascular malformation
- Prolapsed intervertebral disc
- Guillain-Barré syndrome
- Multiple sclerosis
- Spinal hematoma
- Metastases
- Thalassemia
- Infections (e.g., viral)
- Embolic
- Iatrogenic (e.g., hypotension, surgery, positioning, drugs)

an estimate of complication rates in current practice an important objective. A number of large studies have appeared in the last 10 years that attempt to provide contemporary prevalence data for significant neurologic injury following CNB attributable to anesthetic causes. Methodologies include hospital database interrogation, postal questionnaire, hotline reporting, and closed claim analysis of litigation or no-fault insurance systems. This makes comparisons difficult, and significant inaccuracy in numerator, denominator, or both means that the incidence figures quoted must be seen as estimates only. As the following discussion demonstrates, no single figure can be arrived at that describes the inherent "baseline" injury risk for neuraxial anesthetic techniques as a whole.

The importance of considering risk–benefit on a patient-by-patient basis is highlighted in a recent and important retrospective study by Moen and colleagues[10] of serious neurologic complications associated with CNB performed during 1990–1999 in Sweden. The estimated denominator of 1,260,000 spinals and 250,000 epidurals was extrapolated from data from anesthetic departments and sales figures. Although retrospective, the study design aimed to minimize underreporting by comparing multiple data sources and by achieving the participation of 85% of anesthesiology departments in that country. Patients who recovered after successful treatment from anesthetic injury were included.

Although in the general population severe neurologic complications occurred after 1:3600 epidural procedures and 1:20,000 spinal blocks, the rate was far higher in women undergoing total knee arthroplasty who had epidurals (1:1800) and lowest in obstetric patients (1:25,000). The highest rate of major neurologic complications occurred in patients undergoing orthopedic, general, vascular, and urologic surgery. The authors proposed that this is related to the presence in this group of patients of important risk factors including epidural catheter techniques, disordered coagulation, osteoporosis, spinal stenosis, and immunosuppression. This study included some of the cases reported earlier by Dahlgren and Tornebrandt[11] from a single institution where the complication rate was markedly higher. These authors found that irreversible neurologic damage occurred in 1:2834 spinal anesthetics and 1:923 epidurals. In this series, sensory deficits confined to a single nerve root distribution were included, the causal relationship between anesthetic and injury was questionable in some cases, and confidence intervals were not presented, raising the possibility of clustering of rare events.[12] In a retrospective study by Aromaa and colleagues[7] of claims to the no-fault insurance system in Finland between 1987–1993, the incidence of paraplegia or permanent cauda equina syndrome was only 1:91,666 spinals and 1:85,000 epidurals.

In 1997, Auroy and colleagues[13] performed a landmark prospective study of serious complications of 40,000 spinals and 30,000 epidurals (as well as 21,000 peripheral blocks and 11,000 intravenous regional anesthetics) using voluntary reporting by clinicians in France. The incidence of neurologic complications lasting more than 3 months was 1:10,000 spinal and 1:30,000 epidural blocks and a follow-up "hotline" study published by the same author seemed to confirm this incidence.[14] However, both studies probably underestimate the actual risk because of underreporting and volunteer bias.[8]

The most common neurologic complication of CNB is nerve root damage which usually resolves within a year.[13] Generally, only a sensory deficit develops following the same distribution as the painful paresthesia reported during the procedure, although occasionally paresis is seen (most frequently foot drop).[7] Electromyography is helpful to aid localization of the lesion.[11]

## *Obstetric Anesthesia*

The obstetric population represents a relatively homogeneous group at low risk of serious neurologic complications of spinal or epidural.[15] In a multicenter retrospective survey of 505,000 obstetric epidurals by Scott and Hibbard,[16] there were only five serious complications. Only one of 38 single neuropathies lasted longer than 3 months. Six severe neurologic complications were reported in the study by Moen and colleagues in 255,000 obstetric blocks, including two spinal hematomas (both in patients with HELLP syndrome), one abscess, and several traumatic cord lesions. A survey of 300,000 obstetric epidurals performed in France over 5 years reported only one spinal hematoma although the incidence of transient radiculopathy was high at 1:3277.[17] This is supported by several other obstetric reports, in which the incidence of presumed traumatic mononeuropathies was consistently between 1:10,000–1:13,000.[18–20]

Data from the ASA Closed Claims database also supports the impression that significant deficits are rare in the obstetric population.[8]

In a study of complications of neuraxial blockade comparing 368 obstetric closed claims with 453 general closed claims, there was a lower proportion of permanent injuries from obstetric practice (10% versus 26% in nonobstetric files) and a corresponding higher proportion of low-severity and temporary injuries. Significantly, meningitis or intravertebral abscess accounted for 46% of obstetric complications of CNB and was a more common claim than in the general population. However, to put this into perspective, a previous closed claims study found that maternal death or brain damage associated with general anesthesia was reported more frequently than nerve injury caused by regional anesthesia.[21]

## Risk Factors for Neurologic Injury

There are important patient and technique-related factors that increase the chance of severe neurologic complications of epidural, caudal, and spinal anesthesia[22–24] (Table 18-3). Degenerative and other pathologic conditions of the spine are especially important.[22,23] Injection of a large fluid volume into the epidural space has caused transient paraplegia.[25] The study by Moen and colleagues[10] confirmed the importance of spinal stenosis and osteoporosis as risk factors. Thirteen cases of permanent paraparesis or cauda equina syndrome occurred after CNB in patients with spinal stenosis in the absence of any other cause. Degenerative disorders such as spinal stenosis may be asymptomatic and are often only discovered as a result of imaging performed in the

TABLE 18-3. Risk Factors for Severe Neurologic Complications

| |
|---|
| Patient factors |
| Female sex |
| Atherosclerosis |
| Diabetes |
| Advanced age |
| Spinal disorders |
| Osteoporosis |
| Ankylosing spondylitis |
| Spinal stenosis |
| Osteoarthritis |
| Other spinal deformity |
| Neuropathy |
| Coagulation abnormality (including liver disease; bleeding disorder) |
| Technique factors |
| Epidural catheter |
| Traumatic puncture |
| Dysesthesias during insertion |
| Prolonged continuation of block |
| Hypotension |

investigation of an anesthetic complication. However, if the diagnosis is known in advance, other regional techniques such as plexus or peripheral nerve blockade, or spinal anesthesia, can be selected that avoid cord compression risk.[11] The well-recognized risk factors for spinal hematoma and intravertebral abscess are discussed later in this chapter.

## Diagnosis

Because compressive causes such as spinal hematoma and abscess are curable if treated promptly, identification of pathologic lower body motor and sensory deficits must be made as early as possible after the expected regression of neuraxial blockade. Diagnosis may be challenging in this setting and a high index of suspicion is required, particularly when identifiable risk factors are present. For example, detection of the onset of a painless cauda equina syndrome is likely to be difficult in an immobile postoperative patient with a catheterized bladder, perhaps also receiving an epidural infusion of a low-dose local anesthetic/opiate mixture. If new or progressive neurologic symptoms become apparent, the infusion should be discontinued immediately to rule out a local anesthetic or volume effect. The three key management principles are (1) thorough clinical neurologic assessment, (2) magnetic resonance imaging (MRI), and (3) early consultation with colleagues in radiology, neurology, and neurosurgery. MRI allows rapid, high-resolution images of developing intraspinal pathology to be obtained and may be supplemented by other testing such as electromyography should acute compression be ruled out.

Initial presentation as cauda equina syndrome is a feature of several etiologies and it should be readily recognized by all practitioners (Table 18-4). The fine autonomic fibers of the cauda equina are often the first to be affected by compression, ischemia, or neurotoxicity.[26] Damage to S2–S4 roots produces a lower motor neurone lesion with an atonic bladder although continence may be preserved if intravesical pressure is low. Progression of the syndrome leads to weakness of muscles below the knee as well as the hamstrings and gluteal muscles with loss of ankle jerks and preservation of the knee jerk. Sensory loss in the sacral roots produces the characteristic saddle-shaped anesthesia of the perineum, buttocks, and thighs, extending to foot and calf if L5, S1 roots are involved. In the study by Moen and colleagues,[10] cauda equina syndrome occurred in 32 patients and was thought to be related to local anesthetic toxicity or nonspecific compressive effects in patients with spinal stenosis. Complications may also appear as other characteristic patterns such as anterior spinal artery syndrome or arachnoiditis, and these will be discussed later in this chapter.

TABLE 18-4. Causes of Cauda Equina Syndrome

| |
|---|
| Compressive |
| Anesthetic |
| Spinal hematoma |
| Intravertebral abscess |
| Volume effect |
| Nonanesthetic |
| Prolapsed intervertebral disc |
| Spondylolisthesis |
| Positioning (e.g., lithotomy) |
| Noncompressive |
| Arachnoiditis |
| Local anesthetic neurotoxicity |

## Spinal Hematoma

Acute spinal cord compression from a hematoma developing in the subarachnoid, subdural, or extradural space can rapidly produce irreversible paraplegia. A comprehensive neurosurgical review of all 613 cases of spinal hematoma identified in the literature to 2003[27] found that only one in 10 reported cases was related to "a needle in the back" (63 cases), the largest group being idiopathic/spontaneous (38.2%). The majority presented within 24 hours of the presumed triggering event. This disastrous complication of CNB is more likely to occur in the presence of coagulopathy and traumatic insertion procedure as well as other risk factors listed in Table 18-3.[8,28,29] However, spinal hematoma can occur after CNB even in the absence of recognized risk factors. A review of the 61 case reports of spinal hematoma associated with neuraxial anesthetic techniques published between 1906 and 1994 by Vandermeulen and colleagues[28] reported that 13% had no identifiable risk factors at all. In the recent study by Moen and colleagues,[10] coagulation abnormality was documented in only one-third of spinal hematomas. Some of these cases may be caused by puncture of epidural veins or Adamkiewicz's vein (L3-5 level), which lie lateral to the midline. This underlines the importance of vigilance and postoperative neurologic monitoring.

### *Incidence*

Tryba's[30] frequently quoted "baseline" incidence of spinal hematoma of 1 in 150,000 epidurals and 1 in 220,000 subarachnoid blocks (upper 95% confidence limit) now seems to be a serious underestimate in higher risk groups.[15,21,31] Low-molecular-weight heparins (LMWHs) were introduced for routine thromboprophylaxis in 1993 and this is certainly a factor. Tryba and Wedel[3] estimate that spinal hematoma occurred as much as 160 times more frequently in the United States than in Europe during the mid-1990s because of the higher routine daily doses of LMWH. However, a recent study identified 33 cases in Sweden alone during the 1990s and reported that the incidence in the general (nonobstetric) population was 1:10,300 after epidurals versus 1:480,000 after spinal blockade. In a high-risk group (female patients undergoing total knee arthroplasty with an epidural), the incidence was 1:3600.[24] Interestingly, this is in very close agreement with the estimated reporting rate during 1993–1997 in the United States of 1:3100 with epidural indwelling catheters after total hip or knee arthroplasty.[4] In another Scandinavian study, the overall incidence of spinal hematoma causing paraplegia was 1:3077.[11] Thus, despite the lower doses of LMWH used during the 1990s, the incidence of spinal hematoma in Europe is likely to have been higher than previously estimated and this highlights the problem of underreporting error. In their study, Moen and colleagues[10] commented that less strict guidelines were used during the study period and formalized guidelines for CNB in the presence of anticoagulation have subsequently been developed and implemented. These are discussed further below – their effect on the occurrence of spinal hematoma is not yet known and requires ongoing surveillance.

In contrast, the spinal hematoma incidence after obstetric epidurals is probably less than 1:100,000.[16,17] In Moen and colleagues' study,[10] there were two spinal hematomas reported in 255,000 obstetric blocks, but both occurring in patients with the syndrome of hemolysis, elevated liver enzymes, and low platelets (HELLP). The existence of these risk-stratified subgroups in obstetrics reinforces the need for an individual patient approach to risk–benefit decisions regardless of the clinical setting.

### *Diagnosis and Treatment*

Clinical suspicion of the development of spinal hematoma may be aroused by the classic symptoms of progressive lower limb weakness progressing to flaccid paralysis, numbness, and loss of bladder and bowel continence. Onset of cord compression from hematoma may be immediate or take hours or days. From retrospective case report analysis, mean onset time to paraplegia was 14 hours and acute back pain was not a feature in many cases.[29] MRI is the gold standard diagnostic imaging technique and typical appearances are shown in Figure 18-1. MRI should be accompanied by neurosurgical consultation. In the neurosurgical review of 613 cases from all causes discussed above, complete neurologic recovery from spinal hematoma was achieved in about 40% of cases. Comparing prompt surgical intervention (laminectomy and clot evacuation within 12 hours) with treatment delayed beyond 12 hours, the rate of complete recovery was 66% versus 29%. Although recovery after conservative treatment occurred in 25 of 33 cases (76%), these patients were carefully selected. In this series, there was a 5.5% mortality directly related to spinal hematoma.[27] Among spinal hematomas related to neuraxial blockade, recovery seems to be better from lumbosacral hematoma (L2-S1) compared with locations higher in the spinal cord.[28]

With such poor outcomes, it is clear that if there is any risk of hemostatic defect surrounding the use of neuraxial blockade there must be a high index of clinical suspicion of cord compression. Because prognosis is better when preoperative neurologic deterioration is less severe, early diagnosis of spinal hematoma should be a central aim of postoperative surveillance. Serial neurologic examination, allowing blockade to wear off if necessary before reexamination, is often appropriate.

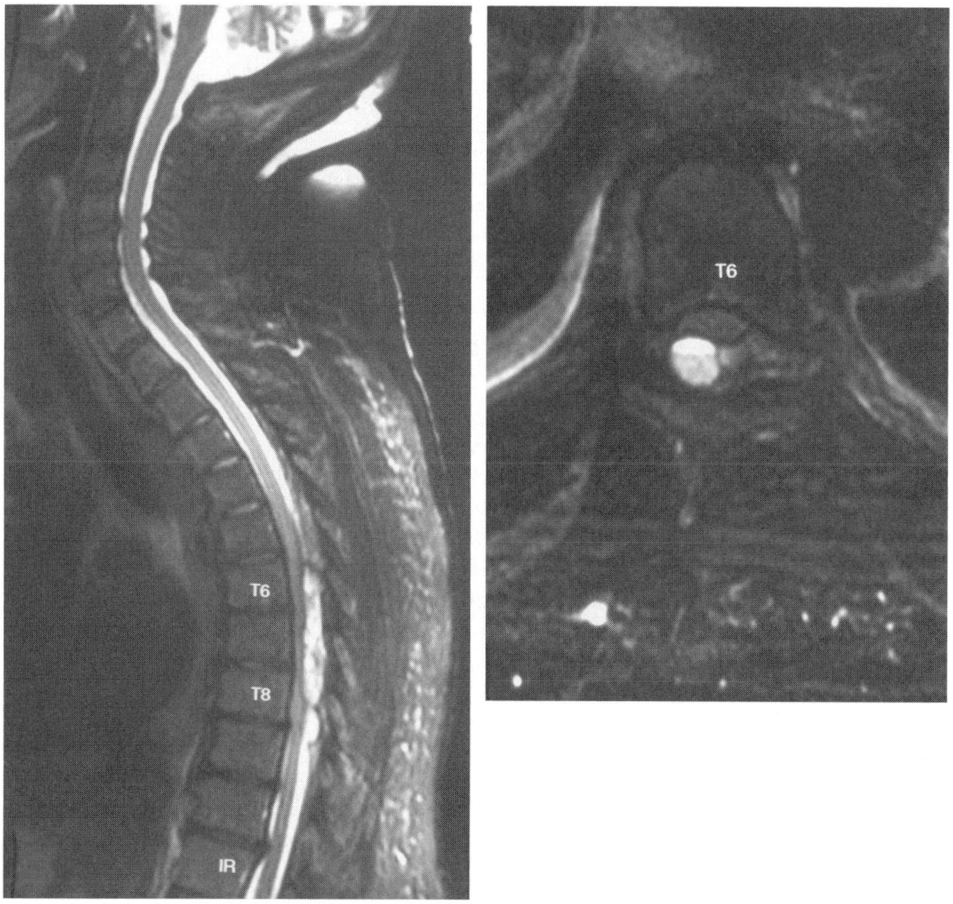


A B

**FIGURE 18-1.** Thoracic epidural hematoma demonstrated by MRI. Sagittal **(A)** and axial **(B)** T2 MR images of cervicothoracic spine showing acute epidural hematoma posterior to the cord at T5–T9 level. Note well-defined layering of blood in **(B)**. (Courtesy Dr. Ayton Hope, Auckland City Hospital.)

TABLE 18-5. 2003 ASRA Guidelines for Neuraxial Anesthesia and Anticoagulation[34]

| Drug class | Recommendation |
|---|---|
| Antiplatelet drugs | |
| (a) Aspirin and NSAIDs* | No contraindication; perform block at any time† |
| (b) Thienopyridine derivatives | Discontinue agent 7 days (clopidogrel) to 14 days (ticlopidine) before CNB‡ |
| (c) GP IIb/IIIa receptor antagonists | CNB contraindicated within 8 hours (eptifibatide, tirofiban) to 48 hours (abciximab) of administration |
| UH | |
| (a) Subcutaneous | No contraindication§ |
| (b) Intravenous | Perform CNB or remove catheter 2–4 hours after last dose and confirm normal coagulation status; delay heparin administration for 1 hour after CNB (e.g., intraoperatively)‖ |
| LMWH | |
| (a) Prophylactic | CNB or catheter removal 10–12 hours after LMWH; administer LMWH 2–4 hours after CNB/catheter removal¶ |
| (b) Therapeutic | Delay CNB at least 24 hours after LMWH; otherwise as above |
| Oral anticoagulants (warfarin) | Document normal INR before CNB; remove catheter when INR still ≤1.5 |
| Thrombolytics | Insufficient data; extreme risk# |
| Herbal medicines | No contraindication; perform block at any time† |

*Including cyclooxygenase-2 inhibitors.
†Caution when combined with other anticoagulants.
‡Insufficient data; actual risk unknown.
§European guidelines recommend withholding CNB for 4 hours after unfractionated subcutaneous heparin and waiting 1 hour after CNB or catheter removal before administration.
‖European guidelines recommend deferring surgery at least 12 hours after traumatic CNB if intraoperative intravenous heparin anticipated.
¶Delay LMWH administration for 24 hours after traumatic CNB.
#Recommend neurologic monitoring at least 2 hourly.

### *Hemostatic Defect*

Clotting abnormalities increase the risk of spinal hematoma after CNB. Partial or complete hemostatic failure from any cause or combination of causes produces a spectrum of risk, which may be negligible in the case of low-dose aspirin, and very high (>1%) in fully heparinized patients[32] or in the presence of thrombolytic therapy.[33] Many drugs have prolonged half-lives and are difficult to reverse. Vessel wall fragility (e.g., treatment with steroids) may also increase the risk of spinal hematoma. The most recent guidelines for CNB in relation to anticoagulant drugs were published by the American Society of Regional Anesthesia (ASRA) in 2003 and are summarized in Table 18-5.[34]

### *Acceptable Laboratory Values for Safe Institution of Neuraxial Blockade*

The minimum platelet count below which it is safe to place a central neuraxial block is not known. It is generally accepted that isolated thrombocytopenia down to a platelet count of $100 \times 10^9$/L does not pose a risk for spinal hematoma, although there is some evidence that the safe level may be as low as $70 \times 10^9$/L in obstetrics.[35] Use of bleeding time as a screening test is not recommended. However, in an individual patient with a history of bleeding or easy bruising, the PFA-100 can be a useful investigation to identify platelet function disorders (e.g., von Willebrand's disease).[36]

Although not currently validated, thromboelastography may become a useful overall test of function of the coagulation system before performing neuraxial blocks.[37] It is probably inadvisable to perform blocks if an abnormality in other coagulation parameters (e.g., prothrombin time or activated partial thromboplastin time) is present. Despite this, where the anticipated benefits are great or if general anesthesia is contraindicated, there is some evidence that minor abnormalities are acceptable.[28,38]

### *Antiplatelet Agents*

The useful antithrombotic effect of low-dose aspirin is a result of irreversible inhibition of platelet cyclooxygenase. This effect lasts for the platelet lifespan (7–10 days) with the relatively less potent and reversible platelet inhibition caused by conventional nonsteroidal antiinflammatory drugs (NSAIDs) lasting approximately 3 days. The minor hemostatic defect caused by the use of these drugs alone does not seem to increase the risk of producing spinal hematoma after neuraxial blockade. A number of case series amounting to many thousands of patients receiving these antiplatelet drugs preoperatively and subsequently given spinal or epidural anesthesia without complication attest to the safety of this combination.[28] However, the evidence from pharmacologic data is that neuraxial blockade is contraindicated in the presence of newer antiplatelet agents. Adenosine diphosphate receptor antagonists such as clopidogrel induce a maximum 40%–50% inhibition of platelet function and this can be achieved after a single dose. This platelet effect is irreversible and recovers completely 7 days after discontinuation of clopidogrel.[39] Although a case of spinal hematoma occurring after a 7-day clopidogrel-free interval has been recently reported, the patient had other risk factors.[40] Near total inhibition of platelet aggregation may be achieved using glycoprotein IIb/IIIa receptor antagonists (e.g., abciximab, eptifibatide). Platelet function normalizes 48 hours after abciximab infusion, and platelet transfusion only partially reverses the effect.[41]

### *Heparin and LMWH*

The presence of therapeutic blood heparin levels is a clear contraindication to epidural or spinal insertion. The situation is less clearcut with therapeutic heparinization shortly after the block procedure. A range of variables such as traumatic procedure, other antiplatelet or anticoagulant therapy, shorter time interval between neuraxial blockade and heparin administration, and unmonitored coagulation state may increase the chance of a spinal hematoma.[24] A number of case series comprising several thousand patients in which attention was given to the sort of risk factors just mentioned point to the relative safety of spinal/epidural anesthesia in patients subsequently heparinized for vascular surgery, although cases of spinal hematoma still occur in this high-risk population.[24] CNB before full systemic heparinization for cardiopulmonary bypass remains very controversial.[42] If performed, then the advice in Table 18-6 should

Table 18-6. Precautions in the Use of Neuraxial Blockade

1. Careful patient selection (assess risk–benefit of CNB)
2. Follow guidelines for anticoagulation and CNB (Table 18-5)
3. Perform in awake patient
4. Consider single-shot intrathecal opioid (±local anesthetic) technique
5. Minimize number of attempts; experienced operator
6. Avoid intraoperative hypotension; care with positioning
7. Avoid epidural local anesthetic solutions that cause motor block
8. Strict neurologic surveillance
9. Communication with postoperative and acute pain teams
10. Advise patients to report back pain and sensorimotor symptoms
11. Ideally MRI should be available

be followed, taking particular care to check lower body neurologic state at regular intervals.

Subcutaneous administration of low-dose unfractionated heparin (UH) and LMWH is effective prophylaxis against venous thromboembolism in surgical patients. These drugs at low doses are not detectable by the usual laboratory tests of coagulation. An unfortunate cluster of nearly 60 cases of spinal hematoma occurred in the United States during the 1990s associated with administration of relatively high doses of LMWH. Those affected were typically older female orthopedic patients undergoing joint replacement surgery with epidural, for whom the estimate of spinal hematoma was 1:3100.[4] As discussed above, the unacceptably high incidence in this important patient subgroup is not isolated to the United States.[10] Overall, UH or LMWH is compatible with neuraxial regional anesthesia if guidelines such as those developed by ASRA are followed (Table 18-5).[34] This does not completely eliminate the risk, as shown in a recent Swedish study in which one-third of hematomas occurred in patients in whom current guidelines were followed.[10] The effects of hepatic disease, renal impairment, and other drugs interfering with coagulation must be assessed, and heparin-induced thrombocytopenia must be excluded. Despite laboratory evidence that a small proportion of patients develop transiently therapeutic heparin levels after UH via the subcutaneous route,[43] the ASRA guideline allows the block to be performed at any time. Pharmacologic differences do exist between individual LMWH preparations, although the rate of spinal hematoma seems to be similar.[34] If a patient unexpectedly requires therapeutic anticoagulation (e.g., myocardial infarction in the postoperative period), at what stage should one remove the epidural catheter? We prefer to remove the catheter before prolonged therapeutic anticoagulation rather than leaving it in situ until treatment is completed.

## Intravertebral Abscess

This section will summarize the complication of intravertebral abscess. For a more detailed discussion of this and other infective complications such as meningitis or the risks of neuraxial blockade in the febrile patient, the reader is referred to Chapter 19.

Although intravertebral infection is thought to be most frequently caused by bacterial migration along the catheter, other possibilities are colonization from hematogenous spread or contamination during the procedure itself; for example, the anesthesiologist's nasal flora has been implicated.[44] The most common organisms are *Staphylococcus* species. The classic symptoms are backache, fever, and radicular pain followed by progressive weakness, which may be delayed for up to several months.[45] Raised inflammatory markers, leucocytosis, and clinical signs of meningism also occur. The mainstay of treatment is decompressive laminectomy, supplemented by antibiotic therapy for 4–6 weeks, although conservative treatment has been used in selected cases.[46] MRI is the investigative procedure of choice (Figure 18-2).

As is the case for spinal hematoma, compression of the spinal cord from an infective process can be causally related to CNB, but can also arise in the total absence of regional anesthesia. In a comprehensive neurosurgical review of 915 cases of intravertebral abscess, only 5.5% were related to CNB or other epidural injections.[46] The review by Kindler et al.[45] of 42 cases associated with CNB reported in the anesthetic literature found that many cases occurred in patients with immunocompromise, including diabetes mellitus (43%). In addition, a relatively high proportion occurred after thoracic epidural catheters (33%) and the authors proposed that difficult insertion and longer duration of use may be implicated. Median duration of epidural catheterization was 4 days, although the range was a few hours to 10 weeks. Eighty percent of patients were treated with surgery, although only 45% made a full recovery. Several subsequent studies have confirmed these risk factors and the poor prognosis of this condition.[47,48]

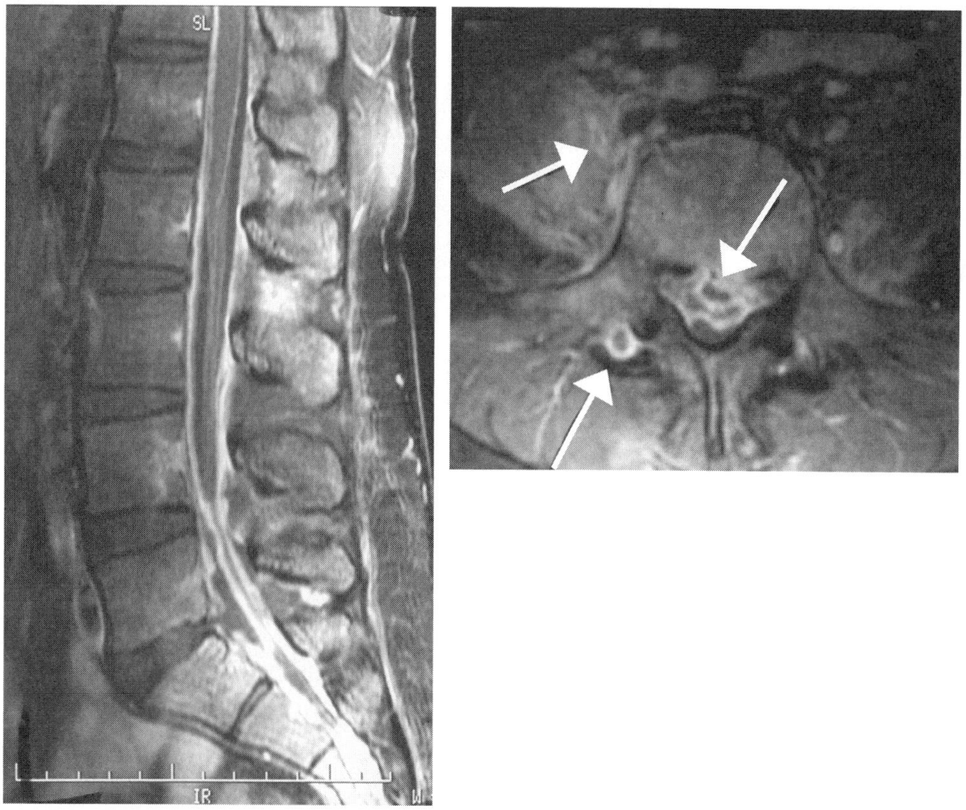


**FIGURE 18-2.** Epidural and paraspinal abscess demonstrated by MRI. Contrast enhanced fat saturated T1 sagittal **(A)** and axial **(B)** MRIs of lumbar spine demonstrating epidural abscess with satellite abscesses in posterior paraspinal tissues and right psoas muscle (see arrows). (Courtesy Dr. Ayton Hope, Auckland City Hospital.)

The incidence is difficult to assess accurately, particularly because presentation may be very late. In a prospective national survey from Denmark during 1997–1998, the overall incidence was 1:1930, although the incidence at non-university hospitals was 1:796.[47] This is significantly higher than in the recent study by Moen and colleagues[10] which reported one abscess in 1,260,000 spinals and 8 in 450,000 epidurals during a 10-year period in Sweden. Spinal abscess is more frequent than hematoma in obstetric patients; the incidence is difficult to define but is certainly significant – Loo and colleagues[15] reported rates of up to 3.7:100,000 in their review. Nine obstetric cases were included in the literature review by Kindler et al.[45]

### *Prevention*

Factors that would be expected to reduce the chance of intravertebral abscess formation after CNB include: meticulous aseptic technique (including obstetric cases) with avoidance of multidose drug vials, use of antibacterial filters for epidural catheters, atraumatic technique, as well as a high index of suspicion (including checking the site regularly), particularly in patients with bacteremia or immunosuppression from any cause. In the neurosurgical review,[46] outcome was no better among anesthesia-related abscesses than in spontaneous cases, suggesting that we need to maintain a higher index of suspicion. There may be a very long interval between the procedure and onset of signs and, as is the case for spinal hematoma, early diagnosis is crucial because outcome is related to degree of neurologic impairment at the time of surgery.

## Spinal Cord Ischemia and Infarction

### *Pattern of Injury*

Patterns of spinal cord injury resulting from inadequate local blood supply are a consequence of the anatomic arrangements (Figure 18-3). The anterior two-thirds of any segment of the spinal cord is supplied by the single anterior spinal artery. This artery

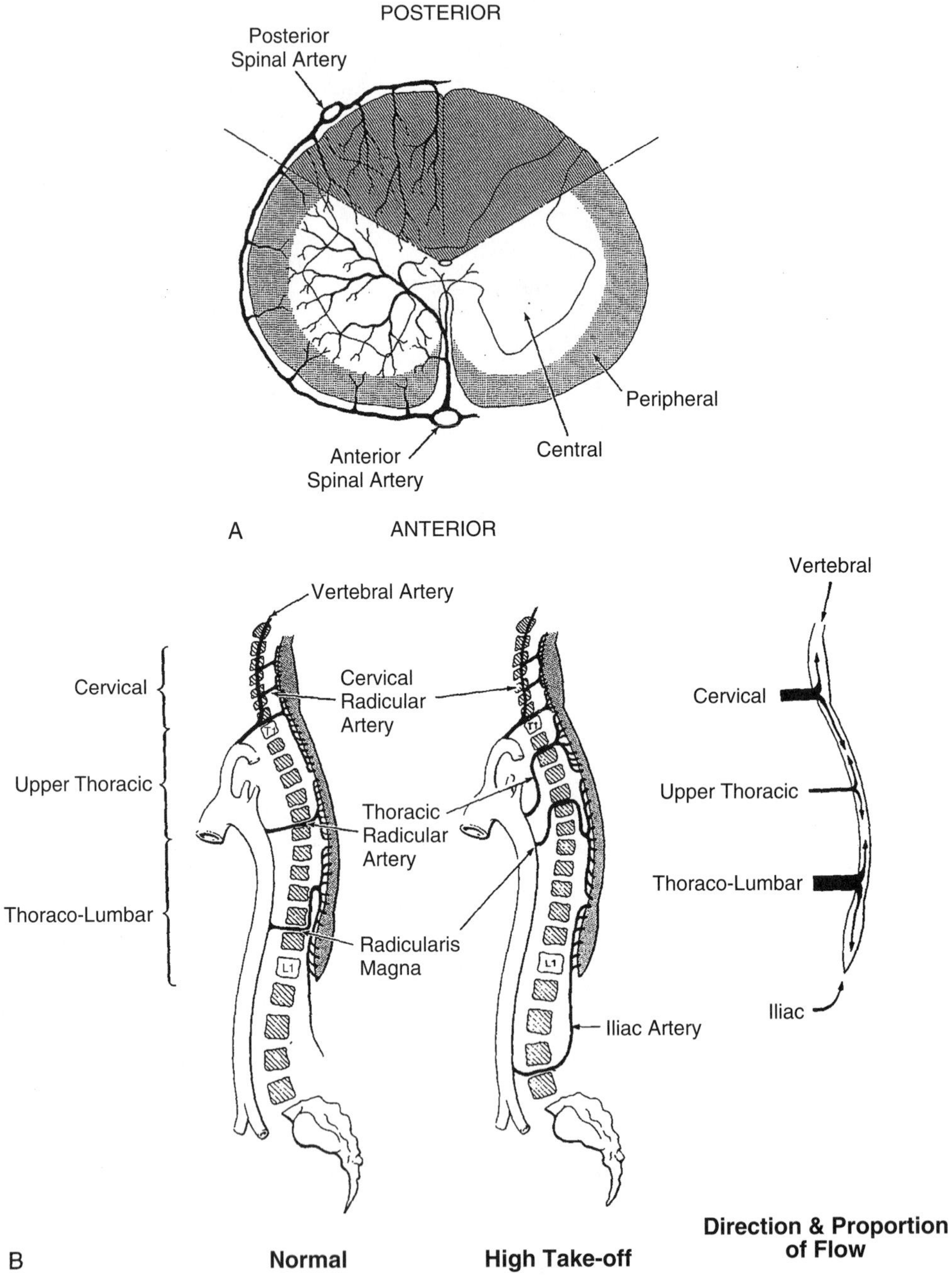


**Figure 18-3.** **(A)** Horizontal section of spinal cord showing territory supplied by anterior and posterior spinal arteries. (From Cousins MJ, Bridenbough PO, eds. Neural Blockade in Clinical Anaesthesia and Management of Pain. 3rd ed. Philadelphia: Lippincott Williams & Wilkins; 1998:255.) **(B)** Vertical arrangement of three zones of aortic blood supply to the anterior spinal artery. High take-off occurs in around 15% of cases. (From Cousins MJ, Bridenbough PO, eds. Neural Blockade in Clinical Anaesthesia and Management of Pain. 3rd ed. Philadelphia: Lippincott Williams & Wilkins; 1998:212. Reprinted with permission from Publisher.)

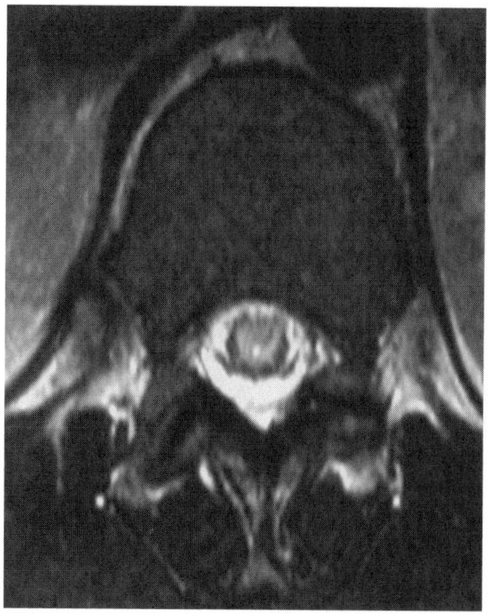

**FIGURE 18-4.** Anterior spinal artery syndrome demonstrated by MRI. Axial T2 MRI of lower thoracic spine. The hyperdense signal in the anterior two-thirds of the spinal cord was present from T7–T11 and is caused by acute infarction in anterior spinal artery territory. (Courtesy Dr. Ayton Hope, Auckland City Hospital.)

receives its blood supply from small paired segmental vessels arising from three distinct aortic origins with poor vertical anastomoses between the cervical, thoracic, and lumbar territories, although there is considerable anatomic variation. The largest of these is usually the radicularis magna (artery of Adamkiewicz), entering on the left between T8 and L3. Damage to this artery from any cause (and needle damage to vessels traversing the intervertebral foramen is possible) can cause ischemia to the entire lumbar cord. It is thought that the midthoracic region comprises a watershed area of the cord and is particularly vulnerable[27] (Figure 18-4). Because the area of spinal cord supplied by the anterior spinal artery contains the anterior and lateral spinothalamic tracts, the anterior horn cells, and the pyramidal tracts, selective loss of perfusion causes the neurologic picture of anterior spinal artery syndrome: below the level of the lesion there is loss of pain and temperature sensation, flaccid paralysis, and later spasticity. Position and vibration sensation are preserved because these modalities are carried in the dorsal columns. Lesser degrees of obstruction to one or more of the segmental radicular arteries supplying the anterior spinal artery may limit weakness and sensory impairment to one limb or asymmetric involvement of the lower limbs, sometimes allowing complete recovery. In contrast, the posterior one-third of the cord is supplied by two anastomosing posterior spinal arteries and is less vulnerable to ischemia.[27]

### *Anterior Spinal Artery Syndrome and Regional Anesthesia*

One case of probable anterior spinal artery syndrome in 30,000 epidurals was described in the prospective survey by Auroy and colleagues.[13] A summary of factors contributing to anterior spinal artery syndrome is presented in Table 18-7. Very similar cases

TABLE 18-7. Important Contributors to Anterior Spinal Artery Syndrome

- Atherosclerosis
- Hypotension
- Positioning (e.g., lithotomy; hyperlordotic)
- Aortic surgery and cross-clamping
- Local vasoconstrictors
- Embolism (thrombus, fat, air, bacterial)
- Dissecting aortic aneurysm
- Vertebral column surgery

have been reported with and without the use of regional techniques,[49] raising the question of whether neuraxial blockade is a major contributor. Usually causation is multifactorial – intraoperative positioning and hypotension seem to be especially important.[50–52] Other factors may contribute such as caval compression and individual anatomic variation in cord blood supply. Damage or irritation to a radicular feeding vessel by needle or epidural catheter as the vessel transverses the intervertebral foramen is postulated as a cause for a case of transient and incomplete anterior spinal artery syndrome.[50,51]

## Spinal Cord and Nerve Root Trauma

Direct trauma by needle or catheter and intraneural injection during anesthetic procedures can cause irreversible damage to neural structures and is usually associated with radicular pain during the procedure. Horlocker and colleagues[53] found that the incidence of persistent sensory symptoms was almost 30 times more common in patients who had experienced dysesthesias during insertion of epidural, spinal, or caudal compared with patients who had no dysesthesias. For this reason, it is widely held that CNB should be performed with the patient awake where possible[54,55], although this is a subject of ongoing debate.[56,57] There have been a disturbing number of cases reported in the literature during the last 5 years of damage to the conus medullaris from spinal anesthesia performed at too high a level resulting in permanent neurologic sequelae.[10,58,59] Many of these cases were young women undergoing obstetric procedures with an incidence in the United Kingdom estimated by Reynolds[60] at approximately 1:20,000. Typical MRI appearances are shown in Figure 18-5. A variety of patient, equipment, and technique-related contributing factors can

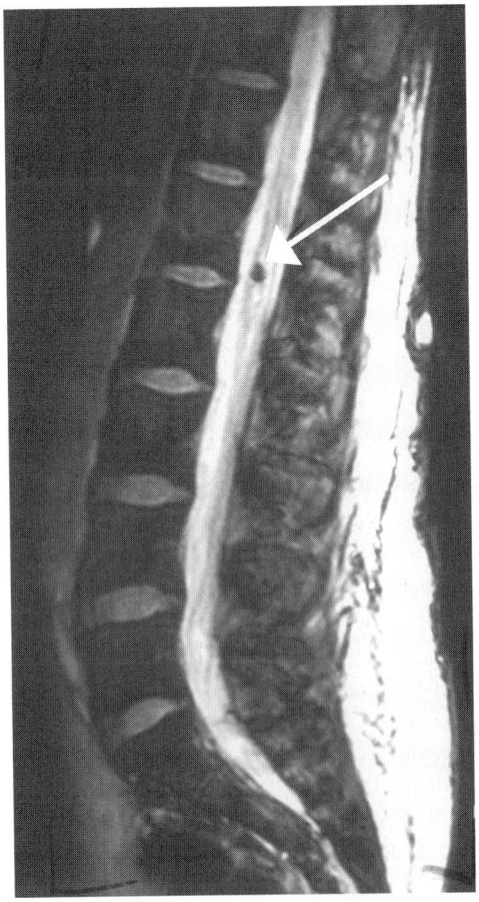

**FIGURE 18-5.** Needle injury to conus medullaris demonstrated by MRI. Sagittal gradient echo T2* MRI of conus medullaris, about 2 weeks after inadvertent needle puncture. T2* sequence accentuates blood products (see arrow). (Courtesy Dr. Ayton Hope, Auckland City Hospital.)

be identified for each case of spinal cord needle trauma.[61] It is important to perform spinal anesthesia at the lower interspace if a choice exists because of the variation in the level of termination of the cord and inaccurate identification of lumbar level.[62] One should also maintain the needle in the midline, obtain good backflow of cerebrospinal fluid, and stop immediately should the patient complain of painful paraesthesias. If multiple attempts are required or persistently blood staining of the cerebrospinal fluid is noted, the procedure should probably be abandoned in favor of another technique.

## Arachnoiditis and Neurotoxicity

Earlier discussion of the Woolley and Roe case serves to introduce this disastrous complication of neuraxial regional anesthesia that has not been eliminated as a rare cause of paraplegia and for which no effective treatment exists. Arachnoiditis now seems to be a less common cause of postoperative paraplegia compared with cord compression by hematoma or abscess and indeed is usually a diagnosis of exclusion.[63,64]

### *Presentation*

Onset of cauda equina syndrome immediately after epidural or spinal anesthesia ("the block never wore off") can be attributable to arachnoiditis but would be more likely from a compressive cause. Adhesive arachnoiditis typically presents as a gradual progressive weakness and sensory loss in the lower extremities beginning days, weeks, or months after a spinal anesthetic. Onset is often accompanied by bladder and bowel symptoms as well as a painful radiculopathy which is usually bilateral, similar in character to the syndrome of transient neurologic symptoms. The course is often progressive, leading to complete paraplegia and occasionally death. The investigation of choice is MRI, and the characteristic appearance is that of edematous nerve roots in the early phase followed later by clumped spinal roots forming bizarre patterns (e.g., "string of pearls") or adherent to the dural sac[65] (Figure 18-6). These radiologic

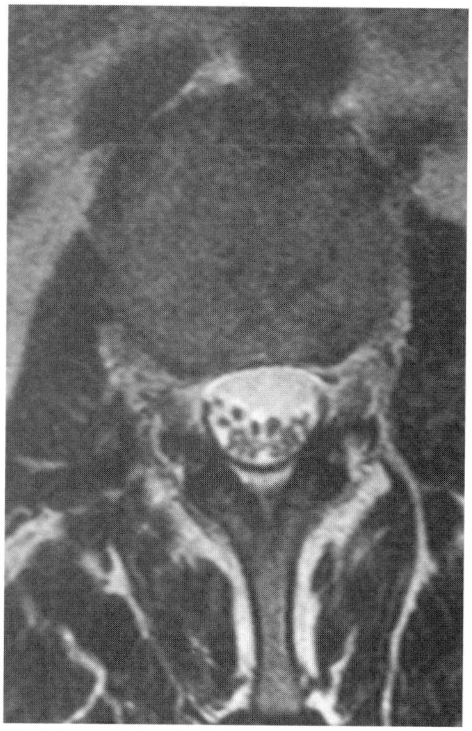

**FIGURE 18-6.** Arachnoiditis demonstrated by MRI. Axial T2 MRI at L2 level in a patient with arachnoiditis demonstrating characteristic clumping of nerve roots of the cauda equina as well as adhesion to the dura. (Courtesy Dr. Ayton Hope, Auckland City Hospital.)

appearances correspond to the typical histologic changes in which an early meningeal inflammatory response leads to chronic arachnoid proliferation, fibrosis, and adhesions constricting the nerve roots and spinal cord.[65] Just how long after epidural, caudal, or spinal anesthesia these techniques can be blamed for subsequent arachnoiditis is unknown, and exclusion of "idiopathic" causes may be impossible.[66]

### *Causes*

It is important to recognize the wide range of causes of inflammation and adhesive scarring of the arachnoid mater, some of which may occur coincidentally with regional anesthesia (Table 18-8). Inherent in CNB is the risk of both drug error and accidental introduction of contaminants into the epidural or subarachnoid spaces. However remote this possibility may seem, it must always be included in the differential diagnosis of postoperative neurologic complications.[65,67] Aldrete's[65] position is that arachnoid inflammation is a pathologic feature common to most mechanisms of injury to intrathecal neural structures including trauma, infection, hematoma, myelography, and other chemical causes.

The intentional use of drugs thought to be safe for CNB has also produced cases of arachnoiditis. Close attention should be given to the licensed or intended route of administration for all agents administered into the epidural or intrathecal spaces. Preservatives have been suggested as a cause in cases of neurologic injury following epidural injection and after inadvertent subarachnoid injection of agents intended for epidural use.[9,68] In one report describing six patients with myelographically confirmed arachnoiditis after epidural anesthesia, detergent contamination of nondisposable glass syringes and the use of multidose vials of local anesthetic containing preservatives were considered possible cause[69] and neither of these practices can be recommended. However, a recent review found no link between obstetric epidurals and chronic arachnoiditis.[64] Early treatment using high-dose steroids and NSAIDs in suspected cases has been suggested by Aldrete in order to reduce progression of the inflammatory process.[65]

### *Local Anesthetic Neurotoxicity*

Evidence from animal studies indicates that local anesthetics are neurotoxic in a concentration-dependent manner.[9,70] The long "dwell time" of hyperbaric 5% lignocaine in contact with neural tissue made possible by the use of spinal microcatheters has led to the abandonment of this combination. This strength of lignocaine has also

TABLE 18-8. Causes of Arachnoiditis

- Idiopathic
- Infection (e.g., meningitis)
- Spinal trauma, surgery, hemorrhage
- Foreign substances introduced into the epidural and subarachnoid spaces (intentional, accidental, drug error)
  - Myelographic contrast agents
  - Antibiotics
  - Corticosteroids
  - Anti-tetanus serum
  - Local anesthetic drugs
  - Detergents
  - Skin antiseptic
  - Unknown contaminant
  - Drug error

been clearly implicated as a cause of cauda equina syndrome in single-shot spinal anesthesia, which is often permanent.[13,14,26,71,72] However, there is no good evidence that lignocaine is more toxic than other agents if used in equipotent concentrations and doses. Lignocaine is approximately 4 times as potent as bupivacaine, so 5% lignocaine equates to 1.25% bupivacaine, not 0.5%, and bupivacaine 15mg equates to lignocaine 60mg. In 1995, Astra USA revised the prescribing information for hyperbaric 5% lignocaine to suggest dilution to 2.5% using saline or cerebrospinal fluid, although it has been suggested that hyperbaric lignocaine should actually be administered in concentrations not greater than 2% and a total dose not greater than 60mg.[26] Bupivacaine has also been implicated in cases of serious neurologic sequelae.[73] Local anesthetic neurotoxicity was thought to be responsible for 23 cases of permanent cauda equina syndrome in the study by Moen and colleagues,[10] occurring predominantly in younger patients. Hyperbaric 5% lignocaine was used in nine cases and 0.5% bupivacaine in 12 cases. It likely that existing polyneuropathy related to diabetes or other diseases as well as concurrent administration of drugs known to be neurotoxic confer a susceptibility to local anesthetic neurotoxicity.[68,72,73]

### *Wrong Drug*

Although iatrogenic medical disasters are very underreported because of medicolegal implications, wrong-drug case reports appear regularly.[74] Epidural catheters expose patients to the risk of accidental wrong drug for several days postoperatively, and potassium chloride via this route seems to be a particular culprit.[67,75–77] Considerable responsibility lies with the anesthetist who places the catheter and subsequently delegates care to nursing staff. Safeguards against drug error include color coding of regional anesthesia equipment and designated infusion pumps. Noninterchangeable "foolproof" connection systems have also been suggested, although these may prove to be prohibitively expensive.[78] Patients should always be told to report neurologic symptoms that develop after they go home.

## Children

Spinal anesthesia in neonates and caudal anesthesia combined with general anesthesia in older children are both widely used techniques (refer to Chapter 13). Overall, no special pediatric risk adjustment for the possibility of severe neurologic injury seems justified when comparing this complication of regional anesthesia with the adult experience. No permanent neurologic damage was reported in 150,000 caudals gathered from 119 pediatric institutions[79] and no serious neurologic complications were reported in three further series reviewed by Badgwell and MacLeod.[80] However, a retrospective French survey[81] of 25,005 caudal, epidural, and spinal anesthetics from 10 institutions reported in 1995 revealed four cases of severe tetraplegia/paraplegia following caudal administration of local anesthetics in male infants under 3 months of age. There were clinical and radiologic features consistent with acute spinal cord ischemia (and in one additional case, brain ischemia) which was irreversible and fatal in three of the five cases. Although the temporal link between caudal and catastrophic outcome is inescapable, a causal link was doubtful in at least two cases. In response to this study, a prospective 1-year survey among pediatric anesthesiologists in France was designed. No neurologic sequelae were detected and the authors concluded that regional techniques "offer a valuable and safe tool for providing high quality analgesia in pediatric patients."[82] Of note, the prospective Auroy hotline study also in France found no complications in 4435 blocks performed in children.[14] With respect to pediatric thoracic epidurals, however, a lack of statistical power limits our ability to draw conclusions.[83]

## References


1. Cope RW. The Woolley and Roe case. 1954. Anaesthesia 1995;50(2):162–173.
2. Maltby JR, Hutter CD, Clayton KC. The Woolley and Roe case. Br J Anaesth 2000; 84(1):121–126.
3. Tryba M, Wedel DJ. Central neuraxial block and low molecular weight heparin (enoxaparin): lessons learned from different dosage regimes in two continents. Acta Anaesthesiol Scand 1997;41:100–103.
4. Schroeder DR. Statistics: detecting a rare adverse drug reaction using spontaneous reports. Reg Anesth Pain Med 1998;23(6 suppl 2):183–189.
5. Dripps RD, Vandam LD. Long term followup of patients who received 10,098 spinal anaesthetics. JAMA 1954;156:1486.
6. Dar AQ, Robinson APC, Lyons G. Postpartum neurological symptoms following regional blockade: a prospective study with case controls. Int J Obstet Anesth 2002;11:85–90.
7. Aromaa U, Lahdensuu M, Cozanitis DA. Severe complications associated with epidural and spinal anaesthesias in Finland 1987–1993. A study based on patient insurance claims. Acta Anaesthesiol Scand 1997;41(4):445–452.
8. Lee LA, Posner KL, Domino KB, Caplan RA, Cheney FW. Injuries associated with regional anesthesia in the 1980s and 1990s: a closed claims analysis. Anesthesiology 2004;101(1):143–152.
9. Borgeat A, Blumenthal S. Nerve injury and regional anaesthesia. Curr Opin Anaesthesiol 2004;17(5):417–421.
10. Moen V, Dahlgren N, Irestedt L. Severe neurological complications after central neuraxial blockades in Sweden 1990–1999. Anesthesiology 2004;101(4):950–959.
11. Dahlgren N, Tornebrandt K. Neurological complications after anaesthesia. A follow-up of 18,000 spinal and epidural anaesthetics performed over three years. Acta Anaesthesiol Scand 1995;39(7):872–880.
12. Renck H. Neurological complications of central nerve blocks. Acta Anaesthesiol Scand 1995;39(7):859–868.
13. Auroy Y, Narchi P, Messiah A, Litt L, Rouvier B, Samii K. Serious complications related to regional anesthesia: results of a prospective survey in France. Anesthesiology 1997; 87(3):479–486.
14. Auroy Y, Benhamou D, Bargues L, et al. Major complications of regional anesthesia in France: The SOS Regional Anesthesia Hotline Service. Anesthesiology 2002;97(5): 1274–1280.
15. Loo CC, Dahlgren G, Irestedt L. Neurological complications in obstetric regional anaesthesia. Int J Obstet Anesth 2000;9(2):99–124.
16. Scott DB, Hibbard BM. Serious non-fatal complications associated with extradural block in obstetric practice. Br J Anaesth 1990;64:537.
17. Palot M, Visseaux H, Botmans C, Pire JC. Epidemiology of complications of obstetrical epidural analgesia [French]. Cah Anesthesiol 1994;42(2):229–233.
18. Paech MJ, Godkin R, Webster S. Complications of obstetric epidural analgesia and anaesthesia: a prospective analysis of 10,995 cases. Int J Obstet Anesth 1998;7(1):5–11.
19. Usubiaga JE. Neurological complications following epidural anaesthesia. Int Anesthesiol Clin 1975;13:1.
20. Holdcroft A, Gibberd FB, Hargrove RL, Hawkins DF, Dellaportas CI. Neurological complications associated with pregnancy. Br J Anaesth 1995;75(5):522–526.
21. Chadwick HS. An analysis of obstetric anesthesia cases from the American Society of Anesthesiologists closed claims project database. Int J Obstet Anesth 1996;5(4): 258–263.
22. Wills JH, Wiesel S, Abram SE, Rupp FW. Synovial cysts and the lithotomy position causing cauda equina syndrome. Reg Anesth Pain Med 2004;29(3):234–236.
23. Stambough JL, Stambough JB, Evans S. Acute cauda equina syndrome after total knee arthroplasty as a result of epidural anesthesia and spinal stenosis. J Arthroplasty 2000;15(3):375–379.
24. Lee BB. Neuraxial complications after epidural and spinal anaesthesia. Acta Anaesthesiol Scand 2003;47(3):371–372.
25. Jacob AK, Borowiec JC, Long TR, Brown MJ, Rydberg CH, Wass CT. Transient profound neurologic deficit associated with thoracic epidural analgesia in an elderly patient. Anesthesiology 2004;101(6):1470–1471.

26. Loo CC, Irestedt L. Cauda equina syndrome after spinal anaesthesia with hyperbaric 5% lignocaine: a review of six cases of cauda equina syndrome reported to the Swedish Pharmaceutical Insurance 1993–1997. Acta Anaesthesiol Scand 1999;43(4):371–379.
27. Kreppel D, Antoniadis G, Seeling W. Spinal hematoma: a literature survey with meta-analysis of 613 patients. Neurosurg Rev 2003;26(1):1–49.
28. Vandermeulen EP, Van Aken H, Vermylen J. Anticoagulants and spinal-epidural anesthesia. Anesth Analg 1994;79:1165.
29. Horlocker TT. What's a nice patient like you doing with a complication like this? Diagnosis, prognosis and prevention of spinal hematoma. Can J Anaesth 2004;51(6):527–534.
30. Tryba M. Epidural regional anesthesia and low molecular weight heparin: Pro [German]. Anasthesiol Intensivmed Notfallmed Schmerzther 1993;28:179–181.
31. Guay J. Estimating the incidence of epidural hematoma – is there enough information? Can J Anaesth 2004;51(5):514–515.
32. Owens EL, Kasten GW, Hessel EA. Spinal subarachnoid hematoma after lumbar puncture and heparinisation: a case report, review of the literature and discussion of anaesthetic implications. Anesth Analg 1986;65:1201.
33. Onishchuk JL, Carlsson C. Epidural hematoma associated with epidural anesthesia: complications of anticoagulant therapy. Anesthesiology 1992;77:1221.
34. Horlocker TT, Wedel DJ, Benzon H, et al. Regional anesthesia in the anticoagulated patient: defining the risks (the second ASRA consensus conference on neuraxial anesthesia and anticoagulation). Reg Anesth Pain Med 2003;28(3):172–197.
35. Beilin Y, Zahn J, Comerford M. Safe epidural analgesia in thirty parturients with platelet counts between 69,000 and 98,000 $mm^{-3}$. Anesth Analg 1997;85:385–388.
36. Franchini M. The platelet-function analyzer (PFA-$100^{R}$) for evaluating primary hemostasis. Hematology 2005;10(3):177–181.
37. Gorton H, Lyons G. Is it time to invest in a thromboelastograph? Int J Obstet Anesth 1999;8(3):171–178.
38. Odoom JA, Sih IL. Epidural analgesia and anticoagulant therapy. Experience with one thousand cases of continuous epidurals. Anaesthesia 1983;38:254.
39. Kam PC, Nethery CM. The thienopyridine derivatives (platelet adenosine diphosphate receptor antagonists), pharmacology and clinical developments. Anaesthesia 2003;58(1):28–35.
40. Litz RJ, Gottschlich B, Stehr SN. Spinal epidural hematoma after spinal anesthesia in a patient treated with clopidogrel and enoxaparin. Anesthesiology 2004;101(6):1467–1470.
41. Kam PC, Egan MK. Platelet glycoprotein IIb/IIIa antagonists: pharmacology and clinical developments. Anaesthesia 2002;96(5):1237–1249.
42. Alston RP, Sinclair CJ, Scott DH. Thoracic epidural analgesia and coronary artery bypass graft surgery. Anaesthesia 1998;53(5):512–513; author reply 513–514.
43. Cooke ED, Lloyd MJ, Bowcock SA, Pilcher MD. Monitoring low-dose heparin prophylaxis. N Engl J Med 1976;294:1066.
44. North JB, Brophy BP. Epidural abscess: a hazard of epidural anaesthesia. Aust NZ J Surg 1979;49:484.
45. Kindler CH, Seeberger MD, Staender SE. Epidural abscess complicating epidural anesthesia and analgesia. An analysis of the literature. Acta Anaesthesiol Scand 1998;42(6):614–620.
46. Reihsaus E, Waldbaur H, Seeling W. Spinal epidural abscess: a meta-analysis of 915 patients. Neurosurg Rev 2000;23(4):175–204; discussion 205.
47. Wang LP, Hauerberg J, Schmidt JF. Incidence of spinal epidural abscess after epidural analgesia: a national 1-year survey. Anesthesiology 1999;91(6):1928–1936.
48. Wang LP, Hauerberg J, Schmidt JF. Long-term outcome after neurosurgically treated spinal epidural abscess following epidural analgesia. Acta Anaesthesiol Scand 2001;45(2):233–239.
49. Bromage PR. Neurological complications of subarachnoid and epidural anaesthesia. Acta Anaesthesiol Scand 1997;41(4):439–444.
50. Linz SM, Charbonnet C, Mikhail MS, et al. Spinal artery syndrome masked by postoperative epidural analgesia. Can J Anaesth 1997;44(11):1178–1181.
51. Mihaljevic T, Belkin M. Anterior spinal cord ischemia after infrainguinal bypass surgery. Ann Vasc Surg 2001;15(6):713–715.
52. Kane RE. Neurologic deficits following epidural or spinal anesthesia. Anesth Analg 1981;60(3):150.

53. Horlocker TT, McGregor DG, Matsushige DK, Schroeder DR, Besse JA. A retrospective review of 4767 consecutive spinal anesthetics: central nervous system complications. Anesth Analg 1997;84:578–584.
54. Rosenquist RW, Birnbach DJ. Epidural insertion in anesthetized adults: will your patients thank you? Anesth Analg 2003;96(6):1545–1546.
55. Bromage PR, Benumof JL. Paraplegia following intracord injection during attempted epidural anesthesia under general anesthesia. Reg Anesth Pain Med 1998;23(1):104–107.
56. Horlocker TT, Abel MD, Messick JM Jr, Schroeder DR. Small risk of serious neurologic complications related to lumbar epidural catheter placement in anesthetized patients. Anesth Analg 2003;96(6):1547–1552.
57. Fischer HB. Regional anaesthesia – before or after general anaesthesia? [see comment]. Anaesthesia 1998;53(8):727–729.
58. Hamandi K, Mottershead J, Lewis T, Ormerod IC, Ferguson IT. Irreversible damage to the spinal cord following spinal anesthesia. Neurology 2002;59(4):624–626.
59. Reynolds F. Damage to the conus medullaris following spinal anaesthesia. Anaesthesia 2001;56(3):238–247.
60. Reynolds F. A reply. Anaesthesia 2001;56(8):799–820.
61. Fettes PDW, Wildsmith JAW. Somebody else's nervous system. Br J Anaesth 2002;88(6): 760–763.
62. Broadbent CR, Maxwell WB, Ferrie R, Wilson DJ, Gawne-Cain M, Russell R. Ability of anaesthetists to identify a marked lumbar interspace. Anaesthesia 2000;55:1106–1126.
63. Talbot L, Lewis C, Hutter CDD, Rice I, Wee MYK. Obstetric epidurals and chronic adhesive arachnoiditis (multiple letters). Br J Anaesth 2004;92(6):902–903.
64. Rice I, Wee MYK, Thomson K. Obstetric epidurals and chronic adhesive arachnoiditis. Br J Anaesth 2004;92(1):109–120.
65. Aldrete JA. Neurologic deficits and arachnoiditis following neuroaxial anesthesia. Acta Anaesthesiol Scand 2003;47(1):3–12.
66. Nogués MA, Merello M, Leiguarda R, Guevara J, Figari A. Subarachnoid and intramedullary cysts secondary to epidural anesthesia for gynecological surgery. Eur Neurol 1992;32:99–101.
67. Kulka PJ, Stratesteffen I, Grunewald R, Wiebalck A. Inadvertent potassium chloride infusion in an epidural catheter [German]. Anaesthesist 1999;48(12):896–899.
68. Al-Nasser B. Toxic effects of epidural analgesia with ropivacaine 0.2% in a diabetic patient. J Clin Anesth 2004;16(3):220–223.
69. Sghirlanzoni A, Marazzi R, Pareyson D, Olivieri A, Bracchi M. Epidural anaesthesia and spinal arachnoiditis. Anaesthesia 1989;44:317.
70. Lambert LA, Lambert DH, Strichartz GR. Irreversible conduction block in isolated nerve by high concentrations of local anesthetics. Anesthesiology 1994;80:1082–1093.
71. Lambert DH, Lambert LA, Strichartz GR, et al. Radicular irritation after spinal anesthesia. Anesthesiology 1996;85(5):1216–1217.
72. Waters JH, Watson TB, Ward MG. Conus medullaris injury following both tetracaine and lidocaine spinal anesthesia. J Clin Anesth 1996;8(8):656–658.
73. Pleym H, Spigset O. Peripheral neurologic deficits in relation to subarachnoid or epidural administration of local anesthetics for surgery. A survey of 21 cases. Acta Anaesthesiol Scand 1997;41(4):453–460.
74. Hew CM, Cyna AM, Simmons SW. Avoiding inadvertent epidural injection of drugs intended for non-epidural use. Anaesth Intensive Care 2003;31(1):44–49.
75. Liu K, Chia YY. Inadvertent epidural injection of potassium chloride. Report of two cases. Acta Anaesthesiol Scand 1995;39(8):1134–1137.
76. Bermejo-Alvarez MA, Cosio F, Hevia A, Iglesias-Fernandez C. Accidental epidural administration of potassium chloride [Spanish]. Rev Esp Anestesiol Reanim 2000; 47(7):323–324.
77. Vercauteren M, Saldien V. Epidural injection of potassium hydrochloride. Acta Anaesthesiol Scand 1996;40(6):768.
78. Wildsmith JA. Alternative coupling systems for regional anaesthetic equipment. Anaesthesia 2002;57(7):726.
79. Gunter J. Caudal anaesthesia in children: a survey. Anesthesiology 1991;75:A936.
80. Badgwell JM, McLeod MM. Complications of epidural and spinal anesthesia in children. Curr Opin Anaesthesiol 1995;8(5):420.

81. Flandin-Blety C, Barrier G. Accidents following extradural analgesia in children. The results of a retrospective study. Paediatr Anaesth 1995;5(1):41–46.
82. Giaufre E, Dalens BJ, Gombert A. Epidemiology and morbidity of regional anesthesia in children: a one-year prospective survey of the French Language Society of Pediatric Anesthesiologists. Anesth Anal 1996;83:904–912.
83. Goresky GV. Thoracic epidural anaesthesia in children – problems with retrospective data. Can J Anaesth 1993;40:810.

# 19 Regional Anesthesia and Infection

Terese T. Horlocker and Denise J. Wedel

Infectious complications may occur after any regional anesthetic techniques, but are of greatest concern if the infection occurs around the spinal cord or within the spinal canal. Possible risk factors include underlying sepsis, diabetes, depressed immune status, steroid therapy, localized bacterial colonization or infection, and chronic catheter maintenance. Bacterial infection of the central neural axis may present as meningitis or cord compression secondary to abscess formation. The infectious source for meningitis and epidural abscess may result from distant colonization or localized infection with subsequent hematogenous spread and central nervous system (CNS) invasion. The anesthetist may also transmit microorganisms *directly* into the CNS by needle/catheter contamination through a break in aseptic technique or passage through a contiguous infection. An indwelling neuraxial catheter, although aseptically sited, may be colonized with skin flora and consequently serve as a source for ascending infection to the epidural or intrathecal space.

Historically, the frequency of serious CNS infections such as arachnoiditis, meningitis, and abscess after spinal or epidural anesthesia was considered to be extremely low – cases were reported as individual cases or small series.[1–3] However, recent epidemiologic series from Europe suggest that the frequency of infectious complications associated with neuraxial techniques may be increasing.[4,5] In a national study conducted from 1997 to 1998 in Denmark, Wang et al.[5] calculated the risk of *persisting* neurologic deficits to be 1:4343 following epidural analgesia. Moen et al.[4] reviewed the Swedish experience from 1990–1999 and reported a low incidence of epidural abscess, but an alarming association of post–spinal block meningitis with α-hemolytic streptococcal cultures, suggesting a nosocomial origin.

This chapter will discuss the clinical presentation of CNS infections, the laboratory and clinical studies evaluating the association between meningitis and dural puncture in bacteremic subjects, and the risk of infection during short-term and chronic epidural catheterization in febrile and immunocompromised patients, including those with herpes simplex virus (HSV) and human immunodeficiency virus (HIV). Finally, the importance and implications of aseptic techniques will be presented.

## Epidemiology of Meningitis and Epidural Abscess

Bacterial meningitis is the most common form of CNS infection, with an annual incidence in the United States of >2.5 cases/100,000 population. The epidemiology of bacterial meningitis has changed significantly in recent years, following the introduction and increasingly widespread use of vaccines for *Haemophilus influenzae* and *Neisseria meningitidis*. Currently, *Streptococcus pneumoniae* accounts for nearly two-thirds of community acquired meningitis; causative organisms of nosocomial meningitis include gram-negative bacilli, *Staphylococcus aureus* and coagulase-negative staphylococci.

Most cases of meningitis are associated with a recent infection (particularly otic or respiratory) or head trauma. Meningitis after spinal anesthesia has been only rarely reported. In a study evaluating the frequency of meningitis in patients undergoing spinal anesthesia, Kilpatrick and Girgis[6] retrospectively reviewed the records of all patients admitted to the meningitis ward in Cairo, Egypt. During a 5-year period from 1975 to 1980, 17 of 1429 patients admitted with a diagnosis of meningitis had a history of recent spinal anesthesia. The patients developed meningeal symptoms 2–30 days (mean 9 days) after spinal anesthesia and were symptomatic for 1–83 days (mean 15 days) before hospital admission. Ten of the 17 had positive cerebrospinal fluid (CSF) cultures; eight were *Pseudomonas aeruginosa*, one was *S. aureus*, and one was *S. mitis*. These organisms were not cultured from patients who had not had spinal anesthesia. Two additional patients with a history of recent spinal anesthesia demonstrated evidence of tuberculous meningitis. The lack of positive CSF cultures was presumed to be a result of oral antibiotic therapy which was present in more than half of patients at the time of admission. However, all patients, including those with negative CSF cultures, were treated with antibiotic therapy. Four of the 17 patients died. These results suggest that meningitis in patients with a history of recent spinal anesthesia is often the result of unusual or nosocomial organisms and that aggressive bacteriologic evaluation and antibiotic coverage are warranted.

Most epidural abscesses are not related to the placement of indwelling catheters, but are believed to be related to infections of the skin, soft tissue, spine, or hematogenous spread to the epidural space.[7] In a large retrospective review, epidural abscess accounted for 2–12 cases per 100,000 admissions to tertiary hospitals.[2] The most frequently identified organisms were *S. aureus* (57%), streptococci (18%), and gram-negative bacilli (13%). The source of infection was most often attributed to osteomyelitis (38%), bacteremia (26%), and postoperative infection (16%). Only one of the 39 cases was related to an epidural catheter. In a more recent review, Ericsson et al.[3] reported 10 cases of epidural abscess. Four of these were associated with invasive spinal procedures including repeated lumbar punctures in the presence of meningitis (two cases), epidural catheter (one case), and a paravertebral anesthetic injection (one case). In a retrospective study, Danner and Hartman[8] reported no spinal infections related to epidural anesthesia/analgesia. These authors were able to characterize the clinical course of epidural abscess, as well as identify risk factors for neurologic recovery. Diagnosis was more difficult and often delayed in patients with chronic epidural abscesses, because these patients were less likely to be febrile or have an increased leukocyte count compared with patients with acute abscesses. However, rapid neurologic deterioration could occur in either group. In addition, earlier diagnosis and treatment improved neurologic outcome. Steroid administration and increased neurologic impairment at the time of surgery adversely affected outcome.

### *Meningitis and Epidural Abscess after Neuraxial Anesthesia*

Neuraxial anesthesia is a rare etiology of CNS infections[4,5,9–18] (Table 19-1). For example, in a combined series of more than 65,000 spinal anesthetics, there were only three cases of meningitis. A similar review of approximately 50,000 epidural anesthetics failed to disclose a single epidural or intrathecal infection.[18] Aromaa et al.[17] reported eight cases of bacterial infections in patients undergoing 170,000 epidural and 550,000 spinal anesthetics (1.1 : 100,000 blocks) from a Finnish database. More

TABLE 19-1. Infectious Complications following regional Anesthesia

| Author, year | No. of patients | Population | Neuraxial techniques | Antibiotic prophylaxis | Duration of indwelling catheter | Complications |
|---|---|---|---|---|---|---|
| Kane,[18] 1981 | 115,000 | Surgical and obstetric | 65,000 spinal 50,000 epidural | Unknown | Unknown | 3 meningitis (all after spinal anesthesia) |
| Du Pen et al.,[9] 1990 | 350 | Cancer and AIDS patients | Permanent (tunneled) epidural analgesia | No | 4–1,460 days | 30 insertion site infections, 19 deep track or epidural space infections; treated with catheter removal and antibiotics, 15 uneventfully replaced |
| Scott and Hibbard,[10] 1990 | 505,000 | Obstetric | Epidural | Unknown | Unknown | 1 epidural abscess; laminectomy with partial recovery |
| Bader et al.,[11] 1992 | 319 | Parturients with chorioamnionitis | General (26), epidural (224), spinal (29), local (50) anesthesia | Yes (13%) | Surgical | None |
| Strafford et al.,[12] 1995 | 1,620 | Pediatric surgical | Epidural analgesia | No | 2.4 days median | 3 positive epidural catheter tip cultures 1 *Candida* colonization of epidural space (along with necrotic tumor) |
| Goodman et al.,[13] 1996 | 531 | Parturients with chorioamnionitis | Spinal (14), epidural (517) anesthesia and analgesia | Yes (23%) | 24 hours (64 patients) | None |
| Dahlgren and Tornebrandt,[14] 1995 | 18,000 | All indications and ages of patients | Spinal (8768) and epidural (9232) | Unknown | Unknown | None |
| Kindler et al.,[15] 1996 | 13,000 | 4,000 obstetric 9,000 surgical | Epidural | Unknown | Unknown | 2 epidural abscess, both requiring laminectomy |
| Auroy et al.,[16] 1997 | 71,053 | Surgical | Spinal (40,640) Epidural (30,413) | Unknown | Unknown | None |
| Aromaa et al.,[17] 1997 | 720,000 | Surgical | Epidural (170,000) Spinal (550,000) | Unknown | Unknown | 4 meningitis 2 epidural abscess 2 discitis 2 superficial skin infections |
| Wang et al.,[5] 1999 | 17,372 | Surgical, cancer, and trauma | Epidural | Unknown | 11 days mean 6 days median | 9 epidural abscess; 7 required laminectomy; complete recovery in 6 of 10 patients 2 subcutaneous infections |
| Moen et al.,[4] 2004 | 1,710,000 | Pain, surgical, and obstetric | Spinal (1,260,000) Epidural (450,000) | Unknown | 2 days–5 weeks | 29 meningitis; partial sequelae in 6 patients 13 epidural abscess, laminectomy performed in six patients; 4 of 5 patients with deficits did not recover |

*Source:* Adapted from Horlocker TT, Wedel DJ. Regional anesthesia and infection. In: Finucane BT, ed. Complications of Regional Anesthesia. Philadelphia: WB Saunders; 1999:170–183. Reprinted with permission from Elsevier.

recent epidemiologic series are alarming. In a national study conducted from 1997 to 1998 in Denmark, Wang et al.[5] reported the incidence of epidural abscess after epidural analgesia was 1:1930 catheters. Patients with epidural abscess had an extended duration of epidural catheterization (median 6 days, range 3–31 days). In addition, the majority of the patients with epidural abscess were immunocompromised. Often the diagnosis was delayed; the time from first symptom to confirmation of the diagnosis was a median of 5 days. *S. aureus* was isolated in 67% of patients. Patients without neurologic deficits were successfully treated with antibiotics, whereas those with deficits underwent surgical decompression (typically with only moderate neurologic recovery). It is difficult to determine why the frequency of symptomatic epidural abscess was so high in this series. Because perioperative antithrombotic therapy was involved in most cases, it is possible that the epidural abscesses were infected epidural hematomas, but this is not strongly supported by the diagnostic imaging studies and neurosurgical findings.

In a retrospective series from Sweden involving 1,260,000 spinal and 450,000 epidural anesthetics (including 200,000 placed for labor analgesia) performed over a decade, Moen et al.[4] reported 42 serious infectious complications. Epidural abscess occurred in 13 patients; nine (70%) were considered immunocompromised as a result of diabetes, steroid therapy, cancer, or alcoholism. Six patients underwent epidural block for analgesia after trauma. The time from placement of the epidural catheter to first symptoms ranged from 2 days to 5 weeks (median 5 days). Although prevailing symptoms were fever and severe backache, five developed neurologic deficits. All seven positive cultures isolated *S. aureus*. Overall neurologic recovery was complete in seven of 12 patients. However, four of the five patients with neurologic symptoms did not recover.

Meningitis was reported in 29 patients for an overall incidence of 1:53,000. A documented perforation of the dura (intentional or accidental) occurred in 25 of 29 cases. Unlike the cases of epidural abscess, which tended to be reported in immunocompromised patients, the patients who developed meningitis following spinal anesthesia were reportedly healthy and undergoing minor surgical procedures. The time interval between neuraxial block and symptoms varied from 8 hours to 8 days (median 24 hours). Importantly, all patients complained of headache, but the classic symptoms of meningitis (fever, headache, and nuchal rigidity) were present in only 14 patients. In the 12 patients in whom positive cultures were obtained, alpha-hemolytic streptococci were isolated in 11 patients and *S. aureus* in one. Meningitis resulted in residual neurologic deficits in six patients.

These large epidemiologic studies represent new and unexpected findings regarding the demographics, frequency, etiology, and prognosis of infectious complications following neuraxial anesthesia. Epidural abscess is most likely to occur in immunocompromised patients with prolonged durations of epidural catheterization. The most common causative organism is *S. aureus*, which suggests the colonization and subsequent infection from normal skin flora as the pathogenesis. Delays in diagnosis and treatment result in poor neurologic recovery, despite surgical decompression. Conversely, patients who develop meningitis following neuraxial blockade typically are healthy and have undergone uneventful spinal anesthesia. Furthermore, the series by Moen et al. validates the findings of individual case reports of meningitis after spinal anesthesia – the source of the pathogen is mostly likely to be the upper airway of the proceduralist.[19–22] Although the frequency of serious infectious complications is much higher than reported previously, the results may be attributable to differences in reporting and/or clinical practice (asepsis, perioperative antibiotic therapy, duration of epidural catheterization).[4,5] Finally, although recent investigations have substantially illuminated the etiology, risk factors, and prognosis of infectious complications after neuraxial blockade, similar information for patients undergoing peripheral regional anesthetic techniques and invasive pain procedures is limited.[23–26]

## Neuraxial Blockade in the Febrile (Bacteremic) or Infected Patient

Few data suggest that spinal or epidural anesthesia during bacteremia is a risk factor for infection of the central neural axis. Although the authors of previous studies[4,5,14,18] did not report how many patients were febrile during administration of the spinal or epidural anesthetic, a significant number of the patients included in these studies underwent obstetric or urologic procedures, and it is likely that some patients had bacteremia after (and perhaps during) needle or catheter placement. Despite the apparent low risk of CNS infection following regional anesthesia, anesthesiologists have long considered sepsis to be a relative contraindication to the administration of spinal or epidural anesthesia. This impression is based largely on anecdotal reports and conflicting laboratory and clinical investigations.

### *Meningitis after Dural Puncture*

Dural puncture has long been considered a risk factor in the pathogenesis of meningitis. Exactly how bacteria cross from the blood stream into the spinal fluid is unknown. The presumed mechanisms include introduction of blood into the intrathecal space during needle placement and disruption of the protection provided by the blood-brain barrier. However, lumbar puncture is often performed in patients with fever or infection of unknown origin. If dural puncture during bacteremia results in meningitis, definite clinical data should exist. In fact, clinical studies are few, and often antiquated.

Initial clinical[27–31] and laboratory[32] investigations were performed more than 80 years ago (Table 19-2). In 1919, Weed et al.[32] demonstrated that lumbar or cisternal

Table 19-2. Meningitis after Dural Puncture

| Author, year | No. of patients | Population | Microorganism (s) | Patients with spontaneous meningitis | Patients with lumbar puncture–induced meningitis | Comments |
|---|---|---|---|---|---|---|
| Wegeforth and Latham,[27] 1919 | 93 | Military personnel | *N. meningitidis* *S. pneumonia* | 38 of 93 (41%) | 5 of 93, including 5 of 6 bacteremic patients | Lumbar punctures performed during meningitis epidemics |
| Pray,[28] 1941 | 416 | Pediatric with bacteremia | *S. pneumonia* | 86 of 386 (22%) | 8 of 30 (27%) | 80% of patients with meningitis <2 years of age |
| Eng and Seligman,[29] 1981 | 1,089 | Adults with bacteremia | Atypical and typical bacteria | 30 of 919 (3.3%) | 3 of 170 (1.8%) | Atypical organisms responsible for lumbar puncture–induced meningitis |
| Teele et al.,[30] 1981 | 271 | Pediatric with bacteremia | *S. pneumonia* *N. meningitidiss* *H. influenza* | 2 of 31 (9%) | 7 of 46 (15%)* | All cases of meningitis occurred in children <1 year of age. Antibiotic therapy reduced risk |
| Smith et al.,[31] 1986 | 11 | Preterm with neonatal sepsis | | 0% | 0% | |

*Source:* Horlocker TT, Wedel DJ. Regional anesthesia and infection. In: Finucane BT, ed. Complications of Regional Anesthesia. Philadelphia: WB Saunders; 1999:170–183. Reprinted with permission from Elsevier.
*Significant association (P < .001).
Spontaneous meningitis = concurrent bacteremia and meningitis (without a preceding lumbar puncture); lumbar puncture–induced meningitis = positive blood culture with sterile CSF on initial examination; subsequent positive CSF culture (same organism present in blood).

puncture performed during septicemia (produced by lethal doses of an intravenously administered gram-negative bacillus) invariably resulted in a fatal meningitis. In the same year, Wegeforth and Latham[27] reported their clinical observations of 93 patients suspected of having meningitis who received a diagnostic lumbar puncture. Blood cultures were taken simultaneously. The diagnosis was confirmed in 38 patients. The remaining 55 patients had normal CSF. However, six of these 55 patients were bacteremic at the time of lumbar puncture. Five of the six bacteremic patients subsequently developed meningitis. It was implied, but not stated, that patients with both sterile blood and CSF cultures did not develop meningitis. Unfortunately, these lumbar punctures were performed during two epidemics of meningitis occurring at a military instillation, and it is possible that some (or all) of these patients may have developed meningitis without lumbar puncture. These two historical studies provided support for the claim that lumbar puncture during bacteremia was a possible risk factor for meningitis.

Subsequent clinical studies reported conflicting results. Pray[28] studied the incidence of pneumococcal meningitis in children who underwent a diagnostic lumbar puncture during pneumococcal sepsis. The incidence of meningitis was no greater among patients who were subjected to lumbar puncture, which produced normal CSF (8 of 30 patients, or 27%), than among those who did not undergo diagnostic spinal tap (86 of 386 patients, or 22%). Eng and Seligman[29] retrospectively reviewed the records of 1089 bacteremic patients, including 200 patients who underwent lumbar puncture. The authors reported that the incidence of meningitis after lumbar puncture did not significantly differ from the incidence of spontaneous meningitis and concluded: "If lumbar puncture induced meningitis does occur, it is rare enough to be clinically insignificant."

However, not all studies have been as reassuring as those described above. In a review of meningitis associated with serial lumbar punctures to treat posthemorrhagic hydrocephalus in premature infants, Smith et al.[31] attempted to identify risk factors. Six of 22 (27%) infants undergoing multiple (2–33) therapeutic dural punctures during a period of 2–63 days developed meningitis. Bacteremia, a risk factor for meningitis in this report, was associated with central venous or umbilical artery catheters. However, 11 septic infants who underwent dural puncture did not develop meningitis. The number of dural punctures, incidence of "difficult or traumatic" procedures, and use of antibiotics did not differ between infants who developed meningitis and those who did not. A causal relationship between the dural puncture and onset of meningitis was not clear. Teele et al.[30] retrospectively reviewed the records of 277 bacteremic children during a 10-year interval from 1971–1980. Meningitis occurred in 7 of 46 (15%) children with normal CSF obtained during a bacteremia. However, only 2 of 231 (1%) children who did not undergo lumbar puncture developed meningitis. These results were significantly different. In addition, children treated with antibiotics at the time of lumbar puncture were less likely to develop meningitis than children who were not treated until after lumbar puncture. The authors admitted that clinical judgment may have allowed the pediatricians to select the child in whom meningitis is developing before the CSF is diagnostic; these patients may appear more ill and thus suggest the performance of a lumbar puncture.

Prevention of lumbar puncture–induced meningitis with antibiotic therapy is supported by a more recent animal study. Carp and Bailey[33] investigated the association between meningitis and dural puncture in bacteremic rats. Twelve of 40 rats subjected to cisternal puncture with a 26-gauge needle during an *Escherichia coli* bacteremia subsequently developed meningitis. Meningitis occurred only in animals with a blood culture result of ≥50 colony forming units/mL at the time of dural puncture, a circulating bacterial count observed in patients with infective endocarditis. In addition, bacteremic animals not undergoing dural puncture, as well as animals undergoing dural puncture in the absence of bacteremia, did not develop meningitis. Treatment of a group of bacteremic rats with a single dose of gentamicin immediately before cisternal puncture eliminated the risk of meningitis; none of these animals developed infection.

This study demonstrates that dural puncture in the presence of bacteremia is associated with the development of meningitis in rats, and that antibiotic treatment before dural puncture reduces this risk. Unfortunately, this study did not include a group of animals that were treated with antibiotics *after* dural puncture. Because many surgeons defer antibiotic therapy until after cultures are obtained, the actual clinical scenario remains unstudied. There are several other limitations to this study. Whereas *E. coli* is a common cause of bacteremia, it is an uncommon cause of meningitis. In addition, the authors knew the sensitivity to the bacteria injected, allowing for appropriate antibiotic coverage. The authors also performed a cisternal puncture (rather than lumbar puncture) and used a 26-gauge needle, producing a relatively large dural defect in the rat compared with humans, and no local anesthetic was injected. Local anesthetic solutions are bacteriostatic, which may theoretically reduce the risk of meningitis in normal clinical settings. Whereas these results may apply to the performance of spinal anesthesia in the bacteremic patient, they do not apply to administration of epidural anesthesia in the febrile patient, which is associated with a higher incidence of vascular injury and typically involves placement of an indwelling foreign body.

### *Meningitis after Spinal and Epidural Anesthesia*

Even when meningitis occurs temporally after spinal anesthesia, it is often difficult to establish a cause-and-effect relationship between spinal anesthesia and meningitis. The following case report describes a probable case of lumbar puncture–induced meningitis.[34] A 60-year-old man underwent kidney stone removal under general anesthesia. On postoperative day six, the patient remained afebrile, but was taken to the operating suite for transurethral clot evacuation. Spinal anesthesia was performed under aseptic technique. CSF was clear. Forty minutes later, shaking chills developed. Initial blood and urine cultures were negative. The following day, the patient became febrile and complained of headache and back pain and appeared confused. CSF examination revealed cloudy CSF with a leukocytosis (80% polymorphonucleocytes), decreased glucose concentration consistent with bacterial infection, but no growth on culture. Three days later, a repeat lumbar puncture was performed with similar results. A third lumbar puncture was performed 2 days later; culture yielded group D streptococcus (enterococci). Group D enterococci are unusual sources of meningitis. In this case it is possible, although unlikely, that the patient was bacteremic before administration of the spinal anesthetic. It is more likely that the bacteria entered the blood stream during bladder irrigation (because bacteremia occurs in perhaps 60% of urologic procedures) and traversed the dura at the puncture site, similar to the animals in the study by Carp and Bailey.[33] However, despite the apparent temporal association, it is difficult to prove that the presence of a prebacteremic dural puncture increased the risk of subsequent meningitis in this patient.

Bacterial meningitis can also present after epidural blockade with or without a localized epidural abscess.[1,35] In a rare report, Ready and Helfer[1] described two cases of meningitis following the use of epidural catheters in parturients. In the first case, a healthy 28-year-old parturient underwent lumbar epidural catheter placement for elective cesarean delivery. The epidural analgesia was provided for 48 hours postoperatively with an opioid. At the time of removal, a 4-cm erythematous indurated area, which was tender to palpation, was noted at the catheter entry site. Three days later, the patient complained of severe headache, nuchal rigidity, and photophobia. An area of cellulitis was present at the epidural insertion site. CSF examinations revealed an increased protein (308 mg/dL), decreased glucose (27 mg/dL), and 3000 leukocytes/μL (73% polymorphonucleocytes). Culture of the CSF was positive for *S. faecalis*. Urine and blood cultures were negative. There was no evidence of epidural abscess on magnetic resonance imaging scan. Antibiotic therapy was initiated and the patient completely recovered. Although it was thought the most likely source of the meningitis was the area of cellulitis surrounding the epidural catheter insertion site, the possibility of alternative causes could not be excluded.

In the second case, a lumbar epidural was placed in a healthy 25-year-old parturient. Delivery occurred uneventfully 50 minutes later, and the catheter was removed. No local inflammation was noted at the catheter insertion site. The patient reported a nonpositional headache and neck stiffness 24 hours later. Lumbar puncture revealed increased protein (356 mg/dL), decreased glucose (5 mg/dL), and 4721 leukocytes/μL (90% polymorphonucleocytes). CSF cultured positive for *S. uberis* (a strain of α-hemolytic streptococcus). However, urine, blood, and vaginal cultures also grew the same organism. Antibiotic therapy was initiated, and recovery was complete. The short duration of the indwelling catheter, the lack of physical findings suggestive of infection at the catheter insertion site, and the presence of the organism in vaginal secretions, blood, and urine suggest that the source of the meningitis was most likely hematogenous spread of the infecting organism from the vagina.[1] The case reported by Berman and Eisele,[34] and the two cases by Ready and Helfer[1] demonstrate how a cause-and-effect relationship should not be assumed between the regional anesthetic and the CNS infection, but rather other possible sources should be investigated.

### *Epidural Abscess after Epidural Anesthesia*

Several relevant studies have specifically examined the risk of epidural abscess in bacteremic patients receiving epidural anesthesia and/or analgesia. The anesthesiologist is frequently faced with the management of the parturient with suspected chorioamnionitis, approximately 8% of whom are bacteremic. Bader et al.[11] investigated the use of regional anesthesia in women with chorioamnionitis. Three hundred nineteen women were identified from a total of 10,047 deliveries. Of the 319 women, 100 had blood cultures taken on the day of delivery. Eight of these had blood cultures consistent with bacteremia. Two hundred ninety-three of the 319 patients received a regional anesthetic; in 43 patients, antibiotics were administered before needle or catheter placement. No patients in the study, including those with documented bacteremias, had infectious complications. In addition, mean temperatures and leukocyte counts in patients who received blood cultures showed no significant differences between bacteremic and nonbacteremic groups. Goodman et al.[13] also retrospectively reviewed the hospital records of 531 parturients who received epidural or spinal anesthesia and were subsequently diagnosed with chorioamnionitis. Blood cultures were drawn in 146 patients; 13 were positive. Antibiotics were administered before the regional block was placed in only 123 patients, whereas nearly one-third of patients did not receive antibiotic therapy in the entire peripartum period. As with the study by Bader et al.,[11] leukocytosis, fever, abdominal tenderness, or foul-smelling discharge were not predictors of positive blood cultures. There were no infectious complications. These authors continue to administer spinal and epidural anesthesia in patients with suspected chorioamnionitis because the potential benefits of regional anesthesia outweigh the theoretical risk of infectious complications. However, the small number of patients with documented bacteremias in both studies defies a definitive statement regarding the risk of CNS infections in patients suspected of chorioamnionitis undergoing regional anesthetic techniques.

Few data exist regarding the placement and maintenance of epidural catheters in patients with an infection at a site distant from the neuraxis. Darchy et al.[36] studied 75 patients in the intensive care unit receiving epidural analgesia (median 4 days), including 21 patients with a known localized concomitant infection. Although five patients had catheter insertion site inflammation/erythema (with or without positive epidural catheter culture), the frequency was not increased by the presence of an infectious source distant to the epidural catheter site. However, the authors recommended a meticulous daily inspection of the catheter insertion site and immediate removal of the catheter if both erythema and local discharge are present, because these two signs of local inflammation are predictors of positive epidural catheter colonization/infection.

### *Factors Affecting Bacterial Colonization During Epidural Catheterization*

Although the epidural catheter tip is frequently colonized, progression to epidural space infection rarely occurs.[9,36] The low frequency of significant epidural infection (1–2 cases per 10,000 hospital admissions)[2] associated with epidural catheter placement is especially notable when compared with the frequency of intravenous catheter-related septicemia, which approaches 1%, or greater than 50,000 cases annually. Several factors may contribute to the low incidence of epidural space infections, including meticulous attention to aseptic technique, careful monitoring of catheter insertion site, antibiotic prophylaxis, and use of bacterial filters. However, because these interventions are frequently initiated in patients with indwelling central venous catheters, additional factors unique to epidural anesthesia and analgesia, such as the bactericidal effect of local anesthetic solutions, may also contribute significantly.

Bupivacaine and lidocaine have been shown to inhibit the growth of a variety of microorganisms in culture.[37] Unfortunately, the bactericidal effect decreases significantly with concentrations of local anesthetic typically used to provide analgesia, whereas opioid solutions do not exhibit *any* ability to inhibit bacterial growth. In addition, growth of *S. aureus* and coagulase-negative staphylococci, the most frequently identified pathogens in epidural infections, is inhibited only at higher concentrations of local anesthetic, such as solutions of 2% lidocaine and 0.5% bupivacaine. Therefore, although it seems that local anesthetic solutions are unlikely to prevent epidural infections in most patients receiving epidural analgesia, it is possible that in immunocompromised patients, local anesthetics may inhibit the growth of more fastidious organisms, even at low concentrations. Further clinical studies are needed to investigate the in vivo bactericidal effects of dilute local anesthetic solutions.

The catheter hub, catheter insertion site, and hematogenous spread are three major routes of entry for microorganisms into the epidural space, with the catheter hub accounting for nearly half of the sources.[9,38,39] A bacterial filter placed at the catheter hub acts as a physical barrier for bacteria present in the infusing solution, and should theoretically reduce the incidence of epidural colonization. However, studies of epidural catheter tip cultures have reported mixed results, and cases of epidural infection after hub colonization despite the use of filters have been reported.[9,39,40] Possible explanations for hub-related epidural infections in patients with bacterial filters include a reduced antimicrobial effectiveness with prolonged use, and direct contamination of the hub during filter-changing techniques. De Cicco et al.[41] reported a positive trend between the number of filter changes and the rate of positive hub cultures. These data suggest that continued attention to aseptic technique is warranted throughout the period of epidural catheterization, and that the use of bacteriologic filters is alone unlikely to be efficacious in preventing epidural colonization and infection.[42]

Controversy exists regarding the conditions under which a disconnected epidural catheter can be safely reconnected. In an in vitro investigation, Langevin et al.[43] inoculated epidural catheters containing a 5 μ/mL fentanyl solution with *S. aureus*, *E. coli*, or *P. aeruginosa*. Eight hours after catheter contamination, providing the fluid in the catheter remained static, no bacteria were detected more than 20 cm from the contaminated catheter hub. Vertical or horizontal positioning of the catheter during incubation did not affect bacterial advancement along the catheter, as long as the fluid was displaced distally less than 20 cm. However, if the fentanyl solution was allowed to drain and advance 33 cm, bacteria were found at the epidural end of the catheter, 88 cm distally. The advancement of bacteria by fluid displacement is clinically significant; in more than two-thirds of patients, fluid will drain by gravity into the epidural space in less than 1 hour after discontinuation of an epidural infusion. The authors concluded that the interior of a disconnected epidural catheter will remain sterile for at least 8 hours if the fluid in the catheter remains static, and the catheter may be aseptically reconnected after removal of the contaminated section. In addition, the presence of a meniscus more than 20–25 cm from the free end of a disconnected catheter may indicate contamination of the catheter tip in the epidural space, and immediate catheter removal was recommended. Unfortunately, the authors did not evaluate the advancement of bacteria in epidural catheters filled with local anesthetic solutions, or investigate the effect of a local anesthetic injected after the bacterial inoculation and incubation.

## Neuraxial Blockade in the Immunocompromised Patient

Large series have demonstrated that patients with altered immune status are at increased risk for infectious complications (Table 19-3).[4,5] Strafford et al.[12] reviewed 1620 pediatric patients who received epidural analgesia for postoperative pain relief. Epidural catheters were left indwelling for a median of 2 days (range, 0–8 days). No patient developed an epidural abscess. One patient with osteosarcoma metastatic spread to spine, chest wall, and lungs became febrile after 10 days of epidural catheterization. The catheter was removed, and a culture demonstrated candidal contamination. A second thoracic epidural catheter was placed 4 days later to provide superior analgesia. Two weeks later, she developed an acute sensory and motor block at T2. Magnetic resonance imaging showed an epidural fluid collection; an emergent laminectomy was performed. A large amount of necrotic tumor as well as fluid containing *Candida tropicalis* was present in the epidural space. Her neurologic deficits resolved postoperatively. Three additional patients with chronic pain syndromes were evaluated for epidural infection, but all were negative. The authors concluded that for terminally ill patients, the risk of infection with long-term epidural catheterization is acceptable, but recommended careful monitoring to avoid serious neurologic sequelae.

Chronic epidural catheterization in immunocompromised patients is also a potential risk for epidural infection. Du Pen et al.[9] studied 350 cancer and HIV-infected patients in whom permanent (tunneled) epidural catheters were placed. The authors examined three areas of the catheter track for evidence of infection: exit site, superficial catheter track, and epidural space. The rate of epidural and deep track catheter-related infections was one in every 1702 days of catheter use in the 19 patients who developed deep track (8) or epidural (15) infections. (Four of the 19 patients had both

Table 19-3. Infectious Complications Following Neuraxial Anesthesia in the Immunocompromised Patient

- The attenuated inflammatory response within the immunocompromised patient may diminish the clinical signs and symptoms often associated with infection and result in a delay in diagnosis and treatment.
- The range of microorganisms causing invasive infection in the immunocompromised host is much broader than that affecting the general population and includes atypical and opportunistic pathogens.
- Initiation of early and effective therapy is paramount in optimizing neurologic outcome – consultation with an infectious disease specialist is advised.
- Prolonged antibiotic therapy (weeks–months) is often required because of persistent and immunologic deficiencies.
- Because eradication of infection is difficult once established, prevention of infection is paramount in caring for immunocompromised patients.

deep track and epidural involvement.) Bacteria cultured were most frequently skin flora. All 19 patients with deep infections were treated with catheter removal and antibiotics; none required surgical decompression or debridement. Catheters were replaced in 15 of the 19 patients who requested them after treatment with no recurrent infections. The authors state recommendations similar to Strafford et al., specifically, long-term epidural catheterization is safe when patients are carefully monitored for signs of infection and receive prompt treatment when the diagnosis is established.

Injection of epidural steroids and underlying disease processes theoretically increase the risk of infection (Figure 19-1).[44–46] Strong[45] described a 71-year-old man with a resolving herpes zoster infection involving the T5-6 dermatome. An epidural catheter was placed at the T6-7 interspace, and 120 mg of methylprednisolone in 5 mL of 0.25% bupivacaine was injected. Three additional doses of bupivacaine were administered, and the catheter was removed intact 26 hours after placement. Four days later, a second epidural catheter was placed at the T5-6 level. Oral antibiotic therapy was initiated. Ten intermittent boluses of 0.25% bupivacaine were made over a 3-day period, and the catheter was then removed. There was no evidence of infection at either catheter insertion site. The patient returned 3 weeks later with a fever, stiff neck, headache, and right-sided flank pain. No neurologic deficits were noted. A thoracic computed tomography (CT) scan revealed an epidural abscess extending from T5-9. An emergency decompressive laminectomy was performed. Cultures at the surgical site were positive for *S. aureus*. The patient was treated with 21 days of intravenous antibiotics, and was discharged without neurologic deficits. Factors contributing to this patient's epidural infection include an immunocompromised host (as suggested by the activation of a latent herpes infection), multiple catheter placement, and decreased immunologic response secondary to steroid administration.

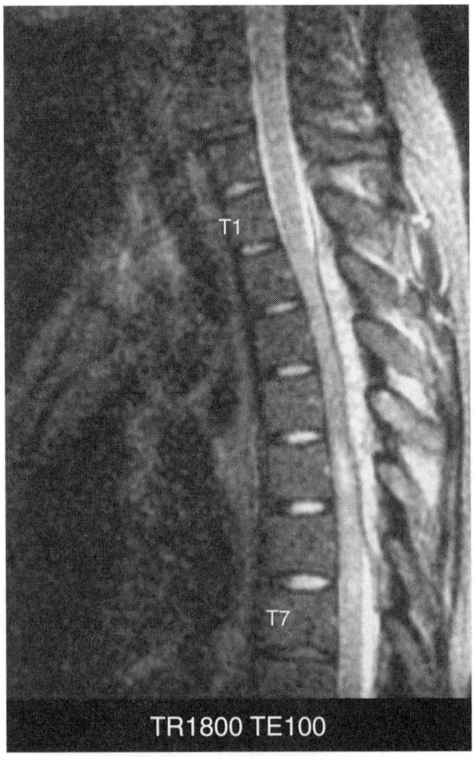


**FIGURE 19-1.** A thoracic epidural abscess is demonstrated by magnetic resonance image in a patient who underwent thoracic epidural placement for management of herpetic neuralgia. (*Source:* Horlocker TT, Wedel DJ. Regional anesthesia and infection. In: Finucane BT, ed. *Complications of Regional Anesthesia*. Philadelphia: WB Saunders; 1999:170–183. Reprinted with permission from Elsevier.)

### *Herpes Simplex Virus*

HSV type-2 (HSV-2) is an incurable, recurrent disease characterized by asymptomatic periods alternating at variable periods with recrudescence of the genital lesions. The primary infection is associated with viremia and can be accompanied by a variety of symptoms including fever, headache, lymphadenopathy, and, in rare cases, aseptic meningitis. In contrast, recurrent or secondary infections present as genital lesions without evidence of viremia. When obstetric patients present for delivery with evidence of active HSV-2 infection, cesarean delivery is usually recommended to avoid exposing the neonate to the virus during vaginal delivery. The use of central neuronal block has been considered controversial by some because of the theoretical concern of introducing the virus into the CNS. Although this issue is usually discussed in the context of obstetric anesthesia, the incidence and prevalence of genital herpes has increased dramatically in the past two decades. Therefore, the theoretical risk of CNS contamination is present in the general surgical population as well.

Bader et al.[47] reviewed management of 169 HSV-2 – infected patients undergoing cesarean delivery. Five were classified as having primary infections with the remaining 164 being secondary. General (59), spinal (75), and epidural (35) anesthetic techniques were used. One patient with primary HSV-2 developed transient unilateral leg weakness following bupivacaine spinal anesthesia. The problem resolved within 1 week. Although this patient was classified by the obstetrician as having a primary infection, genital lesions had appeared 3 weeks before delivery and there was an active lesion at the time of delivery. The number of patients with primary HSV-2 infections was very small in this study; however, the authors suggested that regional anesthesia was safe in cases of secondary infection.

These recommendations are consistent with previous studies. Crosby et al.[48] reviewed a 6-year experience with active HSV-2 infections in obstetric patients in two institutions. Cesarean delivery was performed on 89 affected parturients, all with recurrent herpes disease. There were no neurologic or infectious complications. In a similar retrospective review, Ramanathan et al.[49] reported 43 epidural anesthetics in parturients with HSV-2 infection who had either active lesions (71%) or had at least one recurrence during the pregnancy. Again, no complications were noted in the parturient or neonate. One patient who was treated prenatally with steroids to promote fetal lung maturity developed a lesion in the postnatal period which resolved within 10 days. Neither of these studies included patients with primary infections.

HSV type-1 (HSV-1), the infectious agent for oral herpes, rarely causes genital lesions. However, recurrent HSV-1 has been described in parturients receiving intrathecal and epidural morphine for pain management.[50] The postnatal association is controversial because several other factors such as emotional or physical stress, other infections, and parturition have been cited as causes of recurrent HSV infection. Valley et al.[51] reported a case of thoracic and labial HSV-1 infection in a patient receiving epidural fentanyl. Although surgical stress may have been a factor, this patient had no other known risk factors, and lesions developed near the site of the epidural catheter.

### *Human Immunodeficiency Virus*

The risk of performing regional anesthesia procedures in HIV-infected patients is largely unknown. Hughes et al.[52] reported the safe administration of central neuronal block in 18 HIV-infected parturients. The patients studied showed no postpartum change in immune, infectious, or neurologic status. Avidan et al.[53] and Bremerich et al.[54] also reported a low complication rate for parturients with HIV infection on antiretroviral therapy who underwent spinal anesthesia. However, in all three series (with a combined total of 117 patients), the patients were relatively healthy and in the early stage of their disease. The effects of anesthesia on patients with more advanced disease are unreported.

In a report on the use of epidural blood patch for postdural puncture headache in HIV-positive males, Tom et al.[55] followed nine patients longitudinally for periods ranging from 6 to 24 months. No complications were attributable to the epidural blood patch, although the authors noted the high incidence of neurologic manifestations in this population. Approximately 40% of patients with the diagnosis of acquired immune deficiency syndrome (AIDS) have clinical signs of neurologic disease and at autopsy, patients with AIDS have a 70%–80% incidence of neuropathologic changes. Although many of the neurologic symptoms are unrelated to complications associated with spinal or epidural anesthesia, some such as aseptic meningitis, chronic headaches, and polyneuropathy may be mistaken for problems related to needle placement. A clear understanding of the association of CNS symptoms with HIV infection is important in order to interpret postblock neurologic pathology.

## Aseptic Technique

Although previous publications have repeatedly recommended meticulous aseptic technique, there are no defined standards for asepsis during the performance of regional anesthetic procedures[56] (Table 19-4). Handwashing remains the most crucial component of asepsis; gloves should be regarded as a supplement to – not a replacement for – handwashing.[57] Conversely, the use of gowns and gloves does not further reduce the likelihood of cross-contamination. Surgical masks, initially considered a barrier to protect the *proceduralist* from patient secretions and blood, may be appropriate because of the increasing number of cases of postspinal meningitis, many of which result from contamination of the epidural or intrathecal space with pathogens from the operator's buccal mucosa.[4,20–22] Schneeberger et al.[20] reported four cases of iatrogenic meningitis following spinal anesthesia occurring over a 4-year period. The patients typically presented 24 hours postoperatively with a severe headache (two received an epidural blood patch). All cases involved the same anesthesiologist, who had a history of recurrent pharyngitis and did not wear a mask during the procedure. Interestingly, similar reports have been noted among patients undergoing pain procedures.[58]

### *Antiseptic Solutions*

Controversy still exists regarding the most appropriate and safe antiseptic solution for patients undergoing neuraxial and peripheral techniques. Povidone iodine and chlorhexidine gluconate (with or without the addition of isopropyl alcohol) have been most extensively studied.[59,60] In nearly all clinical investigations, the bactericidal effect of chlorhexidine was more rapid and more effective (extending hours after its application) than povidone iodine. Kinirons et al.[59] compared the rate of epidural colonization using 0.5% chlorhexidine in alcohol with that of 10% povidone iodine. Catheters inserted after skin preparation with chlorhexidine were one-sixth as likely and less quickly colonized as catheters inserted after skin preparation with povidone iodine.

Table 19-4. Variables that May Influence Infectious Complications

- Site of catheter placement (thoracic versus lumbar versus caudal)
- Choice of antiseptic and technique of application
- Choice of barrier protection (masks, gloves, gowns)
- Timing and selection of perioperative antibiotics
- Duration of neuraxial or peripheral catheterization
- Use of bacterial filters
- Dressing type(s) (transparent versus dry gauze dressing; use of antiseptic dressings)

*Source:* Hebl.[56] Reprinted with permission from the American Society of Regional Anesthesia and Pain Medicine.

Although the authors concluded that the use of alcoholic chlorhexidine for cutaneous antisepsis before epidural catheter insertion reduces the risk of catheter colonization, it must be noted that chlorhexidine-alcohol labeling contains a warning against use as a skin preparation before lumbar puncture. Thus, at this time, chlorhexidine is recommended for peripheral and epidural techniques only.

## Infectious Complications of Peripheral Regional Techniques

Although meningitis and epidural abscess are the most significant infectious complications of regional anesthesia, the associate risk following plexus and peripheral techniques remain undefined. Auroy et al.[16] reported no infectious complications in 21,278 single-injection peripheral nerve blocks. This low incidence is supported by Borgeat et al.'s[61] report of no complications in 521 patients undergoing interscalene nerve blockade.

The more frequent placement of catheters for peripheral nerve blockade, often for prolonged periods, might be expected to increase the risk of infectious complications; however, few data are available to support this theoretical assumption. Two studies look more specifically at the infectious risk in continuous peripheral nerve blocks. Capdevila et al.[25] prospectively studied 1416 patients in 10 centers undergoing continuous peripheral nerve blocks for orthopedic procedures. A total of 969 (68%) catheters were cultured when removed, and patients were actively monitored for signs of localized infection or sepsis. A positive bacterial colonization was found in 278 (29%) catheters, most frequently *S. epidermidis*. The incidence of local inflammation was present in 3% of patients. In these patients, 44% of the catheters were colonized, whereas only 19% of catheters were colonized in patients without inflammatory signs. There was no correlation between colonization and the presence of fever. Risk factors for local infection/inflammation were admission to an intensive care unit, male gender, catheter duration exceeding 48 hours, and lack of antibiotic prophylaxis. A study by Cuvillon et al.[26] investigated the incidence of infectious complications in 211 continuous femoral catheters. Colonization of the 208 catheters examined after 48 hours showed a rate of 57% with the most common organism again being *S. epidermidis* (71%). Echography was performed in each instance of positive catheter colonization. No cellulitis or abscess was noted; however, three transitory bacteremias were attributed to the presence of the femoral catheters. There were no long-term sequelae attributable to infectious causes. Although the necessity of antibiotic prophylaxis during placement of permanent epidural catheters and implantable devices to treat chronic pain is well defined,[23,62] the importance of antibiotic prophylaxis during placement and maintenance of neuraxial or peripheral catheters is less clear. In a series of 405 axillary catheters, the single infectious complication occurred in a nonsurgical patient who did not receive the "usual" perioperative antibiotic prophylaxis.[63]

## Anesthetic Management

These studies and epidemiologic data provide guidance in the administration of spinal or epidural anesthesia in the febrile patient. However, as with all clinical judgments, the decision to perform a regional anesthetic technique must be made on an individual basis considering the anesthetic alternatives, the benefits of regional anesthesia, and the risk of CNS infection (which may theoretically occur in any bacteremic patient).

Numerous clinical and laboratory studies have suggested an association between dural puncture during bacteremia and meningitis. The data are not equivocal, however. The clinical studies are limited to pediatric patients who are historically at high risk for meningitis. Many of the original animal studies used bacterial counts that were far in excess of those noted in humans in early sepsis, making CNS contamination more likely.[32,64] Despite these conflicting results, it is generally recommended that, except in the most extraordinary circumstances, central neuronal block should not be performed in patients with untreated systemic infection.

Patients with evidence of systemic infection may safely undergo spinal anesthesia, provided appropriate antibiotic therapy is initiated *before* dural puncture, and the patient has demonstrated a response to therapy, such as a decrease in fever.[33,65] Although few data exist on the administration of epidural anesthesia in the patient with a treated systemic or local (distant) infection, the studies by Bader et al.,[11] Goodman et al.,[13] and Darchy et al.[36] are reassuring. Placement of an indwelling epidural (or intrathecal) catheter in this group of patients remains controversial; patients should be carefully selected and monitored for evidence of epidural infection.

Spinal anesthesia may be safely performed in patients at risk for low-grade transient bacteremia after dural puncture. Once again, little information exists concerning the risk of epidural anesthesia in patients suspected of developing an intraoperative transient bacteremia (such as during a urologic procedure). However, short-term epidural catheterization is likely safe, as suggested by large retrospective reviews which included a significant number of obstetric and urologic patients (Table 19-1).

All patients with an established local or systemic infection should be considered at risk for developing infection of the CNS. Patients should be observed carefully for signs of infection when a continuous epidural catheter is left in place for prolonged periods. In addition, injection of local anesthetic or insertion of a catheter in an area at high risk for bacterial contamination such as the sacral hiatus may also increase the risk for abscess formation.[66,67]

Central neuronal block has been shown to be safe in patients with recurrent HSV infections, although exacerbations of HSV-1 have been reported in association with intrathecal and epidural opioids. There are inadequate data available regarding the safety of spinal and epidural anesthesia in the presence of primary HSV-2 infection; however, viremia, fever, and meningitis have been reported. These findings would suggest a conservative approach.[47–50] Minimal data suggest that regional anesthesia can be performed safely in HIV-infected patients, although underlying neurologic pathology is common in these patients.[51–55]

### *Diagnosis and Treatment*

A delay in diagnosis and treatment of major CNS infections of even a few hours significantly worsens neurologic outcome. Bacterial meningitis is a medical emergency. Mortality is approximately 30%, even with antibiotic therapy. Meningitis presents most often with fever, severe headache, altered level of consciousness, and meningismus. The diagnosis is confirmed with a lumbar puncture. Lumbar puncture should not be performed if epidural abscess is suspected, because contamination of the intrathecal space may result. CSF examination in the patient with meningitis reveals leukocytosis, a glucose level of less than 30 mg/dL, and a protein level greater than 150 mg/dL. In addition, the anesthesiologist should consider atypical organisms in patients suspected of meningitis following spinal anesthesia.

Abscess formation following epidural or spinal anesthesia can be superficial, requiring limited surgical drainage and intravenous antibiotics. Superficial infections present with local tissue swelling, erythema, and drainage, often associated with fever, but rarely causing neurologic problems unless untreated. Epidural abscess formation usually presents days to weeks after neural blockade with clinical signs of severe back pain, local tenderness, and fever associated with leukocytosis (Table 19-5). The clinical course of epidural abscess progresses from spinal ache and root pain, to weakness (including bowel and bladder symptoms) and eventually paralysis.[7,8] The initial back pain and radicular symptoms may remain stable for hours to weeks. However,

TABLE 19-5. Differential Diagnosis of Epidural Abscess, Epidural Hemorrhage, and Anterior Spinal Artery Syndrome

| | Epidural abscess | Epidural hemorrhage | Anterior spinal artery syndrome |
|---|---|---|---|
| Age of patient | Any age | 50% older than 50 years | Elderly |
| History | Infection or immunosuppression* | Anticoagulants | Arteriosclerosis/ hypotension |
| Onset | 1–3 days | Sudden | Sudden |
| Generalized symptoms | Fever, malaise, back pain | Sharp, transient back and leg pain | None |
| Sensory involvement | None or paresthesias | Variable, late | Minor, patchy |
| Motor involvement | Flaccid paralysis, later spastic | Flaccid paralysis | Flaccid paralysis |
| Segmental reflexes | Exacerbated,* later obtunded | Abolished | Abolished |
| Myelogram/CT scan | Signs of extradural compression | Signs of extradural compression | Normal |
| CSF | Increased white cell count | Normal | Normal |

*Source:* Horlocker TT, Wedel DJ. Regional anesthesia and infection. In: Finucane BT, ed. Complications of Regional Anesthesia. Philadelphia: WB Saunders; 1999:170–183. Reprinted with permission from Elsevier.
*Infrequent findings.

the onset of weakness often progresses to complete paralysis within 24 hours. Radiologic evidence of an epidural mass in the presence of variable neurologic deficit is diagnostic. Magnetic resonance imaging is advocated as the most sensitive modality for evaluation of the spine when infection is suspected.[35,68,69] A combination of antibiotics and surgical drainage remains the treatment of choice. As with spinal hematoma, neurologic recovery is dependent on the duration of the deficit and the severity of neurologic impairment before treatment.[4,5,8]

## References


1. Ready LB, Helfer D. Bacterial meningitis in parturients after epidural anesthesia. Anesthesiology 1989;71:988–990.
2. Baker AS, Ojemann RG, Swartz MN, Richardson EP. Spinal epidural abscess. N Engl J Med 1975;293:463–468.
3. Ericsson M, Algers G, Schliamser SE. Spinal epidural abscesses in adults: review and report of iatrogenic cases. Scand J Infect Dis 1990;22:249–257.
4. Moen V, Dahlgren N, Irestedt L. Severe neurological complications after central neuraxial blockades in Sweden 1990–1999. Anesthesiology 2004;101:950–959.
5. Wang LP, Hauerberg J, Schmidt JF. Incidence of spinal epidural abscess after epidural analgesia: a national 1-year survey. Anesthesiology 1999;91:1928–1936.
6. Kilpatrick ME, Girgis NI. Meningitis – a complication of spinal anesthesia. Anesth Analg 1983;62:513–515.
7. Russel NA, Vaughan R, Morley TP. Spinal epidural infection. Can J Neurol Sci 1979;6: 325–328.
8. Danner RL, Hartman BJ. Update of spinal epidural abscess: 35 cases and review of the literature. Rev Infect Dis 1987;9:265–274.
9. Du Pen SL, Peterson DG, Williams A, Bogosian AJ. Infection during chronic epidural catheterization: diagnosis and treatment. Anesthesiology 1990;73:905–909.
10. Scott DB. Hibbard BM. Serious non-fatal complications associated with extradural block in obstetric practice. Br J Anaesth 1990;64:537–541.
11. Bader AM, Datta S, Gilbertson L, Kirz L. Regional anesthesia in women with chorioamnionitis. Reg Anesth 1992;17:84–86.
12. Strafford MA, Wilder RT, Berde CB. The risk of infection from epidural analgesia in children: a review of 1620 cases. Anesth Analg 1995;80:234–238.
13. Goodman EJ, DeHorta E, Taguiam JM. Safety of spinal and epidural anesthesia in parturients with chorioamnionitis. Reg Anesth 1996;21:436–441.

14. Dahlgren N, Tornebrandt K. Neurological complications after anaesthesia. A follow-up of 18,000 spinal and epidural anaesthetics performed over three years. Acta Anaesthesiol Scand 1995;39:872–880.
15. Kindler C, Seeberger M, Siegemund M, Schneider M. Extradural abscess complicating lumbar extradural anaesthesia and analgesia in an obstetric patient. Acta Anaesthesiol Scand 1996;40:858–861.
16. Auroy Y, Narchi P, Messiah A, Litt L, Rouvier B, Samii K. Serious complications related to regional anesthesia: results of a prospective survey in France. Anesthesiology 1997;87: 479–486.
17. Aromaa U, Lahdensuu M, Cozanitis DA. Severe complications associated with epidural and spinal anaesthetics in Finland 1987–1993. A study based on patient insurance claims. Acta Anaesthesiol Scand 1997;41:445–452.
18. Kane RE. Neurologic deficits following epidural or spinal anesthesia. Anesth Analg 1981; 60:150–161.
19. Videira RL, Ruiz-Neto PP, Brandao Neto M. Post spinal meningitis and asepsis. Acta Anaesthesiol Scand 2002;46:639–646.
20. Schneeberger PM, Janssen M, Voss A. Alpha-hemolytic streptococci: a major pathogen of iatrogenic meningitis following lumbar puncture. Case reports and a review of the literature. Infection 1996;24:29–35.
21. Trautmann M, Lepper PM, Schmitz FJ. Three cases of bacterial meningitis after spinal and epidural anesthesia. Eur J Clin Microbiol Infect Dis 2002;21:43–45.
22. Couzigou C, Vuong TK, Botherel AH, Aggoune M, Astagneau P. Iatrogenic Streptococcus salivarius meningitis after spinal anaesthesia: need for strict application of standard precautions. J Hosp Infect 2003;53:313–314.
23. Rathmell JP. Infectious risks of chronic pain treatments. Reg Anesth Pain Med 2006; 31(4):346–352.
24. Bajwa ZH, Ho C, Grush A, Kleefield J, Warfield CA. Discitis associated with pregnancy and spinal anesthesia. Anesth Analg 2002;94:415–416.
25. Capdevila X, Pirat P, Bringuier S, et al. Continuous peripheral nerve blocks in hospital wards after orthopedic surgery. Anesthesiology 2005;103:1035–1045.
26. Cuvillon P, Ripart J, Lalourcey L, et al. The continuous femoral nerve block catheter for postoperative analgesia: bacterial colonization, infectious rate and adverse effects. Anesth Analg 2001;93:1045–1049.
27. Wegeforth P, Latham JR. Lumbar puncture as a factor in the causation of meningitis. Am J Med Sci 1919;158:183–202.
28. Pray LG. Lumbar puncture as a factor in the pathogenesis of meningitis. Am J Dis Child 1941;295:62–68.
29. Eng RHK, Seligman SJ. Lumbar puncture-induced meningitis. JAMA 1981;245: 1456–1459.
30. Teele DW, Dashefsky B, Rakusan T, Klein JO. Meningitis after lumbar puncture in children with bacteremia. N Engl J Med 1981;304:1079–1081.
31. Smith KM, Deddish RB, Ogata ES. Meningitis associated with serial lumbar punctures and post-hemorrhagic hydrocephalus. J Pediatr 1986;109:1057–1060.
32. Weed LH, Wegeforth P, Ayer JB, Felton LD. The production of meningitis by release of cerebrospinal fluid during an experimental septicemia. JAMA 1919;72:190–193.
33. Carp H, Bailey S. The association between meningitis and dural puncture in bacteremic rats. Anesthesiology 1992;76:739–742.
34. Berman RS, Eisele JH. Bacteremia, spinal anesthesia, and development of meningitis. Anesthesiology 1978;48:376–377.
35. Shintani S, Tanaka H, Irifune A, et al. Iatrogenic acute spinal epidural abscess with septic meningitis: MR findings. Clin Neurol Neurosurg 1992;94:253–255.
36. Darchy B, Forceville X, Bavoux E, Soriot F, Domart Y. Clinical and bacteriologic survey of epidural analgesia in patients in the intensive care unit. Anesthesiology 1996;85: 988–998.
37. Feldman JM, Chapin-Robertson K, Turner J. Do agents used for epidural analgesia have antimicrobial properties? Reg Anesth 1994;19:43–47.
38. James FM III, George RH, Naiem H, White GJ. Bacteriologic aspects of epidural analgesia. Anesth Analg 1976;55:187–190.
39. Hunt JR, Rigor BM, Collins JR. The potential for contamination of continuous epidural catheters. Anesth Analg 1977;56:222–224.

40. Barreto RS. Bacteriologic culture of indwelling epidural catheters. Anesthesiology 1962;23:643–646.
41. De Cicco M, Matovic M, Castellani GT, et al. Time-dependent efficacy of bacterial filters and infection risk in long-term epidural catheterization. Anesthesiology 1995;82:765–771.
42. Abouleish E, Amortegui AJ, Taylor FH. Are bacterial filters needed in continuous epidural analgesia for obstetrics? Anesthesiology 1977;46:351–354.
43. Langevin PB, Gravenstein N, Langevin SO, Gulig PA. Epidural catheter reconnection: safe and unsafe practice. Anesthesiology 1996;85:883–888.
44. Mahendru V, Bacon DR, Lema MJ. Multiple epidural abscesses and spinal anesthesia in a diabetic patient. Case report. Reg Anesth 1994;19:66–68.
45. Strong WE. Epidural abscess associated with epidural catheterization: a rare event? Report of two cases with markedly delayed presentation. Anesthesiology 1991;74:943–946.
46. Huang RC, Shapiro GS, Lim M, Sandhu HS, Lutz GE, Herzog RJ. Cervical epidural abscess after epidural steroid injection. Spine 2004;29:E7–E9.
47. Bader AM, Camann WR, Datta S. Anesthesia for cesarean delivery in patients with herpes simplex virus type-2 infections. Reg Anesth 1990;15:261–263.
48. Crosby ET, Halpern SH, Rolbin SH. Epidural anaesthesia for caesarean section in patients with active recurrent genital herpes simplex infections: a retrospective review. Can J Anaesth 1989;36:701–704.
49. Ramanathan S, Sheth R, Turndorf H. Anesthesia for cesarean section in patients with genital herpes infections: a retrospective study. Anesthesiology 1986;64:807–809.
50. Crone LL, Conly JM, Storgard C, et al. Herpes labialis in parturients receiving epidural morphine after cesarean section. Anesthesiology 1990;73:208–213.
51. Valley MA, Bourke DL, McKenzie AM. Recurrence of thoracic and labial herpes simplex virus infection in a patient receiving epidural fentanyl. Anesthesiology 1992;76:1056–1057.
52. Hughes SC, Dailey PA, Landers D, Dattel BJ, Crombleholme WR, Johnson JL. Parturients infected with human immunodeficiency virus and regional anesthesia. Anesthesiology 1995;82:32–37.
53. Avidan MS, Groves P, Blott M, et al. Low complication rate associated with cesarean section under spinal anesthesia for HIV-1-infected women on antiretroviral therapy. Anesthesiology 2002;97:320–324.
54. Bremerich DH, Ahr A, Buchner S, et al. Anesthetic regimen for HIV positive parturients undergoing elective cesarean section [German]. Anaesthesist 2003;52:1124–1131.
55. Tom DJ, Gulevich SJ, Shapiro HM, Heaton RK, Grant I. Epidural blood patch in the HIV-positive patient. Anesthesiology 1992;76:943–947.
56. Hebl JR. The importance and implications of aseptic techniques during regional anesthesia. Reg Anesth Pain Med 2006;31(4):311–323.
57. Saloojee H, Steenhoff A. The health professional's role in preventing nosocomial infections. Postgrad Med J 2001;77:16–19.
58. Molinier S, Paris JF, Brisou P, Amah Y, Morand JJ, Alla P, Carli P. Two cases of iatrogenic oral streptococcal infection: meningitis and spondylodiscitis [French]. Rev Med Int 1998;19:568–570.
59. Kinirons B, Mimoz O, Lafendi L, Naas T, Meunier J, Nordmann P. Chlorhexidine versus povidone iodine in preventing colonization of continuous epidural catheters in children: a randomized, controlled trial. Anesthesiology 2001;94:239–244.
60. Birnbach DJ, Stein DJ, Murray O, Thys DM, Sordillo EM. Povidone iodine and skin disinfection before initiation of epidural anesthesia. Anesthesiology 1998;88:668–672.
61. Borgeat A, Ekatodramis G, Kalberer F, Benz C. Acute and nonacute complications associated with interscalene block and shoulder surgery: a prospective study. Anesthesiology 2001;95:875–880.
62. Mangram AJ, Horan TC, Pearson ML, Silver LC, Jarvis WR. Guideline for prevention of surgical site infection, 1999. Hospital Infection Practices Advisory Committee. Infect Control Hosp Epidemiol 1999;20:250–278.
63. Bergman BD, Hebl JR, Kent J, Horlocker TT. Neurologic complications of 405 consecutive continuous axillary catheters. Anesth Analg 2003;96:247–252.
64. Petersdorf RG, Swarner DR, Garcia M. Studies on the pathogenesis of meningitis. II. Development of meningitis during pneumococcal bacteremia. J Clin Invest 1962;41:320–327.

65. Chestnut DH. Spinal anesthesia in the febrile patient. Anesthesiology 1992;76:667–669.
66. McNeely JK, Trentadue NC, Rusy LM, Farber NE. Culture of bacteria from lumbar and caudal epidural catheters used for postoperative analgesia in children. Reg Anesth 1997;22:428–431.
67. Kost-Byerly S, Tobin JR, Greenberg RS, Billett C, Zahurak M, Yaster M. Bacterial colonization and infection rate of continuous epidural catheters in children. Anesth Analg 1998;86:712–716.
68. Mamourian AC, Dickman CA, Drayer BP, Sonntag VKH. Spinal epidural abscess: three cases following spinal epidural injection demonstrated with magnetic resonance imaging. Anesthesiology 1993;78:204–207.
69. Curling OD, Gower DJ, McWhorter JM. Changing concepts of spinal epidural abscess: a report of 29 cases. Neurosurgery 1990;27:185–192.

# 20 Regional Anesthesia in the Presence of Neurologic Disease

Andrea Kattula, Giuditta Angelini, and George Arndt

Performing regional anesthesia in patients with preexisting neurologic or neuromuscular disease remains controversial. Numerous anecdotal reports describe the successful use of regional techniques in a variety of neuromuscular disorders including multiple sclerosis, amyotrophic lateral sclerosis (ALS), muscular dystrophies, myotonias, and others.[1] However, a study of significant size to confirm or support the safety of regional anesthesia in these patients continues to remain scarce. Specific guidelines regarding the use of regional techniques in the setting of neurologic disease are difficult to define because of these limitations. Therefore, the goal of this chapter is to review several of the more common neurologic disorders that an anesthesiologist may encounter and outline what information currently exists to help guide the use of regional anesthesia.

Two characteristics of the neuromuscular system that continue to be considered as a contraindication to regional anesthesia include the following: increased intracranial pressure with respect to epidural or spinal anesthesia and evolving or unstable neuromuscular disease. In the background, it is difficult to ignore the literature surrounding cauda equina syndrome in patients who received continuous spinal anesthesia through small-gauge catheters in the past. From this information, higher concentrations of local anesthetics for a longer duration have the potential to be toxic to nerves. More recently, lidocaine more than other local anesthetics has been shown to be neurotoxic in clinically available concentrations, even in short durations. However, there are several disadvantages to general anesthesia that could be detrimental as well. For instance, these patients may have decreased respiratory reserve which may be compromised by even small amounts of narcotics and muscle relaxants. Therefore, judicious use of local anesthetics, especially at lower concentrations, may achieve a middle ground of safety with potentially fewer side effects. This chapter will review some of these disorders and the information available on the use of regional anesthetic techniques in their presence.

## General Considerations

Evaluation of the patient with neuromuscular disease must consider not only the neuromuscular deficits, but also the effects the disease may have had on other organ systems, particularly respiratory and cardiovascular. These secondary effects may have a significant impact on the administration and course of both general and regional anesthesia in these patients.

Evaluation and documentation of preexisting neurologic deficits is a vital part of the preoperative anesthesia workup for any patient with an underlying neurologic disorder. This is imperative whether regional or general anesthesia is planned. Changes in neurologic status are frequently seen in the perioperative period in these patients, and the documentation of preexisting deficits facilitates the interpretation of any changes seen postoperatively.

The patient with generalized neurologic/neuromuscular disease may be at risk for respiratory compromise in the perioperative period. In particular, impaired ventilatory reserve with reduced ability to respond to hypercapnia and hypoxia may result in an increased risk of respiratory failure.[2,3] The site of surgical incision affects the risk of respiratory complications, with a higher incidence in patients undergoing upper abdominal and thoracic procedures. The method of perioperative analgesia may have a significant influence on this risk of respiratory compromise, providing the anesthesiologist with an opportunity to positively influence the patient's course.

In addition to hypoventilation, dysfunction of the pharyngeal muscles and the potential of aspiration add to the possibility of pneumonia postoperatively. Maintenance of an awake patient can only aid in the prevention of aspiration. Additionally, an endotracheal tube can be protective at the expense of further loss of muscle tone of both the respiratory and pharyngeal muscles. Finally, patients with advanced neurologic disorders can have a degree of restrictive lung disease which makes mechanical ventilation higher risk for barotraumas.[4]

Preoperative assessment of respiratory function and reserve is important and may include measurement of oxygen saturation, arterial blood gas, pulmonary function, and maximum negative inspiratory force. History of swallowing evaluations can be helpful to highlight additional risks in the perioperative period.

Similarly, the cardiovascular effects of neuromuscular disorders must also be considered in the preoperative evaluation. Autonomic dysfunction occurs with many neurologic disorders and constitutes the major contributor to complications related to this organ system. ALS, Guillain-Barré syndrome, multiple sclerosis, and spinal cord lesions above the level of T6 can all have alteration of the autonomic nervous system. In addition, diabetes mellitus, amyloidosis, uremia, and connective tissue disorders are systemic diseases associated with autonomic dysfunction which may coexist in these patients as well.[5,6]

Several findings in the preoperative evaluation may guide the clinician to an increased suspicion for the presence of autonomic dysfunction.[7] The absence of beat-to-beat heart rate variability with deep breathing is one of the most sensitive signs of autonomic dysfunction. Additional characteristic signs include resting tachycardia, orthostatic hypotension, cardiac dysrhythmias, and impotence.

Because of the presence of autonomic dysfunction, these patients have shortening of the Q-T interval which puts them at risk for cardiac conduction abnormalities. In addition, wide fluctuations in blood pressure leads to the frequent need for intraoperative vasopressor therapy. Required avoidance of oral intake makes the presence of relative hypovolemia common. A sympathectomy from neuraxial blockade, but potentially a variable amount from narcotics and inhalational anesthetics as well, can result in exaggerated hypotension in this setting. Finally, unexpected intraoperative cardio-respiratory arrests have been reported in patients with autonomic dysfunction which is second in frequency only to respiratory failure.[8,9]

Myocardial dysfunction and arrhythmias caused by changes in the cardiac muscle and conduction pathways are associated with numerous myopathic diseases including the muscular dystrophies, Guillain-Barré syndrome, and polio. A high index of suspicion must be maintained in the preoperative evaluation of these patients, as exercise tolerance is likely to be very limited by underlying neuromuscular disease. Screening by historical assessment is often inadequate.

## Regional Anesthesia and Multiple Sclerosis

Multiple sclerosis is an acquired central nervous system disease characterized by multiple sites of demyelination in the brain and spinal cord. The periventricular white matter, optic nerves, and brainstem are most often affected. Multiple sclerosis does not affect the peripheral nervous system. Demyelination of axons results in a slowing of sensory and motor conduction which leads to widely variable clinical signs and symptoms specific to the sites of demyelination. Examples of the spectrum of symptomatology include the following: visual disturbances because of involvement of the optic nerve, gait disturbances and incoordination secondary to cerebellar changes, and spinal cord demyelination resulting in paresthesias, weakness, and bowel/bladder incontinence.

The diagnosis of multiple sclerosis is made on clinical grounds because there are no specific diagnostic tests. Supportive information may be gained from evoked potential studies with visual, brainstem, and somatosensory potentials revealing slowed conduction. Magnetic resonance and computed tomographic imaging are used to identify plaques throughout the central nervous system. Seventy percent of patients will exhibit a nonspecific increase in protein on cerebrospinal fluid examination.[10]

The clinical course of multiple sclerosis is characterized by a series of remissions and exacerbations over years. Eventually, however, residual symptoms begin to persist between relapses. Extreme variability is seen among individuals, and the waxing and waning course makes it difficult to evaluate the effects of therapeutic interventions. Treatment is mainly supportive with avoidance of stress, excessive fatigue, and marked changes in temperature. Increasing evidence is accumulating that multiple sclerosis is most likely an autoimmune disease involving T cells. Research is directed at treating inflammatory damage to myelin as well as remyelination techniques. Corticosteroids may induce remission during an acute attack[11] but likely do not affect the long-term course of the disease. Interferon β may augment natural disease suppression mechanisms. A decoy similar to the structure of myelin for the autoantibodies has been used. It is called glatiramer, and studies so far are unclear if it is more efficacious alone or in combination with interferon. Intravenous immunoglobulins can reduce the relapse rate, but not likely disease progression. Nonspecific immune suppressants including azathioprine and methotrexate have variable effects. Symptomatic treatment of muscle spasms is also indicated.[12]

There are some case reports that indicate that even intravenous lidocaine has been associated with unmasking the symptoms of multiple sclerosis in a previously undiagnosed patient. Recently, endogenous oligopeptides capable of sodium channel blockade have been discovered in higher concentrations in the cerebrospinal fluid of multiple sclerosis patients compared with normal controls. In fact, these peptides may be active at sites of demyelination and produce some of the negative symptoms of multiple sclerosis, including weakness. Areas of damaged myelin in which ectopic foci of depolarization are capable of producing some of the positive symptoms of multiple sclerosis including spasticity.[13] Furthermore, there is some literature indicating that lidocaine and mexiletine can be used to treat some of the positive symptoms of multiple sclerosis.[14]

The exacerbating factors of stress, fatigue, changes in temperature, and infection are potentially associated with the perioperative period for more than one reason.[15] Delineating the natural course of the disease from the effects of surgery and anesthesia can be very difficult. The purported effects of anesthesia on the course of multiple sclerosis continue to be controversial. There also continues to be a very small number of studies in this area. However, it is the neurologic disease that has the most information about the effects of regional anesthesia. Because of a continuing lack of evidence of safety, reluctance to utilize regional techniques in multiple sclerosis patients persists.

Many of the studies and case reports available involve obstetric patients with multiple sclerosis, which constitutes a subset of patients likely to be considered for regional anesthesia. The natural history of multiple sclerosis in pregnancy is characterized by remission during gestation[16,17] because of a presumed immunomodulatory protective effect.[18] This is also seen in other parturients with autoimmune disorders such as rheumatoid arthritis. In fact, patients who have had a full-term pregnancy have a tendency toward an increased time interval to sustained disability. Patients are likely to have more multiple sclerosis relapses in the first 3 months postpartum regardless of whether they received an epidural.[18]

Neuraxial, and in particular spinal, anesthesia has been implicated as a potential cause of exacerbations in these patients[19] even though contradictory retrospective studies and case reports exist.[20,21] Theories to explain any exacerbation of multiple sclerosis symptoms by spinal anesthesia focus on the potential for an increased susceptibility of demyelinated areas of nerves to the neurotoxic effects of local anesthetics.[20] The three to four times higher concentration of local anesthetic reaching the spinal cord white matter with subarachnoid as opposed to epidural anesthesia could explain the higher risk of exacerbation posed by this modality.[22] Schapira[23] demonstrated that diagnostic lumbar puncture alone did not appear to induce relapses in patients with multiple sclerosis, lending support to the theory that any effects of spinal anesthesia on multiple sclerosis are related to local anesthetic neurotoxicity. In addition, intrathecal morphine has also been used successfully without exacerbation anecdotally in patients with multiple sclerosis.

Bader et al.[20] performed a retrospective and partially prospective review of all obstetric multiple sclerosis patients at the Brigham and Women's Hospital between 1982 and 1987 and noted no significant difference in exacerbation rates between patients receiving epidural anesthesia and local infiltration for vaginal delivery. The total number of pregnancies in patients with multiple sclerosis in this study was 32. However, all of the women who did experience a relapse within 3 months postpartum had received epidural anesthesia with a concentration of bupivacaine greater than 0.25%. This was a total of three patients. The authors proposed that the use of higher bupivacaine concentrations over a longer period of time (i.e., labor epidurals) may affect the rate of postpartum multiple sclerosis relapse, particularly if multiple local anesthetic boluses are required. Warren et al.[24] also reported minor exacerbations in a patient following two separate epidurals (years apart) for vaginal delivery, although a relatively large total dose of bupivacaine was used on the second occasion only. Of note, although these incidents suggest that local anesthetics may potentially produce neurologic symptoms in demyelinated areas of patients with multiple sclerosis, these effects have not been permanent and generally gradual recovery over time is the rule.[25]

Despite these concerns, there are many reports of successful use of epidural anesthesia in multiple sclerosis patients without evidence of relapse. Capdeville and Hoyt[26] performed a retrospective review of all obstetric patients with multiple sclerosis admitted to University Hospitals of Cleveland from 1986 to 1993. Over this 7-year period, eight women with multiple sclerosis underwent eight vaginal deliveries, one cesarean delivery, and five obstetric-related procedures. The anesthetic techniques used were five epidurals, two general anesthetics, one pudendal block, and one narcotic technique. Only two exacerbations of multiple sclerosis were noted by chart review. One of these occurred after a general anesthetic, and the other was noted in a patient receiving a pudendal block. No exacerbations were seen in patients receiving epidural anesthesia.

Crawford et al.[21] documented only one perioperative relapse in 50 nonobstetric and seven obstetric patients with multiple sclerosis receiving lumbar epidural anesthesia. Again, the numbers are too small to lead to generalized recommendations but do indicate anecdotal success without complication involving the use of regional anesthesia in patients with multiple sclerosis.

Confavreux et al.[27] published in 1998 one of the largest prospective studies on the rate of pregnancy-related multiple sclerosis relapses. It included 269 pregnancies in 254 women from 12 European countries from 1993 to 1995. A total of 42 patients received epidural analgesia. The rate of relapse per year was not different when compared with those who did not receive an epidural.

A significant concern in patients with multiple sclerosis is the presence of autonomic dysfunction and the potential for chronic hypovolemia in these immobilized patients. Both factors increase the risk of hemodynamic instability during anesthesia. Kytta and Rosenberg[28] evaluated 56 adult patients with documented multiple sclerosis undergoing a total of 71 anesthetics at the University Central Hospital, Helsinki, Finland, from 1973 to 1982. A retrospective evaluation was made of the different anesthetic techniques used – 42 general anesthetics, five regional anesthetics, and 24 infiltrative techniques. All five patients receiving regional anesthesia (three epidurals and two spinals) had marked hypotension with significant sympathetic blocks. The authors subjectively observed a reduced response to intravenous fluids and vasopressor therapy. They proposed that this may be related to autonomic dysfunction in patients with multiple sclerosis which had been exacerbated by a chronic volume-depleted state.

The use of regional anesthesia in patients with multiple sclerosis remains unclear. Multiple case reports support its successful use, particularly in obstetric patients. Other case reports suggest a risk of perioperative symptom exacerbation and hemodynamic instability. If regional anesthesia is considered, the risk and benefits must be fully discussed with the patient. Special note during these discussions must be made of the potential for exacerbations of multiple sclerosis related to stress and temperature changes associated with the perioperative period regardless of the anesthetic technique used. In addition, parturients have a particular issue with increased incidence of multiple sclerosis relapse early in their postpartum period.

## Regional Anesthesia and Amyotrophic Lateral Sclerosis

ALS is a degenerative disease of lower motor neurons, motor nuclei of the brainstem, and descending pathways of upper motor neurons.[29] It results in clinical features of both upper and lower motor neuron lesions with variability depending on the muscle groups involved. ALS limited to brainstem nuclei is referred to as pseudobulbar palsy. Symptoms limited to the motor cortex are then usually referred to as primary lateral sclerosis.[30] The etiology remains unclear, and the disease most frequently affects males in their fifth to seventh decade of life.

The clinical features of ALS involve progressive muscular atrophy with weakness and fasciculations of skeletal muscles. Bulbar muscle weakness often predominates with an associated risk of aspiration. A characteristic emotional lability is seen.[30] Autonomic nervous system dysfunction is common with the associated risk of exaggerated hemodynamic responses during anesthesia. Death from myocardial or respiratory failure ensues, often within 6 years of the onset of symptoms.

Epidural anesthesia has been successfully used in patients with ALS.[31] Kochi et al.[31] reported three cases in which lumbar epidural anesthesia was used, emphasizing the advantage of avoiding tracheal intubations. In this patient population, any duration of mechanical ventilation could accelerate the loss of muscle tone, and weaning from the ventilator could be quite a challenge. However, a high epidural or spinal block can affect intercostals muscle function with detrimental effects in patients with minimal ventilatory reserve.

## Regional Anesthesia and Spinal Cord Injuries

Spinal cord injury has classically been divided into two distinct stages. Initial injury is classified as spinal shock which consists of a 1- to 3-week period of flaccid paralysis including loss of sensation temperature regulation, and spinal cord reflexes below the level of injury.[32] Hypotension, bradycardia, and changes in the electrocardiogram (premature ventricular contractions, nonspecific ST-T wave changes) are characteristic. Regional anesthesia is not frequently used during this stage of spinal shock because of the evolving neurologic injury. It is necessary to be able to follow the examination and the above-mentioned potential of neurotoxicity of local anesthetics in extremely susceptible nerves. There is also a risk of hemodynamic instability as well as hypothermia.

The chronic stage of spinal cord injury is characterized by skeletal muscle spasticity and the return of spinal and autonomic reflexes below the level of injury. Autonomic hyperreflexia is seen in approximately 85% of patients with lesions at or above T6.[33] In this setting, a reflex response may be produced by a cutaneous (incision) or visceral (bladder distension, uterine contraction) stimulus below the level of injury. This afferent stimulus activates preganglionic sympathetic nerves, resulting in severe hypertension because of intense vasoconstriction below the level of the lesion. Under normal conditions, this response is modulated by inhibitory impulses from higher central nervous system centers. With a spinal cord lesion, this inhibitory input is lost and the vasoconstriction proceeds unimpeded. The resulting hypertension stimulates the carotid sinus baroreceptors, leading to reflex bradycardia and vasodilation above the level of injury.[32] As the cord level rises above T6, the potential for compensatory vasodilation decreases and the potential for severe injury can include acute left ventricular failure with pulmonary edema, dysrhythmias, cerebrovascular hemorrhage, retinal bleeding, seizures, and an increasing number of deaths.

Prevention and early treatment of autonomic hyperreflexia is critical. Both general and regional anesthesia have been used effectively. Broecker et al.[34] noted that spinal and epidural anesthesia were logical choices to prevent autonomic hyperreflexia because the afferent limb of the reflex would be blocked. Spinal anesthesia has been shown to be particularly useful,[35] but epidural blocks are less reliable.[34] Parturients at risk for autonomic hyperreflexia from uterine contractions are likely to benefit from the early use of continuous lumbar epidural analgesia after the onset of labor.[36] Baraka[37] reported the successful use of epidural meperidine in a laboring patient at risk for autonomic hyperreflexia. In addition to its prophylactic use, regional anesthesia has been used therapeutically in patients with autonomic hyperreflexia.[36]

Regardless of the anesthetic technique used, medications should be available to treat severe hypertension in the patient with autonomic hyperreflexia. Sodium nitroprusside, ganglionic blockers (i.e., trimethoprim), and alpha blockers (i.e., phentolamine, phenoxybenzamine) have been used.

Concerns often raised regarding the use of spinal anesthetics in this group of patients with spinal cord injury include potential difficulty in placement, difficulty in control or examination of block level, and a potential increased risk of hypotension. Lambert et al.[35] performed a retrospective review of 78 procedures in 50 spinal cord–injured patients considered "at risk" for autonomic hyperreflexia. No significant differences were seen in intraoperative blood pressure between those receiving spinal or general anesthesia. Both techniques seemed to protect equally against intraoperative hypertension.

## Regional Anesthesia and Peripheral Neuropathies

Peripheral neuropathies result from either the disruption of axons with distal degeneration or segmental demyelination caused by Schwann cell degeneration.[38] They classically start distally and spread proximally resulting in a "glove and stocking" distribution of decreased sensation, weakness, and reduced reflexes. Some, such as diabetic and alcoholic neuropathy, can be associated with tender muscles. The etiologies of peripheral neuropathies are considerable, including metabolic disorders (diabetes mellitus, renal failure, hepatic failure, porphyria, and nutritional deficiencies), connective tissue disorders, infection, toxins, malignancy, endocrine disorders, and Guillain-Barré syndrome. Diagnosis depends on metabolic screening tests, serology, infection, and autoimmune evaluations. Electromyogram studies reveal evidence of denervation and a reduction in nerve conduction velocity.

Diabetic peripheral and autonomic neuropathies are encountered frequently in patients presenting for anesthesia and surgery. Clinically, the peripheral neuropathy predominantly affects the lower extremities with paresthesias, weakness, and sensory loss more distally and often worse at night. Occasionally, the neuropathy of diabetes may present as a mononeuropathy causing transient pain and weakness in an isolated nerve distribution. The associated autonomic neuropathy may be significant, with anesthetic implications related to an increased risk of intraoperative hemodynamic instability[39] and an increased risk of unexplained intraoperative cardiac arrest.

The use of regional anesthesia in patients with preexisting peripheral neuropathies depends on a thorough analysis of the risks and benefits for each individual patient. The diabetic patient with a propensity toward perioperative cardiovascular complications[39] might benefit from a regional, particularly spinal, technique that allows the awake patient to report episodes of angina. Another purported advantage of epidural or spinal anesthesia in diabetic patients relates to an improved ability to maintain blood glucose control with the inhibition of the surgical stress response.[40] Certainly, some patients may have exaggerated hypotension with respect to their preexisting autonomic neuropathy. This must be weighed against other risks and benefits that would affect the patient. Furthermore, large doses of local anesthetics have been associated with myocardial depression in diabetic patients.[41]

Guillain-Barré syndrome is an acute inflammatory demyelinating disease of the peripheral nervous system with an incidence of approximately 1:100,000 persons per year.[42] It is postulated to have an autoimmune process directed at myelin similar to multiple sclerosis. Although there may be a correlation with a history of surgery, vaccination, recent respiratory or gastrointestinal tract infection, the etiology is considered to remain unknown. Patients present with the acute onset of lower motor neuron paralysis including flaccid paralysis and reduced reflexes. It begins in the lower extremities and progresses cephalad over hours to days.[43] Bulbar dysfunction and intercostals muscle weakness may ensue, with resultant respiratory failure and the patient's inability to protect their airway. Painful distal extremity paresthesias are common. Autonomic dysfunction occurs in a significant number of patients[44], which results in hemodynamic instability, tachycardia, and cardiac conduction disturbances. Ninety percent of patients will have the most progressive symptoms within 2 weeks.

The treatment of Guillain-Barré is mainly supportive and nonspecific. Many patients will require endotracheal intubation and mechanical ventilation secondary to the respiratory weakness and bulbar dysfunction. Plasmapheresis and intravenous immunoglobulin have been used as treatments during the acute phase and are considered to be equally efficacious. Steroids have been studied and may actually have a deleterious effect. Management of hemodynamic variability associated with autonomic dysfunction can be very challenging. Guillain-Barré usually resolves spontaneously over weeks to months, but approximately 20% of patients will have residual neurologic deficits. The mortality rate is estimated at 5%.[25]

Regional anesthesia has been used successfully in patients with Guillain-Barré syndrome. In particular, epidural anesthesia has been used in parturients with Guillain-Barré without adverse effects.[45] These patients had some residual effects from an episode of Guillain-Barré in the past, but did not have an acute episode of the disease. Epidural narcotics have been used without complication in the acute phase of the disease in an attempt to control painful paresthesias.[46,47] Although the case reports are infrequent, this is another example that narcotics have not been shown to cause toxicity administered neuraxially in patients with neurologic disease[48,49] – even in the setting of acute demyelination. However, no patients received local anesthetics in the acute phase of Guillain-Barré. When considering regional techniques, patients can have exaggerated responses to indirect vasopressors because of their autonomic dysfunction.

## Regional Anesthesia and Muscular Dystrophy

Muscular dystrophies are primary disorders of muscle without clearly evident proximal cause, resulting in progressive weakness. Of the several types, Duchenne's is the most common and most severe.

Duchenne's muscular dystrophy is a sex-linked recessive trait usually only clinically expressed in males. It involves a degeneration of skeletal muscle with atrophy and increased fat and fibrous tissue, but no evidence of denervation. The result is progressive symmetric weakness culminating in death by 15–25 years of age usually attributable to congestive heart failure or pneumonia. Diagnosis is based on muscle biopsy, and increase of serum creatine kinase may be followed to track progression of the disease.

Cardiovascular involvement, although not predominant, may result in significant morbidity and mortality. Congestive heart failure, mitral regurgitation secondary to papillary muscle dysfunction, and sinus tachycardia are common.[50] Dysrhythmias have resulted in cardiac arrest during induction of general anesthesia[51] or in the immediate perioperative period.[52]

Patients with muscular dystrophy are at increased risk for pneumonia and respiratory failure in the perioperative period. Kyphoscoliosis and skeletal muscle weakness produce a restrictive pattern on pulmonary function testing. In addition, depressed laryngeal reflexes and reduced gastric emptying combine to predispose these patients to pulmonary aspiration. Careful monitoring of pulmonary function and attention to clearance of secretions and chest physical therapy are important.

Regional anesthesia may offer significant advantages in these patients. The use of agents known to trigger malignant hyperthermia can be avoided in this population of patients who have an increased risk of this complication.[53] The risk of pulmonary aspiration may be decreased provided that regional anesthesia allows sedation to be minimized. Finally, regional techniques are not without problems. Kyphoscoliosis may lead to technically difficult placement of spinal or epidural blocks. Paralysis of intercostals muscles from regional anesthesia may predispose to respiratory insufficiency.

## Regional Anesthesia and Myotonic Dystrophy

Myotonic dystrophy is the most common of the myotonic disorders which include myotonia congenital and the paramyotonias. The disorders are characterized by persistent contraction and delayed relaxation following muscle stimulation which is unrelieved by denervation or paralysis.[54] Myotonic dystrophy is inherited as an autosomal dominant trait with symptoms becoming chronically evident in the second or third decade.[55] There is progressive deterioration of skeletal, cardiac, and smooth muscle function. Initially, involvement of the intrinsic hand and facial muscles progresses to proximal limb musculature as well as bulbar dysfunction with weakness of pharyngeal and laryngeal muscles. Diaphragmatic involvement is common. Cardiomyopathy is common as well. The cardiac conduction system is particularly affected with a significant risk of dysrhythmias and atrioventricular block.[56,57] Bulbar dysfunction and delayed gastric emptying make these patients at high risk for pulmonary aspiration. Associated endocrine disorders also occur, including diabetes mellitus, adrenal, and thyroid dysfunction. Ultimately, death occurs as a result of dysrhythmias, respiratory, or cardiac failure. Treatment is mostly supportive, but can involve the use of quinine or procainamide for myotonic symptoms.[56]

When patients with myotonic dystrophy present for anesthesia, the preoperative evaluation of pulmonary function is critical. Pulmonary function tests usually reveal a restrictive deficit with mild arterial hypoxemia on a blood gas. A preoperative measurement of baseline negative inspiratory force may be a useful guide to perioperative management. A baseline electrocardiogram should be obtained to assess for cardiac conduction abnormalities. Any underlying respiratory infection should be treated.

General anesthesia presents unique problems in the patient with myotonic dystrophy. Succinylcholine may result in exaggerated contraction of muscles resulting in more difficulty with the placement of an endotracheal tube as well as ventilation. The use of neostigmine to reverse neuromuscular blockade may precipitate myotonic contractions. Patients tend to be extremely sensitive to the respiratory depressant effects of sedatives, opioids, and general anesthetics.[58] An underlying component of central sleep apnea is often present, which further complicates airway management and necessitates added caution in the use of sedatives.

The use of regional anesthesia in patients with myotonic dystrophy is attractive because of the avoidance of neuromuscular blocking agents and their reversal drugs. In addition, the use of sedatives and other anesthetics that may produce respiratory depression can be minimized. Finally, avoidance of triggering agents for malignant hyperthermia can be achieved even though only an association, not a definite risk, has been demonstrated between myotonic dystrophy and this genetic disease.[57] Regional anesthetics can present a different set of concerns. Myotonic contractions are not relieved by spinal or epidural anesthesia – only direct infiltration of an affected muscle with local anesthetic will relieve myotonia. In patients with marginal ventilatory reserve, the effect of high epidural or spinal blockade on intercostals muscle function must be considered, especially because many of these patients may have diaphragmatic dysfunction. When performing regional anesthesia, additional sedatives and anxiolytics should be used with caution. Respiratory status should be continuously assessed for signs of hypoventilation or apnea.

Pregnant patients with myotonic dystrophy may require anesthesia for labor and delivery. General, spinal, and epidural anesthetics have been used successfully in these patients for caesarean delivery.[59,60] However, myotonia and weakness may be exacerbated during pregnancy. Patients with myotonic dystrophy are at increased risk for caesarean delivery because of prolonged labor, as well as postpartum hemorrhage from uterine smooth muscle dysfunction.[59,60]

Cold is a well known trigger for myotonic contractions. Therefore, no matter what technique is used, normothermia is required throughout the perioperative period.[61]

## Regional Anesthesia and Myasthenia Gravis

Myasthenia gravis is an autoimmune disorder of unknown etiology affecting the neuromuscular junction with a decrease in the number of acetylcholine receptors and the presence of antireceptor antibodies in 70%–90% of patients.[62] Skeletal muscle weakness is characteristically worsened by activity. Although smooth and cardiac muscle are uninvolved, myocarditis and dysrhythmias may be present.[63] Treatment modalities include cholinesterase inhibitors, corticosteroids, immunosuppressants, plasmapheresis, and thymectomy. Progressive weakness may be associated with progression of the disease (myasthenic crisis) or may reflect excessive muscarinic effects of anticholinesterase drugs (cholinergic crisis). Evaluation of the patient's response to the administration of edrophonium allows differentiation between the two phenomena.

The major anesthetic consideration in myasthenia gravis relates to the use of neuromuscular blockers with affected patients displaying extreme sensitivity to nondepolarizing blockers is unpredictable. Preexisting skeletal muscle weakness, which is present in varying degrees in these patients, may be potentiated by the relaxant effects of volatile anesthetic agents. Finally, ester local anesthetics may display a prolonged elimination half-life because of reduced plasma cholinesterase activity in patients treated with anticholinesterases,[64] suggesting that amide local anesthetics may be preferable when high or repeated doses are anticipated.

Patients with myasthenia gravis need preoperative assessment of both pulmonary function and aspiration risk because of bulbar dysfunction. Patients with preexisting respiratory compromise are predisposed to significant respiratory depression from anesthetic agents. Therefore, sedatives should be used with caution.

Patients should be monitored closely throughout the perioperative period for myasthenic or cholinergic crisis as well as for gradual deterioration in respiratory function precipitated by stress, infection, missed or excessive anticholinesterase doses, electrolyte abnormalities, or aminoglycoside antibiotics. Identifying patients at particular risk for perioperative compromise and the need for postoperative ventilation was delineated by Leventhal et al.[65] as the following:

1. A history of myasthenia gravis for more than 6 years.
2. A history of unrelated chronic obstructive airway disease.
3. A pyridostigmine dose greater than 750mg/day during the 48 hours immediately preoperative.
4. A vital capacity of less than 2.9L.

Regional anesthesia has been used successfully in patients with myasthenia gravis. It is the preferred analgesic technique in laboring parturients with the disease who are planning a vaginal delivery.[66] The use of regional anesthesia may reduce respiratory risk by avoiding the depressant effects of opioids as well as inhaled agents and neuromuscular blockers. In addition, postoperative analgesia and chest physical therapy can also be managed better with neuraxial analgesia. Once again, there is the potential risk of intercostal blockade resulting in respiratory compromise. As is also present in some of the preceding disease states, the combination of bulbar dysfunction with respiratory compromise makes securing the airway with an endotracheal tube somewhat advantageous to avoid potential aspiration.

## Conclusion

Regional anesthesia has been used successfully in patients with neurologic disease. The literature is scarce and limited. There are distinct benefits in avoiding the side effects of neuromuscular blockers, general anesthetics, and opioids. The whole patient should be evaluated and examined before any type of anesthetic to document disease progression and effects on other organ systems. An informed decision should be made by the patient and clinician. A regional technique should probably be avoided in the setting of an acute inflammation of the nerves. If a regional technique is used, lower concentrations of local anesthetics should be considered. Lidocaine should be avoided. Neuraxial narcotics with careful attention to dosing and postoperative monitoring may be a safe alternative.

## References

1. Johnson ME. Potential neurotoxicity of spinal anesthesia with lidocaine. Mayo Clin Proc 2000;75(9):921–932.
2. Ferguson IT, Murphy R, Lascelles R. Ventilatory failure in myasthenia gravis. J Neurol Neurosurg Psych 1982;45:217–222.
3. Loh L. Neurological and neuromuscular disease. Br J Anaesth 1986;58:190–200.

4. Klingler W, Lehmann-Horn F, Jurkat-Rott K. Complications of anaesthesia in neuromuscular disease. Neuromuscul Disord 2005;15:195–206.
5. Stoelting RK, Dierdorf SF. Endocrine disease. In: Anesthesia and Coexisting Disease. 3rd ed. New York: Churchill Livingstone; 1993:342.
6. Borel C. Evaluation of the patient with neuromuscular disease. In: Rogers MC, Tinker JH, Covino BG, Longnecker DE, eds. Principles and Practice of Anesthesiology. St. Louis: Mosby; 1993:266–275.
7. Persson A, Solders G. R-R variations in Guillain-Barré syndrome: a test of autonomic dysfunction. Acta Neurol Scand 1983;67:294–300.
8. Kahn JK, Sisson JC, Vinik AI. Prediction of sudden cardiac death in diabetic autonomic neuropathy. J Nucl Med 1988;29:1605–1606.
9. Watkins PJ. Diabetic autonomic neuropathy. N Engl J Med 1990;322:1078.
10. Ellison GW, Visscher BR, Graves MC, et al. Multiple sclerosis. Ann Intern Med 1984; 101:514–526.
11. Compston DAS. The management of multiple sclerosis. Q J Med 1989;70:93–101.
12. Tselis A, Lisak RP. Multiple sclerosis: therapeutic update. Arch Neurol 1999;56(3): 277–280.
13. Perlas A, Chan VWS. Neuraxial anesthesia and multiple sclerosis. Can J Anaesth 2005;52: 457–458.
14. Sakurai M, Kanagawa I. Positive symptoms in multiple sclerosis: their treatment with sodium channel blockers, lidocaine and mexiletine. J Neurol Sci 1999;162: 162–168.
15. McDonald WI, Silberberg DH. Multiple Sclerosis. London: Butterworth; 1986.
16. Abramsky C. Pregnancy and multiple sclerosis. Ann Neurol 1994;36:S38–41.
17. VanWalderveen MAA, Tas MW, Barkhof F, et al. Magnetic resonance evaluation of disease existing during pregnancy in multiple sclerosis. Neurology 1994;44:327–329.
18. Damek DM, Shuster EA. Pregnancy and multiple sclerosis. Mayo Clin Proc 1997;72(10): 977–989.
19. Bamford C, Sibley W, Laguna J. Anesthesia in multiple sclerosis. Can J Neurol Sci 1978;5: 41–44.
20. Bader AM, Hunt CO, Datta S, et al. Anesthesia for the obstetric patient with multiple sclerosis. J Clin Anesth 1988;1(1):21–24.
21. Crawford JS, James FM III, Nolte H, et al. Regional anesthesia for patients with chronic neurological disease and similar conditions. Anaesthesia 1981;36:821.
22. Stoelting RK, Dierdorf SF. Diseases of the nervous system. In: Anesthesia and Coexisting Disease. 3rd ed. New York: Churchill Livingstone; 1993:217.
23. Schapira K. Is lumbar puncture harmful in multiple sclerosis? J Neurol Neurosurg Psych 1959;22:238.
24. Warren TM, Datta S, Ostheimer GW. Lumbar epidural anesthesia in a patient with multiple sclerosis. Anesth Analg 1982;61:1022–1023.
25. Varner PD. Anesthesia for the patient with neurologic disease. 46th Annual ASA Refresher Course Lectures 146, 1995.
26. Capdeville M, Hoyt MR. Anesthesia and analgesia in the obstetric population with multiple sclerosis: a retrospective review. Anesthesiology 1994;81(3A):1173.
27. Confavreux C, Hutchinson M, Hours MM, et al. Rate of pregnancy related relapse in multiple sclerosis. N Engl J Med 1998;339:285–291.
28. Kytta J, Rosenberg PH. Anesthesia for patients with multiple sclerosis. Ann Chir Gynaecol 1984;73:229–303.
29. Campbell MJ. Motor neuron diseases. In: Walton J, ed. Disorders of Voluntary Muscle. London: Churchill-Livingstone; 1988:759–792.
30. Stoelting RK, Dierdorf SF. Diseases of the nervous system. In: Anesthesia and Coexisting Disease. 3rd ed. New York: Churchill-Livingstone; 1993:209.
31. Kochi T, Oka T, Mizuguchi T. Epidural anesthesia for patients with amyotrophic lateral sclerosis. Anesth Analg 1989;68:410–412.
32. Warren T, Fletcher M. Anesthetic management of the obstetric patient with neurologic disease. Clin Anaesth 1986;4(2):291–304.
33. Stoelting RK, Dierdorf SF. Diseases of the nervous system. In: Anesthesia and Coexisting Disease. 3rd ed. New York: Churchill-Livingstone; 1993:226.
34. Broecker BH, Hranowsky N, Hackler RH. Low spinal anesthesia for the prevention of autonomic dysreflexia in the spinal cord injury patient. J Urol 1979;122:366.

35. Lambert DH, Deane RS, Mazuzan JE. Anesthesia and the control of blood pressure in patients with spinal cord injury. Anesth Analg 1982;61:344–348.
36. Ravindan RS, Cummins DF, Smith IE. Experience with the use of nitroprusside and subsequent epidural analgesia in a pregnant quadriplegic patient. Anesth Analg 1981;60: 61–63.
37. Baraka A. Epidural meperidine for control of autonomic hyperreflexia in a paraplegic parturient. Anesthesiology 1985;62:688–690.
38. Stoelting RK, Dierdorf SF. Diseases of the nervous system. In: Anesthesia and Coexisting Disease. 3rd ed. New York: Churchill-Livingstone; 1993:218.
39. Burgos LG, Ebert TJ, Asiddao C, et al. Increased intraoperative cardiovascular morbidity in diabetics with autonomic neuropathy. Anesthesiology 1989;70:591–597.
40. Stoelting RK, Dierdorf SF. Diseases of the nervous system. In: Anesthesia and Coexisting Disease. 3rd ed. New York: Churchill-Livingstone; 1993:346.
41. Lucas LF, Tsueda K. Cardiovascular depression after brachial plexus block in two diabetic patients with renal failure. Anesthesiology 1990;73:1032–1035.
42. Adams RD, Victor M. Diseases of the peripheral nerves. In: Principles of Neurology. 4th ed. New York: McGraw-Hill; 1989:1035.
43. Barash PG, Cullen BF, Stoelting RK. Rare and coexisting disease. In: Clinical Anesthesia. 3rd ed. Philadelphia: JB Lippincott; 2001:491–520.
44. Lichtenfeld P. Autonomic dysfunction in the Guillain-Barré syndrome. Am J Med 1971; 50:772–780.
45. McGrady EM. Management of labour and delivery in a patient with Guillian-Barré syndrome. Anaesthesia 1987;42:899.
46. Connelly M, Shagrin J, Warfield C. Epidural opioids for the management of pain in a patient with the Guillain-Barré syndrome. Anesthesiology 1990;72:381–383.
47. Rosenfeld B, Borel C, Hanley D. Epidural morphine treatment of pain in Guillain-Barré syndrome. Arch Neurol 1986;43:1194–1196.
48. Berger JM, Ontell R. Intrathecal morphine in conjunction with a combined spinal and general anesthetic in a patient with multiple sclerosis. Anesthesiology 1987;66:400–402.
49. Leigh J, Fearnley SJ, Lupprian KG. Intrathecal diamorphine during laparotomy in a patient with advanced multiple sclerosis. Anaesthesia 1990;45:640–642.
50. Stoelting RK, Dierdorf SF. Diseases of the nervous system. In: Anesthesia and Coexisting Disease. 3rd ed. New York: Churchill-Livingstone; 1993:436.
51. Chalkiadis GA, Branch KG. Cardiac arrest after isoflurane anaesthesia in a patient with Duchenne's muscular dystrophy. Anaesthesia 1990;45:22–25.
52. Sethna NF, Rockoff MA, Worthen HM, et al. Anesthesia related complications in children with Duchenne's muscular dystrophy. Anesthesiology 1988;68:462–465.
53. Wang JM, Stanley TH. Duchenne muscular dystrophy and malignant hyperthermia – 2 case reports. Can Anaesth Soc J 1986;33:492–497.
54. Duncan PG. Neuromuscular diseases. In: Katz J, Steward DJ, eds. Anesthesia and Uncommon Pediatric Diseases. Philadelphia: WB Saunders; 1987:509–525.
55. Adams RD, Victor M. The muscular dystrophies. In: Principles of Neurology. 4th ed. New York: McGraw-Hill; 1989:1124.
56. Adams RD, Victor M. Disorders of muscles characterized by cramp, spasm, pain, and localized masses. In: Principles of Neurology. 4th ed. New York: McGraw-Hill; 1989: 1172–1174.
57. Stoelting RK, Dierdorf SF. Skin and musculoskeletal diseases. In: Anesthesia and Coexisting Disease. 3rd ed. New York: Churchill-Livingstone; 1993:438.
58. Mudge BJ, Taylor PB, Vanderspek AFL. Perioperative hazards in myotonic dystrophy. Anaesthesia 1980;35:492–495.
59. Cope DK, Miller JN. Local and spinal anesthesia for caesarean section in a patient with myotonic dystrophy. Anesth Analg 1986;65:687–690.
60. Paterson RA, Tousignant M, Skene DS. Caesarean section for twins in a patient with myotonic dystrophy. Can Anaesth Soc J 1985;32:418–421.
61. Bader A. Neurologic and neuromuscular disease. In: Chestnut DH, ed. Obstetric Anesthesia: Principles and Practice. St. Louis: Mosby; 1994:930.
62. Marchiori PE, DosReis M, Quevedo ME, et al. Acetylcholine receptor antibody in myasthenia gravis. Acta Neurol Scand 1989;80:387–389.
63. Hofstad H, Ohm O-J, Mork SJ, et al. Heart disease in myasthenia gravis. Acta Neurol Scand 1984;70:176–184.

64. Bader A. Neurologic and neuromuscular disease. In: Chestnut DH, ed. Obstetric Anesthesia: Principles and Practice. St. Louis: Mosby; 1994:927.
65. Leventhal SR, Orkin FK, Hirsh RA. Prediction of the need for postoperative mechanical ventilation in myasthenia gravis. Anesthesiology 1980;53:26–30.
66. Rolbin SH, Levinson G, Shnider SM, et al. Anesthetic considerations for myasthenia gravis and pregnancy. Anesth Analg 1978;57:441–447.

# 21 Evaluation of Neurologic Injury Following Regional Anesthesia

Quinn H. Hogan, Lloyd Hendrix, and Safwan Jaradeh

Modern anesthesia is a highly predictable undertaking with a very low failure rate. The ability to produce successful anesthesia is a less important characteristic of excellent anesthetic practice than the ability to recognize and treat adverse perioperative events. Recognition of myocardial ischemia or prompt treatment of catastrophic bleeding are examples of the situations requiring careful diagnosis and calm, decisive action. This same approach should prevail when the adverse event is a neurologic complication of regional anesthesia, only there is an added difficulty. At few other times in the practice of anesthesia will a practitioner be so directly confronted with responsibility for an adverse outcome as with a complication from neural blockade, because in a sense the "smoking gun" is clearly in our hands. Additional opprobrium may stem from the common misconceptions that complication rates should be zero in the practice of anesthesiology, and that the complication would not have occurred if only a general anesthetic had been performed.

The goal for this chapter is to provide a framework for evaluation of neurologic injury during regional anesthesia. Because other chapters address the details of various types of injury, diagnosis of specific complications will not be addressed here. Rather, the means of diagnosis are discussed, principally: gathering of pertinent history; physical examination, especially of the neurologic system; clinical neurophysiologic analysis, including nerve conduction study and electromyography; and radiologic imaging. Only rarely are other methods used to determine the presence or cause of neurologic injury, such as surgical exploration, or biopsy. Occasionally, blood tests may be necessary, including blood count (to identify leukocytosis from infection), glucose (to test for diabetes mellitus), erythrocyte sedimentation rate (indicative of infection or connective tissue disease if elevated), and blood serology (syphilis, lyme disease, human immunodeficiency virus).

Knowledge of the patient's baseline neurologic status before anesthesia is a key element that is often missing and impossible to recover at the time of evaluation of a neurologic injury. A missing reflex or an anesthetic patch of skin, for instance, have ominous implications only if they are absent before neural blockade. It is therefore absolutely essential to do a brief neurologic examination focused on the area of blockade before performing regional anesthesia.

## History

### *Identifying the Complication*

The initial step in diagnosis of neural injury is identification and delineation of neural dysfunction. This is often vexing in the context of regional anesthesia because temporary nerve blockade is the desired goal of uncomplicated regional anesthesia. Therefore, a distinction must be made between unexpectedly prolonged effects of local anesthetic and a pathologic event.

The duration of local anesthetic effect is often confusingly specified without consideration of the site of blockade. Whereas lidocaine may produce only an hour of anesthesia in the subarachnoid space, peripheral neural blockade can be expected to last much longer, particularly if high volumes are administered and epinephrine is coinjected. Another source of confusion comes from the definition used in published sources for anesthetic duration. Whereas the duration of predictable surgical anesthesia after a peripheral nerve block may be specified as perhaps 3 hours for 0.5% bupivacaine, a residual component of block may persist for more than 8 hours. The duration of neuraxial blockade is usually specified as the time before the upper limit of skin analgesia recedes two dermatomal segments. Sensory changes may be expected to persist for a much greater time at lower sites, especially about the level of epidural injection. Paresis from etidocaine neural blockade may outlast sensory changes. In all these cases, continued anesthetic effect may mistakenly be interpreted as neural injury.

Certain features of neural change may suggest injury rather than anesthetic effect. Resolving anesthesia should show a pattern of steady regression of block, so that any new or intensifying neural dysfunction in the absence of further anesthetic injection must be considered to represent neural injury. Sensory or motor defects produced by neural injury are usually patchy rather than uniform in distribution because of uneven damage among the components of a plexus or nerve roots. Mechanical damage by catheter or needle is typically restricted to a single nerve root or peripheral nerve.

### *Preexisting Conditions*

If neural damage is suspected, information obtained preoperatively about the patient's baseline neurologic status should be supplemented by a thorough postoperative inquiry. Any earlier episode of similar neural dysfunction, even if subsequently resolved, may indicate ongoing neurologic disease such as multiple sclerosis. Reactivation of reflex sympathetic dystrophy or herpetic neuralgia is another example that may be revealed by thorough questioning. Spinal stenosis, which is a risk factor for neurologic sequelae after epidural anesthesia,[1] may be discerned by a history of neurogenic claudication.

### *Surgical Events*

Discussion with the surgeon of possible etiologies for a new neural deficit may be revealing. Nerve injury in the wound may not have been mentioned to the anesthetist, or long-acting local anesthetic may have been injected by the surgeon. Compression by dressings or casts may compromise neural function, as may a compartment syndrome from edema or bleeding around the wound. Vascular injury during the operation could result in neurologic complications, most dramatically with spinal cord injury after thoracic aneurysm repair. Because of this, it is probably desirable to let the local anesthetic blockade abate after aortic surgery and before continuous postoperative blockade to allow confirmation of normal intact neurologic function. Neuraxial opioid analgesia can be continued during this period of observation.

Positioning of the patient should be reviewed because direct pressure (e.g., peroneal nerve at the fibular head) or tension on nerves (e.g., traction on the brachial plexus from hyperextension of the shoulder during thoracotomy) may produce nerve injury that might otherwise be attributed to a regional anesthetic mishap.

### *Anesthetic Events*

The details of anesthetic management should be thoroughly reviewed, especially if portions of the anesthetic care were delivered by other anesthetists. Drug choice, dose, and last time of administration are of obvious importance. Long duration of blockade and high concentration of agents probably increases the risk of neural complications. The development of hypotension, which itself is a source of neurologic injury, should be identified.

Blood return through the block needle, although sometimes sought, indicates the possibility of hematoma as mechanism of neural compromise. Injection into an unintended space may not have been evident at the time of the block procedure. Undesired entry into the subarachnoid space may be evident only after doses suitable for epidural anesthesia have been injected, increasing the risk of local anesthetic toxicity. Attempted aspiration of cerebrospinal fluid (CSF) before each epidural injection should be a standard maneuver. Observation of a gradual development and expected sequence of blockade and hemodynamic changes offers some reassurance that the proper site of drug deposition has been achieved. Conversely, maldistribution will not only lead to possible toxic results but also fail to produce desired anesthetic effects. Examples include accumulation of hyperbaric subarachnoid lidocaine in the terminal dural sack, or injection through a catheter intended for the epidural space but placed in or adjacent to a spinal nerve in the intervertebral foramen.

The presence of paresthesia or pain during needle placement may herald mechanical injury or injection within a nerve fascicle. Because sedation or general anesthesia precludes the observation of pain and paresthesiae, the exact timing of needle placement and injections relative to systemic medication may be critical, and the depth of sedation or presence of general anesthesia at the time of neural blockade should be noted. Injection into the spinal cord is unlikely to take place in a patient who is awake and can report the accompanying intense sensory event. However, injection into the cord, or even into a peripheral nerve with longitudinal passage of solution into the cord,[2] may go unrecognized in an unresponsive patient, resulting in catastrophic myelopathy. Sudden hypotension may accompany the cord injury. Such events are most likely to occur during thoracic epidural injections or subarachnoid injections in obese patients in whom the surface landmarks mistakenly lead to high lumbar needle placement.

### *Development of Neurologic Dysfunction*

The sequence and timing of the onset of symptoms related to the nerve injury should be determined to provide clues to the etiology and best treatment. The onset of pain, weakness, sensory deficit, and changes in sphincter control may be obtained from the patient, although sedation in the early postoperative period may compromise recollection of the details. Nurses are important sources of information, as are family members if the patient has already been discharged home. The ideal is frequent and complete postoperative visits by the anesthetist.

## Physical Examination

### *General Examination*

Elements of the general physical examination are important to check routinely at postoperative rounds, even if a neurologic injury is not suspected. Hematoma or ecchymosis at the injection site and peripheral ischemia for extremity blocks have obvious implications. Systemic manifestations of inadequate hemostasis may be a clue to epidural bleeding. Signs of infection at the block site may be early evidence of a developing deep infection. The presence of a fever, especially in the absence of another obvious source, should raise the question of a deep infection such as in the epidural space, although fevers are often absent. Tenderness and spasm of the muscles may result from bleeding, infection, or neural injury. A distended bladder may indicate a dysfunctional sphincter.

### *Neurologic Examination*

Determining neurologic function is essential for identification and monitoring of the progress of neurologic injury after regional anesthesia. Full analysis requires care and attention to details in the neurologic examination. For instance, the authors have observed transient myelopathy (spinal cord injury) following lumbar epidural catheter placement, which resulted in a deficit mainly of joint position sense and vibration sense. The examination need not necessarily include the entire neurologic system, but may be focused on the involved area. Central concerns are the presence or absence of muscle weakness, muscle atrophy, sensory loss, changes in the reflexes, and vasomotor/trophic changes. Rectal examination should be done if there are sphincter complaints. The observation of muscle atrophy a few days after regional anesthesia almost always indicates a preexisting condition.

Injury to a component of the peripheral nervous system, including the cranial nerves, spinal nerve roots, brachial and lumbosacral plexus, and peripheral nerves, will present with findings limited to the area of innervation. The dysfunction may involve the sensory fibers, motor fibers, autonomic fibers, or a combination of these. Dysfunction of the afferent fibers results in sensory loss, and should be sought by sensory testing with more than one modality. Nociceptive afferents can be stimulated by scratch (corner of a foil wrapper of an alcohol swab, or a broken tongue blade), whereas touch can be tested by contact with a gauze pad or the examiner's finger. The patient's ability to ascertain joint position change can be quickly determined. Motor nerve damage causes weakness, wasting, and hyporeflexia. For most purposes, comparison of these features against the uninvolved side is adequate to reveal a deficit. Involvement of the autonomic system leads to altered sweating and trophic changes involving the bone and skin, but these are unlikely soon after an injury.

Neurologic complications after regional anesthesia about the vertebral column may cause neural dysfunction and pain that can be attributable to injury of either the roots or the cord itself. With radicular injury, there are associated reflex, sensory, and motor changes as outlined in Table 21-1, and evidence of irritation such as pain with straight

TABLE 21-1. Clinical Manifestations of Common Radiculopathies

| Root | Pain/sensory loss | Reflex arc | Motor deficit |
|---|---|---|---|
| C5 | Shoulder | Biceps | Shoulder abduction |
| C6 | Lateral arm, forearm, thumb | Biceps, brachioradialis | Elbow flexion |
| C7 | Dorsal arm and forearm, middle finger | Triceps | Elbow flexion |
| C8 | Medial arm and forearm, little finger | Finger flexion | Finger flexion, hand intrinsics |
| L3 | Anterior and medial thigh | Adductor, patellar | Thigh adduction |
| L4 | Medial leg | Patellar | Leg extension |
| L5 | Lateral calf and leg, posterior thigh, dorsum of foot | Hamstring | Ankle dorsiflexion |
| S1 | Posterior calf and leg, plantar surface | Achilles | Ankle plantar flexion |

leg raising. Local anesthetics may be sufficiently toxic to produce inflammatory radiculopathy. With damage to the spinal cord, the level of the lesion is likewise determined by the pattern of sensory and motor abnormalities. The location of a cord lesion may be one to two levels higher than found by dermatomal sensory examination. Acute damage to the cord causes areflexia and hypotonia at and below the level of the lesion. In about 2–3 days, upper motor neuron signs (spasticity, hyperreflexia, extensor plantar responses) develop below the level of the lesion, whereas lower motor neuron signs (atrophy, hyporeflexia, fasciculations) evolve at the level of the lesion.

Injury to the cord or compression of neuraxial structures from adjacent masses such as hematoma or abscess in the epidural space may be distinguished by the pattern of neural deficit evident on examination. Early and severe midline vertebral pain followed later by weakness is the hallmark of an epidural process, whereas early weakness and sensory symptoms in association with a mild and rather vague pain is more characteristic of spinal cord damage. Bowel and bladder dysfunction are hallmarks of spinal cord lesions. Injury of the conus medullaris and cauda equina should be suspected with early sphincter dysfunction, saddle anesthesia, or radicular pain of the lower extremities. Spinal cord infarction is typically caused by the occlusion of the anterior spinal artery, particularly when the nerve blood supply is premorbidly compromised, such as in diabetes or in uremia. This artery supplies all areas of the cord except the posterior columns, so injury leads to severe sensory and motor dysfunction below the level of lesion that spares touch, vibration, and joint position senses.

The neurologic examination may be supplemented by diagnostic lumbar puncture in certain cases. If meningitis is suspected, white blood cells will be evident and cultures of CSF may show a pathogen, whereas CSF protein is increased and glucose is decreased. Toxic myelitis or radiculitis may be accompanied by eosinophils in the CSF and an increased protein content. An undiagnosed preexisting tumor may be revealed by a positive CSF cytology, and CSF serology may reveal evidence of syphilis, lyme disease, or herpetic infection. A lumbar puncture is probably most helpful if the condition is progressive and imaging is negative.

## Physiologic Study

Iatrogenic injuries to the spinal cord, spinal roots, or peripheral nerves can be evaluated electrophysiologically. Electrodiagnostic techniques include evoked potentials, nerve conduction studies, and needle electrode examination of muscles (electromyography or "EMG"). Their use should complement the clinical examination, not replace it. Their importance increases when the clinical information cannot be obtained or when the patient is noncooperative.

### *Techniques in Electrodiagnosis*

A complete discussion of electrophysiologic testing is beyond the scope of this chapter, and the reader is referred to a basic text.[3] Table 21-2 summarizes some of these techniques and their anatomic correlates.

#### Motor Conductions

Motor conductions are performed by placing recording electrodes over the muscle, and stimulating electrodes over the respective nerve (Figure 21-1). A brief stimulus that elicits a maximal response of the muscle is applied to the nerve. The latencies, amplitudes, and conduction velocities of the direct evoked responses (M waves) are recorded from muscle. Needle electrode or magnetic stimulation of the proximal peripheral nerve ("near-nerve root stimulation") is possible but rarely necessary.

The stimulus also causes an impulse that travels proximally. This leads to late responses that include F and H waves (Figure 21-1). The F wave results from the

TABLE 21-2. Anatomic Structures and Their Electrodiagnostic Correlates

| Anatomic structure | Electrodiagnostic method of assessment |
|---|---|
| Sensory axons, distal segments | Sensory nerve conductions (distal latencies and amplitudes) |
| Sensory axons, proximal segments | H waves, somatosensory evoked potentials |
| Sensory axons, central pathways | Somatosensory evoked potentials |
| Motor axons, distal segments | Motor nerve conductions (distal latencies and amplitudes) |
| Motor axons, proximal segments | F waves, H waves |
| Neuromuscular junction | Repetitive motor nerve stimulation, single-fiber EMG |
| Motor units | Needle EMG |

depolarization of anterior horn cells in response to the proximal impulse of a supramaximal stimulus along motor axons. The H wave results from the depolarization of anterior horn cells in response to the proximal impulse of a low-intensity stimulus along sensory axons and sensorimotor monosynapses in the cord and therefore is a reflex. The F waves can be recorded from any muscle, whereas the H reflex is recorded at rest from the soleus or flexor carpi radialis muscles only.

### Repetitive Stimulation

Repetitive stimulation of a peripheral nerve while recording the M responses allows the evaluation of neuromuscular junction integrity and fatigability. In myasthenia, stimulation rates of 2–3 Hz produce a progressive decrease in the amplitude of the first few M responses called decrement, analogous to the finding after partial

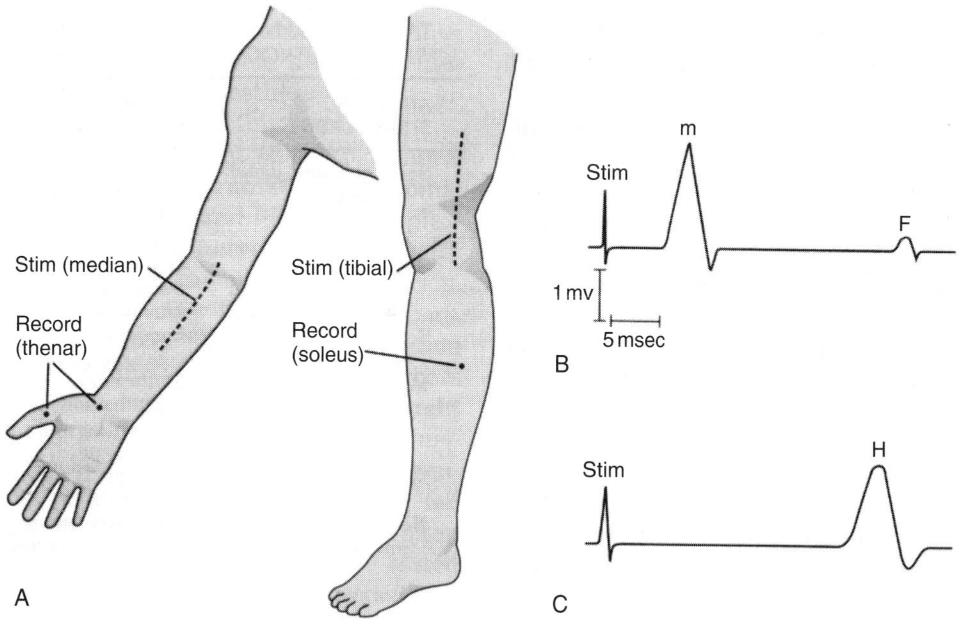


**FIGURE 21-1.** Evoked motor responses during nerve conduction studies. **(A)** Stimulation of a peripheral nerve, such as the median or tibial, produces a response in the innervated muscle (thenar or soleus). Surface electrodes detect the evoked muscle electrical activity as various waves **(B and C)**. The M wave is produced by direct activation by motor nerves. The F wave results from activation of anterior horn cells by antidromic motor nerve impulses, followed by orthodromic muscle activation, leading to a long latency (about 30–50 μs). The H wave is caused by stimulation of sensory fibers that synaptically activate motor neurons (about 17–35 μs). Disease states are identified by changes in amplitude and latency of the various waves.

nondepolarizing pharmacologic neuromuscular blockade. After 10–15 seconds of strong voluntary contraction of the muscle, there is partial or complete repair of the decrement called postactivation facilitation, analogous to posttetanic facilitation in the setting of pharmacologic neuromuscular blockade. Facilitation wears off over 90–240 seconds, at which time the decrement returns and may worsen, leading to postactivation exhaustion.

#### Sensory Conductions

Sensory conductions are obtained using recording electrodes along the sensory nerve of interest. Sensory responses usually have small amplitudes and can be difficult to record, particularly in disease.

#### Needle EMG

Needle EMG records changes of voltage generated by the firing of motor units using a small needle electrode inserted into the muscle (Figure 21-2A). The motor unit action potentials are sampled by moving the needle slowly in the muscle. The examiner first evaluates insertional and spontaneous activity while the muscle is at rest. Next, the motor units are examined during minimal and then increasing effort.

At rest, normal muscle has no spontaneous or insertional activity outside the endplate region. At low voluntary activation, few motor units are recruited and their corresponding motor unit action potentials (MUAPs), distinguished by the particular morphology of their depolarization, are recorded. Recruitment refers to the number and firing rate of different activated MUAPs at a given voluntary effort. At maximal effort, the MUAPs overlap, resulting in interference pattern. Other MUAPs measured parameters are amplitude, duration, and configuration. The number and size of muscle fibers within a motor unit determine its MUAP amplitude and duration. The configuration depends on the number of phases (voltage changes from baseline) and turns in the MUAP (any waveform polarity change). By convention, a MUAP with more than four phases or five turns is polyphasic, or complex. The MUAP complexity derives from differences in conduction times for the various muscle fibers within the motor unit. Normal MUAPs are stable, showing minimal variability with repetitive firing. Variability of interpotential intervals between muscle fiber action potentials belonging to the same motor unit is termed jitter. This increases in neuromuscular transmission disorders.

### *Diagnostic Value of Electrodiagnosis*

Nerve conduction studies can reveal various abnormalities. Reduced amplitudes of the evoked responses indicate axonal loss (e.g., following injection into a nerve fascicle) or demyelination (e.g., following injection adjacent to a fascicle or compression from a tourniquet) of the nerve portion distal to the stimulator. The response latency changes little in the former, and increases excessively in the latter. Stimulation of the same nerve further proximally may help differentiate the two conditions. In pure axonopathies, the amplitudes of both proximal and distal responses are similarly and proportionately decreased compared with the normal values. In demyelinating nerve lesions, in which the axons remain intact, proximal stimulation leads to additional decrease in the amplitude exceeding that found normally, a phenomenon termed partial conduction block. This is often associated with slowing of the nerve conduction velocity secondary to myelin changes. In chronic neuropathies, both axonal and demyelinating, there is sometimes an increase in the duration of the evoked responses termed temporal dispersion. With proximal nerve (plexus, root) lesions, the F and H waves show delayed latencies or inconsistency in demyelination, and inconsistency or absence in axonal loss. Repetitive motor nerve stimulation allows the evaluation of neuromuscular junction dysfunction as described above.

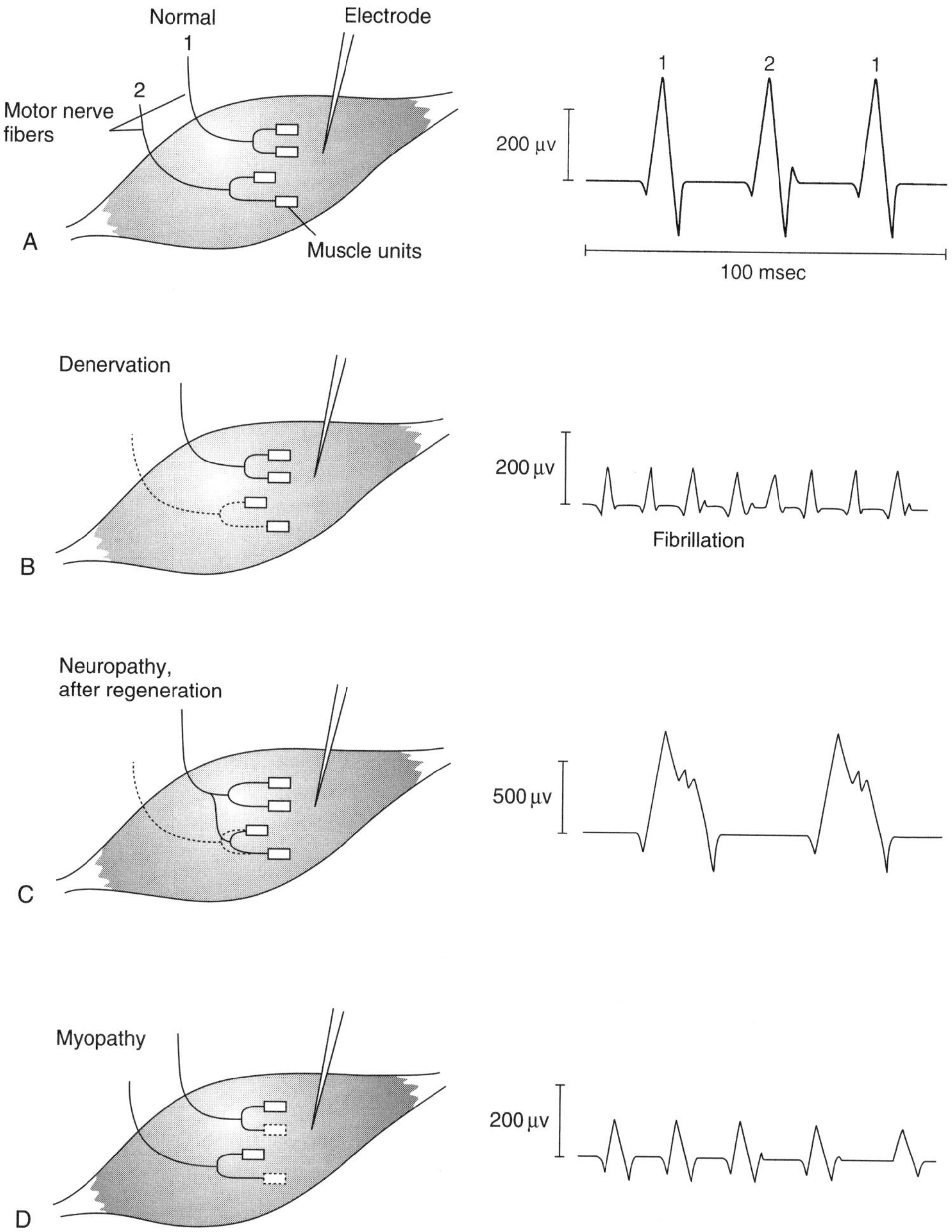


**FIGURE 21-2.** Needle EMG, in which muscle depolarization is detected by a needle electrode inserted into the muscle. The drawings show two motor units, each consisting of a single motor neuron and the fibers it innervates (small boxes). Activity at rest is shown. **(A)** In the normal state, the electrode may pick up complexes produced by several different motor units (identified here as 1 and 2), each with a somewhat different action potential configuration. **(B)** After injury to the motor nerve (dotted line), individual denervated muscle fibers spontaneously depolarize, producing fibrillations, seen as high-frequency, low-amplitude potentials. **(C)** With reinnervation of muscle fibers by sprouts from adjacent motor neurons, large and complex potentials are seen. Spontaneous activation of the entire motor unit produces fasciculation potentials. **(D)** In myopathic conditions, loss of muscle fibers (dotted boxes) leads to diminished amplitude of potentials.

Needle EMG abnormalities can be divided into three categories.

1. Excessive response of the muscle to needle insertion or movement. This usually takes the form of trains of rhythmic "positive waves." These are frequently seen in denervated muscle fibers, and sometimes in active myopathic processes. A peculiar form of rhythmic discharges that tends to wax and wane is termed "myotonic discharges." This is the main abnormality in myotonic dystrophy and myotonia congenita. The insertional activity becomes reduced when muscle fibers are replaced by connective tissue.

2. Abnormal spontaneous activity, in the form of "fibrillation" or "fasciculation" potentials (Figure 21-2B). Fibrillations are rhythmic potentials emanating from denervated single muscle fibers, and are the hallmark of active, ongoing axonopathies. They appear when degeneration of the axon progresses peripherally to cause destruction of the motor endplate. This takes about 2–3 weeks after injury and is maximal 1–3 months after injury (Table 21-3). Fasciculations are nonrhythmic potentials originating from single motor units, and although they can be seen in health and various neurogenic diseases, they are prominent in motor neuron disease.

3. Abnormalities of the MUAPs, involving their recruitment, amplitude, duration, complexity, or any combination of these. In neurogenic diseases, the number of motor axons in a given muscle decreases, resulting in reduced number of MUAPs for the level of voluntary effort, referred to as decreased recruitment. The degree of reduction parallels the severity of the lesion. As muscle fibers are reinnervated from adjacent motor neurons, the number of muscle fibers per motor unit increases several months after injury. This leads to the appearance 1–3 months after injury of MUAPs that are increased in amplitude, duration, and complexity (Figure 21-2C). In myopathic conditions, the number of muscle fibers within the motor unit decreases. This leads to MUAPs of small amplitude and short duration (Figure 21-2D). The variability of the myofibers results in asynchrony of the impulses from individual myofibers, and the MUAP may be complex. The smaller size of affected motor units increases the number of MUAPs firing at a given voluntary effort, or increased recruitment. Evaluation of MUAP stability provides information about the neuromuscular transmission within the corresponding unit as mentioned before.

### *Limitations of Electrodiagnosis*

Nerve conduction studies test mainly the function of large sensory and motor nerve fibers. Therefore, disorders confined to the small myelinated or unmyelinated fibers will not be detected by these techniques. Another limitation is when the neurologic abnormality involves a nerve that is not accessible to practical testing. An example would be an injury to sensory branches of the lumbar or femoral plexus that can be

TABLE 21-3. Chronology of EMG Abnormalities after Axonal Injury

| | | | Motor unit action potentials | | |
|---|---|---|---|---|---|
| Time after lesion | Insertional activity | Fibrillation potentials | Recruitment | Amplitude/ duration | Shape |
| Acute (<14 days) | Normal | Absent | Reduced | Normal | Normal |
| Subacute (14–21 days) | Increased | Present | Reduced | Normal | Normal |
| Recent (1–3 months) | Increased | Present (maximal) | Reduced | May increase | Polyphasic |
| Chronic (>6 months) | May be increased | Present but fewer | Reduced | Increased | Polyphasic |

variable in their location and branching patterns. When proximal nerve (plexus, root) lesions are small, the F and H waves elicited from the intact majority of fibers would neutralize the expected delay. Nerve conductions and somatosensory evoked potentials are less useful in timing lesions with respect to chronicity. When an axon is injured, the segment distal to the injury site remains excitable for several days, and then becomes inexcitable until reinnervation occurs. Because there are no features indicating duration of denervation, loss of nerve responses does not provide any chronologic information in the absence of a prior baseline study.

Needle EMG preferentially evaluates smaller MUAPs because they are recruited first. With increasing effort, larger units appear, but the tracing approaches the full interference pattern and these units become difficult to distinguish. Therefore, disorders affecting mainly larger MUAPs, such as disuse atrophy, cause little impairment of the EMG. Another limitation is the lag between a nerve injury and the sequence of EMG abnormalities, outlined in Table 21-3.

### *Interpretative Value of Electrodiagnosis*

The sampling of nerves and muscles will depend on the clinical question. When a radiculopathy is suspected, neurogenic abnormalities should be seen in at least two muscles supplied by that root but by different motor nerves (e.g., supraspinatus and deltoid for a C5 radiculopathy). There is overlap of myotomal innervation of the paraspinal muscles that lessens their segmental localizing value. However, it is important to study these muscles. They are innervated by the posterior primary ramus of the segmental spinal nerve, which branches from the anterior ramus just lateral to the intervertebral foramen. An abnormality involving both the paraspinous and other muscles, and therefore both posterior and anterior primary rami, must be attributable to a lesion proximal to their branching, i.e., the nerve root. An injury to the plexus (anterior primary rami) will show no abnormalities in the paraspinous muscles. Because of their short axons, examination of the paraspinous muscles is also helpful in estimating the timing of nerve injury, because peripheral progression of axonal destruction affects these muscles first.

EMG can also quantitate the severity of neurologic injury and determine whether axonal damage has occurred. This is particularly important when the patient is noncooperative with the clinical examination. When ordering an EMG, it is usually helpful to wait a few weeks until definite evidence for denervation has appeared. However, if the patient's condition is complicated by the presence of other neurologic disorders (e.g., polyneuropathy), or if litigation is suspected, it is preferable to obtain a baseline study immediately after injury because subacute or chronic changes would indicate a preexisting condition.

When sensory nerve action potentials cannot be obtained peripherally, either because of near-complete nerve section or because the nerves are less accessible to conventional testing (lateral femoral cutaneous nerve in meralgia paresthetica, dorsal nerve of the penis in saddle numbness, trigeminal cutaneous branches in facial numbness), somatosensory evoked potentials may provide information about remaining nerve function. They can be useful in traumatic brachial plexus lesions or if subclinical myelopathy is suspected, and can demonstrate that somatosensory pathways are preserved in hysterical patients who present with sensory loss.

## Imaging

Topics discussed here may be more thoroughly explored in standard texts.[4]

### *Plain Films*

Plain radiography is a simple, relatively inexpensive method of imaging the bony, and to some extent, the soft tissue components of the spine. Spatial resolution is good, whereas contrast resolution is generally inferior to that of computed tomography (CT) or magnetic resonance imaging (MRI). It provides a gross screening method for assessing presence of pneumothorax, alignment and mineralization of bony structures, and degenerative disease. Acute osteomyelitis and discitis are generally evident earlier with radionuclide imaging and MRI. Myelography with plain films and fluoroscopy of intrathecal contrast has largely been supplanted by CT imaging after contrast injection or MRI. Where these more costly options are unavailable, myelography may be necessary to identify space-occupying lesions in the vertebral canal such as abscess or hematoma.

## *Computed Tomography*

### Technology

CT has been used for imaging the spine for more than 25 years. Over that time, there has been a steady refinement of the technology resulting in improved spatial and contrast resolution, decreased scan time, and increased flexibility through the use of image reformatting. Although MRI is being used increasingly for spine imaging, CT continues to have advantages in some circumstances.

The underlying principle behind CT is that the internal structure of an object can be reconstructed from multiple projections of the object. The CT gantry contains an array of X-ray detectors and an X-ray tube that rotates about the patient. A pulsed X-ray beam is passed through the patient repeatedly and the detectors measure the radiation in many different projections at any given axial level in the patient. The data are used to reconstruct a cross-sectional display.

Each pixel, or picture element, of a CT image is assigned a CT number or Hounsfield unit based on the X-ray attenuation of the corresponding voxel, or volume element, in the patient. The densest body tissue, compact bone, and the least-dense body tissue, air, have the highest and lowest values, respectively. To display this digital information as an image, the CT numbers must be "mapped" onto a gray scale of 8–12 shades ranging from white to black. The way in which the digital scale is matched to the display gray scale is termed *window*. The window *width* is the range between the highest and lowest CT number to be displayed; the window *level* is the median number in the range. By adjusting the window width and level, various tissues may be optimally displayed.

### Limitations

Artifacts are generally related to patient motion, high-density foreign objects, detector malfunction, and the inherent limitations of reconstruction algorithms for portraying objects of geometric complexity. Images degraded by motion typically reveal vertical streaks. Motion is generally less of a problem with CT than with MRI; each image is obtained sequentially, and any single slice can be repeated with minimal additional time. Metallic foreign objects (aneurysm clips, bullet fragments, etc.) produce radially oriented streak artifact. Beam hardening artifact may be seen when dense structures in the field attenuate the lower energy portions of the X-ray beam; this artifact is seen as dark streaks in the image. Partial volume artifact is generated by complex, irregular interfaces between structures of very high and very low attenuation. The result is both light and dark streaks in the image, which can be reduced by decreasing the slice thickness.

Statistical noise refers to imprecision in CT number measurements and is the single most significant factor limiting image quality. The problem can be diminished by increasing the scan time and the magnitude of the beam, but this results in greater radiation exposure to the patient. Properly positioning the patient in the center of the gantry can help to minimize noise.

Tissues with similar X-ray density will show low contrast differences between them. The difference in X-ray attenuation of various soft tissues (excluding fat) is only about 4%. In spine imaging, contrast between the spinal cord, nerve roots, disc margins, and CSF can be improved by the use of iodinated contrast material placed in the thecal sac by lumbar or C1-2 puncture. An additional limitation is that only axial views are produced by CT imaging. Reconstruction in other planes is possible but with diminished resolution.

CT utilizes the same ionizing radiation used for conventional radiography. Precautions should be made to minimize the dose to the fetus, lens of the eye, and gonads.

## Indications

CT imaging is well adapted to evaluation of neurologic trauma. The contrast resolution of CT is significantly greater than that of conventional radiography. Soft tissues such as intervertebral discs, the spinal cord, ligaments, hematomas, and paraspinous soft tissue planes can be more readily demonstrated. The axial plane is generally excellent for evaluation of the spinal canal. Fracture lines and displaced bone fragments are generally well demonstrated, with the possible exception of nondisplaced fractures oriented in the transverse plane.

Degenerative changes in the vertebral column are clearly evident by CT imaging. As the intervertebral disc ages, there is loss of axial height and radial bulging of the annulus fibrosus occurs. CT readily shows the margins of the disc extending uniformly beyond those of the adjacent vertebral bodies. Marginal osteophyte and gas within the disc space, if present, are readily identified. The focal, asymmetric bulging of a herniated disc is generally well demonstrated with CT. Intrathecal contrast material can improve identification of the disc margin in difficult cases. The use of intravenous contrast to differentiate recurrent/residual disc herniation from postoperative scarring has largely been replaced by MRI with intravenous paramagnetic contrast material.

Stenosis of the vertebral canal and intervertebral foramina can be optimally evaluated with CT, whether secondary to bony encroachment, abnormal soft tissue such as herniated disc material, or both. In general, hypertrophic bone changes, subtle subarticular bony erosions, defects of the pars interarticularis, and soft tissue calcification are seen better with CT than MRI.

Masses in the vertebral column may occur within the spinal cord (intramedullary), intradural but extramedullary, or epidural. Most intramedullary tumors differ little in attenuation from normal spinal cord but may distort or expand the cord. Intrathecal contrast improves CT visualization of the spinal cord margins, although the spinal cord and any intramedullary abnormality is generally demonstrated to significantly better advantage with MRI. Arachnoiditis can be diagnosed with CT, although the findings may be subtle without intrathecal contrast material. Thickening and bunching of the roots are pathognomonic of arachnoiditis when clearly identified (Figure 21-3).

Intrathecal contrast also improves visualization of intradural masses. Because of CSF pulsations, intradural lesions in the thoracic spine may be better seen with intrathecally enhanced CT than with MRI. Hematoma and loculated infection within the dura are extremely rare, but would be evident. Masses in the epidural space include tumors (usually malignant), abscesses, and hematomas. CT imaging can distinguish between them by density and pattern of tissue involvement. Fresh blood is often more radiodense than tumor or abscess and tends to conform to the boundaries of the canal. Tumor or infection may readily spread to the paraspinous tissues. CT can identify infection and inflammation by demonstration of both osteolysis and any soft tissue mass effect. Destruction of the vertebral endplates and disc space is more typical of infection than tumor.

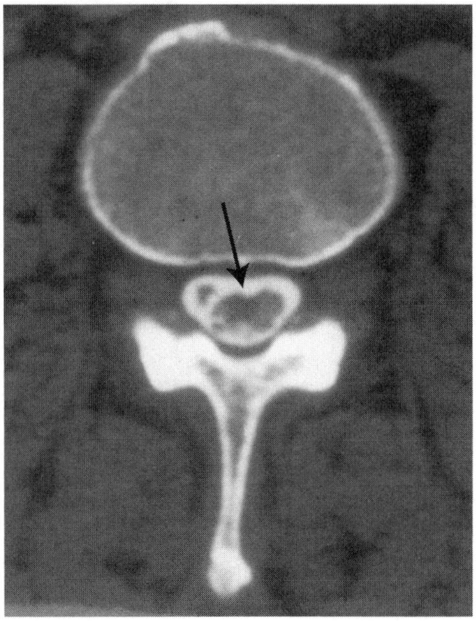

**FIGURE 21-3.** CT image through the second lumbar vertebra after intrathecal contrast injection (CT myelogram), showing arachnoiditis. The nerve roots are thickened and clumped together in a mass (arrow).

## Magnetic Resonance Imaging

### Technology

MRI is based on the phenomenon of nuclear magnetic resonance. This phenomenon can be observed with certain nuclei such as hydrogen, tritium, carbon 13, fluorine 19, and phosphorus 31, among others. Of these, hydrogen, with its single proton nucleus, is by far the most abundant in living organisms and has a large magnetic moment. At present, virtually all clinical MRI is based on magnetic resonance of the hydrogen nucleus.

When placed in a magnetic field, the hydrogen nucleus (a proton) will precess like a gyroscope about the axis of the magnetic field, and it will do so at a frequency specific for the nuclear species and the particular magnetic field strength. Each individual proton will align itself such that its own magnetic moment is parallel to the magnetic field, either with or directly opposite in direction. From the perspective of quantum mechanics, all protons will be found in one of two energy states, either positive or negative, each with the same absolute value. Protons placed in a magnetic field may absorb a photon of energy when exposed to a pulse of electromagnetic radiation (RF pulse) and be elevated to a higher energy state, and emit a photon when they fall to the lower state, a process known as relaxation. This results in a resonant exchange of energy between the protons and the electromagnetic field known as nuclear magnetic resonance. During relaxation, the energy emitted may be detected as a radiosignal with components longitudinal and transverse to the magnetic field. Relaxation can be resolved into two separable processes of longitudinal and transverse relaxation, with rates measured by time constants T1 and T2, respectively. The different rates of relaxation affect the intensity of the signal emitted by a particular tissue and its appearance in the final image.

For clinical imaging, the subject is placed within the bore of a large magnet. Field strength generally ranges between 0.2 and 1.5 Tesla, much greater than the earth's magnetic field that measures approximately $0.5 \times 10^{-4}$ Tesla. A specific sequence of electromagnetic radiation in the radiofrequency range is used to excite the tissues. A

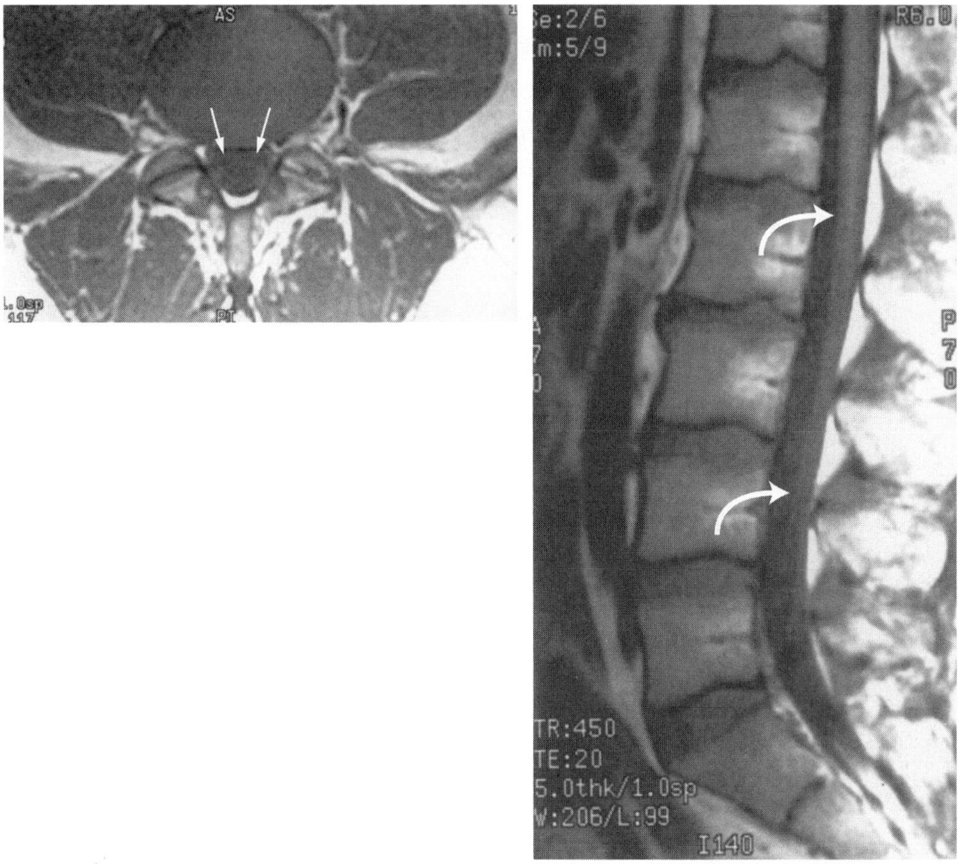


A

B

**FIGURE 21-4.** Normal T1-weighted MRIs. **(A)** In the axial plane through a lumbar disc (anterior up). **(B)** In the midline sagittal plane of normal lumbar vertebrae (anterior left). Fat has a high signal intensity (appears bright), whereas muscle and disc have intermediate signal intensity. Low signal intensity (dark) is characteristic of water (e.g., CSF, straight arrows) and fast-flowing blood (vena cava, aorta). Cortical bone has no signal (appears black) but marrow has low signal intensity. Roots and cord appear as intermediate signal intensity(curved arrows). Note the signal fall-off (darker image) at greater distances from the posterior surface coil.

receiver then detects the signal subsequently emitted by the relaxing hydrogen protons within the subject. This signal is digitized, and the data are used to construct a set of cross-sectional images. The brightness of a particular tissue in clinical images is proportional to the signal intensity emitted by that tissue after excitation with the RF pulse.

A pulse sequence is a pattern of RF pulses designed with the strategy of differentiating tissues from one another based on the differences in tissue relaxation rates. The difference in brightness, or contrast between two particular tissues, is significantly affected by the timing parameters of the particular pulse sequence used. Currently, the most frequently used pulse sequence is the spin-echo pulse sequence. Generally, two series are obtained: one with T1 weighting (Figure 21-4), and the other with T2 weighting (Figure 21-5). A T1-weighted series provides contrast based largely on longitudinal relaxation rate differences between tissues, and the contrast in a T2-weighted series is based largely on differences in transverse relaxation rates. Tissues with a short T1 such as fat will appear bright in T1-weighted images, and those tissues with a long T2 such as homogeneous fluid will appear bright in T2-weighted images.

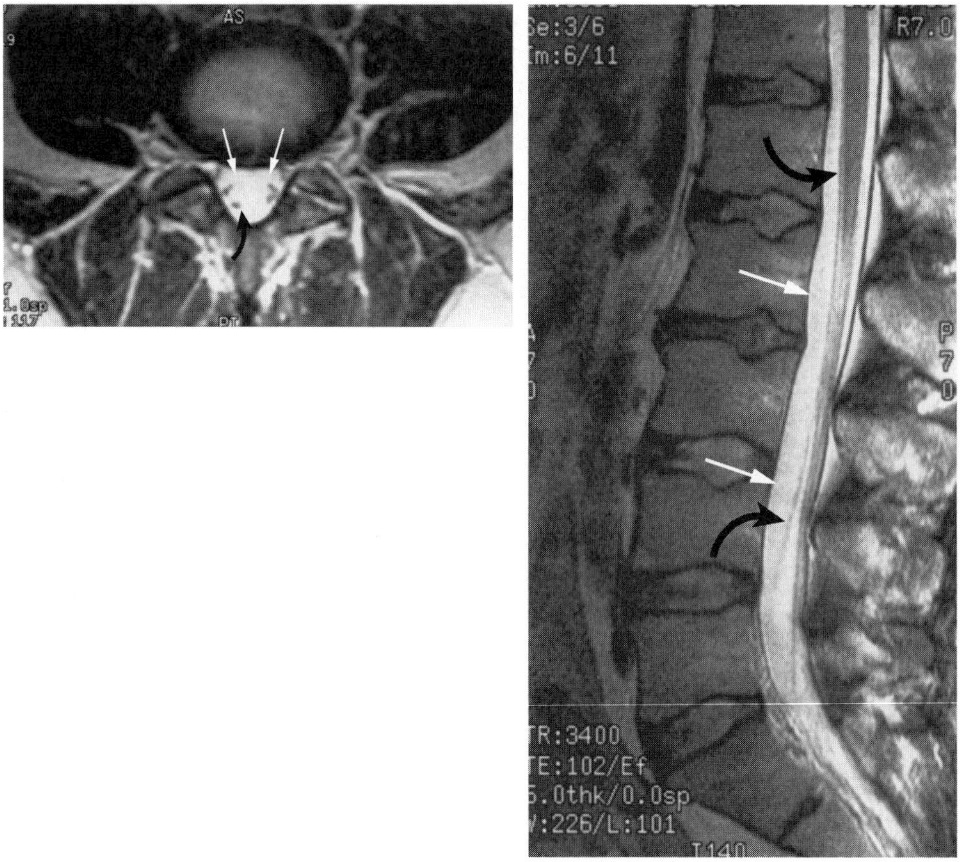


A B

**FIGURE 21-5.** Normal T2-weighted MRIs. **(A)** In the axial plane through a lumbar disc (anterior up). **(B)** In the midline sagittal plane of normal lumbar vertebrae (anterior left). CSF (white arrows) has a high signal intensity, especially where stationary, whereas fat is not as bright as in T1 images. Other tissues have intermediate signal intensity. Roots and cord (black arrows) are of intermediate signal intensity, so contrast with CSF. The disc nucleus is bright if it has not become desiccated from degenerative disease.

In certain situations, the contrast between tissues can be increased through the intravenous administration of a gadolinium chelate. Gadolinium, with its unpaired electrons, is paramagnetic and preferentially promotes relaxation of tissues in which it accumulates. This results in the increased brightness in T1-weighted images of tissues in which gadolinium has accumulated, because of increased vascularity or vessel permeability, such as infection, tumor, or breakdown of the blood-brain barrier.

### Limitations

No definite ill effects of magnetic fields on human beings have been documented to date from exposure to MRI. However, certain devices and ferromagnetic objects pose potential dangers to patients and others in the scanning area. Patients with a wide variety of implanted prostheses, including cardiac pacemakers, cochlear implants, neurostimulators, certain heart valves, and certain aneurysm clips, should not be examined by MRI, because these devices may malfunction or be displaced by the magnetic field. Objects such as oxygen tanks, wheelchairs, and other loose items such as scissors and jewelry are potential missiles. Specially designed wheelchairs, oxygen tanks, and other items have been developed for use in proximity to strong magnetic fields. Rapidly changing magnetic fields in clinical MRI scanners may potentially lead to the generation of electric currents within a subject with implanted wires such as a cardiac pacemaker or nerve stimulator. No significant problems have been reported, but a burn is possible.

The radiofrequency transmitter of an MRI scanner can generate several kilowatts of peak power that is partially deposited as heat in the body of the subject. This also has not been a practical limitation. To date, there is no evidence to suggest that an embryo is adversely affected by magnetic or radiofrequency fields at the intensities used in clinical MRI scanners. Nonetheless, many centers have a policy excluding pregnant females for all but urgent studies, particularly during the first trimester of pregnancy. As much as 10% of the population experiences some degree of claustrophobia upon being placed in the magnet bore. Most of these patients will tolerate the study with mild oral or intravenous sedation.

Successful MRI generally requires a cooperative, near-motionless subject. The MRI process is prone to several artifacts most of which relate to either inhomogeneity in the magnetic field or movement of tissue. Inhomogeneity of the magnetic field is most often attributable to paramagnetic substances (surgical wires and clips, pedicle screws, dental fillings, makeup, etc.) that lead to distortion or deletion of portions of images, particularly noticeable in T2-weighted images. Certain regions, even with cardiac gating, are prone to motion artifact from breathing, cardiac motion, and CSF pulsations.

For most clinical applications, the spatial resolution of MRI is slightly less than that of CT or plain radiography. However, contrast resolution is often superior. Cortical bone is often better visualized with CT or plain radiography. CSF pulsations in the thoracic spine may be particularly troublesome both by obscuring subtle pathology and masquerading as abnormal vessels on the surface of the cord that may be seen with certain vascular malformations. The appearance of flowing blood may be confusing. Rapidly flowing blood, such as that in arteries and large veins, may appear as a signal void. Slow-flowing blood, particularly when the direction of flow is perpendicular to the imaging plane, may appear bright in T1-weighted images. The intravenous administration of gadolinium generally tends to increase the signal intensity of flowing blood.

### Indications

A survey of the axial skeleton by CT is time consuming and impractical. MRI, however, is an excellent method of performing screening examinations of the spine, because a relatively large number of levels can be studied simultaneously and in virtually any desired plane.

Despite some difficulties in demonstrating cortical bone, most major spinal fractures and dislocations can be identified with MRI. Disc and ligament injury are typically better identified with MRI than CT. The spinal cord is better seen with MRI than with any other current imaging modality. Intramedullary hematoma, syrinx, cord edema and swelling, and myelomalacia can be well demonstrated with MRI. Compression of the thecal sac and spinal cord by bone or soft tissue can be easily recognized.

MRI is generally sensitive for focal collections of blood, whether acute, subacute, or chronic. Acute blood in the central nervous system is usually most apparent in T2-weighted images, and appears as an area of significantly decreased signal intensity. Subacute blood (1 week to 1 month) gradually becomes high in signal intensity in T1-weighted images. This always precedes the subsequent change from low to high signal intensity seen in T2-weighted images. In the spine, epidural hematomas may appear intermediate in signal intensity in both T1- and T2-weighted images, and may mimic herniated disc material or other epidural soft tissue. Nonetheless, epidural blood and its resultant mass effect in the vertebral canal are generally well seen with

MRI (Figures 21-6 and 21-7). Unlike an abscess, blood should not show enhancement following gadolinium administration. Hematomas in the soft tissues at the site of needle insertion will also be evident.

For degenerative disease, the morphologic data provided by CT and MRI are largely comparable. Both can identify disc bulging or herniation, loss of disc height, and reactive changes in the adjacent vertebral bodies. Additionally, MRI can detect desiccation of the disc, an early manifestation of degeneration, by signal intensity changes (loss of signal intensity in T2-weighted images). The two modalities are roughly comparable in evaluation of the lumbar disc levels. MRI is generally superior to CT without intrathecal contrast in the evaluation of cervical or thoracic disc levels.

Hypertrophic, degenerative changes of the facet joints, synovial cysts, and thickening of the ligamentum flavum can be well seen with MRI, although small osteophytes, subchondral erosions of the facet joints, and ligamentous calcification are generally better demonstrated with CT. Defects of the pars interarticularis (spondylolysis) are often better appreciated with CT.

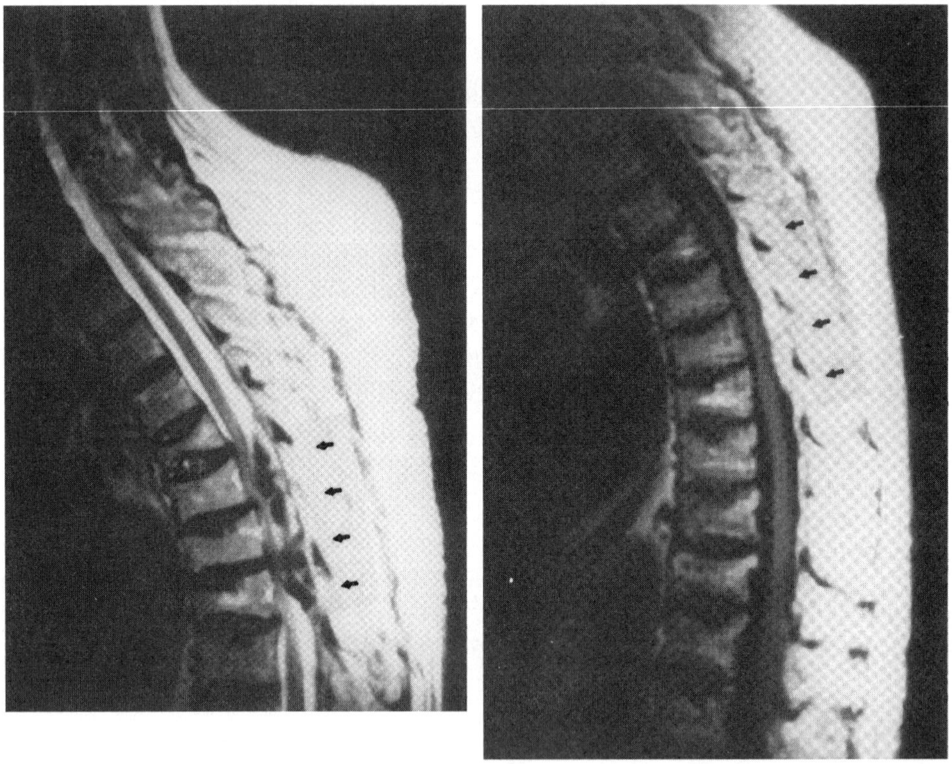

A B

**Figure 21-6.** **(A)** T2-weighted magnetic resonance midline sagittal image of the thoracic vertebral column, showing epidural hematoma (arrows). The patient had a thoracic epidural catheter placed 2 days previously for thoracotomy, and developed lower extremity weakness and sensory loss. The hematoma at this stage appears heterogeneous, with dark and bright areas, because of blood products undergoing various degrees of clot lysis. The CSF is bright, and therefore contrasts well with the posterior hematoma and the cord as it is displaced anteriorly. **(B)** T1-weighted image of the same patient in A, 12 days later, at which time the neurologic condition was improving without decompressive surgery. The hematoma (arrows) appears uniformly bright, contrasting with the dark CSF of T1 images, and is smaller in size, with less displacement of cord (intermediate intensity). It would be similarly bright on T2-weighted images at this stage, but would then contrast poorly with bright CSF. (From Morisaki H, Doi J, Ochiai R, Takeda J, Fukushima K. Epidural hematoma after epidural anesthesia in a patient with hepatic cirrhosis. Anesth Analg 1995;80:1033–1035.)

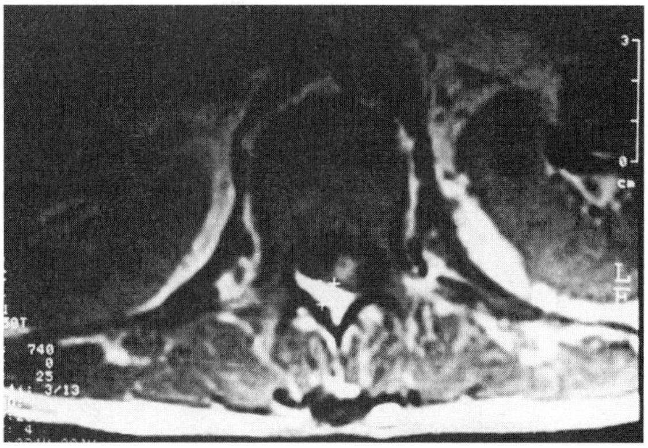

**FIGURE 21-7.** T1-weighted magnetic resonance axial image through the first lumbar vertebra, demonstrating a dorsal epidural hematoma (between the two "+" marks). Two days after placement of a lumbar epidural catheter for revascularization surgery upon the leg, progressive bilateral lower extremity weakness and sensory loss was noted. CT examination at that time was interpreted as normal, but persistent deficit led to this MRI 14 days later. The hematoma appears as a uniform high signal intensity by this time, contrasting with the dark CSF. The cord (intermediate signal) is displaced to the anatomic left. Decompressive surgery provided no recovery of function. (From Tekkok IH, Cataltepe O, Tahta K, Bertan V. Extradural haemotoma after continuous extradural anaesthesia. Br J Anaesth 1991;67:112–115.)

Postoperative scarring associated with discectomy will generally appear as epidural soft tissue of similar signal intensity to residual or recurrent disc material. Differentiation of fibrous tissue or scar from recurrent or residual disc material is made easier by intravenous administration of a gadolinium chelate. Fibrous tissue generally enhances uniformly, whereas disc material, with the possible exception of the periphery, generally does not enhance.

MRI has particular advantages for imaging infectious and inflammatory lesions. Osteomyelitis is generally readily apparent, and MRI is very sensitive for destructive or inflammatory process involving marrow or disc. Abscess adjacent to nerve plexuses or at other sites of needle insertion will be apparent by MRI. Any epidural or paraspinous soft tissue inflammation or mass effect is usually identifiable, and generally demonstrates enhancement with administration of intravenous paramagnetic contrast agent (Figure 21-8). Arachnoiditis may reveal thickening and clumping together of nerve roots of the cauda equina. Alternatively, the involved nerve roots may be adherent to the inner surface of the thecal sac and give the appearance of an empty sac. After intravenous paramagnetic contrast agent administration, there may be enhancement of nerve roots affected by arachnoiditis.

MRI is the best imaging modality for evaluation of intramedullary masses, because the internal architecture and not merely the contour of the cord is demonstrated. Similarly, intradural extramedullary masses are well demonstrated, particularly with the use of intravenous paramagnetic contrast agent, although CSF pulsation artifact in the thoracic spine can occasionally obscure lesions in the spinal canal. The bone destruction and/or soft tissue mass associated with malignant epidural tumors are generally readily apparent with MRI. These lesions usually show decreased signal intensity in T1-weighted images and increased signal intensity in T2-weighted images relative to normal bone. Most such lesions show varying degrees of contrast enhancement.

## *Radionuclide Bone Scan*

### Technology

The most widely used radiopharmaceuticals for skeletal imaging are technetium-labeled phosphate analogs. Tc-99m-labeled skeletal radiopharmaceuticals rapidly

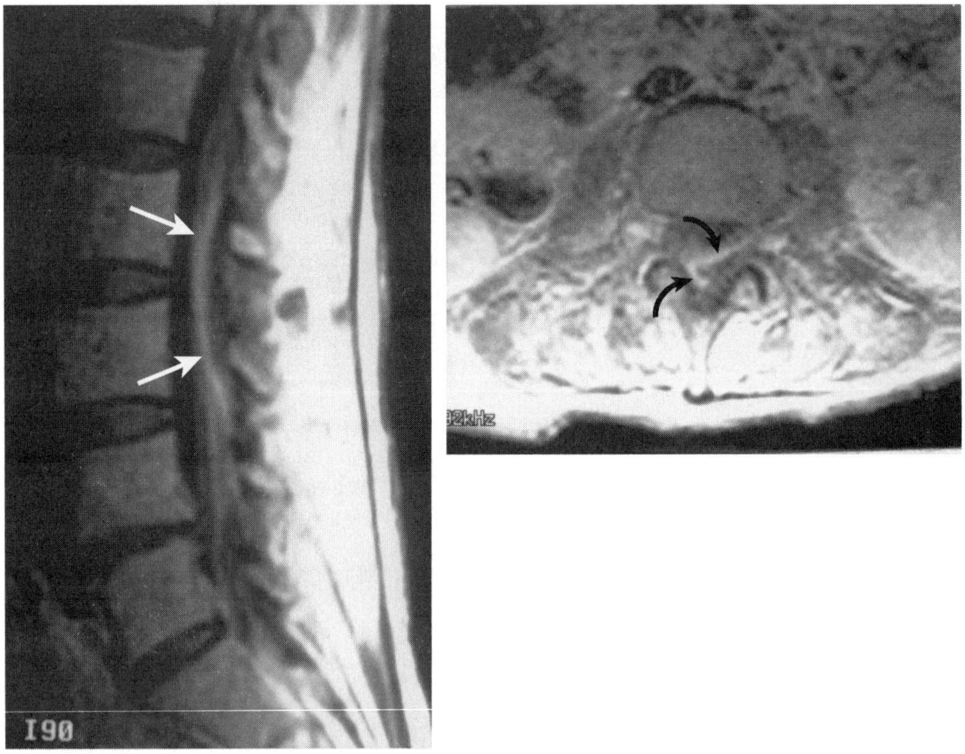


A B

**FIGURE 21-8.** T1-weighted magnetic resonance lumbar vertebral images after intravenous gadolinium injection, showing epidural abscess. The patient had tibial osteomyelitis treated with intravenous antibiotics and eventually amputation, leading to phantom limb pain treated by lumbar epidural catheter. Midline sagittal image **(A)** shows a lenticular mass (arrows) in the posterior vertebral canal of the second and third lumbar vertebrae. The anterior rim of the mass is bright because of gadolinium enhancement, whereas the area enclosed by this rim has lower signal intensity, probably indicative of purulent material. Axial image **(B)** shows dark CSF and the abnormal soft tissue posterior and to the left (patient's) of the dural sac. The rim of inflamed tissue enhances (becomes bright) with gadolinium, especially on the anterior and right aspects of the abscess (arrows).

distribute throughout the extracellular fluid space. Uptake in bone is rapid and is primarily related to blood supply. Increased osteogenesis, among other factors, results in increased tracer uptake. Decreased uptake, or "cold" lesions, may be seen in areas of decreased blood flow or bone destruction.

Imaging is normally done with a gamma scintillation camera 2–4 hours after injection of the radiotracer. Generally, the entire skeleton is imaged in both anterior and posterior projections, and spot views of particular regions are typically included as dictated by the clinical picture. "Dynamic" imaging immediately after injection may be performed in cases of suspected osteomyelitis versus cellulitis. Bone single photon emission CT (SPECT) imaging may be used for high-contrast regional imaging and is of value in the evaluation of complex bony structures such as the spine.

### Limitations

Broadly speaking, the limitations of radionuclide bone scanning are modest spatial resolution and lack of specificity. Although modern gamma cameras and SPECT scanning have significantly improved the resolution of skeletal radionuclide studies, the spatial resolution does not approach that of plain films, CT, or MRI. Lack of specificity is arguably the major limitation of skeletal scintigraphy. Because any cause of altered bone formation will result in abnormal tracer localization, it is imperative to take the clinical findings into account when evaluating the bone scan.

#### Indications

Skeletal scintigraphy is a very frequently performed imaging procedure that provides a means of surveying the entire skeleton quickly and at a reasonable cost. It is extremely sensitive and usually detects skeletal lesions earlier than other imaging modalities. Although the presence of a single lesion on a bone scan taken out of the clinical context is nonspecific, the anatomic location of a lesion and whether it is single or multiple often provides important information for forming a differential diagnosis.

The vast majority of bone scans are abnormal by 24–72 hours after a fracture. Most fractures will remain abnormal on bone scan for a minimum of 5–7 months, and most will appear normal after 2 years. Skeletal scintigraphy is very sensitive in the detection of subtle trauma such as stress fractures and can therefore help to assure the earliest diagnosis and treatment of such lesions.

The radionuclide bone scan almost always shows abnormal increased tracer uptake by the time there are clinical symptoms from osteomyelitis. The axial skeleton is infected more often than the extremities in adults. An organism may be disseminated via the paraspinous venous plexus, leading to discitis as well as involvement of other vertebral levels. In some cases it may be difficult to distinguish osteomyelitis from increased bone activity secondary to hyperemia accompanying cellulitis of the overlying soft tissues. Dynamic, or three-phase, scintigraphy is a technique used to differentiate osteomyelitis from cellulitis. The standard tracer is given as a bolus injection and imaging is performed immediately and at 5 minutes, in addition to the routine imaging at 2–4 hours after injection. Osteomyelitis shows arterial phase hyperemia and progressive focal skeletal uptake. Cellulitis shows venous hyperemia with persistent soft tissue activity. Any increased skeletal uptake tends to be mild and nonfocal. Lesions that may mimic osteomyelitis include osteoarthritis, gout, fractures, and reflex sympathetic dystrophy.

Skeletal scintigraphy is very sensitive for detecting the presence and extent of metastatic disease to bone. The rate of false-negative skeletal scintigraphy for the most common neoplasms may be as low as 2%.

### *Radionuclide Infection/Inflammation Imaging*

#### Technology

Gallium-67 is a cyclotron-produced radiopharmaceutical that binds strongly to plasma proteins, primarily transferrin, whereby it is transported to the site of inflammation or infection. It may also accumulate at the site of certain neoplasms. Indium-111 is a cyclotron-produced radionuclide with a 67-hour half-life and two photopeaks. It is used to label white blood cells, which takes approximately 2 hours. Imaging is routinely performed at 18 and 24 hours after tracer injection.

#### Limitations

From an imaging standpoint, gallium-67 is not optimal, resulting in a high degree of scatter and inefficient detection by current gamma cameras. The indium-111 leukocyte labeling process is time consuming and difficult in patients with depressed white cell counts. White blood cells must be separated from erythrocytes and platelets because they are much more numerous.

#### Indications

In the evaluation of bone and soft tissues, gallium-67 scintigraphy is used primarily to detect infection. Increased uptake in bone can also occur in patients with previous surgery, fractures, and prostheses. Because standard bone imaging does not return to normal soon after improvement, gallium-67 scanning is often used for evaluating the effectiveness of therapy. Relative to gallium-67 imaging, indium-111–labeled leukocyte scintigraphy shows both less activity in background tissues and greater concentration in infected tissue. Overall, imaging with indium-111–labeled white blood cells appears to be superior to gallium-67 imaging for the detection of osteomyelitis. However, indium-111 leukocyte scintigraphy seems to have a low sensitivity for osteomyelitis of the spine.

### *Angiography*

#### Technology

State-of-the-art digital subtraction angiography systems use computerized image processing, resulting in superior contrast resolution. Vascular anatomy is delineated by intravenous injection of an iodine-containing contrast agent during simultaneous rapid sequence filming. It is generally regarded as the "gold standard" for blood vessel imaging. Intravascular injection of contrast material requires placement of a catheter within the vascular tree of interest, generally via percutaneous puncture of the common femoral or brachial artery.

#### Limitations

Catheter angiography is an invasive procedure, and as such it carries with it a small but definite possibility of adverse events, including arterial injury, infection, renal or cardiac toxicity, infarction, bleeding, and idiopathic reaction to contrast media.

#### Indications

If transarterial needle placement for nerve block has resulted in symptomatic vascular damage, angiography is the optimal means of evaluating compromise of the lumen resulting from subintimal hematoma or creation of an arteriovenous fistula. Angiography of the spine may be necessary if other, less-invasive imaging modalities leave significant questions unanswered. Arteriovenous malformations of the spinal cord, for example, can be recognized with MRI, but the detailed anatomy can be best appreciated with angiography. Spinal dural arteriovenous fistulas or perimedullary arteriovenous fistulas are generally not well seen with MRI, because they typically occur in the thoracic region where CSF pulsation artifact is greatest. However, MRI may demonstrate accompanying signal change in the spinal cord secondary to ischemia from venous hypertension and stasis.

### *Imaging of Complications of Regional Anesthesia*

Appropriate use of imaging techniques is an important aid in the evaluation of neural complications of nerve blocks. Imaging may not only confirm the presence of a mass such as abscess or hematoma, but may also help in resolving more confusing diagnostic dilemmas. For instance, concurrent conditions such as spinal stenosis or herniated disc are readily apparent on CT and MRI. When possible, images from before the onset of neurologic complaints should be compared with postinjury images.

Choice of the best imaging modality is ideally made through consultation with a radiologist. CT is ideal for identifying bone abnormalities, and MRI excels in delineating soft tissue abnormalities, especially within the spinal canal. In most cases in which complaints originate in multiple neural segments and when neuraxial injury is suspected, MRI is optimal. The exception is the evaluation of arachnoiditis, which is best identified using CT imaging after subarachnoid contrast injection. More peripheral lesions and complications arising from blockade of a nerve plexus or peripheral nerve are less likely to be evident on imaging. Even so, accumulation of edema fluid

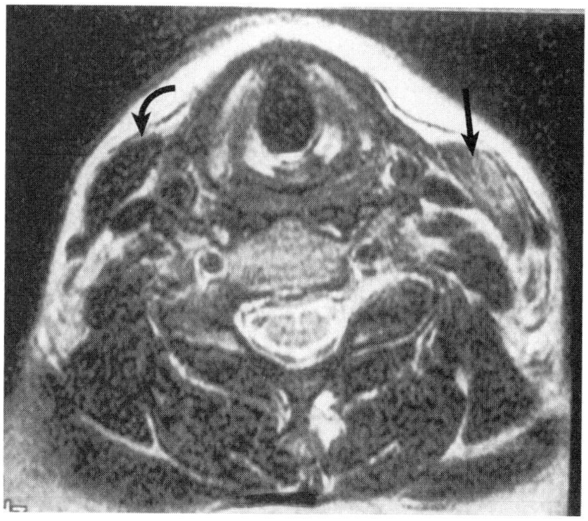

**FIGURE 21-9.** T2-weighted axial image at the level of the sixth cervical vertebra, demonstrating local anesthetic myotoxicity. The patient had received intercostal bupivacaine 45 days before and complained of left neck pain. The left sternocleidomastoid muscle (straight arrow) is enlarged and shows uniformly increased signal intensity indicative of the elevated fluid content from edema.

in areas of inflammation may be evident on MRI or the extremities, as with muscle injury from local anesthetic injection (Figure 21-9), or swelling which produces a compartment syndrome and neural compression.

Cost may be a factor that limits the use of MRI, because CT is typically less than half as expensive to perform. However, obtaining the correct information is almost always the predominating issue, and the cost of missing an important finding is high, so cost should rarely be an important factor in selecting the type of image. A factor favoring the use of MRI is the lack of ionizing radiation. Because the radiation dose for CT is low, this also should not be a consideration in choice of imaging.

## Integration

The components of evaluation enumerated above need to be assembled into diagnostic and therapeutic decisions that can benefit the patient. Information gathered from these various sources is usually processed intuitively, and formulae or well-established decision pathways are not available for rare conditions such as neural injury from regional anesthesia. It is especially difficult to know when to consult other physicians or obtain elaborate tests and images. A general sequence for solving diagnostic problems[5] begins with combining the set of positive observations into aggregate findings: for example, lower extremity sensory loss and motor weakness with defective bowel and bladder control can be consolidated into the single aggregate finding of cauda equina injury. There may be a number of these aggregate findings (e.g., there might also be evidence of infection or bleeding), so the clinician must pick the most plausible condition as a hypothesis and seek confirmation of it. At this point, if the data are not persuasive or there is more than one equally possible diagnosis, testing and consultation are considered. A final diagnosis can usually be validated by examining whether it can explain all the data.

A detailed history and physical examination are mandatory when a neural injury is discovered after regional anesthesia, and often results in a more reliable diagnosis. The decision of when to obtain consultation and diagnostic studies, however, is often unclear. Tests and consultations are only helpful if the information would change treatment, and the nature of the suspected diagnosis usually dictates whether studies should be obtained. Diagnoses with critical therapeutic implications should be pursued with the greatest intensity. A case in point is when the possibilities include epidural abscess or hematoma, which if not surgically relieved can lead to permanent and extensive neural injury and threaten life. Therefore, consultation and imaging are strongly recommended early in the workup if severe polyradiculopathy or myelopathy are evident. In contrast, identification of a mild neural injury to a peripheral nerve, or a mild monoradiculopathy following neuraxial injection, does not have as clear a therapeutic implication, so circumstances in which these are suspected might be pursued with less urgency, particularly with regard to intensive or invasive examination. If a neural defect is persistent or intense, studies may need to be pursued.

It is necessary to avoid focusing on only anesthetic causes of injury to the exclusion of alternative causes. If vascular occlusion is the cause of neural dysfunction but has been neglected as an etiologic possibility, an opportunity for successful treatment may be missed. A sense of responsibility may ironically lead the anesthesiologist astray. Finally, there may be social reasons for obtaining diagnostic consultation or tests. The patient may only be satisfied by detailed workup, and legal considerations are an unavoidable fact of medical life.

Clarity and completeness of communication directly affects the quality of the information gained from consultation and tests. This usually requires discussion with the consultant (e.g., neurologist, neurosurgeon, neuroradiologist) because details may be incompletely available from the medical record, and few clinicians know how to interpret (or even find) anesthesia and recovery room notations. The key issue of accurate and complete communication is illustrated by a case:

> An elderly man received epidural anesthesia as a component of his anesthetic for retropubic prostatectomy and node excision that lasted 7 hours. The blockade, initiated before induction of general anesthesia, was uneventful, but dense and uniform sensory and motor dysfunction of the lower extremities persisted 12 hours after the final 0.5% bupivacaine injection. Fearing an epidural hematoma, MRI of the lumbar vertebral column was requested with the reason for imaging stated as "neurologic abnormality, rule out hematoma." The image (Figure 21-10A) was interpreted as showing an abnormality, possibly hematoma or artifact. The epidural catheter was removed and surgical consultation pursued. Further imaging 3 hours later (Figure 21-10B) confirmed that the area of increased signal intensity was flow artifact by CSF motion; by this time, the block was beginning to recede.

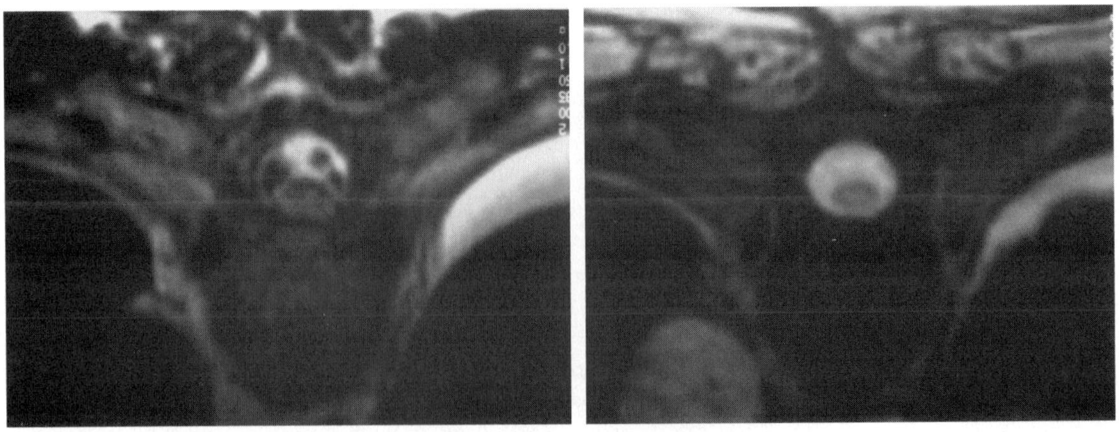

A B

**FIGURE 21-10.** **(A)** T2-weighted axial image through a thoracic vertebra, showing bright CSF and areas in the CSF of uncertain origin (see text). **(B)** Repeat image of same patient and level, using a different T2-weighted pulse sequence technique (gradient echo) less susceptible to flow artifact. The CSF is now uniform and without masses, and the cord appears normal.

Had the radiologist more completely understood the indication for imaging, it would have been clear that epidural bleeding was the suspected condition and that an intrathecal abnormality was only a remote diagnostic consideration. The images would have been interpreted as not supportive of hematoma as the etiology of the neurologic condition, and artifact would have been the more strongly suspected source of the abnormal image. Similarly, direct discussion between the anesthesiologist and radiologist after obtaining the initial images would have made clear the strong likelihood that the study was normal, avoiding consternation and disruption of care. The consultation should indicate what is being looked for, rather than simply specifying the test to be done. Finally, discussion can indicate the necessary degree of urgency, and because an iatrogenic condition is being sought, direct discussion may avoid injudicious wording of the written report.

There are adverse consequences from obtaining excessive diagnostic studies. Apart from the obvious considerations of complications from the procedures and cost, identification of more minor defects as resolution of tests is improved leads to the risk of overtreating insignificant conditions.[6] Additionally, false-positive results can lead to pursuit of an irrelevant diagnosis. Despite these concerns, imaging and neurophysiologic study are helpful in most cases when neurologic injury follows regional anesthesia.

## References

1. Yeun EC, Layzer RB, Weitz SR, Olney RK. Neurologic complications of lumbar epidural anesthesia and analgesia. Neurology 1995;45:1795–1801.
2. Moore DC, Hain RF, Ward A, Bridenbaugh LD. Importance of the perineural spaces in nerve blocking. JAMA 1954;156:1050–1053.
3. Kimura J. Electrodiagnosis in Diseases of Nerve and Muscle. 2nd ed. New York: Oxford University Press; 1989.
4. Osborn AG. Diagnostic Neuroradiology. St. Louis: Mosby; 1994.
5. Eddy DM, Clanton CH. The art of diagnosis: solving the clinicopathological exercise. N Engl J Med 1982;306:1263–1268.
6. Black WC, Welch HG. Advances in diagnostic imaging and overestimation of disease prevalence and the benefits of therapy. N Engl J Med 1993;328:1237–1243.

# 22 Case Studies of Regional Anesthesia

William F. Urmey

This chapter presents some of the known complications of regional anesthetics through illustrative case reports. Although the case reports are not those of actual patients, they are representative of real cases and incorporate features from actual reports or clinical experiences. Care has been taken to make certain that the depiction of presenting signs and symptoms are true to those actually reported in the literature. Reports are followed by relevant discussion, which includes our present understanding of underlying mechanisms and etiologic factors that are believed to contribute to the development of the complications. Diagnosis and management of complications are briefly covered as well. It is not possible to discuss all known regional anesthetic complications here. Therefore, five clinically important, well-recognized syndromes complicating routine regional anesthetics have been chosen. These should be appreciated and understood by all practitioners in this subspecialty.

## Case 1: Permanent Cervical Spinal Cord Injury Following Interscalene Brachial Plexus Block Performed During General Anesthesia

A 17-year-old healthy adolescent girl with a diagnosis of recurrent shoulder dislocation presented for arthroscopic stabilization of her left shoulder. Following the administration of midazolam and propofol in divided doses, the patient was unarousable but breathing spontaneously. Her oxygen saturation ($Spo_2$) was 100% by pulse oximetry. The left interscalene groove was palpated and a 5-cm insulated stimulating needle was inserted at the standard level corresponding to C6. The needle was advanced until a motor response (wrist flexion) was observed at a current amplitude of 0.41 mA, pulse duration of 0.1 ms. After negative aspiration, 40 mL 0.25% bupivacaine with 5 μg/mL epinephrine was injected in divided doses, with negative aspiration before each 5-mL aliquot. Within 20 seconds of the local anesthetic injection, the patient became apneic and her $Spo_2$ decreased to 74%. Positive pressure ventilation with 100% oxygen returned her $Spo_2$ to 100% and the patient was endotracheally intubated following intravenous propofol and vecuronium. After the surgical procedure and discontinuation of general anesthesia, the patient was unable to be extubated and was noted to have dilated pupils bilaterally. She was transferred to the postanesthetic care unit where she required mechanical ventilation for several hours. After extubation, it was recognized that she had a dense left-sided hemiparesis. She devel-

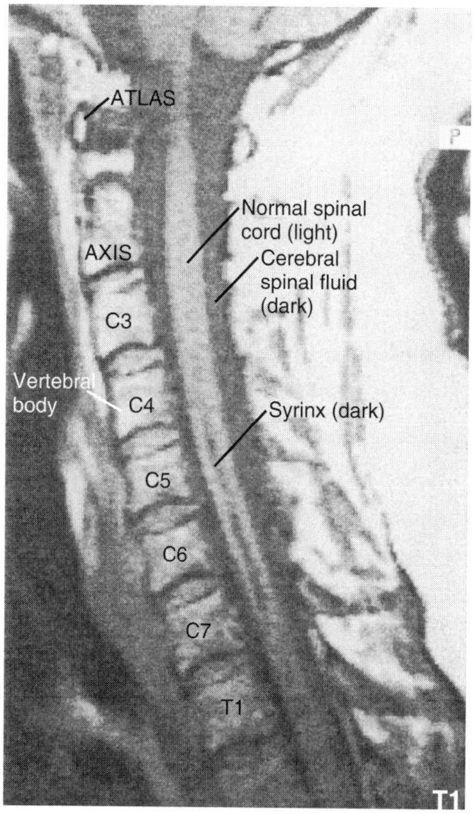


**FIGURE 22-1.** Scan of the T1-weighted sagittal section of the cervical spinal cord magnetic resonance imaging performed 9 months after interscalene block in a patient who received an interscalene block under general anesthesia. A syrinx or cavity is present in the central portion of the right half of the cervical spinal cord. (From Benumof,[2] reprinted with permission.)

oped bowel and bladder dysfunction and a postdural puncture headache was noted the following day. Magnetic resonance imaging was performed which revealed syringomyelia of the left side of the lower cervical and upper thoracic spinal cord, extending from C6-7 to T1 (see Figure 22-1).

## *Discussion*

This patient received an injection of local anesthetic into the substance of the cervical spinal cord. Intraneural injection of local anesthetic under pressure has been shown experimentally to spread along the longitudinal axis of nerves.[1] Therefore, theoretically, injection into a proximal nerve root could spread directly into the spinal cord. However, Benumof[2] reported four cases in which interscalene block, performed on patients during general anesthesia, resulted in permanent injury to the cervical spinal cord. Imaging studies of the cervical spinal cords of these patients showed varying degrees of vacuolization or a syrinx of the spinal cord. Benumof cited the pattern of injury and lack of damage to structures outside of the cervical spinal cord as providing convincing evidence that injection in each case was made directly into the substance of the spinal cord. Similar medicolegal cases have been reviewed by this author. In each case, the interscalene injection was performed during general anesthesia, which prevented the patient from being able to withdraw from the needle in the event of a painful paresthesia or painful injection. Although performance of interscalene block during general anesthesia is, at present, within the accepted standard of care, general anesthesia should be viewed as a relative contraindication to interscalene block. By contrast to the interscalene block by paresthesia, as originally described by Winnie,[3] the ability to use a nerve stimulator to elicit an appropriate motor response eliminates the necessity for patient feedback or cooperation. Furthermore, profound sedation or general anesthesia can be administered without compromising the ability to elicit a motor response to electrical stimulation. Finally, the length of the needle should be appropriate. The brachial plexus is very superficial at the interscalene groove. The plexus can be located and blocked in the majority of patients by using a 2.5-cm needle. Needles longer than 3.75 cm are not necessary for the performance of an interscalene block.

## Significant Neuropraxia Associated with Regional Anesthesia

Significant neurologic injuries associated with regional anesthesia are indeed rare. Although incidents of significant neuropraxia are, in all likelihood, not underestimated by practicing anesthesiologists, they are certainly grossly underreported. Major neuropraxia usually follows departure from accepted technique, administration of brachial plexus block under general anesthesia, or failure to heed a patient's reaction or complaint of severe pain upon injection.

Several large-scale multicenter clinical investigations support the safety of regional anesthesia.[4–7] In a recent excellent prospective investigation from France, Auroy et al.[5] studied 103,730 regional anesthetics. Of 34 serious neurologic complications (radiculopathy, cauda equina syndrome, or paraplegia), 21 (62%) were associated with paresthesia or pain upon injection. Thirteen patients did not have associated paresthesia. Of these, 12 were spinal anesthetics, nine of which were with 5% hyperbaric lidocaine. One can generalize that for the most part these serious injuries were either paresthesia-associated or 5% intrathecal lidocaine-associated. Although brachial plexus blocks were not discussed separately, peripheral nerve blocks had an exceptionally low incidence of neurologic complications.

It has been shown, in animals, by Selander et al.[8] that histologic evidence of nerve damage can result when nerves are pierced by needles or when local anesthetic is injected into the nerve.[9] Short beveled needles cannot be counted on to prevent nerve injury, as was shown by Rice and McMahon[10] in a rat model. These investigators found that rat sciatic nerve impaled by short-beveled needles had more frequent lesions that were more severe and took longer to heal than those induced by conventional long-beveled needles. In a study comparing short bevel to conventional beveled needles with regard to postblock neuropraxias, Selander et al. found no significant differences in minor neuropraxias. They reported that all neuropraxias resolved over a 6-month period.

## Should Regional Anesthesia Be Performed on the Anesthetized Patient?

The above referenced large-scale multicenter clinical investigations support the safety of regional anesthesia[4–7]; however, if we as anesthesiologists continue to "run red lights" by placing needles in close proximity to the nerves of unconscious patients, we are bound to have an occasional serious, albeit rare, "accident." Regional anesthesia is frequently performed in patients who are under general anesthesia or heavy sedation. Spinal or epidural anesthesia does not require patient participation for a successful anesthetic. The advent of the nerve stimulator has allowed for high success rates of peripheral nerve or plexus blockade without absolute need of an awake patient who is able to report a paresthesia. The practice of performing regional blocks during general anesthesia has become an accepted standard of care for the pediatric patient.[11,12] Until recently, there have been no compelling clinical data that absolutely support the hypothesis that regional anesthesia is unsafe in the heavily sedated or fully anesthetized patient.[11] Nevertheless, conventional wisdom, backed by the clinical experiences of experts,[13,14] has supported the contention that regional anesthesia in an unconscious or anesthetized patient is contraindicated.

Bromage wrote that "Sudden severe pain during placement of a spinal or epidural (or severe pain upon injection during peripheral nerve block) is a time-honored signal that nerve tissue is endangered and that the needle should be promptly withdrawn and then resited."[13] It does not require more than common sense to see that this crucial patient feedback is lost once the patient is rendered unconscious. That is, the patient loses his only defense against your needle! Regional anesthetic complications are in all probability highly underreported.[15] Nevertheless, there are numerous case reports that support the notion that regional anesthetic complications are frequently associated with painful paresthesias or other sensations. These symptoms will certainly be missed in the unconscious patient. New data strongly question the routine use of the nerve stimulator in the anesthetized patient.

Moore,[14,15] another expert regional anesthesiologist, who also had clinical experience that spanned several decades, has written editorials in support of accepted paresthesia techniques of regional anesthesia. In one editorial, Moore wrote, "It is unfortunately the case that using the nerve stimulator while attempting to locate a nerve, particularly in unconscious patients, has not avoided neuropathy. We have reviewed six medico-legal cases in which permanent brachial plexus neuropathy occurred and in which the nerve stimulator was used." In a different editorial,[14] Moore warned to stop injecting if, upon injection of 0.5–1 mL of local anesthetic, the patient complains of cramp-like pain. Urmey has reviewed a case in which brachial plexus block by nerve stimulator in an anesthetized patient was implicated in ipsilateral phrenic paralysis.

Trentman et al.[16] reported a case of brachial plexus neuropathy that followed an attempt at subclavian vein catheterization. During multiple attempts, the patient noticed the sudden onset of a "hot, electrical" sensation down her arm which resulted in a "severe lower trunk (brachial) plexopathy" as documented by electromyography. It is likely that if anesthetized, this patient may have had several more attempts and potentially further nerve injury.

Barutell et al.[17] reported on an obese patient who had an interscalene block administered with an 8.8-cm needle. The patient noted a sharp paresthesia in her right arm when the needle was inserted and, at the same time, a "brisk jerk of the head occurred." The paresthesia worsened upon injection. Despite this warning, injection was continued and the patient had a respiratory arrest after 8 mL and pupils were noted to be fixed and dilated. The patient subsequently was found to have a permanent and complete denervation of C8 and T1 nerve roots. It is probable that, if injection had been stopped, no permanent injury would have occurred.

Urmey and Stanton[18] reported that they were unable to consistently elicit a motor response following sensory paresthesia during interscalene block administration. These investigators designed a study to determine if nerve contact by a needle as evidenced by a clear sensory paresthesia was necessarily associated with a motor response upon nerve stimulation up to 1.0 mA.

Twenty interscalene block patients were prospectively studied using the paresthesia technique of Winnie with a 22-gauge, 3.8-cm (1-1/2″) needle. In 10 patients, a short-beveled insulated needle was used (Stimex, B-D) and in the following 10 patients a long-beveled noninsulated needle (B-D) was used. Immediately after the report of a paresthesia and before local anesthetic injection, the nerve stimulator power was turned on and amperage slowly increased from 0 to 1.0 mA maximal amperage. Presence and location of upper extremity motor response, if any, were recorded. After this, 50 mL mepivacaine 1.5% with epinephrine was injected. Interscalene block was carefully evaluated by a single observer.

All 30 patients had easily elicited paresthesias, 22 to shoulder, six to arm, and two to the hand. Only 9 of 30 patients (30%) had visible or reported motor response. All blocks had good evidence of sensory and motor blockade and 26 were judged "excellent" by blinded orthopedic surgeons. The remaining block was judged as "good." No patient required general anesthesia. This study showed that evidence of sensory response (paresthesia), presumably caused by nerve contact, was not associated with ability to elicit a motor response in 70% of patients, despite stimulation at milliamperage that exceeds the minimal accepted by most anesthetists. Conversely, this study provided evidence that, if patients are under general anesthesia, a lack of motor response does not guarantee that contact with a sensory nerve fascicle has not occurred.

This was the first clinical study that examined the relationships between a sensory response (paresthesia) and a motor response to electrical stimulation in peripheral nerve or plexus block. Subsequent to the original report of the above data, these findings were confirmed in the axilla in a study by Choyce et al.[19] These investigators studied 72 patients during axillary block, using a similar protocol to that published by Urmey and Stanton. Paresthesia was associated with a motor response to electrical stimulation up to 0.5 mA, pulse duration of 0.1 ms in only 77% of the patients studied. Therefore, 23% lacked a motor response.

Mulroy and Mitchell[20] reported four cases in which a mechanical paresthesia ("presumed nerve contact") was obtained before motor response to electrical stimulation during brachial plexus block performance with a nerve stimulator.

All of these reports confirm what experienced clinicians believe, that is, that neither paresthesia nor use of a peripheral nerve stimulator completely rule out the possibility of the needle's tip being intraneural.[21] In fact, in all the devastating cases presented by Benumof using a nerve stimulator, minimal amperage was $\geqslant$0.81 mA.

Bollini et al.[22] further researched the relationship between a paresthesia and a motor response to electrical stimulation in a study of 22 patients undergoing interscalene brachial plexus block. Interscalene block was performed with an insulated needle coupled to a peripheral nerve stimulator. A motor response was obtained at 0.5 mA in all patients. The nerve stimulator was then turned off and the needle further advanced in the same direction. A mechanical paresthesia was elicited in 21 of the 22 patients. The most likely explanation was that a motor response to electrical stimulation occurred with the needle's tip at a small distance from the nerve, whereas mechanical paresthesia required nerve contact.

### Conclusion

Regional anesthesia is extremely safe. As physicians, we have an obligation to do everything possible to minimize complications when we perform regional blocks. Without doubt, most nerve injuries following regional anesthesia go unreported. Nevertheless, many of the complications that have been reported were associated with sensory and/or motor response warnings. Oversedation, general anesthetics, and muscle relaxants obliterate to certain degrees such warnings, and therefore are not part of what constitutes an optimally safe scenario for regional blockade. It is true that heeding a single warning paresthesia may not always prevent nerve injury in the awake patient. However, the unconscious patient could theoretically have several such injuries that occur during search for a nerve or during intraneural injection without any valuable warning or ability to defend themselves against your needle.

## Case 2: Respiratory Failure Following Interscalene Block

A 66-year-old man with a torn rotator cuff presented for right rotator cuff repair. His medical history was only remarkable for a 30-pack-year smoking history and chronic obstructive pulmonary disease. Preoperative pulmonary function testing showed a forced vital capacity (FVC) of 1.8 L (40% predicted). The surgeon called the anesthesiologist 2 days preoperatively to request regional anesthesia, in view of the patient's pulmonary disease.

The anesthesiologist administered an interscalene block with 30 mL 0.5% bupivacaine with epinephrine. Approximately 7 minutes after the interscalene injection, the patient became dyspneic and progressively cyanotic, requiring intubation. Attempts to wean and extubate the patient repeatedly failed. Only 12 hours after the interscalene block was the patient finally able to be extubated.

### *Discussion*

Respiratory failure as a complication of interscalene block is very rare. However, respiratory failure can occur secondary to brachial plexus–related pneumothorax,[23] inadvertent subarachnoid or epidural injection of local anesthetic,[24–27] or as in this case, from diaphragmatic paresis.[28] With proper technique, the incidence of pneumothorax or epidural/spinal[24,25,27] anesthesia following interscalene block should be virtually nonexistent. However, diaphragmatic paresis with resultant respiratory impairment has been shown to occur with an incidence of 100%. In one study, this incidence was not reduced by decreasing anesthetic volume to 20 mL.[29] Reductions in routine pulmonary function tests of 20%–40% can be expected within 15 minutes of interscalene block administration. These reductions persist 3–5 hours after mepivacaine interscalene block and at least 9 hours after bupivacaine interscalene block when epinephrine is added.[30]

#### Anatomic Basis for Phrenic Nerve Paresis

Phrenic nerve paralysis has been reported to occur following supraclavicular block. Various incidences have been reported which may depend on the sensitivity of the diagnostic test used. Nevertheless, it is a frequent accompaniment of supraclavicular block, with reported incidences up to 80%.[31] Urmey et al.[32] reported a 100% incidence of ipsilateral hemidiaphragmatic paresis following interscalene block. This finding has been supported by numerous subsequent studies.[29,33,34]

Two anatomic theories have been proposed to explain diaphragmatic paresis. Originally, phrenic paresis was attributed to spread of local anesthetic solution into the space between the anterior and middle scalene muscles.[35] Presently, diaphragmatic paresis is believed to occur by local anesthetic action on the cervical nerve roots C3–C5, which form the phrenic nerve.[34] The brachial plexus is characterized by free communication with the cervical plexus above it. Both plexuses are surrounded by the same fascial confines, the fascia arising from the anterior and middle scalene muscles. Local anesthetic labeled with radiographic contrast has been shown by Winnie et al.[36] to spread freely into the cervical plexus following interscalene injection. Sensory studies by Urmey et al.[29,34] support that sensory dermatomal levels of C3 and often C2 occur routinely. Thus, motor anesthesia of these same nerve roots can be expected as well and this is the most likely anatomic explanation for phrenic nerve paresis. Another fact that supports this concept is that the timing of sensory anesthesia of these cervical nerve roots coincides with the onset and maximal degree of diminution in pulmonary function associated with interscalene block.

The extremely rare complication of permanent phrenic nerve paralysis can occur from trauma to the phrenic nerve during exploration or injection. The phrenic nerve runs anterior to the interscalene groove. This complication has been reported following interscalene block.[37,38]

#### Pulmonary Function Alterations

Consistent reductions in pulmonary function occur following interscalene block. Whereas reductions of 20%–40% in forced expiratory volume in 1 second ($FEV_1$) and FVC have been found in several studies,[29,33,34,39] diminutions of more than 60% have been observed in isolated cases.[29] These results indicate complete or near complete phrenic nerve paresis. The magnitude of the pulmonary function reductions are similar to those that have been reported following surgical phrenic nerve ablation[40] or complete phrenic nerve paralysis of a pathologic etiology.[41] In a study of direct phrenic nerve infiltration with 1% mepivacaine in healthy volunteers, Gould and coworkers[42] demonstrated a 27% reduction in vital capacity.

The decreases in pulmonary function seem to be largely independent of local anesthetic volume or concentration. Doses of 20–28 mL of 0.75% bupivacaine were found by Pere to result in pulmonary function decreases of 20%–40%.[39] These decreases in pulmonary function as well as altered diaphragmatic motility persisted for at least 24 hours when an infusion of 5–9 mL bupivacaine 0.125% was administered. A mean reduction in FVC of 32.0% ± 8.9% was found in a group of patients following a 20-mL injection of 1.5% mepivacaine for interscalene block.[29]

### Contraindications to Interscalene Block

Absolute contraindications to interscalene brachial plexus block include a history of contralateral pneumonectomy or preexisting contralateral hemidiaphragmatic paresis. Relative contraindications include severe chronic obstructive pulmonary disease or any neuromuscular disorder in which a 25% decrease in FVC would not be tolerated. A preblock FVC of 1 L or less is a contraindication to interscalene block. Conditions such as ankylosing spondylitis, in which rib cage motion is restricted, may also place a patient at increased risk of respiratory failure following the diaphragmatic paresis associated with this regional anesthetic.

Another relative contraindication involves patient positioning in the lateral position (with the functionally intact diaphragm down) or any positioning or strapping that will inhibit contralateral chest wall expansion. Respiratory failure has been reported following extubation in a patient who had surgery in the lateral position, with the unblocked side dependent, during combined interscalene block and general anesthesia.[28]

### Diagnosis of Hemidiaphragmatic Paresis and Treatment of Associated Respiratory Dysfunction

There are several methods of diagnosing hemidiaphragmatic paresis. These include fluoroscopy,[43] double-exposure chest X-ray,[44] and ultrasonography.[45] The sensitivity of fluoroscopy has been challenged[46] and this criticism also applies to the double-exposure radiographic technique. Ultrasonography of the zone of apposition of diaphragm to rib cage is simple and very sensitive. This technique, in addition to pulmonary function testing, may be used for preoperative evaluation of the patient if preexisting diaphragmatic disease is suspected.

Pulse oximetry is advocated for patients undergoing interscalene block or any brachial plexus injection above the clavicle. Supplemental oxygen is also recommended for such patients. Supplemental sedation should be carefully given and patients observed closely after the block. Equipment to assist or control ventilation should be immediately available, for the rare instances when it is necessary.

Dyspnea developing after interscalene block is rare in the otherwise healthy patient. In studies, we have found that pulmonary function changes occur early after completion of interscalene block and that these changes are essentially complete within 15 minutes. This is reassuring because maximal pulmonary alterations occur when the anesthesiologist is present and therefore fears of progression of dysfunction upon discharge to the floor or home are unfounded.

If a patient develops difficulty breathing following interscalene block, he or she should be reassured and closely observed. In this author's experience, most patients complaining of dyspnea have more than adequate pulmonary function. Symptoms of dyspnea may be somewhat relieved by placing the patient in the upright or sitting position as tolerated. This position optimizes diaphragmatic geometry and utilizes favorable gravitational effects on the diaphragm to help expand the lungs, increasing functional residual capacity. The sitting position has been found to significantly increase FVC compared with the supine position in patients who underwent interscalene block.[30]

Auscultation of the ipsilateral lung field often reveals diminished (or almost silent) breath sounds. One should be careful not to automatically assume that this implies pneumothorax. Pneumothorax is an extremely unusual complication of interscalene block if the block is performed correctly with a needle of proper length. Chest radiography may be obtained if pneumothorax is suspected. Finally, positive pressure ventilation may be needed in some patients. Assisted or controlled ventilation by face mask, laryngeal mask airway, or endotracheal intubation should be done if clinically indicated.

#### Conclusion

Hemidiaphragmatic paresis is an expected side effect of brachial plexus block performed above the clavicle. An understanding of the onset and duration of the associated pulmonary function changes is crucial to safe management, especially in patients with significant pulmonary disease.

## Case 3: Bradycardia During Spinal Anesthesia

A 20-year-old female athlete was scheduled for elective knee arthroscopy. Medical history was notable only for the history of fainting. A spinal anesthetic with 60 mg lidocaine 2% plain was administered at the L4-5 interspace. The patient elected to watch the video monitor and remained completely alert, refusing sedation. Thirty minutes after the spinal was injected, the patient complained of nausea. Her baseline heart rate of 50 bpm was now 28 bpm. Suddenly, the patient was asystolic. She quickly turned cyanotic despite positive pressure ventilation with 100% oxygen by mask.

### *Discussion*

This patient experienced sudden bradycardia during spinal anesthesia. Bradycardia during spinal anesthesia is a potentially dangerous event. All anesthesiologists must have a strategy for identifying patients at risk and should institute immediate treatment when bradycardia occurs. Danger of sudden bradycardia progressing to cardiac arrest was clearly illustrated in a closed claims analysis of unexpected cardiac arrest during spinal anesthesia published by Caplan et al.[47] in 1988. Unfortunately, although all 14 patients analyzed in this study were resuscitated intraoperatively, six of the 14 patients experienced severe neurologic deficits and subsequently died in the hospital. The remaining eight had serious neurologic sequelae. This analysis demonstrated that, although spinal anesthesia is widely regarded as very safe, sudden cardiac arrest may occur rarely. Despite the fact that all patients were healthy, difficult resuscitation with poor neurologic outcomes ensued. Thus, although rare, this complication may be unheralded and disastrous.

#### Physiologic Factors in Sudden Bradycardia During Spinal or Epidural Anesthesia

An imbalance between parasympathetic and sympathetic nervous systems has been proposed to occur in the setting of epidural or spinal anesthesia. With a significant sensory anesthetic level, the patient may be devoid of sympathetic output but have normal parasympathetic innervation. The normal response to sudden bradycardia, for example during fainting, is a reflex increase in sympathetic output. The patient with high-level spinal anesthesia may be unable to mount such a response. This also may explain the reports of difficult resuscitation in bradycardic patients who were otherwise healthy.

Asystole has been described during both spinal and epidural anesthesia.[48,49] Inadequate filling pressures, decreased vascular resistance, a relatively empty ventricle, and an unaltered or heightened vagal output are often part of a physiologic scenario where sudden bradycardia or asystole occurs. Caplan et al.,[47] in the closed claims analysis referred to above, cited the early use of intravenous epinephrine as a factor in those patients who had more successful resuscitation. Exogenously administered epinephrine acts to restore some of the sympathetic balance, inhibiting bradycardia, increasing cardiac filling pressures, and preserving cardiac output. It also acts directly on the cardiac conduction system with a chronotropic effect on the heart.

### Bezold-Jarisch Reflex

Much attention has been focused on the Bezold-Jarisch reflex as the cause of sudden acute bradycardia during spinal or epidural anesthesia.[49] The basis of this reflex is a decrease in stretch tension on mechanoreceptors located in the left ventricle. A suddenly empty left ventricle triggers this paradoxical reflex which results in increased parasympathetic activity. Sympathetic output is also inhibited. Anything that decreases left ventricular end-diastolic volume suddenly, such as spinal anesthesia, may trigger this reflex.

By contrast, bradycardia that is slow in onset, developing after administration of spinal anesthesia, has long been recognized and attributed to decreased activity of the cardioaccelerator nerves to the heart.[50] This is a different phenomenon than the sudden bradycardia or asystole in the patient presented above. Complete sympathectomy of the heart itself only reduces heart rate by about 20%.[51]

### Precipitating Factors in the Development of Sudden Bradycardia During Spinal or Epidural Anesthesia

#### *Sedatives*

There are many theoretical and real factors that may be associated with the development of bradycardia during spinal or epidural anesthesia. Use of sedatives leading to hypoventilation and hypoxia during spinal anesthesia has been implicated as a possible contributing factor in sudden cardiac arrest in the patient with spinal anesthesia.[47] However, this author has witnessed patients *without any sedation* experience sudden asystole.

#### *Neurocardiogenic Bradycardia*

Lack of adequate sedation in an overly anxious patient may contribute to development of sudden bradycardia in the patient during spinal or epidural anesthesia. The single most important identifiable predisposing factor for bradycardia during regional anesthesia in this author's practice has been a history of fainting or syncope. More than one patient with a history of fainting has been observed to develop sudden asystole during spinal or epidural anesthesia. This author has observed an unsedated patient who upon removal of surgical drapes and viewing the surgical dressing, at the end of his procedure, suddenly become asystolic and cyanotic, requiring cardiorespiratory resuscitation. Frerichs et al.[52] have described a similar psychogenic cardiac arrest during epidural anesthesia for knee arthroscopy in a young athletic patient. Increased vagal tone in young or athletic patients may contribute to this syndrome. Often bradycardia is preceded by complaints of nausea, dizziness, or anxiety. Diaphoresis, yawning, or sighing are sometimes noted as well.

In the study by Carpenter et al.,[51] factors concluded to be associated with side effects of spinal anesthesia included peak block height, use of hyperbaric preparations of local anesthetics, administration of spinal anesthesia above the L3-4 interspace, and use of procaine. Patients receiving β-blockers had a significantly higher incidence of bradycardia. However, it is this author's opinion, based on experience, that this represents a different phenomenon and that these patients are at no increased risk of development of sudden severe bradycardia. Indeed β-blockers may be protective in patients prone to syncope because they have been used to decrease the incidence of bradycardia and syncope in patients during tilt-table testing.[53]

Tarkkila and Isola[54] analyzed the predictive value of several variables with regard to hypotension, bradycardia, and nausea. They found that anesthetic sensory levels above T6 and age younger than 50 years were associated with bradycardia during spinal anesthesia.

Cardiac arrest during neuraxial block occurs at a rate of 1.3–18 per 10,000.[55] In a retrospective analysis at the Mayo Clinic, Kopp et al.[55] recently examined the frequency of cardiac arrest during neuraxial anesthesia and examined the factors associated with survival. They found an incidence of cardiac arrest of 1.8 per 10,000 patients. Interestingly, spinal anesthesia was associated with an incidence of 2.9 compared with 0.9 per 10,000 for epidural anesthesia. In 46% of the patients who arrested, the cardiac arrest was associated with a specific surgical event, such as the cementing of an orthopedic prosthesis. Importantly, survival of the arrest was significantly and favorably affected by rapid resuscitation ($9 \pm 20$ versus $34 \pm 12$ minutes, $P < .001$).

### Treatment of Bradycardia during Spinal or Epidural Anesthesia

The predominant form of bradycardia that occurs during spinal or epidural anesthesia is nonthreatening, slow in onset, is not associated with major hemodynamic changes, and is easy to treat. Atropine or ephedrine will result in heart rate increases in most patients with this form of bradycardia. Bradycardia is often made worse when phenylephrine or any isolated α-agonist is used to treat hypotension.[56]

Bradycardia that is more precipitous or severe should be treated immediately. A direct-acting β-agonist is necessary and usually effective if administered early, before cardiac output decreases substantially. As discussed above, Caplan et al.[47] alluded to the importance of early administration of intravenous epinephrine in bradycardia cardiac arrest. Sharrock et al.[56] have also discussed use of epinephrine to treat or prevent bradycardia. In a study comparing epinephrine to phenylephrine during epidural anesthesia, epinephrine resulted in higher cardiac output, stroke volume, cardiac index, and a more effectively maintained heart rate.[57]

Asystole occurring during spinal or epidural anesthesia must be treated immediately. One must keep in mind that this event is primarily a circulatory phenomenon and therefore treatment should be aimed at restoring cardiac function. This is not always a simple task in the setting of a high sympathetic block. Precordial thump-pacing has been used in several patients by this author with concomitant administration of intravenous epinephrine (8 µg is a good starting dose) and atropine (0.8–1.0 mg) with excellent and dramatic effect. Precordial thump-pacing has been reported in case reports of resuscitation following asystole during spinal anesthesia.[49,58] If sudden asystole occurs during spinal or epidural anesthesia, every second that passes without treatment is crucial. Prolonged asystole diminishes cardiac output and leads to cyanosis in these patients very quickly. Decreased cardiac output rapidly results in an inability to effectively treat with intravenous pharmacologic support. Precordial thump-pacing often results in 1:1 capture and helps to maintain an effective cardiac output allowing definitive pharmacologic support. What begins as a pure circulatory event can quickly become a respiratory problem as well. Oxygen and positive pressure ventilation should be quickly added in the cyanotic patient or if a decrease in oxygen saturation occurs. Availability of transcutaneous pacing or transvenous pacing equipment can also be helpful in some situations. Finally, in rare patients in whom treatment is not quickly instituted, conventional cardiopulmonary resuscitation and advanced life-support measures are needed.

The importance of immediate availability and institution of pharmacologic therapy cannot be overemphasized. At the author's institution, epinephrine is routinely diluted to 4 µg/mL and drawn up in a syringe for immediate availability. Atropine, ephedrine, and isoproterenol should also be available. Finally, as when performing any major regional anesthetic, equipment for airway management and positive pressure ventilation should be at hand.

### Conclusion

Sudden and severe bradycardia or asystole have been associated with routine spinal or epidural anesthesia. Prospective, controlled studies are needed to identify variables placing patients at added risk. These include clinical, demographic, and anesthetic variables. It seems that younger patients with high vagal tone, patients with a history of syncope or fainting, and patients with higher sensory levels of spinal or epidural anesthesia may be at added risk. However, this complication can occur with any patient. Treatment, initially directed at the cardiovascular system, must be instituted immediately upon onset of symptoms or as soon as the occurrence of bradycardia or asystole is recognized. Even a short delay in providing proper therapy may result in a resuscitation with poor outcome.

## Case 4: Epidural Hematoma

A 68-year-old woman without significant medical history presented for an outpatient knee arthroscopy and debridement. The anesthesiologist discussed spinal anesthesia with the patient, who accepted. A 25-gauge pencil-point needle was used. The anesthesiologist attempted the spinal needle insertion at L4-5, L3-4, and L2-3. After marked technical difficulty, successful subarachnoid access and injection was done at L2-3. The surgery and intraoperative anesthetic course were uneventful. However, 1 hour postoperatively, the patient complained of chest pain and she was noted to be in atrial fibrillation. An angiogram revealed a pulmonary embolism. The medical consultant recommended admission of the patient and anticoagulation with heparin. That evening the patient complained of back and leg pain and was started on patient-controlled analgesia with morphine. This resulted in some relief, but the following morning, a motor and sensory neural deficit was discovered in both legs. Emergency magnetic resonance imaging of the lumbar spine revealed an epidural hematoma at L5 extending to L1.

### *Discussion*

Many patients who present for elective or emergency surgery are receiving or will receive drugs that alter coagulation for treatment of coexisting diseases. This is important and something that all practicing regional anesthesiologists must have a strategy for handling. However, what makes this issue a growing concern is the fact that many of the surgical procedures for which we routinely administer regional anesthetics are associated with postoperative thromboembolic events, and our patients typically receive drugs to help prevent these events. Orthopedic, obstetric, urologic, and many general surgical procedures are associated with high incidences of deep venous thrombosis. We are now aware that pulmonary embolism is the leading cause of perioperative mortality in patients who have undergone elective total hip arthroplasty.[59] Because of this, we are becoming more aggressive and successful in reducing the incidence of postoperative thromboembolic events through the use of perioperative, prophylactic anticoagulant and antiplatelet drugs.

One of our most potent means of reducing postoperative deep venous thrombosis (DVT) and pulmonary embolism is the use of epidural or spinal anesthesia. This has been clearly demonstrated in orthopedic patients undergoing repair of fractures or joint-replacement surgery.[60,61] Regional anesthesia can reduce the incidence of DVT by approximately 50%. Numerous pharmacologic techniques have also been used and combined with regional anesthesia in attempts to further this reduction in DVT. These include antiplatelet drugs, warfarin, and heparin. Most recently, fragments of the heparin molecule called low-molecular-weight heparins (LMWHs) have been produced and are being used in a more widespread manner.

It is important for us to understand the risk to our patients of using such anticoagulant regimens if they are also to receive axial regional anesthetics. The problem is that the scientific literature presently cannot answer the question. In fact, the incidence of spinal or epidural hematoma associated with regional anesthesia has been estimated as less than 1 in 10,000.[62] Thus, to get an adequate power for appropriate statistical analysis, it is necessary to study hundreds of thousands of patients in order to estimate the risk of our practice. This has added importance following the reports of development of hematomas secondary to withdrawal of epidural catheters. Therefore, we may not be safe even in the postoperative period with epidural analgesic infusions.

Some authors have cited articles as being definitive studies that show or argue that there is no heightened risk of epidural or spinal hematoma with concomitant anticoagulant use.[63] One must be careful in making conclusions based on available scientific publications. One example is the claim made by Odoom and Sih[64] from their study of regional anesthesia and perioperative warfarin use. They performed a retrospective review of only 1000 patients. There may have been underreporting of serious complications. In the published report, they stated, "It is concluded that, provided adequate precautions are taken, epidural anesthesia can be safely used in patients receiving anticoagulant therapy." This irresponsible conclusion is simply unfounded based on this study of grossly inadequate power to answer such a question. This is a potentially devastating complication and practitioners can be falsely reassured by such publications.

### Are Anticoagulants Associated with an Increased Risk of Spinal or Epidural Hematoma During Regional Anesthesia?

Association of the development of spinal or epidural hematoma with anticoagulant use has been based on either theory or sporadic case reports. In one review of case reports, Mayumi and Dohi[65] identified 13 cases of spinal hematoma (Table 22-1). Of these case reports, five were associated with the use of heparin. In one case report, the patient had been given an antiplatelet drug. This article may be misleading, however, because there may have been selective reporting of cases.

In a comprehensive review of the literature by Vandermeulen et al.,[77] the experience from 1906 to 1994 was analyzed. Forty-two of 61 patients with reported spinal or epidural hematoma had hemostatic abnormalities. Placement of either the needle or catheter was cited as being difficult in 25% and bloody in 25%. Thus, of the 61 reported cases, 53 (87%) had some associated abnormality.

It is important to recognize that regional anesthesia is a technical specialty. Technique seems to be a factor in many of the reported cases of spinal or epidural hematoma. One typical case was detailed in Mayumi and Dohi's review. A 70-year-old woman had a toe amputation. Ticlopidine (an antiplatelet drug) was started 10 days before surgery. Several laboratory indices of coagulation, including bleeding time, were within normal limits. However, several attempts were made to perform a lumbar spinal anesthetic, and postoperatively a spinal hematoma was identified at the T10 level.

Rao and El-Etr[78] performed a study that is frequently quoted in the anesthesia literature. During the period from 1973 to 1978, 3164 epidurals and 847 continuous spinal anesthetics were studied. Fifty to sixty minutes after placement of the epidural or spinal, 5000 units of heparin were administered to each patient every 3 minutes to achieve therapeutic anticoagulation, defined by an activated clotting time that was twice the normal value. There were no epidural or spinal hematomas identified.

Horlocker and Wedel[79] published a retrospective analysis of 188 patients who received postoperative warfarin after epidural catheters were in place. No incidents of spinal hematoma were identified. But this study was retrospective and only a small number of patient charts were reviewed.

TABLE 22-1. Spinal Subarachnoid Hematoma after Lumbar Puncture: A Review of Case Reports

| Reference | Age of patient (years) | Site of puncture | Underlying disease | Etiologic factors |
|---|---|---|---|---|
| Courtin[66] | 20 | ? | Syphilis | ? |
| Hammes[67] | 34 | L3-4 | Meningitis | Multiple puncture |
| King and Glas[68] | 63 | ? | Cirrhosis, diabetes mellitus, hypertension | ? |
| Joosten et al.[69] | 74 | L4-5 | ? | Anticoagulant therapy |
| Rengachary and Murphy[70] | 64 | L1-2 | Fractured femur | ? |
| Kirkpatrick and Goodman[71] | 56 | L3-4 | T12 compression fracture | ? |
| Sadjadpour[72] | 61 | ? | Pulmonary embolism, TIA | Heparin |
| Collmann and Rimpau[73] | 36 | ? | Chronic renal failure | Heparin, difficult lumbar puncture |
| Diaz et al.[74] | 55 | ? | Cerebrospinal fluid blockade | Heparin |
| Masdeu et al.[75] | 61 | L4-5 | Leukemia | Thrombocytopenia |
| | 29 | ? | Diabetes mellitus, frontal subdural hematoma | Multiple lumbar punctures |
| Brem et al.[76] | 81 | ? | TIA | Heparin |
| | 63 | ? | TIA | Heparin |

*Source:* Reproduced from Mayumi and Dohi,[65] with permission from Lippincott Williams & Wilkins.
TIA, transient ischemic attack.

### Antiplatelet Drugs

Because of the difficulty of studying sufficient patient numbers to identify a risk of spinal hematoma, in the subsequent study, Horlocker et al.[62] instead looked at the incidence of *minor* hemorrhagic complications (blood in needle or catheter). They found no documented spinal hematomas or serious neurologic sequelae. There was, however, blood noted in the catheter or needle in 22% of patients. Preoperative antiplatelet therapy did *not* increase the incidence of bloody needles or catheters. Although the term "minor hemorrhagic complication" was coined by these authors, I am not certain if these occurrences can be correctly termed "complications." The meaning of their findings is unclear because the appearance of blood in the needle or catheter is a predictable event and has never been linked to serious sequelae.

### Low-molecular-weight Heparin

LMWHs are being used on an increasing basis for surgical thromboprophylaxis. The increasing popularity can be attributed to increased bioavailability of the drugs compared with conventional unfractionated heparin. The drug preparations are also characterized by longer half-lives and less antiplatelet activity. According to a Danish survey, 60% of anesthetic departments in Denmark used spinal or epidural anesthesia with LMWH. A 10-year European experience with LMWH has identified six cases of spinal hematomas. Recently, LMWH was approved in the United States. Based on efficacy studies, higher doses than those used routinely in Europe were approved by the Food and Drug Administration. This has resulted in a longer active drug half-life which is more likely to extend the drug activity to the time of postoperative epidural catheter removal. These may be the reasons that in the first 18 months of the United States experience, the same number of spinal hematomas, six, as were reported in Europe were identified in a mere 18 months. This translates to a very significant approximate incidence of spinal hematoma of 0.1%.

According to the most recent guidelines developed at the ASRA Consensus Conference on Neuraxial Anesthesia and Anticoagulation,[80] patients receiving preoperative LMWH thromboprophylaxis should have needle placement deferred for at least 10–12 hours after the last dose. Higher-dose regimens of LMWH (e.g., enoxaparin 1 mg/kg daily) require delays of at least 24 hours before needle placement.

### Conclusion

Regional anesthesia is deliberately used in patients at risk for postoperative deep venous thrombosis for its demonstrated benefits. Increasingly, these same patients are receiving concomitant drugs with anticoagulant effects. Although it has not been and may never be definitively demonstrated that these patients are at an increased risk for serious spinal hematoma, there is considerable evidence in isolated case reports of an association of spinal hematoma and anticoagulant use. There is a theoretical and case report–based link of anticoagulant use with spinal or epidural hematoma. Trauma during epidural needle, spinal needle, or epidural or spinal catheter insertion has been associated with hematoma formation. In all likelihood, technical difficulty in block placement places patients at an increased risk of this serious complication.

If necessary to administer spinal or epidural anesthesia to patients receiving heparin, warfarin, or LMWH, careful monitoring of prothrombin time and partial thromboplastin time should be done. Care in placement and removal of the epidural catheter should be taken. If symptoms or signs of epidural hematoma occur, aggressive diagnostic and therapeutic measures must be taken without delay. A delay of a few hours can lead to irreversible neurologic deficit.

## Case 5: High Epidural/Total Spinal

A 54-year-old man was scheduled for femoropopliteal bypass grafting. His medical history was notable for hypertension and chronic obstructive pulmonary disease attributed to a 50-pack-year smoking history. Because of his chronic obstructive pulmonary disease, an epidural anesthetic was chosen. Epidural anesthesia was administered at the L3-4 interspace with 0.5% bupivacaine with added epinephrine. Fifteen milliliters of the local anesthetic was injected through the 17-gauge epidural needle with the patient in the lateral decubitus position. Upon turning the patient supine, an additional 10 mL was injected through the catheter in 5-mL aliquots. Within 1 minute, the patient had difficulty speaking and the $Spo_2$ decreased to 82%. The anesthesiologist found that he could aspirate fluid freely from the epidural catheter. He intubated the patient but was unable to wean the patient from the ventilator until the following day.

### *Discussion*

High epidural or spinal anesthesia results in significant changes in cardiovascular and pulmonary physiology. It is predominately through effects on these two physiologic systems that high spinal or epidural anesthesia can pose such an immediate threat to patient well-being, capable of causing rapid morbidity or mortality if not recognized or treated expeditiously. The cardiovascular effects include precipitous decreases in blood pressure, heart rate, and cardiac output. The effects on heart rate secondary to block of cardioaccelerator nerves or rapid vasodilation causing reflex bradycardia are discussed above under Case 3. Pulmonary changes are dependent on the level of spinal or epidural anesthesia. Changes increase in magnitude as anesthetic level progresses from abdominal and thoracic respiratory muscle paralysis to diaphragmatic paralysis. With total spinal or massive epidural anesthesia, function of the medullary respiratory control center may be blocked, leading to respiratory failure.

### Pulmonary Effects of High Spinal Anesthesia

With more cephalad levels of epidural or spinal anesthesia, the chest wall muscles (rib cage and abdominal) are blocked – in extreme cases leaving the diaphragm to work alone. This approximates the situation in the quadriplegic patient. Under routine epidural anesthesia, the main muscle of respiration, the diaphragm, remains intact and therefore pulmonary function is little changed in most studies. This is in contrast to other regional anesthetics, for example, interscalene block and interpleural block, that affect the diaphragm by phrenic nerve paralysis and may have more profound effects on pulmonary function and chest wall mechanics.[32,34,81] Nevertheless, rib cage muscular contraction and diaphragmatic contraction coordinate during normal breathing to move the rib cage in a homogeneous manner.[82,83] If this coordination is interrupted, the characteristics of normal breathing will change.

In terms of their effects on respiration, epidural and spinal anesthesia can be considered similar entities. However, with lower doses or weaker local anesthetics (e.g., for obstetric analgesia), an epidural may result in a differential block with motor nerve function relatively preserved.[84] Indeed, one study by Freund et al.[85] found reductions in expiratory reserve volume of 48% with spinal compared with only 21% with epidural anesthesia to similar anesthetic sensory levels.

### Pulmonary Function

Conventional pulmonary function tests are relatively insensitive in detecting changes in the respiratory system caused by epidural anesthesia. Most studies to date suggest that routine spinal and epidural anesthesia have little effect on pulmonary function tests.[50] Urmey and McDonald[86] confirmed this in a recent study on 30 patients during high-dose (25–30mL lidocaine 2%) lumbar epidural anesthesia. Despite the large local anesthetic doses that resulted in a mean sensory level to pinprick of T-5.6, the mean decrease in FVC was only 176mL ($P < .05$) and peak expiratory flow rate decreased by just 0.34L/second ($P < .05$). Although these reductions were statistically significant, they are hardly of any clinical import. This is attributable to the fact that routine pulmonary function tests are much more dependent on lung mechanics than expiratory muscle activity. Indeed, $FEV_1$ is a clinically useful measurement in diagnosing lung pathology because of this dependence on the lung. The $FEV_1$ is therefore highly reproducible despite variations in expiratory effort. Conversely, $FEV_1$ is a relatively insensitive means of assessing changes in expiratory effort when this effort is compromised by epidural anesthesia.

This is supported by recent studies. Sundberg et al.[87] found that high thoracic epidural anesthesia that blocked T-1 through T-5 had little effect on FVC which decreased by about 300mL. $FEV_1$ had a similar diminution of only 200mL. Takasaki and Takahashi[88] found similar small reductions in respiratory function with cervical and thoracic epidural anesthesia.

### Expiratory Muscle Compromise and Diminished Cough

By contrast to the subtle changes that occur in pulmonary function tests, cough strength is markedly diminished by epidural anesthesia. We recently found that

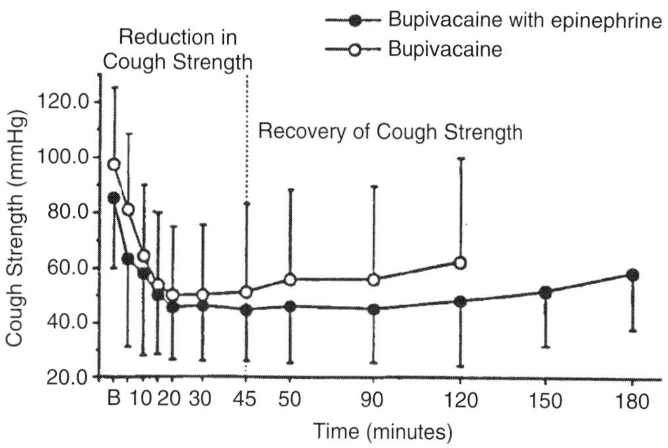


**FIGURE 22-2.** Reduction of cough strength as a function of time after epidural local anesthetic injection. (Reprinted from Finucane BT, ed. Complications of Regional Anesthesia. Philadelphia: Elsevier; 1999, with permission from Elsevier; adapted from Mineo R, Sharrock NE, Castellano P, Urmey WF. Effects of adding epinephrine to epidural bupivacaine assessed by thoraco-abdominal muscle strength. Reg Anesth 1990;15:S1.)

patients receiving 0.75% bupivacaine lumbar epidural anesthesia had an approximate 50% reduction in peak intrathoracic pressure during maximal cough[89] within 20 minutes of epidural injection (Figure 22-2). This is similar to the findings of Egbert et al.[90] who found a 53% reduction in intraabdominal pressure change with cough during spinal anesthesia. This occurs because of thoracoabdominal muscle paralysis during epidural anesthesia. Normal contraction of these muscles causes a rapid increase in intrathoracic pressure that produces acute turbulent airflow in the lung.[91] Therefore, the ability to cough effectively may be compromised by epidural anesthesia.

### Ventilatory Control

Normal ventilation is altered very little by epidural anesthesia. Only small changes occur in tidal volume, respiratory rate, minute ventilation, or arterial $P_{CO_2}$. Transient decreases in respiratory rate immediately after epidural injection have been reported. These transient changes may be attributable to increases in cerebrospinal fluid pressure.

Steinbrook et al.[92,93] studied $CO_2$ response in unpremedicated patients during spinal anesthesia. They found a small increase in the ventilatory response to $CO_2$. Anxiety, chest wall afferent neural blockade, and sedation all may contribute to altered minute ventilation during routine epidural anesthesia. Interruption of the medullary respiratory control center may occur during massive epidural or total spinal anesthesia. This will lead to rapidly progressive respiratory failure requiring immediate intervention and positive pressure ventilation.

### Cardiovascular Effects

Effects of high spinal or epidural anesthesia on the cardiovascular system can be largely attributed to interruption of preganglionic sympathetic nerves. This predictably results in arterial and venous vasodilation which decreases preload and afterload to the heart. Degree of systematic hypotension is dependent on the level of anesthesia; with more cephalad levels, increasing sympathetic denervation occurs. Change in blood pressure may also depend on preanesthetic volume status and supplemental drugs. Very early studies demonstrated that neuroaxial blockade resulted in diminutions in arterial blood pressure, cardiac output, stroke volume, and total peripheral resistance in volunteers.[94]

Carpenter et al.[51] prospectively studied 952 patients undergoing spinal anesthesia. The incidences of hypotension (defined as systolic blood pressure less than 90 mm Hg) and bradycardia (heart rate less than 50 beats per minute) with routine spinal anesthesia were investigated. These investigators found a 33% incidence of hypotension and a 13% incidence of bradycardia. These incidences were for a group of patients with a mean spinal anesthetic sensory level of T5 ± 3. With higher levels or total spinal anesthesia, hypotension and bradycardia would be more prevalent.

The effect of massive epidural or total spinal is to cause venous and arterial vasodilation. The result is a decrease in total peripheral resistance as well as cardiac preload. Without pharmacologic support, a significant decrease in stroke volume occurs. Cardiac output decreases despite the reduction in afterload. Sharrock and colleagues[56] characterized some of the changes in cardiovascular physiology in patients with epidural anesthesia levels at or above T4. Heart rate, mean arterial pressure, pulmonary artery diastolic pressure, cardiac index, stroke volume, and systemic vascular resistance all decreased in a statistically and clinically significant manner.

## Conclusion

Without vasopressor therapy, massive epidural or total spinal anesthesia will inevitably lead to circulatory collapse and cardiac arrest. It is therefore mandatory to diagnose the complications early and treat them aggressively. Combination $\alpha$- and $\beta$-agonists are recommended. Pure $\alpha$-agonists such as phenylephrine may cause further decreases in cardiac output[56] and may precipitate or worsen bradycardia. It is important to maintain preload at preanesthetic levels in these patients. Patient positioning can attenuate the effects of venodilation because of sympathectomy. Patients with conditions that inhibit effective venous return such as intraabdominal masses or pregnancy are more susceptible to large decreases in venous return during spinal or epidural anesthesia. Likewise, these patients may be very difficult to treat or resuscitate. Proper positioning, including lateral uterine displacement in the parturient, may be crucial in managing these patients.

## References

1. Selander D, Sjostrand J. Longitudinal spread of intraneurally injected local anesthetics. An experimental study of the initial neural distribution following intraneural injections. Acta Anaesthesiol Scand 1978;22(6):622–634.
2. Benumof J. Permanent loss of cervical spinal cord function associated with interscalene block performed under general anesthesia [case report]. Anesthesiology 2000;93: 1541–1544.
3. Winnie AP. Interscalene brachial plexus block. Anesth Analg 1970;49:455–466.
4. Aromaa U, Lahdensuu M, Cozanitis D. Severe complications associated with epidural and spinal anaesthesias in Finland 1987–1993. A study based on patient insurance claims. Acta Anaesthesiol Scand 1997;41:445–452.
5. Auroy Y, Narchi P, Messiah A, Litt L, Rouvier B, Samii K. Serious complications related to regional anesthesia. Anesthesiology 1997;87:479–486.
6. Horlocker T, McGregor D, Matsushige D, Schroeder D, Besse J. A retrospective review of 4767 consecutive spinal anesthetics: central nervous system complications. Anesth Analg 1997;84:578–584.
7. Kroll D, Caplan R, Posner K, Ward R, Cheney F. Nerve injury associated with anesthesia. Anesthesiology 1990;73:202–207.
8. Selander D, Dhumer K, Lundborg G. Peripheral nerve injury due to injection needles used for regional anesthesia. An experimental study of the acute effects of needle point trauma. Acta Anaesthesiol Scand 1977;21:182–188.
9. Selander D, Brattsand R, Lundborg G, Nordborg C. Local anaesthetics: importance of mode of application, concentration and adrenaline for the appearance of nerve lesions. Acta Anaesthesiol Scand 1979;23:127–136.

10. Rice A, McMahon S. Peripheral nerve injury caused by injection needles used in regional anaesthesia: influence of bevel configuration, studied in a rat model. Br J Anaesth 1992;69(5):433–438.
11. Broadman L. Where should advocacy for pediatric patients end and concerns for patient safety begin? [Editorial]. Reg Anesth 1997;22:205–208.
12. Giaufre E, Dalens B, Grombert A. Epidemiology and morbidity of regional anesthesia in children: a one-year prospective survey of the French-Language Society of Pediatric Anesthesiologists. Anesth Analg 1996;83:904–912.
13. Bromage P. Nerve injury and paralysis related to spinal and epidural anesthesia. Reg Anesth 1993;18:481–484.
14. Moore D. No paresthesias–no anesthesia, the nerve stimulator or neither? [Letter]. Reg Anesth 1997;22:388–390.
15. Moore D. Peripheral nerve damage and regional anesthesia [Editorial]. Br J Anaesth 1994;73:435–436.
16. Trentman T, Rome J, Messick J. Brachial plexus neuropathy following attempt at subclavian vein catheterization. Reg Anesth 1996;21:163–165.
17. Barutell C, Vidal F, Raich M, Montero A. A neurological complication following interscalene brachial plexus block. Anaesthesia 1980;35:365–367.
18. Urmey W, Stanton J. Inability to consistently elicit a motor response following sensory paresthesia during interscalene block administration. Anesthesiology 2002;96(3):552–554.
19. Choyce A, Chan V, Middleton W, Knight P, Peng P, McCartney C. What is the relationship between paresthesia and nerve stimulation for axillary brachial plexus block? Reg Anesth Pain Med 2001;26(2):100–104.
20. Mulroy MF, Mitchell B. Unsolicited paresthesias with nerve stimulator: case reports of four patients. Anesth Analg 2002;95(3):762–763.
21. Neal JM. How close is close enough? Defining the "paresthesia chad." Reg Anesth Pain Med 2001;26(2):97–99.
22. Bollini CA, Urmey WF, Vascello L, Cacheiro F. Relationship between evoked motor response and sensory paresthesia in interscalene brachial plexus block. Reg Anesth Pain Med 2003;28(5):384–388.
23. Brown D, Cahill D, Bridenbaugh L. Supraclavicular nerve block: anatomic analysis of a method to prevent pneumothorax. Anesth Analg 1993;76:530–539.
24. Scammell SJ. Case report: inadvertent epidural anaesthesia as a complication of interscalene brachial plexus block. Anaesth Intensive Care 1979;7(1):56–57.
25. Kumar A, Battit GE, Froese AB, Long MC. Bilateral cervical and thoracic epidural blockade complicating interscalene brachial plexus block: report of two cases. Anesthesiology 1971;35(6):650–652.
26. Cook LB. Unsuspected extradural catheterization in an interscalene block. Br J Anaesth 1991;67(4):473–475.
27. Ross S, Scarborough CD. Total spinal anesthesia following brachial-plexus block. Anesthesiology 1973;39(4):458.
28. Gentili M, Lefoulon-Gourves M, Mamelle J, Bonnet F. Acute respiratory failure following interscalene block: complications of combined general and regional anesthesia [letter]. Reg Anesth 1994;19:292–293.
29. Urmey W, Gloeggler P. Pulmonary function changes during interscalene block: effects of decreasing local anesthetic injection volume. Reg Anesth 1993;18:244–249.
30. Urmey W, Gloeggler P. Effects of bupivacaine 0.5% compared with mepivacaine 1.5% used for interscalene brachial plexus block [abstract]. Reg Anesth 1992;17:13.
31. Knoblanche GE. The incidence and aetiology of phrenic nerve blockade associated with supraclavicular brachial plexus block. Anaesth Intensive Care 1979;7(4):346–349.
32. Urmey W, Talts K, Sharrock N. One hundred percent incidence of hemidiaphragmatic paresis associated with interscalene brachial plexus anesthesia as diagnosed by ultrasonography. Anesth Analg 1991;72:498–503.
33. Pere P, Pitkanen M, Rosenberg PH, et al. Effect of continuous interscalene brachial plexus block on diaphragm motion and on ventilatory function. Acta Anaesthesiol Scand 1992; 36(1):53–57.
34. Urmey W, McDonald M. Hemidiaphragmatic paresis during interscalene brachial plexus block: effects on pulmonary function and chest wall mechanics. Anesth Analg 1992;74: 352–357.

35. Shaw W. Paralysis of the phrenic nerve during brachial plexus anesthesia. Anesthesiology 1949;10:627–628.
36. Winnie AP, Radonjic R, Akkinemi S, Durrani Z. Factors influencing the distribution of local anesthetics in the brachial plexus sheath. Anesth Analg 1979;58:225–234.
37. Robaux S, Bouaziz H, Boisseau N, Raucoules-Aime M, Laxenaire MC. Persistent phrenic nerve paralysis following interscalene brachial plexus block. Anesthesiology 2001;95(6): 1519–1521.
38. Bashein G, Robertson HT, Kennedy WF Jr. Persistent phrenic nerve paresis following interscalene brachial plexus block. Anesthesiology 1985;63(1):102–104.
39. Pere P. The effect of continuous interscalene brachial plexus block with 0.125% bupivacaine plus fentanyl on diaphragmatic motility and ventilatory function. Reg Anesth 1993;18:93–97.
40. Fackler CD, Perret GE, Bedell GN. Effect of unilateral phrenic nerve section on lung function. J Appl Physiol 1967;23(6):923–926.
41. Arborelius M Jr, Lilja B, Senyk J. Regional and total lung function studies in patients with hemidiaphragmatic paralysis. Respiration 1975;32(4):253–264.
42. Gould L, Kaplan S, McElhinney AJ, Stone DJ. A method for the production of hemidiaphragmatic paralysis. Its application to the study of lung function in normal man. Am Rev Respir Dis 1967;96(4):812–814.
43. Kreitzer SM, Feldman NT, Saunders NA, Ingram RH Jr. Bilateral diaphragmatic paralysis with hypercapnic respiratory failure. A physiologic assessment. Am J Med 1978; 65(1):89–95.
44. Hickey R, Ramamurthy S. The diagnosis of phrenic nerve block on chest X-ray by a double-exposure technique. Anesthesiology 1989;70(4):704–707.
45. Diament MJ, Boechat MI, Kangarloo H. Real-time sector ultrasound in the evaluation of suspected abnormalities of diaphragmatic motion. J Clin Ultrasound 1985;13(8): 539–543.
46. Loh L, Goldman M, Davis JN. The assessment of diaphragm function. Medicine (Baltimore) 1977;56(2):165–169.
47. Caplan RA, Ward RJ, Posner K, Cheney FW. Unexpected cardiac arrest during spinal anesthesia: a closed claims analysis of predisposing factors. Anesthesiology 1988;68(1): 5–11.
48. Reiz S. Pathophysiology of hypotension induced by spinal/epidural analgesia. In: Wust H, Stanton-Hicks M, eds. Anaesthesiology and Intensive Care Medicine: New Aspects in Regional Anesthesia. 4th ed. Berlin: Springer-Verlag; 1986.
49. Mackey DC, Carpenter RL, Thompson GE, Brown DL, Bodily MN. Bradycardia and asystole during spinal anesthesia: a report of three cases without morbidity. Anesthesiology 1989;70(5):866–868.
50. Greene N. Physiology of Spinal Anesthesia, Pulmonary Ventilation and Hemodynamics. Baltimore: Williams and Wilkins; 1981.
51. Carpenter RL, Caplan RA, Brown DL, Stephenson C, Wu R. Incidence and risk factors for side effects of spinal anesthesia. Anesthesiology 1992;76(6):906–916.
52. Frerichs RL, Campbell J, Bassell GM. Psychogenic cardiac arrest during extensive sympathetic blockade. Anesthesiology 1988;68(6):943–944.
53. Gold BS, Weitz SR, Lurie KG. Intraoperative "syncope": evaluation with tilt-table testing. Anesthesiology 1992;76(4):635–637.
54. Tarkkila P, Isola J. A regression model for identifying patients at high risk of hypotension, bradycardia and nausea during spinal anesthesia. Acta Anaesthesiol Scand 1992;36(6): 554–558.
55. Kopp SL, Horlocker TT, Warner ME, et al. Cardiac arrest during neuraxial anesthesia: frequency and predisposing factors associated with survival. Anesth Analg 2005;100(3): 855–865.
56. Sharrock NE, Mineo R, Urquhart B. Hemodynamic response to low-dose epinephrine infusion during hypotensive epidural anesthesia for total hip replacement. Reg Anesth 1990;15(6):295–299.
57. Sharrock NE, Go G, Mineo R. Effect of i.v. low-dose adrenaline and phenylephrine infusions on plasma concentrations of bupivacaine after lumbar extradural anaesthesia in elderly patients. Br J Anaesth 1991;67(6):694–698.
58. Chester WL. Spinal anesthesia, complete heart block, and the precordial chest thump: an unusual complication and a unique resuscitation. Anesthesiology 1988;69(4):600–602.

59. Huo M, Salvati E, Sharrock N, et al. Intraoperative heparin thromboembolic prophylaxis in primary total hip arthroplasty. A prospective, randomized, controlled, clinical trial. Clin Orthop 1992;274:35–46.
60. Tuman KJ, McCarthy RJ, March RJ, DeLaria GA, Patel RV, Ivankovich AD. Effects of epidural anesthesia and analgesia on coagulation and outcome after major vascular surgery. Anesth Analg 1991;73(6):696–704.
61. Sorenson R, Pace N. Anesthetic techniques during surgical repair of femoral neck fracture: a meta analysis. Anesthesiology 1992;77:1095–1104.
62. Horlocker TT, Wedel DJ, Schroeder DR, et al. Preoperative antiplatelet therapy does not increase the risk of spinal hematoma associated with regional anesthesia. Anesth Analg 1995;80(2):303–309.
63. Pham J, Montefiore A, Deschamps A. Low-molecular-weight heparin and epidural/spinal anaesthesia – is there a risk? Acta Anaesthesiol Scand 1994;38(3):303–304.
64. Odoom JA, Sih IL. Epidural analgesia and anticoagulant therapy. Experience with one thousand cases of continuous epidurals. Anaesthesia 1983;38(3):254–259.
65. Mayumi T, Dohi S. Spinal subarachnoid hematoma after lumbar puncture in a patient receiving antiplatelet therapy. Anesth Analg 1983;62(8):777–779.
66. Courtin RF. Some practical aspects of lumbar puncture. Postgrad Med 1952;12(2): 157–161.
67. Hammes E. Hemorrhage in the cauda secondary to lumbar puncture. Arch Neurol Psych 1920;3:595.
68. King OJ Jr, Glas WW. Spinal subarachnoid hemorrhage following lumbar puncture. Arch Surg 1960;80:574–577.
69. Joosten EM, Hommes OR, Meijer E. Spinal arachnoid blood clot as a complication following lumbar puncture in the course of anticoagulant therapy [Dutch]. Ned Tijdschr Geneeskd 1970;114(33):1364–1366.
70. Rengachary SS, Murphy D. Subarachnoid hematoma following lumbar puncture causing compression of the cauda equina. Case report. J Neurosurg 1974;41(2):252–254.
71. Kirkpatrick D, Goodman SJ. Combined subarachnoid and subdural spinal hematoma following spinal puncture. Surg Neurol 1975;3(2):109–111.
72. Sadjadpour K. Hazards of anticoagulation therapy shortly after lumbar puncture. JAMA 1977;237(16):1692–1693.
73. Collmann H, Rimpau W. Spinal subarachnoid haematoma following lumbar puncture. On the pathogenesis of postpuncture spinal bleeding (author's transl) [German]. Nervenarzt 1978;49(10):605–608.
74. Diaz FG, Yock DH Jr, Rockswold GL. Spinal subarachnoid hematoma after lumbar puncture producing acute thoracic myelopathy: case report. Neurosurgery 1978;3(3): 404–406.
75. Masdeu JC, Breuer AC, Schoene WC. Spinal subarachnoid hematomas: clue to a source of bleeding in traumatic lumbar puncture. Neurology 1979;29(6):872–876.
76. Brem SS, Hafler DA, Van Uitert RL, Ruff RL, Reichert WH. Spinal subarachnoid hematoma: a hazard of lumbar puncture resulting in reversible paraplegia. N Engl J Med 1981;304(17):1020–1021.
77. Vandermeulen EP, Van Aken H, Vermylen J. Anticoagulants and spinal-epidural anesthesia. Anesth Analg 1994;79(6):1165–1177.
78. Rao TL, El-Etr AA. Anticoagulation following placement of epidural and subarachnoid catheters: an evaluation of neurologic sequelae. Anesthesiology 1981; 55(6):618–620.
79. Horlocker TT, Wedel DJ, Schlichting JL. Postoperative epidural analgesia and oral anticoagulant therapy. Anesth Analg 1994;79(1):89–93.
80. Horlocker TT, Wedel DJ, Benzon H, et al. Regional anesthesia in the anticoagulated patient: defining the risks (the second ASRA Consensus Conference on Neuraxial Anesthesia and Anticoagulation). Reg Anesth Pain Med 2003;28(3):172–197.
81. Kowalski SE, Bradley BD, Greengrass RA, Freedman J, Younes MK. Effects of interpleural bupivacaine (0.5%) on canine diaphragmatic function. Anesth Analg 1992;75(3): 400–404.
82. De Troyer A, Estenne M. Coordination between rib cage muscles and diaphragm during quiet breathing in humans. J Appl Physiol 1984;57(3):899–906.
83. Urmey W, Loring S, Mead J, et al. Upper and lower rib cage deformation during breathing in quadriplegics. J Appl Physiol 1986;60(2):618–622.

84. Fink BR. Mechanism of differential epidural block. Anesth Analg 1986;65(4):325–329.
85. Freund FG, Bonica JJ, Ward RJ, Akamatsu TJ, Kennedy WF Jr. Ventilatory reserve and level of motor block during high spinal and epidural anesthesia. Anesthesiology 1967; 28(5):834–837.
86. Urmey W, McDonald M. Changes in pulmonary function tests (PFT) during high-dose epidural anesthesia [abstract]. Anesthesiology 1990;73:A1154.
87. Sundberg A, Wattwil M, Arvill A. Respiratory effects of high thoracic epidural anaesthesia. Acta Anaesthesiol Scand 1986;30(3):215–217.
88. Takasaki T, Takahashi T. Respiratory function during cervical and thoracic extradural analgesia in patients with normal lungs. Br J Anaesth 1980;52:1271–1276.
89. Sharrock NE, Castellano P, Sanborn K, Mineo R. Correlation of cough strength and hemodynamics with recovery from sensory block during epidural anesthesia [abstract]. Reg Anesth 1989;14(suppl):S87.
90. Egbert LD, Tamersoy K, Deas TC. Pulmonary function during spinal anesthesia: the mechanism of cough depression. Anesthesiology 1961;22:882–885.
91. McCool FD, Leith DE. Pathophysiology of cough. Clin Chest Med 1987;8(2):189–195.
92. Steinbrook RA, Topulos GP, Concepcion M. Ventilatory responses to hypercapnia during tetracaine spinal anesthesia. J Clin Anesth 1988;1(2):75–80.
93. Steinbrook RA, Concepcion M. Respiratory effects of spinal anesthesia: resting ventilation and single-breath $CO_2$ response. Anesth Analg 1991;72(2):182–186.
94. Ward RJ, Bonica JJ, Freund FG, Akamatsu T, Danziger F, Englesson S. Epidural and subarachnoid anesthesia. Cardiovascular and respiratory effects. JAMA 1965;191(4): 275–278.

# 23 International Morbidity Studies on Regional Anesthesia

Lorri A. Lee, Karen B. Domino, Kari G. Smedstad, Nils Dahlgren, Yves Auroy, Dan Benhamou, and Albert H. Santora

Morbidity studies concerning regional anesthesia have been published by authors in many countries. The purpose of the studies is to document the types of complications that are associated with the practice of regional anesthesia. The studies examine the causes and mechanisms leading to injury, the severity of the injury, the outcome with respect to recovery and survival, and the physician's culpability in relation to the morbid event.

By design, this chapter is multiauthored. The morbidity studies presented in this chapter are written by recognized authorities from various countries (except for the Australian data that are summarized by Santora). Each section of this chapter is referenced by authors' names and by country. References specific to each study are listed at the end of each section.

Interestingly, many of the larger morbidity studies compile and analyze data obtained from medicolegal sources. Information from this chapter will be analyzed and summarized in the book's final chapter that deals with the medicolegal aspects of regional anesthesia.

# Section 1

# Complications Associated with Regional Anesthesia: An American Society of Anesthesiologists' Closed Claims Analysis

Lorri A. Lee and Karen B. Domino

## Introduction

The American Society of Anesthesiologists' (ASA) Closed Claims Project is designed to systematically evaluate adverse anesthetic outcomes derived from detailed information from the closed claim files of 35 professional liability insurance companies in the United States since its inception.[1] Some companies may insure anesthesiologists in more than 40 states. Other sources are mainly statewide organizations that include both physician-owned and private companies. These organizations currently insure approximately 40% of the practicing anesthesiologists in the United States. There are currently more than 7000 claims for adverse outcomes that originated between 1970 and 2003 in the database. Approximately 2–5 years elapse between the occurrence of an adverse event and the closure of its associated claim, so there may be a significant time lag for analyses of specific events.

Trained practicing anesthesiologists visit each insurance company office to review claims files against anesthesiologists at periodic intervals and collect detailed information from standard data collection forms. Claims with enough information to reconstruct the sequence of events and to determine the nature and causation of injury are included. Claims without sufficient information and dental injury claims are excluded from the database. The closed claim files usually contain relevant hospital and medical records, depositions from involved healthcare personnel, expert and peer reviews, deposition summaries, outcome reports, and the cost of settlement or jury award. Reviewers assess the overall appropriateness of anesthetic care based on the standard of care at the time of the event, and its contribution to the injury. A severity of injury score is assigned to each claim that is designated by the onsite reviewer using the insurance industry's 10-point scale, where 0 = no injury and 9 = death. A score of 1 represents emotional injury; 2–4 reflect temporary injuries; 5 reflects permanent, nondisabling injuries; and 6–8 reflect permanent and disabling injuries. Onsite reviewers provide a summary of events. Data collection forms and summaries are then sent to practicing anesthesiologists of the Closed Claims Project Committee in Seattle,

Washington, U.S.A., where a minimum of two committee members review each claim, and any discrepancies between members regarding claims are resolved by a third member.

Data are then analyzed according to variables of interest including damaging event, patient demographics, procedure, severity of injury, etc. Specific limitations of this type of data analysis have been detailed elsewhere, but briefly include lack of denominator data, lack of a complete set of adverse anesthetic events, outcome bias, retrospective collection of data with information obtained from direct participants who may be biased, and somewhat low interrater reliability for assessment of standard of care.[2–4] However, the ASA closed claims database does allow analysis of rare events that would otherwise require impractical large multicenter long-term studies, and provides an overview of medical liability for anesthesiologists.[5]

## Complications Associated with Regional Anesthesia

Data for this analysis of the regional anesthesia claims were derived from the ASA Closed Claims Project database with date of claim event from 1980 to 1999, and have been described in detail elsewhere.[6] For purposes of analysis and comparison, inclusion criteria were: 1) any claim that involved regional anesthesia used for surgical or obstetric procedures (regional anesthesia group); and 2) any claim that involved general anesthesia or monitored anesthesia care for surgical or obstetric procedures (other surgical anesthesia group). Claims involving administration of both regional and general anesthesia were included in the group from which the complication resulted. Claims involving eye blocks for ophthalmic surgery were included in the regional anesthesia group if the block was administered by an anesthesia care provider. Claims resulting from eye blocks administered by surgeons (with monitored anesthesia care by the anesthesia personnel) were included in the group of other surgical anesthesia claims. Claims for chronic and postoperative pain management (n = 360) and obstetric claims involving only injuries to the baby (n = 131) were excluded from this analysis. The final analysis compared 1006 regional anesthesia claims to 3551 other surgical anesthesia claims.

Claims in this analysis were categorized according to damaging events (mechanisms of injury) and complications (injuries). Primary damaging events are the predominant mechanism of injury for any claim. Broad categories for damaging events include respiratory system events, cardiovascular system events, regional block–related events, equipment problems, drug administration errors, other anesthesia events, surgical events or patient condition, and none or unknown events. Specific damaging events included in the broad category of regional block–related damaging events were unintentional intravascular injection or absorption of local anesthetic, shearing or breaking of an epidural catheter, high block, inadequate analgesia from block, dural puncture, block needle trauma, and neuraxial cardiac arrest. Neuraxial cardiac arrest was defined for this analysis as the sudden onset of severe bradycardia or cardiac arrest during neuraxial block with relatively stable hemodynamics preceding the event without an apparent alternative causation.

Complications are the injuries for which the patient (plaintiff) is seeking compensation, and multiple complications may be involved in one claim. Death was considered the complication whenever it was associated with other injuries. Complications were categorized as nerve damage if there were clinical, anatomic, or laboratory findings consistent with damage to discrete elements of the spinal cord or peripheral nervous system.[7] Low back pain or muscle aches without specific neuroanatomic lesions were categorized as other complications, and were not included as nerve damage. Injuries of the neuraxis were defined as temporary or permanent insults to the spinal cord or neuraxis.

TABLE 23-1-1. Demographics of Regional versus Other Surgical Anesthesia Claims

| | Regional anesthesia (n = 1006) | | Other surgical anesthesia (n = 3551) |
|---|---|---|---|
| Age (years) | | | |
| Mean | 44 | * | 42 |
| Range | 0.25–94 | | 0–89 |
| | [n (% of 1006)] | | [n (% of 3551)] |
| ASA | | | |
| 1–2 | 548 (54%) | * | 1576 (44%) |
| 3–5 | 158 (16%) | * | 918 (26%) |
| Gender | | | |
| Female | 651 (69%) | * | 1949 (55%) |
| Male | 310 (31%) | * | 1579 (44%) |
| Obesity | 206 (20%) | | 670 (19%) |
| Emergency | 186 (18%) | | 610 (17%) |
| Obstetrics | 366 (36%) | * | 113 (3%) |

Percentages do not sum to 100% because of missing data (not shown).
*$P \leq .05$ between regional anesthesia and other surgical anesthesia groups.

### *Regional (n = 1006) Versus Other Surgical Anesthesia Claims (n = 3551)*

The demographics for the regional anesthesia group were heavily influenced by the large contribution (n = 366, 36%) from obstetric patients resulting in more ASA 1–2 and female patients, compared with the other surgical anesthesia group (Table 23-1-1; $P < .05$). Similarly, the overall technique in regional anesthesia claims (Figure 23-1-1) was significantly influenced by obstetrics, which involved predominately epidural anesthetics (70%, data not shown). In contrast, nonobstetric claims were associated with subarachnoid blockade (40%) more frequently than epidural anesthesia (27%, data not shown). Other techniques used in the nonobstetric group consisted primarily of upper extremity blocks, eye blocks, and intravenous regional anesthesia.

The proportion of claims with death or brain damage was significantly lower in the regional anesthesia group compared with the other surgical anesthesia group (22%

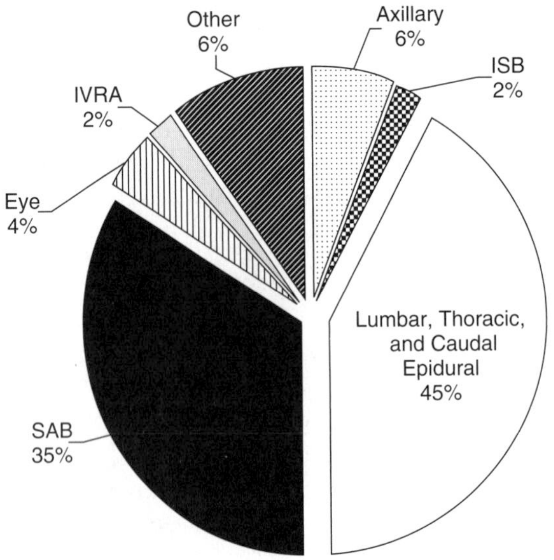


**FIGURE 23-1-1.** Type of technique for regional anesthesia claims 1980–1999 (n = 1006). Obstetric claims (n = 366) significantly influence the percentages, and resulted in more claims from epidural anesthesia than subarachnoid block. SAB, subarachnoid block; IVRA, intravenous regional anesthesia; ISB, interscalene block.

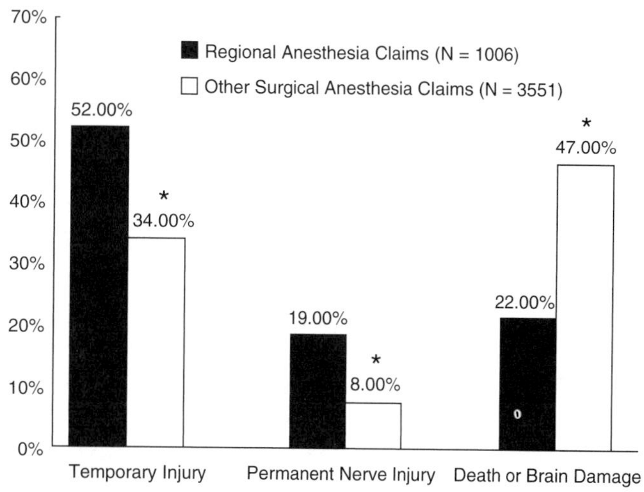


**FIGURE 23-1-2.** Outcomes in regional versus other surgical anesthesia claims 1980–1999. Claims for regional anesthesia (n = 1006) and other surgical anesthesia (n = 3551) are grouped according to severity of injury. Regional anesthesia had a greater proportion of claims for permanent nerve injury and temporary injury, and a lower proportion of claims for death or brain damage, than claims for general anesthesia. Other permanent injuries accounted for 7% (n = 72) of regional anesthesia claims and 11% (n = 386) of other surgical anesthesia claims (data not shown). *$P \leq .05$ regional versus other surgical anesthesia claims.

versus 47%, $P < .05$; Figure 23-1-2). Permanent nerve injuries (paraplegia, quadriplegia, peripheral nerve injuries) and temporary injuries (headache, back pain, temporary nerve damage, etc.) were significantly more common in the regional anesthesia claims compared with the other surgical anesthesia claims ($P < .05$).

Nearly half of the damaging events (n = 483) for regional anesthesia claims were block-related, which included block technique, neuraxial cardiac arrests, inadequate anesthesia and analgesia, high spinal/epidural, epidural/spinal catheter breakage, and unintentional intravascular injections or absorption (Table 23-1-2). Respiratory events

TABLE 23-1-2. Primary Damaging Events in Regional versus Other Surgical Anesthesia Claims

| | Regional anesthesia (n = 1006) n (% ) | | Other surgical anesthesia (n = 3551) n (%) |
|---|---|---|---|
| Block-related | 483 (48) | * | 1 (0) |
| Block technique | 249 (25) | | 1 (0) |
| Neuraxial cardiac arrest | 81 (8) | | |
| Inadequate anesthesia/analgesia | 48 (5) | | |
| High spinal/epidural | 40 (4) | | |
| Epidural/spinal catheter | 35 (3) | | |
| Unintentional intravenous injection | 30 (3) | | |
| Other anesthetic event | 123 (12) | * | 393 (11) |
| Cardiovascular event | 46 (5) | | 486 (14) |
| Respiratory event | 43 (4) | * | 1071(30) |
| Equipment | 18 (2) | * | 442 (12) |
| Surgical event | 40 (4) | | 139 (4) |
| Wrong drug or dose | 29 (3) | | 136 (4) |
| No event | 148 (15) | | 639 (18) |
| Unknown | 73 (7) | | 239 (7) |
| Multiple events | 3 (0) | | 4 (0) |

Surgical events include complications of surgical technique or patient condition, with no anesthetic contribution to the complication.
*$P \leq .05$ between regional anesthesia and other surgical anesthesia groups.

comprised the largest category of damaging events in the other surgical anesthesia group (30%), whereas only 4% of regional anesthesia claims had respiratory damaging events ($P < .05$).

### *Death or Brain Damage in Regional Anesthesia Claims (n = 217)*

The most common damaging events in regional anesthesia claims for death or brain damage were neuraxial cardiac arrest (n = 73, 34%) and unintentional intravascular injection (n = 12, 6%) [Figure 23-1-3]. Other block-related or anesthesia-related damaging events (high spinal/epidural) accounted for an additional 16 claims (7%). The remainder of these high-severity injury claims (n = 115, 53%) were associated with non-block-related damaging events. Claims for death or brain damage in the regional anesthesia group involved predominately neuraxial blocks [subarachnoid blocks (n = 108, 50%) and epidural blocks (n = 90, 41%)]. The remaining death or brain damage claims for the regional anesthesia group involved interscalene (n = 5, 2%), axillary (n = 3, 1%), and miscellaneous blocks (n = 11, 5%).

## Neuraxial Cardiac Arrest

Neuraxial cardiac arrest accounted for the largest category of block-related regional anesthesia claims with death or brain damage (34%). Of the 81 claims for neuraxial cardiac arrest collected from the 1980s and 1990s, 73 (90%) resulted in death or permanent brain damage. No significant difference was found between decades for age, ASA status, or severity of injury for neuraxial cardiac arrest. The most common regional technique in neuraxial cardiac arrest claims was subarachnoid blockade (n = 57), followed by lumbar epidurals (n = 20), caudal epidurals (n = 2), thoracic epidural (n = 1), and combined subarachnoid/epidural (n = 1). Eleven of 21 neuraxial cardiac arrest claims with lumbar or thoracic epidurals developed an unintentional subarachnoid block. These findings demonstrate that 68 of 81 neuraxial cardiac arrest claims (84%) were associated with either an intentional or unintentional subarachnoid block.

To examine potential risk factors for neuraxial cardiac arrest, associated factors for the 31 claims from the 1990s were examined when both capnography and pulse

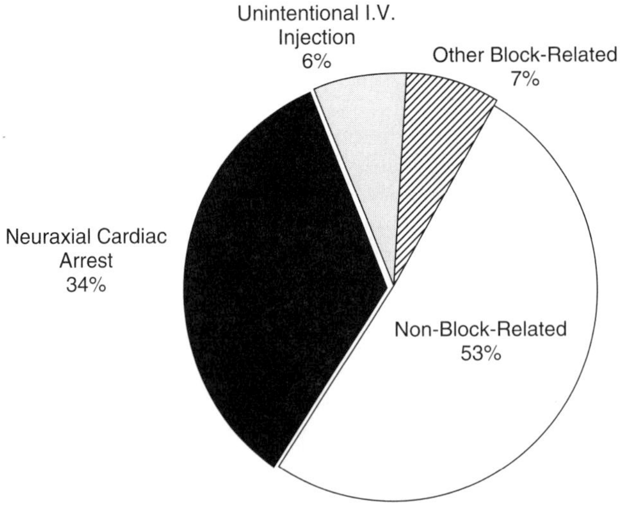


**FIGURE 23-1-3.** Regional anesthesia death or brain damage claims 1980s and 1990s: primary damaging events (n = 217). Other block/anesthesia-related events include high spinal/epidural block and regional block technique. Non-block-related events include other cardiovascular event (such as pulmonary/air/amniotic embolus, stroke, hypotension, myocardial infarction), n = 36; inadequate ventilation, n = 24; wrong drug or dose, n = 10; surgical event/error, n = 9; bronchospasm, n = 7; allergic reaction, n = 7; and miscellaneous causes, n = 22.

oximetry monitoring were widely available and recommended as part of standard monitoring. Thirty-five percent (n = 11) of these cases occurred outside the operating room (nine cases in obstetrics and two cases in the recovery room). Pulse oximetry was used in 74% of these 31 neuraxial cardiac arrest claims (n = 23) and capnography was used in 35% (n = 11). Sedation was administered in 52% of these cases (n = 16). Recognition of neuraxial cardiac arrest was delayed in 26% of claims (n = 8) and resuscitation was delayed in 58% (n = 18).

Almost three-quarters of the block-related claims with death or brain damage in regional anesthesia claims were associated with neuraxial cardiac arrest. Recovery from this event remains poor in the ASA closed claims database. Only one of 14 neuraxial cardiac arrest cases described by Caplan et al.[5] in 1988 had a moderate to good neurologic recovery. At that time, oversedation during neuraxial anesthesia leading to cyanosis was thought to contribute to these cardiac arrests. Consequently, pulse oximetry was recommended for routine use when sedation was administered during neuraxial anesthesia. Early use of epinephrine in the treatment of sudden severe bradycardia with neuraxial anesthesia, and immediate treatment of cardiac arrest with a full resuscitation dose of epinephrine, were additional recommendations.

Although the 1990s claims more frequently mentioned utilization of capnography and pulse oximetry, outcomes were not significantly improved over the 1980s in our database. Despite the frequent identification of cardiac arrest by the presence of cyanosis, there is little evidence to suggest that inadequate oxygenation and/or ventilation is a common precipitating event for neuraxial cardiac arrest.[8,9] Utilization of pulse oximetry and/or capnography monitoring did not prevent an outcome of death or brain damage in most cases. These findings likely result from two factors. First, as described above, delays in recognition and treatment of neuraxial cardiac arrest continue to occur. Anesthesiologists must be vigilant for this complication and promptly utilize appropriate resuscitative maneuvers if monitors are to be of any benefit at prevention. Second, some cases of neuraxial cardiac arrest are known to occur with almost instantaneous onset of bradycardia/asystole without preceding arterial desaturation, leaving insufficient time for treatment before full cardiac arrest ensues. Therefore, monitoring may not avert all cases of neuraxial cardiac arrest. Because cases that recover completely are unlikely to result in claims, the success and failure rates of prompt resuscitation and monitoring cannot be determined from this database.

Although timely institution of appropriate treatment for neuraxial cardiac arrest has been associated with full recovery in several case studies, many patients are refractory to rescue.[8,10] These results may be explained by studies in dogs demonstrating that cardiac arrest during total spinal anesthesia is difficult to treat because of the intense sympathetic blockade which decreases circulating blood volume and reduces coronary perfusion pressure, thereby rendering cardiopulmonary resuscitation (CPR) ineffective.[11] Moreover, other studies in dogs have shown that neuraxial anesthetic blockade prevents an increase in epinephrine and norepinephrine catecholamine levels during cardiac arrest compared with controls without neuraxial blockade.[12] Consequently, both severe vasodilation and lack of an appropriate catecholamine response to stress make resuscitation during neuraxial cardiac arrest more difficult. These studies support recommendations regarding early use of epinephrine. In the 1990s neuraxial cardiac arrest claims, adequate resuscitation with epinephrine was delayed in 58% of claims. All cases of unintentional subarachnoid block involved a delay in either recognition or treatment of neuraxial cardiac arrest. However, the remaining 42% of cases did not seem to have a delay in treatment with epinephrine, and indicate that even early administration of epinephrine will not guarantee a good outcome during neuraxial cardiac arrest.

These findings are consistent with Rosenberg et al.'s dog study measuring coronary perfusion pressure during cardiac arrest under total spinal anesthesia with CPR after epinephrine administration.[11] Seven of eleven dogs demonstrated a coronary perfusion pressure ≥15 mm Hg, a strong predictor of myocardial resuscitation,[13] after 0.01 mg/kg epinephrine administration at 4 minutes after arrest, whereas 9 of 11 dogs had a coronary perfusion pressure ≥15 mm Hg when the dose of epinephrine was increased to 0.1 mg/kg at 6 minutes after arrest. Cardiac arrest studies in humans without total spinal blockade also indicate that high-dose epinephrine (0.2 mg/kg) administration is more likely to achieve coronary perfusion pressures ≥15 mm Hg, compared with standard-dose epinephrine, but it has had limited success in human trials.[14] It is unclear whether or not high-dose epinephrine would benefit neuraxial cardiac arrest patients. However, heightened awareness of the potential for neuraxial cardiac arrest during an unintentional subarachnoid block may decrease the time to appropriate treatment.

Two frequently suggested mechanisms to explain neuraxial cardiac arrest are: 1) left ventricle hypovolemia causing a paradoxical bradycardic response via stretch/mechanoreceptors (the Bezold-Jarisch reflex); and 2) blockade of the cardiac accelerator fibers with high sympathetic blockade >T4.[9] Baseline bradycardia and male gender have been shown to predispose patients to an increased occurrence of severe bradycardia (<40 beats per minute) under neuraxial blockade. These bradycardic episodes are widely distributed throughout the time course of cases of variable duration.[9] Therefore, patients undergoing a neuraxial anesthetic should be monitored with electrocardiogram and pulse oximetry for the entire duration of the case, and resuscitation drugs and equipment should be readily available.

#### Unintentional Intravenous Injections

Unintentional intravenous injection was the second most common mechanism of injury resulting in death or brain damage for regional anesthesia claims (n = 12). The vast majority of these cases occurred in the 1980s (n = 11) compared with the 1990s (n = 1). The anesthetics involved were all epidural blocks, and cardiac arrest occurred in 9 of 12 cases. Test doses were used in 10 of these blocks, but only three test doses contained epinephrine. Most claims (n = 9) were associated with obstetrics.

Surprisingly, there were no cases of direct intravascular injection during peripheral blockade for claims resulting in death and brain damage in our database. The higher frequency of unintentional intravenous injections observed in France during peripheral blockade compared with neuraxial anesthetics was associated with seizures only, and not death or brain damage.[15,16] Seizures, which subside with full recovery, are less likely to result in claims, and may explain the low number of peripheral nerve block claims (n = 3) associated with unintentional intravenous injections in the ASA closed claims database. The preponderance of obstetric patients developing this complication with epidural anesthesia may be explained by 1) an increased frequency of unintentional intravenous injections caused by the dilated epidural veins during labor, and/or 2) their physiologic vulnerability to the hemodynamic consequences of an unintentional intravenous injection. The use of epinephrine in test doses in laboring patients has been controversial in the past, and may explain the low proportion of cases where it was used (25%).[17,18]

### *Permanent Nerve Injuries in Regional Anesthesia Claims (n = 193)*

Permanent nerve injuries accounted for 19% (n = 193) of regional anesthesia claims compared with only 8% (n = 273) of other surgical anesthesia claims ($P \leq .05$). Lumbosacral nerve root injuries and paraplegia were the most common injuries encountered in the regional anesthesia group (Table 23-1-3), and significantly higher proportions of these nerve injuries were present in the regional anesthesia group compared with the other surgical anesthesia group ($P \leq .05$). In contrast, the proportions of ulnar nerve and brachial plexus injuries and quadriplegia were significantly increased in the other surgical anesthesia group ($P \leq .05$; Table 23-1-3).

TABLE 23-1-3. Permanent Nerve Injuries in Regional versus Other Surgical Anesthesia Claims

| | Regional anesthesia (n = 193) n (%) | | Other surgical anesthesia (n = 273) n (%) |
|---|---|---|---|
| Lumbosacral nerve root | 66 (34) | * | 6 (2) |
| Paraplegia | 49 (25) | * | 16 (6) |
| Brachial plexus | 22 (11) | * | 62 (23) |
| Ulnar nerve | 17 (9) | * | 106 (39) |
| Median nerve | 13 (7) | | 9 (3) |
| Femoral/sciatic nerves | 15 (8) | | 31 (12) |
| Radial nerve | 3 (2) | | 4 (1) |
| Quadriplegia | 0 | * | 20 (7) |

*$P \leqslant .05$ between regional anesthesia and other surgical anesthesia claims.

## Injuries to the Neuraxis (n = 84)

Hematoma was the most common cause of neuraxial complications in regional anesthesia claims (43%), and had poor neurologic recovery, with 89% of cases resulting in permanent deficit (Figure 23-1-4). Injuries of the neuraxis caused by anterior spinal artery syndrome and spinal cord infarct also had poor neurologic recovery. Unknown causes of injury to the neuraxis accounted for 12 of 13 cases with permanent injury. Other causes of injury to the neuraxis (e.g., cervical fracture after fall from table, arachnoiditis, transverse myelitis, intrathecal catheter, and direct needle trauma without hematoma) also resulted in 4 of 5 cases with permanent neurologic disability. Injuries that resulted in few permanent deficits included epidural abscess (25%),

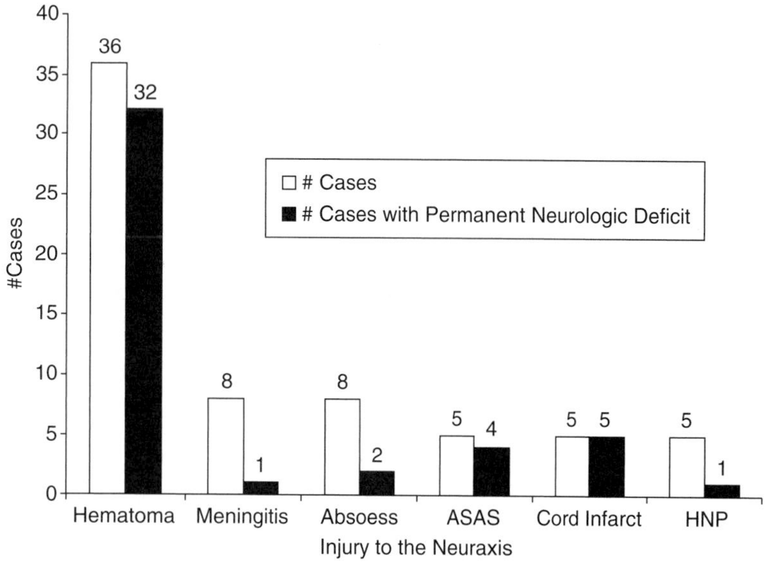


**FIGURE 23-1-4.** Injuries to the neuraxis from regional anesthesia claims 1980–1999 (n = 84). Hematoma was the most common cause of injury to the neuraxis with poor neurologic recovery. Infectious complications and herniated disc (HNP) had good neurologic recovery. Unknown causes of injury to the neuraxis accounted for 12 of 13 cases with permanent injury (data not shown). Other causes of injury to the neuraxis (e.g., cervical fracture after fall from table, arachnoiditis, transverse myelitis, intrathecal catheter, and direct needle trauma without hematoma) also resulted in 4 of 5 cases with permanent neurologic disability (data not shown). ASAS, anterior spinal artery syndrome; HNP, herniated nucleus pulposus.

herniated disc (20%), and meningitis (13%). Not surprisingly, hematoma cases (n = 36) were associated primarily with vascular (56%) and orthopedic (22%) procedures in which the use of anticoagulant therapy is high. Other procedures associated with hematoma were general surgery (11%), obstetrics (8%), and urologic (3%). Nonhematoma injuries to the neuraxis (n = 45) were most often associated with obstetrics (44%), followed by orthopedic (20%), urologic (16%), vascular (13%), and general surgical (7%) procedures.

Almost three-quarters (n = 26, 72%) of regional anesthesia claims with epidural or intraspinal hematomas had evidence of either an intrinsic or iatrogenic coagulopathy. Epidural catheters were removed in the presence of anticoagulation in six patients. Six of the 10 cases without a coagulopathy had signs of direct needle trauma in the cord above L1. Back pain was present in 25% of hematoma cases, increased sensory block in 53% of cases, and increased motor block was present in 83% of these claims. Mean number of days for diagnosis (postoperative day 2) was significantly longer than the mean number of days for the onset of symptoms (postoperative day 1, $P \leq .05$).

Injuries to the neuraxis caused by herniated discs and infectious complications (epidural abscess and meningitis) had a better neurologic recovery than injuries caused by hematoma, anterior spinal artery syndrome, and spinal cord infarction (Figure 23-1-4). The high proportion of cases in our database associated with hematoma and perioperative coagulopathy (intrinsic or iatrogenic) are consistent with Vandermeulen et al.'s[19] review of the literature in which they found that 42 of 61 (68%) neuraxial hematomas were associated with a coagulopathy. Intraoperative administration of heparin for vascular procedures was used in over half of our neuraxial hematoma claims. Three cases were given additional medications that can impair coagulation (aspirin, urokinase, Toradol, dextran, coumadin, and subcutaneous heparin) either preoperatively or postoperatively. The small number of hematoma cases (n = 2) associated with low-molecular-weight heparin may reflect the lag time from date of incident to date of entry into the ASA closed claims database. The two cases of intrinsic coagulopathy were caused by severe preeclampsia and von Willebrand's disease.

Despite these significant complications, neuraxial anesthesia for vascular surgery has been associated with significant patient benefits including reduced graft thrombosis and improved graft blood flow.[20–22] Moreover, the safety of regional anesthesia for vascular surgery with anticoagulation has also been demonstrated with no epidural hematomas reported in approximately 6000 patients from three studies.[23–25] Because of the demonstrated benefits and safety, regional anesthesia will continue to be used for vascular surgery with anticoagulation. Careful risk–benefit assessments and appropriate informed consent should be made preoperatively. Coagulation parameters should be normalized before removal of indwelling neuraxial catheters in the postoperative period. Vigilance for this rare, but devastating complication must be maintained with prompt recognition of the symptoms of an epidural hematoma. Our data are consistent with other published studies demonstrating that an increased motor block out of proportion to the infused local anesthetic is the most common presenting symptom for epidural hematomas.[19,26] Concentrated local anesthetic infusions may diminish symptoms of back pain. Other less common symptoms include increased sensory block, and bowel and bladder dysfunction. Patients with increasing neuraxial blockade without changes in the local anesthetic infusion, or with neuraxial blocks out of proportion to the local anesthetic being used (especially increased motor block), should be evaluated immediately for the presence of a neuraxial hematoma. Magnetic resonance imaging (MRI) is the most sensitive radiologic study for diagnosing these lesions. Neurologic recovery from epidural hematomas is thought to be primarily dependent on the time from symptom onset to decompression. Waiting until the next morning for resolution of the block after discontinuation of the local anesthetic infusion can waste valuable time. Prompt diagnosis and treatment are essential to a good outcome.

Direct needle trauma continues to be a significant source of spinal cord injury. Some of these cases may be explained by the anatomic variability among patients in the location of the end of the spinal cord (T12 to L3),[27] and in the iliac crest alignment with lumbar interspaces (L4-5 to L3-4).[28] The study by Broadbent et al.[29] demonstrated that anesthetists were able to identify the correct lumbar interspace by palpation in only 29% of 100 patients undergoing MRI scans. Anesthetists in this study labeled the lumbar interspace one level higher (cephalad) than the correct location in half of these cases. In some cases, the labeled interspaces were up to four levels higher than the correct location. Moreover, the spinal cord terminated below L1 in 19% of patients. Based on these studies, needle insertion at the most caudad suitable interspace may reduce direct needle trauma to the cord, particularly in obese patients where landmarks may be difficult to palpate.

### *Temporary Injuries in Regional Anesthesia Claims (n = 521)*

Obstetrics was associated with 50% (n = 259) of temporary injury claims in the regional anesthesia group, compared with 3% (n = 35) in the other surgical anesthesia group. The most common temporary injuries in obstetric patients in the regional anesthesia group were headache (32%), back pain (22%), nerve damage (17%), inadequate analgesia (17%), and emotional distress (14%). The most common temporary injuries in nonobstetric patients in the regional anesthesia group (n = 265) were nerve damage (36%), headache (14%), back pain (11%), and emotional distress (7%).

The majority of claims in the regional anesthesia group were associated with temporary injuries, such as headache, back pain, inadequate analgesia, and emotional distress, primarily from obstetrics. A higher proportion of minor injuries were present in obstetric patients (83%) compared with nonobstetric patients (35%). In contrast, nonobstetric patients had a higher proportion of claims associated with nerve damage (36%) compared with the obstetric group (17%). These differences may partially be explained by the physiology of laboring females who are at increased risk for postdural puncture headache and back pain,[30,31] and by the limitations in administering systemic intravenous or inhalational anesthesia in the obstetric population. In addition to these physiologic and safety issues, the high expectations of some women for childbirth to be a beautiful experience may make them less tolerant of minor complications compared with the group of nonobstetric patients who primarily receive anesthesia for surgery for pathologic conditions.

### *Eye Injuries in Regional Anesthesia Claims (n = 48)*

Eye injuries after blocks performed by anesthesiologists comprised 4% of all regional anesthesia claims (Chapter 6). Cataract extraction and/or intraocular lens implant was the most common procedure associated with eye injury claims (n = 39, 81%), followed by other or unknown eye surgery (n = 6, 13%). Three claims (6%) were for nonocular procedures associated with lumbar epidurals (two claims were unrelated to the regional anesthetic, and one claim was for a cerebrovascular accident causing visual deficits with postoperative lumbar epidural analgesia). There were significantly more claims involving eye surgery from the 1990s (n = 35) compared with the 1980s (n = 10, $P \leq .01$). Retrobulbar blocks were the most frequently utilized anesthetic for the 45 eye surgery claims (64%) followed by peribulbar blocks (27%), and other or unspecified eye blocks (9%). Eye injuries associated with blocks were predominately high severity with 82% of claims associated with permanent injury, and 62% of claims associated with blindness of the injured eye. Regional block technique was the most common damaging events (n = 40, 89%) with few claims associated with patient movement (n = 3, 7%). There was no identifiable damaging event in the remainder of claims (n = 2, 4%).

Claims associated with eye blocks have significantly increased during the 1990s compared with the 1980s, and their severity of injury is generally high and associated

Table 23-1-4. Payment Factors for Regional versus Other Surgical Anesthesia Claim

| | % Payment | Median payment (range) | % Appropriate care | % Payment in cases with appropriate care |
|---|---|---|---|---|
| Regional (n = 1,006) | 44* | $90,000* ($134.00–$6M) | 61* | 29* |
| Other surgical (n = 3,551) | 55 | $120K ($25.00–23.2M) | 47 | 36 |

*$P \leq .05$ between regional anesthesia and other surgical anesthesia groups.

with the block technique. Some studies have suggested that the sub-Tenon's block is a safer block compared with retrobulbar and peribulbar eye blocks, but large randomized controlled trials are currently lacking.[32] The increased use of topical anesthetics for cataract procedures may reduce complications associated with eye blocks to a greater extent than a change in block technique.

### *Liability*

Cases associated with regional anesthesia had a significantly lower percentage of claims with payment to the plaintiff compared with the other surgical anesthesia group, a lower median payment, a higher percentage of claims judged with appropriate care standards, and a lower percentage of payment of cases with appropriate standard of care (Table 23-1-4). These differences may reflect the greater proportion of regional anesthesia claims with temporary injury compared with other surgical anesthesia claims.

## Conclusion

Most injuries associated with regional anesthesia claims are temporary, and related to obstetrics. However, block-related complications, including neuraxial cardiac arrest, inadvertent intravenous injections, and neuraxial hematomas, continue to result in significant patient injury and death. Delay in recognition of a neuraxial cardiac arrest and/or resuscitation occurred in more than half of the cases, and contributed to poor outcome. Most cases were associated with either intentional or unintentional subarachnoid blockade. Almost all regional anesthesia claims associated with inadvertent intravenous injections were related to epidural anesthetics for obstetrics, and only one quarter of claims utilized epinephrine in the test doses. There was a significant delay from symptom onset to diagnosis for neuraxial hematomas, and almost all of these claims resulted in permanent neurologic injury. Anesthesiologists must be vigilant for these high-severity injuries and adequately monitor patients undergoing regional anesthesia.

## References

1. Cheney FW. The American Society of Anesthesiologists Closed Claims Project. What have we learned, how has it affected practice, and how will it affect practice in the future? Anesthesiology 1999;91:552–556.
2. Caplan RA, Posner KL, Cheney FW. Effect of outcome on physician judgments of appropriateness of care. JAMA 1991;265:1957–1960.
3. Cheney FW, Posner K, Caplan RA, et al. Standard of care and anesthesia liability. JAMA 1989;261:1599–1603.

4. Lee LA, Domino KB. The Closed Claims Project. Has it influenced anesthetic practice and outcome? Anesthesiol Clin North Am 2002;20:485–501.
5. Caplan RA, Ward RJ, Posner KL, et al. Unexpected cardiac arrest during spinal anesthesia: A closed claims analysis of predisposing factors. Anesthesiology 1988;68:5–11.
6. Lee LA, Posner KL, Domino KB, et al. Injuries associated with regional anesthesia in the 1980s and 1990s. Anesthesiology 2004;101:143–152.
7. Cheney FW, Domino KB, Caplan RA, et al. Nerve injury associated with anesthesia: a closed claims analysis. Anesthesiology 1999;90:1062–1069.
8. Lovstad R, Granhus G, Hetland S. Bradycardia and asystolic cardiac arrest during spinal anaesthesia: a report of five cases. Acta Anaesthesiol Scand 2000;44:48–52.
9. Lesser JB, Sanborn KV, Valskys R, et al. Severe bradycardia during spinal and epidural anesthesia recorded by an anesthesia information management system. Anesthesiology 2003;99:859–866.
10. Geffin B, Shapiro L. Sinus bradycardia and asystole during spinal and epidural anesthesia: a report of 13 cases. J Clin Anesth 1998;10:278–285.
11. Rosenberg J, Wahr J, Sung C, et al. Coronary perfusion pressure during cardiopulmonary resuscitation after spinal anesthesia in dogs. Anesth Analg 1996;82:84–87.
12. Rosenberg J, Wortsman J, Wahr J, et al. Impaired neuroendocrine response mediates refractoriness to cardiopulmonary resuscitation in spinal anesthesia. Crit Care Med 1998;26:533–537.
13. Paradis N, Martin G, Rivers E, et al. Coronary perfusion pressure and the return of spontaneous circulation in human cardiopulmonary resuscitation. JAMA 1990;263:1106–1113.
14. Paradis N, Martin G, Rosenberg J, et al. The effect of standard- and high-dose epinephrine on coronary perfusion pressure during prolonged cardiopulmonary resuscitation. JAMA 1991;265:1139–1144.
15. Auroy Y, Narchi P, Messiah A, et al. Serious complications related to regional anesthesia: results of a prospective survey in France. Anesthesiology 1997;87:479–486.
16. Auroy Y, Benhamou D, Bargues L, et al. Major complications of regional anesthesia in France: The SOS Regional Anesthesia Hotline Service. Anesthesiology 2002;97:1274–1280.
17. Dain S, Rolbin S, Hew D. The epidural test dose in obstetrics: is it necessary? Can J Anaesth 1987;34:601–605.
18. Norris M, Ferrenbach D, Dalman H, et al. Does epinephrine improve the diagnostic accuracy of aspiration during labor epidural analgesia? Anesth Analg 1999;88:1073–1076.
19. Vandermeulen E, Van Aken V, Vermylen J. Anticoagulants and spinal-epidural anesthesia. Anesth Analg 1994;79:1165–1177.
20. Christopherson R, Beattie C, Frank S, et al. Perioperative morbidity in patients randomized to epidural or general anesthesia for lower extremity vascular surgery. Perioperative Ischemia Randomized Anesthesia Trial Study Group. Anesthesiology 1993;79:422–434.
21. Hickey N, Wilkes M, Howes D, et al. The effect of epidural anaesthesia on peripheral resistance and graft flow following femorodistal reconstruction. Eur J Vasc Endovasc Surg 1995;9:93–96.
22. Tuman K, McCarthy R, March R, et al. Effects of epidural anesthesia and analgesia on coagulation and outcome after major vascular surgery. Anesth Analg 1991;73:696–704.
23. Rao T, El-Etr A. Anticoagulation following placement of epidural and subarachnoid catheters: an evaluation of neurologic sequelae. Anesthesiology 1981;55:618–620.
24. Odoom J, Sih I. Epidural analgesia and anticoagulant therapy: experience with one thousand cases of continuous epidurals. Anesthesia 1983;38:254–259.
25. Baron H, LaRaja R, Rossi G, et al. Continuous epidural analgesia in the heparinized vascular surgical patient: a retrospective review of 912 patients. J Vasc Surg 1987;6:144–146.
26. Wysowski D, Talarico L, Bacsanyi J, Botstein P. Spinal and epidural hematoma and low-molecular-weight heparin. N Engl J Med 1998;338:1774.
27. Saifuddin A, Burnett S, White J. The variation of position of the conus medullaris in an adult population. Spine 1998;23:1452–1456.
28. Render C. The reproducibility of the iliac crest as a marker of lumbar spine level. Anaesthesia 1996;51:1070–1071.
29. Broadbent CR, Maxwell WB, Ferrie R, et al. Ability of anaesthetists to identify a marked lumbar interspace. Anaesthesia 2000;55:1122–1126.

30. Lybecker H, Moller J, May O, et al. Incidence and prediction of postdural puncture headache. A prospective study of 1021 spinal anesthesias. Anesth Analg 1990;70:389–394.
31. Howell C, Dean T, Lucking L, Dziedzic K, Jones P, Johanson R. Randomised study of long term outcome after epidural versus non-epidural analgesia during labour. BMJ 2002;325:357–360.
32. Guise PA. Sub-Tenon anesthesia: a prospective study of 6,000 blocks. Anesthesiology 2003;98:964–968.

# Section 2
## American Society of Anesthesiologists' Closed Claims Project: Chronic Pain Management

Albert H. Santora

Fitzgibbon et al.[1] analyzed data "... to identify and describe issues and trends in liability related to chronic pain management by anesthesiologists."[1]

Data from 5475 claims collected between 1970 and 1999 were examined. Acute pain management claims were excluded from the study. Two categories of claims were analyzed and compared:

1. Surgical/obstetric: 5125
2. Chronic pain management: 284.

The following tables and figures summarize the study.

Table 23-2-1 lists the procedures administered in the chronic pain management claims. Note that of the 276 claims involving invasive procedures, 216 involved a block or injection (78%).

Table 23-2-2 lists injuries related to various chronic pain interventions.

Figure 23-2-1 documents common adverse outcomes associated with epidural injections. Note that death or brain damage was reported only when a local anesthetic with or without an opioid had been added to a steroid injection.

Table 23-2-3 presents a comparison of the chronic pain group with the surgical/obstetric group with respect to various parameters.

Figure 23-2-2 presents median payment data over two epochs.

### Summary of the Chronic Pain Management Closed Claims Analysis

1. Chronic pain management claims increased from 2% in the 1970s and 1980s to 10% of all claims analyzed in the 1990s.
2. There were no pediatric patients in the chronic pain management group.

TABLE 23-2-1. Procedures in Chronic Pain Management Claims (n = 284)

| | Claims | |
|---|---|---|
| | No. | % |
| Invasive procedures | 276 | 97 |
| Injections | 138 | 49 |
| Epidural steroids ± associated agents | 114 | |
| Trigger point | 17 | |
| Facet | 4 | |
| Other | 3 | |
| Blocks | 78 | 27 |
| Peripheral | 28 | |
| Stellate ganglion | 19 | |
| Other autonomic | 9 | |
| Neuraxial | 9 | |
| Upper/lower extremity | 7 | |
| Axial | 4 | |
| Head and neck | 2 | |
| Ablative procedures | 17 | 6 |
| Agent | 13 | |
| Technique | 4 | |
| Implantation or removal of devices | 12 | 4 |
| Implantable pump | 5 | |
| Nerve stimulator | 4 | |
| Catheter | 3 | |
| Device maintenance | 20 | 7 |
| Other interventions* | 11 | 4 |
| Noninvasive pain management | 8 | 3 |
| Medication prescription | 5 | |
| Opinion/diagnosis | 2 | |
| Cupping procedure | 1 | |

*Source:* Fitzgibbon, et al.[1] Reprinted from Anesthesiology. Used with permission from Lippincott Williams & Wilkins.
Total does not sum to 100% because of rounding.
*Includes three claims involving multiple procedures associated with complications. One of these claims involved invasive plus noninvasive pain management.

3. Most chronic pain management claims resulted in temporary or nondisabling injuries (76%).
4. During the 1990s, the size of payment for chronic pain management claims and surgical/obstetric claims was not significantly different.
5. Sixty-four percent of the chronic pain management claims resulted from injuries that were not apparent until after discharge from the treatment facility.
6. "Blocks and injections together accounted for 78% of claims related to invasive pain management."[1]
7. "Epidural steroid injections (±associated agents) accounted for 83% of injections and 40% of all chronic pain management claims."[1]
8. "Peripheral blocks and autonomic blocks each accounted for 36% (total 72%) of the 78 block claims."[1]
9. The most common complications for all invasive procedures were nerve injury and pneumothorax. Pneumothorax was the most common complication of trigger point injection.

TABLE 23-2-2. Primary Outcome for Invasive Pain Management Claims

| | All invasive procedures (n = 276) | | Blocks (n = 78) | | Injections (n = 138): Epidural steroid + agents (n = 114) | | Injections (n = 138): Trigger, facet, other (n = 24) | | Ablative (n = 17) | | Implant/removal (n = 12) | | Maintenance (n = 20) | | Other/multiple (n = 11) | |
|---|---|---|---|---|---|---|---|---|---|---|---|---|---|---|---|---|
| Outcome | No. | % | No. | % | No. | % | No. | % | No. | % | No. | % | No. | % | No. | % |
| Nerve injury | 63 | 23 | 14 | 18 | 28 | 25 | 2 | 8 | 8 | 47 | 2 | 17 | 4 | 20 | 5 | 45 |
| Pneumothorax | 59 | 21 | 40 | 51 | 0 | 0 | 18 | 75 | 1 | 6 | 0 | 0 | 0 | 0 | 0 | 0 |
| Infection | 35 | 13 | 2 | 3 | 24 | 21 | 0 | 0 | 0 | 0 | 3 | 25 | 4 | 20 | 2 | 18 |
| Death/brain damage | 26 | 9 | 4 | 5 | 9 | 8 | 0 | 0 | 1 | 6 | 0 | 0 | 9 | 45 | 3 | 27 |
| Headache | 21 | 8 | 1 | 1 | 20 | 18 | 0 | 0 | 0 | 0 | 0 | 0 | 0 | 0 | 0 | 0 |
| Increased pain/no relief | 21 | 8 | 7 | 9 | 10 | 9 | 0 | 0 | 0 | 0 | 2 | 17 | 1 | 5 | 1 | 9 |
| Retained catheter | 9 | 3 | 1 | 1 | 4 | 4 | 1 | 4 | 0 | 0 | 3 | 25 | 0 | 0 | 0 | 0 |
| None | 7 | 3 | 1 | 1 | 4 | 4 | 0 | 0 | 1 | 6 | 1 | 8 | 0 | 0 | 0 | 0 |
| Other | 42 | 15 | 8 | 10 | 18 | 16 | 3 | 13 | 6 | 35 | 1 | 8 | 4 | 20 | 2 | 18 |

*Source:* Fitzgibbon et al.[1] Reprinted from Anesthesiology. Used with permission from Lippincott Williams & Wilkins.
Epidural injection of steroids (±local anesthetic and opioids) and injections, including trigger point, facet, and others, are listed separately, with percentage shown for each separate category. Otherwise, the percentage of claims implies the percentage in each invasive procedure group. Totals sum to more than 100% because of multiple complications in some claims.

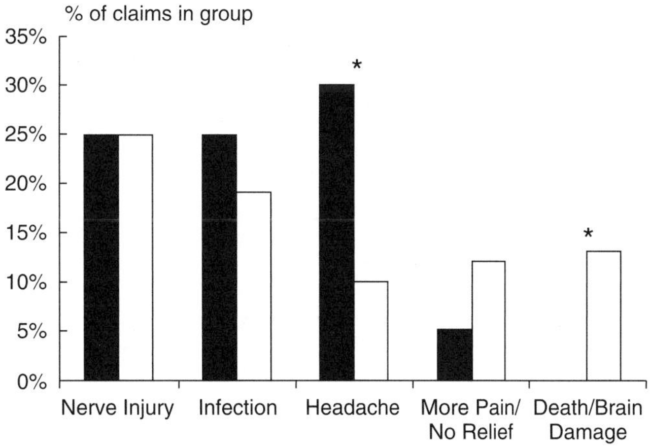


**FIGURE 23-2-1.** Most common outcomes in epidural injections. Solid bars represent injections with steroids only. Open bars indicate injections in which local anesthetic or opioid (or both) were added to the steroid. $^*P \leq .05$ between proportion of injection group with that outcome. (From Fitzgibbon et al.[1] Reprinted from Anesthesiology. Used with permission from Lippincott Williams & Wilkins.)

TABLE 23-2-3. Payment, Standard of Care, and Prevention: Chronic Pain Management versus Other Claims

| | Chronic pain (n = 284) | | Surgical/obstetric (n =5125) | | |
|---|---|---|---|---|---|
| | No. | % | No. | % | *P* value |
| Payment made to plaintiff | 142 | 53 | 2777 | 59 | NS |
| No payment | 126 | 47 | 1891 | 41 | NS |
| Standard care | 155 | 65 | 2501 | 56 | ≤.01 |
| Substandard care | 84 | 35 | 1934 | 44 | ≤.01 |
| Injury became apparent in anesthesia facility | 71 | 36 | 2166 | 83 | ≤.01 |
| Injury became apparent after discharge | 127 | 64 | 443 | 17 | ≤.01 |
| Complication preventable by better preanesthetic evaluation | 15 | 7 | 395 | 9 | NS |
| Not preventable by better preanesthetic evaluation | 213 | 93 | 4080 | 91 | NS |
| Complication preventable by better postanesthetic care | 26 | 12 | 431 | 11 | NS |
| Not preventable by better postanesthetic care | 195 | 88 | 3592 | 89 | NS |
| Appropriate informed consent documented | 141 | 66 | 2404 | 72 | NS |
| Appropriate informed consent not documented | 74 | 34 | 959 | 29 | NS |

*Source:* Fitzgibbon et al.[1] Reprinted from Anesthesiology. Used with permission from Lippincott Williams & Wilkins.
Claims in which items could not be assessed were excluded from analysis on an item-by-item basis. *P* values were calculated by % test.
NS = not statistically significant.

## Analysis of More Severe Outcomes

Some of the claims were associated with catastrophic outcomes.

1. Half of the 63 nerve injury claims involved the spinal cord.
   a. Fourteen were associated with epidural steroid injection (six resulting in paraplegia, one in quadriplegia)
   b. Five after blocks (two with paraplegia)
   c. One after cervical facet block
2. "Of the 18 claims for paraplegia or quadriplegia, 4 were associated with epidural abscess, 8 with chemical injury in which the anesthetic or neurolytic agent was injected into the spinal cord, and 4 with hematoma. Two of the claims for

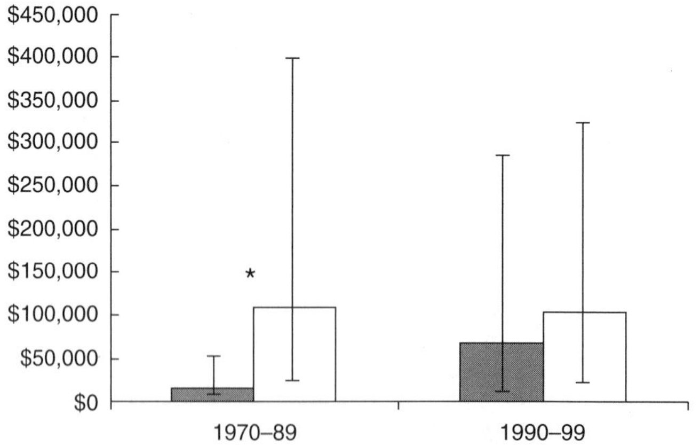


**FIGURE 23-2-2.** Median payment over different time periods. Bar heights indicate median payment (solid bars: chronic pain claims; open bars: surgical/obstetric claims); lines indicate 25th and 75th percentile payment ranges. Payment in chronic pain management claims was lower than payment in surgical/obstetric claims in 1970–1989. Payments between these groups did not differ in 1990–1999. $*P \leq .01$ between pain management and surgical/obstetric payments. (From Fitzgibbon et al.[1] Reprinted from Anesthesiology. Used with permission from Lippincott Williams & Wilkins.)

hematoma involved administration of epidural steroids in patients who received anticoagulants."[1]

3. Thirty-five claims involving infection were reported. Infection was most often associated with epidural steroid injection. Many of the infections reported were serious:
   a. Meningitis: 34%
   b. Epidural abscess: 20%
   c. Osteomyelitis: 9%
4. Nine of 26 claims resulting from death or brain damage involved an epidural steroid injection. Interestingly, only epidural steroid injections that contained local anesthetics with or without an opioid resulted in death or brain damage.
5. Use of a "test dose" was not standard practice.
6. "3 severe outcomes were the result of a delayed respiratory depression from epidural morphine administered along with the [epidural] steroid."[1]

## Conclusion

Fitzgibbon et al.[1] offered or implied relevant clinical suggestions based on the findings of their study:

1. A test dose should be used when administering a regional block.
2. The volume of solution injected into the epidural space [for pain blocks] should not exceed that of a typical intrathecal test dose.
3. The addition of local anesthetics and opioids to epidural steroid injections can lead to more severe outcomes (death and brain damage). Are these adjunctive drugs really necessary?
4. ". . . It is important to establish a monitoring system for pneumothorax and to instruct patients as to the symptoms and signs of a pneumothorax after intercostal nerve blocks, stellate ganglion blocks, trigger point injections, and brachial plexus blocks."[1]

## Reference

1. Fitzgibbon DR, Posner KL, Domino KB, Caplan RA, Lee LA, Cheney FW. Chronic pain management. Anesthesiology 2004;100:98–105.

# Section 3

## Complications of Regional Anesthesia Leading to Medical Legal Action in Canada

Kari G. Smedstad

Regional anesthesia is used frequently in Canadian operating rooms, labor suites, and pain clinics. Complications are not frequent, but do occur. Measures of complications are published reports, anecdotal evidence, and medial legal actions. This chapter describes the latter in the Canadian setting.

In Canada, all anesthesia services are provided by physicians. All legal actions against physicians are defended by the Canadian Medical Protective Association (CMPA). The CMPA is a Canada-wide medical mutual defense association for physicians. It is not an insurance company. Established in 1901, the CMPA is funded and operated on a not-for-profit basis by physicians and for physicians. More than 65,000 Canadian physicians are members of the CMPA, comprising about 95% of doctors licensed to practice in Canada. The medical legal situation in Canada is unique, and one cannot discuss litigation against anesthesiologists without describing briefly how CMPA works.[1]

Membership fees are set annually through a review of experience with claims and costs. The fees and income from investments fund a reserve to handle the cost of present and future claims. The CMPA is fully funded to pay for all claims related to the current and past years. Because the organization operates on an occurrence basis, members are eligible to receive assistance regardless of when a claim is made, including protection in retirement and against a member's estate. This protection also ensures that compensation is available for injured patients when they are eligible to receive a settlement or court award. The CMPA defense philosophy holds professional integrity first and foremost. The association will vigorously defend a member as long as there is good expert support for their medical care. Cases are not settled against physicians in Canada because of expedience or cost savings.

The CMPA Risk Management Services provides seminars and educational sessions for physicians of all specialties across Canada. Statistics and analyses of closed claims can be made available for study and educational purposes within the framework of the educational mission of the organization. Thus, the results published in this chapter are comprehensive and accurate. A review of closed claims in regional anesthesia in Canada has previously been published.[2] The cases that form the basis of this discussion have been updated to include closed claims from 1990 to 2002.

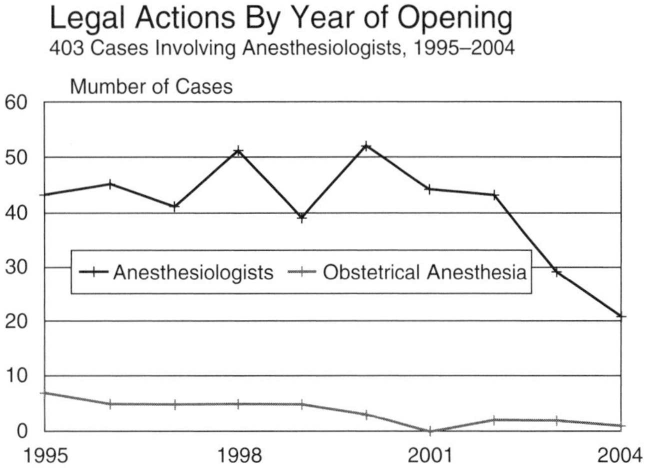


**FIGURE 23-3-1.** Anesthesia-related legal actions in Canada have decreased over the last 10 years. Legal actions related to obstetric anesthesia are very few in the same time period.

## Legal Cases Against Anesthesiologists

The risk of a legal action against an anesthesiologist in Canada is similar to the risk for the average physician; about 1 in 65 (2003) is sued every year. When threatened about a legal action or worried about a bad outcome or occurrence, anesthesiologists contact the CMPA and receive help with a variety of matters. These include advice, help with hospital privileges, complaints to provincial/territorial regulatory authorities, involvement in coroner's inquests, billing matters, and civil and criminal legal action related to the professional practice of medicine. Thus, only a very small proportion of files opened relate to civil legal actions. To put the figures related to regional anesthesia in context, the statistical review for 2003 shows that CMPA opened 15,127 new files, of which 1117 were legal actions. Only a small proportion of these cases actually proceed to trial.[3]

In 2003 there were 39 new legal actions commenced involving anesthesiologists. Most legal actions against anesthesiologists arise from general anesthesia cases. Twenty percent of all anesthesia claims in Canada are related to regional anesthesia, and only 13%, or 2–5 cases per year, come from obstetric anesthesia (see Figure 23-3-1).

In Canada, about 60% of cases that arise from anesthesia practice are dismissed, and approximately 30% of claims against anesthesiologists are settled. Cases are settled when expert support is lacking. Experts are peers who are familiar with the practice of anesthesiology relevant to the claim. The remaining 10% go to trial. When going to court, anesthesiologists win about 80% of cases, but the courts find against the doctor in the remaining 20%. CMPA protection provides no limit to the cost of legal help which the member is eligible to receive. Similarly, there is no dollar limit on damages paid to patients, but structured settlements are encouraged.

## Disabilities and Legal Outcome

Not all harm suffered by patients during anesthesia is attributable to negligent anesthetic care. Therefore, the severity of physical disabilities suffered by patients may not be related to the legal outcome of claims. Physical disabilities for the purpose of legal action in Canada can be classified as: minor: pain, scarring; major: disabilities that interfere with the activities of daily living; catastrophic: resulting in severe neurologic impairment; and death.

Legal outcomes are divided into four categories: 1. consent dismissal – plaintiff(s) withdraws or abandons the legal action before trial. 2. Settlement – legal action is resolved by way of a payment by CMPA on behalf of the defendant member before trial. 3. Judgment for the defendant – the court decides in favor of the defendant at trial (case won). 4. Judgment for the plaintiff at trial (case lost).

## Claims Experience in Regional Anesthesia

Twenty percent of medical legal actions in anesthesia are related to regional anesthesia. The legal outcome is overall better in these cases than in cases related to anesthesia in general – in that 80% are dismissed and only 11% are settled. Should the case go to court, the outcome is the same: 8 of 10 cases are won.

If the patient experiences a complication, even resulting in a significant disability, but there is no fault in the standard of care, the case is usually dismissed or won in Canada. Vigorous defense of doctors who practice within the standard of care results in fewer lawsuits. Good plaintiffs' lawyers in Canada know this, and most investigate the validity of a claim before taking the case.

Neuraxial blocks (spinal and epidural blocks) comprise the majority of cases that lead to medical legal difficulties. Peripheral nerve blocks also give rise to complications that may trigger complaints and lawsuits. Regional anesthesia is increasingly used in postoperative pain management, and recently we have seen cases arise from both acute and chronic pain management.

Cases arising after spinal and epidural anesthesia can fall into any of the four categories of outcome. Paraplegia is a catastrophic outcome. Postdural puncture headache (PDPH) is a "minor" outcome and, to date, no such case has been settled against a Canadian anesthesiologist. In contrast, in 3 of 4 cases of paraplegia resulting from an epidural anesthetic, the legal outcome was unfavorable to the physician.

Overall, the patient outcome from malpractice claims related to regional anesthesia was similar to that of all anesthesia claims, with a slightly higher percentage of patients suffering minor or major disabilities, but fewer catastrophic outcomes and deaths.

## Analysis of Regional Anesthesia Claims over a 20-year Period

The CMPA database allowed for analysis of closed claims related to litigation against anesthesia practitioners who performed regional anesthesia in Canada. The cases closed in the years 1990–2002, but the actual medical care or procedures that gave rise to these claims happened from 1977–2000. The average claim can take between 3 and 4 years to process and complete.

There were 77 cases related to regional anesthesia performed in operating suites or pain clinics across the country. The procedures were for intraoperative anesthesia, postoperative pain relief, or treatment of chronic pain. In addition, there were 41 cases arising from obstetric anesthesia and analgesia in the same period. These will be discussed separately.

Patients who sue doctors or hospitals do so for many reasons, but usually litigation arises when the patient or the family believes that the outcome of the procedure has caused damage. Unsatisfactory outcome will not in itself lead to legal actions; there are usually a number of factors that may influence the patient or family to launch a legal complaint. These include communication failure, lack of consent, permanent disability, unexpected catastrophic outcome, or death.

### *Neuraxial Blocks*

Epidural or spinal analgesia and anesthesia is frequently used in the operating setting and in the pain clinic. We do not know how many such procedures are performed daily in Canada, but the trend is to use neuraxial blocks as an adjuvant to anesthesia for thoracic, abdominal, and lower body surgery. Spinal anesthesia is frequently used for pelvic and urologic procedures. Combined spinal and epidural anesthesia is also used frequently. The denominator is therefore probably very large, and the number of cases leading to legal problems very small. We cannot put a number on this ratio.

### *Epidural Blocks*

There were 25 cases involving epidural injections. Of these, nine were epidural steroid injections, three epidural blocks for chronic pain relief, seven cases of epidural catheters inserted for postoperative pain relief, and six cases of epidural anesthesia for surgery. The complications associated with these epidural procedures varied widely. There was one broken catheter, where the tip could not be found. Other minor outcomes (see above) were two cases of PDPH and one case of lipolysis of the back. Numbness, temporary weakness, and ongoing back pain led to complaints in some cases. One patient complained of awareness! There was a case of "vasomotor instability" and one case of intravascular injection with seizures. Viral hepatitis, contracted months after the epidural, led to a complaint against the anesthesiologist. Two patients developed foot-drop, one after an epidural steroid injection and one after attempted epidural anesthesia for hernia repair. Total or high spinal anesthesia necessitating resuscitation occurred in three cases, one after an epidural steroid injection and two after epidural analgesia for postoperative pain relief. Even though one of these patients had a cardiac arrest, the resuscitation was successful in all cases, and no permanent sequelae resulted. All the cases mentioned above were dismissed.

More serious outcomes were four cases of paraplegia and one case of organic brain damage. These cases are instructive, in that all except one case were settled on behalf of the doctors involved because they could not be defended. However, one case of paraplegia was dismissed, because the lesion occurred well above the insertion of the epidural and the etiology of the cord damage could not be ascertained. The four cases that could not be defended hinged on lack of consent for the procedure, lack of monitoring during hypotensive anesthesia, and use of a nonapproved drug for epidural injection. In the fourth case, the epidural steroid injection was not related to the development of paraplegia; it resulted from a sequestered disc, but the case could not be defended because the doctors involved did not adequately assess the patient before going ahead with the injection. There were no deaths in the epidural group.

### *Spinal Anesthesia*

Eleven legal actions arose from spinal anesthesia for surgery. That is a remarkably small number over a 20-year period considering the commonality of spinal anesthesia. All these actions were dismissed. Two complaints were for PDPH. Persistent back pain or sciatica occurred in several cases; one of these was thought to be attributable to aseptic meningitis, the others to preexisting conditions. One complainant had had multiple attempts at insertion of the spinal needle. One patient developed persistent tinnitus and hearing loss. There was one case of cauda equina syndrome of unproven origin, and a complaint of leg weakness that presented 6 months after the spinal anesthetic and was found to be caused by disc disease.

Only one case had a serious outcome, namely, paraplegia as a result of a cord bleed. The patient was anticoagulated, and the bleed occurred 12 days postoperatively and was thought to be spontaneous and not related to the spinal anesthetic.

### *Other Types of Anesthetic Blocks*

The remaining 41 cases span the spectrum of anesthesia pain management.

Seven cases were associated with cataract surgery, in which anesthesia staff performed retrobulbar or peribulbar blocks (Chapter 6). Global perforation occurred in five cases, two were settled, and two won in court. There was one case of vitreous hemorrhage and one of acute glaucoma postoperatively. Both were dismissed.

There were eight cases of sympathetic plexus blocks, including celiac plexus (1), stellate ganglion (4), and lumbar sympathetic chain (3).

A phenol neurolytic block of the celiac plexus, resulting in paraplegia, was settled. Also settled was a case of paraplegia and incontinence resulting from a neurolytic lumbar sympathetic block. The other cases arose from pneumothorax, septicemia, or pain issues, some preexisting, and these were all dismissed.

Four cases involved damage to nerves: sacral nerve-root, femoral, obturator, and ulnar. Two were neurolytic blocks with phenol or alcohol, both resulting in paralysis. These were settled. Two cases arose from persistent or aggravated pain; these were dismissed.

Intercostal nerve blocks caused complications in four actions, two for serious injuries and two for pneumothorax. One patient fainted and sustained fractures; this case was settled. One patient with a preexisting condition developed aspiration pneumonia after the procedure and died. This case was won in court.

Regional blocks of the brachial plexus, paravertebral nerves, and supraclavicular plexus caused pneumothorax. All were dismissed.

Injection of the cervical plexus of nerves for chronic neck pain caused three legal actions, two of them dismissed. In both cases, the patient had dyspnea and temporary paralysis, treated with appropriate airway management and resuscitation. The third patient developed cardiac arrest and sustained permanent neurologic damage. The case was settled because of inadequate resuscitation and failure to monitor appropriately.

Two cases arose from acupuncture treatment, and both centered on consent discussions. One case was settled, the other dismissed. A patient developed pneumothorax from trigger-point injections, and again the case was dismissed. Thus, all 11 cases of pneumothorax as a complication of different regional blocks were dismissed.

In the miscellaneous category, a case of septic arthritis from an intraarticular injection of steroid was dismissed. After the insertion of a spinal cord stimulator, the patient developed weakness and hemiparesis, which was found to be related to the preexisting condition and thus dismissed.

Bier block for surgery of the upper limb is frequently used. Two legal cases came to light. One case had a catastrophic outcome because the local anesthetic was mistakenly diluted with concentrated saline, resulting in serious tissue damage. This case was settled. The other case alleged development of sympathetic dystrophy; this allegation was dismissed.

Three cases of facet joint injections led to legal actions. One patient had dural puncture and worse pain, one patient developed a paraspinal abscess, and the third had seizures after an inadvertent intraarterial injection. Two cases were dismissed, the third won in court. This case went to court because of deficient discussion of material risk.

### *Obstetric Anesthesia and Analgesia (Chapter 14)*

The annual number of legal actions from obstetric anesthesia has been stable since 1980 (see Figure 23-3-1). During that time, obstetric analgesia including epidural and combined spinal-epidural analgesia has become more prevalent, and there has been a change to regional anesthesia for operative delivery.[4] The prevalence of epidural analgesia for labor is about 30% overall in Canada.[5]

We analyzed 41 cases from CMPA's closed files. Thirty-one cases were dismissed, five settled, four won in court, and one case judged against the physician. There were 10 incidents of PDPH, all dismissed. Accidental total spinal anesthesia occurred in two cases. One was dismissed, the other had a catastrophic outcome and the case was settled on the grounds that the care was inadequate. Two sheared epidural catheters led to complaints that were dismissed. Four instances of nerve root irritation or damage were also dismissed, as were all six cases in which the patient complained of pain, either during cesarean delivery or after the delivery.

One case of pain in labor received much attention in the national and international press[6] and this case was won in court.

Preexisting conditions can lead to medical legal actions. A patient who was found to have neurologic deficits was diagnosed with syringomyelia, unrelated to epidural pain relief in labor. Another patient developed a postdelivery cavernous sinus thrombosis. Dense hemiplegia 3 days after delivery was found to result from cerebral hemorrhage secondary to pregnancy-induced hypertension. These cases were dismissed, as were two others, one related to consent discussion and one to the wrong drug injected, but without sequelae.

Two patients developed epidural abscesses after labor analgesia. Both resulted in neurologic deficits. One case was settled, the other dismissed when the action was not pursued.

There were three cases of amniotic fluid embolism leading to major or catastrophic outcome or death. The cases in the two former categories were both won in court.[7] The case of the patient who died was settled, because vigilance was found wanting. That settlement was shared between anesthesia and obstetrics.

Remaining in the "catastrophic" outcome category were two cases of paraplegia and one of hypotension causing perinatal asphyxia. One case of paraplegia was settled, the other was the only case in this entire series of regional anesthesia legal cases that was lost in court. Although the paraplegia was thought to be caused by a decrease in blood pressure and lack of blood supply to the fetus during cesarean delivery, the judge found the anesthesia staff liable because of inadequate monitoring and record keeping.

A last case was also related to hypotension in labor after epidural analgesia. Lack of monitoring, lack of adequate fluid therapy, and failure to appreciate the effect on the fetus resulted in a large settlement for lifetime care of the child. One patient died. Death was not deemed related to the anesthetic.

## Cost of Litigation

Medical legal actions are costly for the plaintiff and for the defense.

The cost of the 77 regional anesthesia claims discussed above depended on the outcome. Sixty cases were dismissed. The average cost of a dismissed case was 13,000 Canadian dollars. There were 12 settled cases. The cost of settling a case averaged $520,000. The high cost reflects the serious disabilities in some of these cases. Five cases went to court and were won in favor of the doctor with an average cost of $110,000. No regional anesthesia cases were lost in court.

Obstetric anesthesia costs differ somewhat. Although there are few cases, the cost may be very high if the case includes care for a compromised baby. The average of the settled cases in regional obstetric anesthesia was $190,000, but one claim for a compromised baby was for 4.6 million dollars. The mean cost for the cases that were won in court was almost double that of the regional claims, around $190,000. Dismissing the cases in obstetric anesthesia costs around $15,000, similar to the regional claims. If a case is lost in court, as was one case in the obstetric anesthesia series, the cost may run into millions of dollars, reflecting catastrophic outcome.

The costs of CMPA fees have increased significantly for many "high risk" specialists in Canada. At the top of the scale are obstetricians, followed closely by neurosurgeons and orthopedic surgeons. The costs have remained relatively stable for anesthesia practitioners over the last 25 years, reflecting the risk-management initiatives taken in our specialty, particularly with regard to airway management and monitoring.

Doctors in Canada are reimbursed by the provincial governments for most of their malpractice premiums.

## Legal Issues

What can we learn from these cases? We should not practice "defensive medicine." We should practice regional anesthesia to the best of our ability, keeping up to date, and perform according to the standard of care that is expected of a trained anesthesiologist. We cannot avoid getting sued occasionally even if all goes well. As can be seen from the cases discussed, minor complications can lead to legal action even if no bad outcome results. But we can minimize the risk of lawsuits.

Consent discussion: We know what the common risks are in regional anesthesia. We are obligated to mention common risks and serious risks regardless of frequency when discussing a procedure. It is estimated that the risk of dural puncture and PDPH is about 1% in teaching hospitals.[8] Similarly, pneumothorax is a known complication of many different blocks, and this should be mentioned in the consent discussion. Questions have been raised regarding the consent for obstetric anesthesia. This has been well explained in two publications in recent years.[9,10] Material risk should be put in the context of the planned procedure, bearing in mind that paralysis and nerve damage is exceedingly rare but can occur. This is particularly important when performing neurolytic blocks. As is seen from our series, most cases are dismissed when the consent discussion was adequate.

Record keeping is very important. To properly defend a legal claim, the CMPA must depend on the written record. In all cases, the record should be complete and legible! The consent discussion can be mentioned briefly, or ticked off on a preprinted record.

If an unexpected or untoward outcome has occurred, it is wise to write a note in the chart. This should be factual and state the procedure, the clinical findings and outcome, and the plan for further action. The best defense is a complete clinical record.

Take note of preexisting conditions. Certain patients are more prone to complications from regional anesthesia, for instance, those with diabetes or obesity. We are aware of the problems associated with anticoagulation, and are very vigilant about blocks in such patients. It is interesting that there were no legal cases associated with epidural hematomas related to the performance of blocks. Only one case occurred, and that was found to be spontaneous. Patients with neurologic diseases such as amyotrophic lateral sclerosis and Klippel Feil deformity presented in this series. It is important to note the presence of such abnormalities. Similarly, take note of common conditions such as scoliosis and previous back surgery. These patients are more likely to present difficulties with regional anesthesia.

Monitoring vital signs before and during procedures is clearly part of the standard of care. It is very difficult to defend the practitioner if monitoring is inadequate. Monitoring should be documented. Know what to do if complications arise. Regional anesthesia should be performed in an environment where resuscitation can be properly performed.

Wrong drugs are sometimes administered by mistake. Usually this is a systems failure, and hospitals are working hard to provide safeguards to minimize this risk. We are accustomed to checking all drugs before we give them, but should a mistake be made, it must be documented and the patient must be followed adequately. It is also necessary to disclose such errors, to prevent recurrence and ensure adequate care in follow-up.

## Conclusion

We have discussed 77 cases of regional anesthesia and 41 obstetric anesthesia legal actions which comprise the closed claims that occurred in Canada in the time period 1980–2002. The complications that led to legal action are those that are frequently associated with regional anesthesia. Although rare, legal action cannot always be avoided, but a favorable outcome of the action is influenced by good practice. That includes appropriate consent discussion, good record keeping, good communication strategies, and adherence to the standard of care.

## References

1. Duranceau A. The Canadian Medical Protective Association. Bull Am Coll Surg 1998; 83:23–28.
2. Peng P, Smedstad K. Litigation in Canada against anesthesiologists practicing regional anesthesia. A review of closed claims. Can J Anaesth 2000;47:105–112.
3. The Canadian Medical Protective Association. 2003 Annual Report. Ottawa, ON.
4. Morley-Forster P. Regional techniques for cesarean section. Tech Reg Anesth Pain Manage 2001;5:24–29.
5. Oyston J. Obstetrical anesthesia in Ontario. Can J Anaesth 1995;42:1117–1125.
6. Morrison S. Mother of twins sues for $2.4 million. The Spectator, Hamilton, ON. Tuesday, August 9, 1994.
7. St-Amand J. Medicolegal nightmare: a tragic case, a needless trial. Can Med Assoc J 1993;148:806–809.
8. Norris M, Leighton B, DeSimone C. Needle bevel direction and headache after inadvertent dural puncture. Anesthesiology 1989;70:729–731.
9. Jackson A, Henry R, Avery N, et al. Informed consent for labour epidurals: what labouring women want to know. Can J Anaesth 2000;47:1068–1073.
10. Smedstad K. Informed consent for epidural analgesia in labour. Can J Anaesth 2000; 47:1055–1059.

# Section 4

## Neurologic Complications of Regional Anesthesia in the Nordic Countries

Nils Dahlgren

The Hippocratic oath states that the main obligation in medicine is to not hurt the patient. This statement is much easier said than done and as noble as this goal is, it is impossible to achieve, because all medical interventions carry undesired side effects. So, medical practice always includes a balance of risks that should be based on solid facts to avoid subjective thinking, misleading recommendations, and faulty decisions.

Why look at the Nordic countries when discussing complications of regional anesthesia? It must be taken for granted that Nordic doctors performing regional anesthesia are just as skilled as any other group of anesthesiologists, and that complications of regional anesthesia are the same irrespective of the country where they occur.

What makes the Nordic countries of special interest is that an overwhelming part of their healthcare systems are nonprivate, without influence of economic reasons for clean medical results. But also, the Nordic societies are characterized by a severe bureaucratic order. For example, each individual carries a personal identification number, thus eliminating the risk of double recording when searching different data files. Cases of medical malpractice are peer reviewed and handled by special institutions, not ordinary criminal courts, and all Nordic countries have insurance policies granting economic compensation to any patient suffering damage through medical treatment, without the necessity of finding a guilty party. Reporting of complications is encouraged and mishaps in medical treatment are looked upon mainly with the idea of finding ways to avoid a repetition of similar accidents.

Most regional anesthetic techniques have been used for more than three-quarters of a century. Despite this vast experience, uncertainties regarding the frequency of complications still burden some of them. This is attributable to ever-changing opinions about indications for the various methods, changes in concurrent medical therapy, and the continuing sophistication of regional anesthetic equipment and local anesthetic drugs. However, inaccuracies also find their source in the literature through statements extracted from materials of irrelevant composition or studies of insufficient size to determine the frequency of these uncommon mishaps.

Regional anesthetic techniques are excellent ways to provide analgesia, not only during surgery, but also for postoperative comfort. Fortunately, severe complications of neural blockades are very infrequent and their study in a prospective design would demand huge numbers of patients in order to obtain relevant statistics. An easier way to approach the truth is through retrospective studies. However, this study design is hampered by other inaccuracies.

Incidences are calculated from two figures, the number of accidents under study (the nominator) and the number of treatments administered using the technique under investigation (the denominator). Inaccuracies in any of these figures give faulty results. These elements were applied to severe neurologic complications of central blockades from a recent study, hence the following text primarily refers to this material.[1] This Swedish study, covering the whole country for 10 years (1990–1999), was based on a mailed enquiry confirmed through search of adequate administrative files dealing with malpractice or insurance matters, in all 127 cases. The investigators were specifically interested in patients with the following problems: cauda equina syndrome, spinal hemorrhage, epidural abscess, and meningitis. It was found that the anesthesia departments reported only half of the severe complications that were documented to have taken place. Information about the remaining half was obtained from administrative files with an overlap in 17 cases. The main reason for this lack of accuracy was explained by inadequate recording practices in the departments. But more importantly, 30 departments had denied any knowledge of these complications. Twelve of these departments were subsequently found to be responsible for 13 severe neurologic complications. Obviously, underreporting is a major obstacle in retrospective studies.

Regarding the determination of the denominator, nationwide records are not available, even in Sweden. However, information was obtained from 85% of the Swedish anesthesiology departments (72 of 85), and through follow-up in official records for specific operations, where the use of central neuraxial blockade was accurately described,[2] an estimate of 1,710,000 blockades was determined to constitute the denominator, comprising 1,260,000 spinal blockades and 450,000 epidural blockades, of which 200,000 were obstetric. So far, this is the largest collection of central neuraxial blocks that has been analyzed for major neurologic complications worldwide.

Complications of regional anesthesia can be explained on the basis of five different actions, outlined below, with reference to the delivery of a local anesthetic drug, or a mixture of drugs (if it ever came about).

**A. The deposition is correct**, however, the effects of the ensuing blockade gives rise to damage.

*For example: hypotension and bradycardia, uncontrolled respiratory insufficiency and uncontrolled neural traction*

In 1988 Caplan et al.[3] reported 14 cases of cardiac arrest under spinal anesthesia. Two analogous cases were also reported by Aromaa et al.[4] in a recent Finnish study based on insurance claims over 6-1/2 years. The Finns concluded that oversedation in combination with obesity were causative factors. Their study comprised 550,000 spinal blockades. No analogous cases were reported in the Swedish study; however, this was not specifically asked for. The paravertebral deposition of local anesthetics might result in epidural spread resulting in hypotension. See also D.

An example of neural traction is when the patient's paralyzed arm accidentally falls off the operating table causing a stretch of the brachial plexus. Peripheral nerves can be stretched by up to 5% of their original length without disruptive damage.

**B. The deposition is correct**, however the manipulation results in complications.

*For example: toxic, infectious, and allergic reactions*

These types of complications are most frustrating. Severe neural defects ensue even though everything appeared normal during the procedure. The Swedish study revealed 32 cases of toxic cauda equina syndrome, i.e., sensory-motor loss in the legs and pelvis, usually after an otherwise uncomplicated central neural blockade. This syndrome occurs irrespective of age or gender, usually following a spinal anesthetic. Maldistribution of the local anesthetic is the most likely cause of this problem following continuous spinal blockade with microcatheters.[5] Hyperbaric solutions predispose to this kind of lesion regardless of the local anesthetic used. Spinal stenosis seems to be a risk factor for cauda equine syndrome and the prognosis is poor.

Meningitis is a feared complication of central neural blockade. Of 29 cases, 25 had had dural perforation. Age or gender does not influence the incidence of this problem. Symptoms usually appear within 24 hours of the procedure. Absentmindedness, malaise, and urinary retention are some of the subtle symptoms observed and it is difficult to link these symptoms to meningitis. Also, the symptoms and signs of meningitis might be very similar to those associated with PDPH. Classic symptoms of meningitis including headache, stiff neck, and fever were observed in only 14 of the 29 reported cases. Prevention of this complication requires the obligatory use of a cap, face mask, and sterile gloves by the anesthesiologist and strict observation of sterile technique. The literature contains cases in which the microbial agent identified in the patient's liquor was also identified in the nose of the anesthesiologist.[6] Given the correct diagnosis and rapid treatment of meningitis, the prognosis is good; however, five of 29 cases developed minor neurologic problems that were ongoing.

Epidural abscess was seen in 13 patients, 12 of whom had had continuous epidural blockade. This complication probably occurs more frequently, because these patients are usually referred to infectious disease specialists, and are thus outside control of the anesthesia department. Symptoms of spinal abscess usually appear about 1 week after the introduction of an epidural catheter (range 2 days to 5 weeks). These symptoms usually comprise severe backache, fever, and malaise. Neurologic symptoms developed in five patients. The indication for epidural cannulation was acute pain treatment in six of them. This group of patients was seriously ill and receiving terminal pain treatment. Laminectomy was performed in six patients and complete resolution occurred in three.

**C. The deposition is correct**, but the neural tissue is mechanically damaged by the procedure.

*For example: compressive damage from bleeding following or pressure caused by the volume of the injectate or dural puncture*

Intraspinal bleeding, if not treated within 12 hours of the first symptoms, often results in permanent neurologic damage. The cause of the neurologic deficit is mechanical pressure or impaired perfusion. Vascular disruption is caused by needles and catheters, but may also be caused by high pressure from injected solutions. Compression from bleeding most likely results from an arterial bleed because cerebrospinal fluid pressure usually exceeds central venous pressure in the supine patient.[7] An intrathecal bleed is contained by the dural sac while the pressure generated by epidural bleeding is dependent on the capacitance of the epidural space. Degenerative angiopathy is seen in severe atherosclerosis and in inflammatory conditions. Vulnerable vessels could be found at the site of a fractured vertebra and in patients given chronic steroid medication. Sclerotic derangement in the mesenchymal tissue of the spine closes the epidural space resulting in high pressures during and after injections of local anesthetics. To conclude, it is easily understood that spinal bleeding disorders are age dependent. Risk is further increased with deficient coagulation, either spontaneous or iatrogenic. Three of four patients with this severe complication are female.[1,8] The Swedish study found 33 cases of spinal hemorrhage of which 25 were epidural hematomas. Bleeding occurred as a result of manipulation of the catheter in some of these cases. In 11 cases, anticoagulant treatment was closely linked to the bleeding. Motor weakness was the most prominent symptom in 18 cases, whereas six patients complained of sensory disturbances and all of these symptoms occurred usually within 24 hours of central neuraxial blockade. One patient developed symptoms of bleeding 2 weeks after a technically problematic spinal blockade. There were no risk factors for bleeding in 11 of these patients. The prognosis in these cases depended heavily on how quickly problems were detected. Twenty-seven of 33 patients in this series developed neurologic deficits. Eleven of these patients were surgically decompressed. Among the six patients who recovered, one had a laminectomy. Early detection of neurologic compression of the spinal cord is crucial in the postoperative period.

In obstetrics, about one epidural cannulation in 100 results in a perforation of the dura.[9] This could well pass unnoticed. In fact, five patients in the Swedish series who sustained dural punctures developed intracranial subdural hematomas. Four of these patients required craniotomy. Symptoms were mistaken for PDPH in these cases. When a patient develops a headache following central neural blockade, one cannot assume that all of these headaches are related to cerebrospinal fluid leakage. Rarely, these symptoms are the harbinger of a serious intracranial event. The anesthesiologist must always consider serious intracranial pathology in patients with persistent headache following central neural blockade.

**D. The deposition is incorrect** and thus causes damage.

*For example: intravascular injection, unintentional spinal or epidural injection, and intraneural injection*

Unbound, unionized molecules of any local anesthetic rapidly penetrate the membranes of excitable cells (neuronal or cardiac) and exert their pharmacologic action. Intraarterial injections of fractions of a milliliter of local anesthetics moving intracranially result in seizure activity. The amount of local anesthetic required to cause seizure activity when injected intravenously is much greater because of plasma protein binding and binding in the tissues; however, serious problems still arise. Obstetric patients are particularly vulnerable because of the large venous channels with intermittently high flow in the epidural space and a number of cases of cardiogenic toxicity have been reported.[10] In a French study involving 100,000 regional anesthetics, there were 23 cases of seizures with no fatalities.[11] In the Swedish study, there were no seizures reported.

A feared complication is traumatic lesions of the spinal cord as a result of needle trauma during attempts at central neural blockade attributable to inaccurate apprehension of lumbar anatomy.[12] Needle placement above the L2-3 interspace increases the risk of serious neurologic damage because of the presence of the spinal cord. Some patients complain of lancinating pain when there is encroachment on the spinal cord and therefore local anesthetics are usually not injected under these circumstances. However, this warning sign is not consistent and is not present if the patient is anesthetized and more serious damage can occur when local anesthetics are injected. In the Swedish series, nine patients sustained spinal cord damage and eight of these occurred during attempts at epidural anesthesia. The prognosis in these patients was poor.

Paravertebral injections of local anesthetics in the cervical region may spread into the intrathecal space from the root sleeve, which may extend several millimeters outside the intervertebral foramen. The dose of local anesthetic used for interscalene block is usually around 30 mL which is sufficient to cause a massive total spinal block. See also paragraph A.

Severe pain is a consistent symptom of intraneural injection of local anesthetics. Intraneural injections of local anesthetics result in pressures as high as 700 mm Hg when using a 10-mL syringe[13] and this is usually associated with severe pain. This warning sign is lost in the anesthetized patients.

**E. The deposition is incorrect** and the lack of effect causes damage.

*For example: cardiac damage attributed to pain reaction*

In a study by Auroy et al.,[12] three patients experienced a cardiac arrest attributed to pain at the start of surgery because the block was not working effectively. One case was fatal. Obviously, the patient must be well anesthetized before surgery starts. The author recommends that all patients be appropriately sedated while undergoing regional anesthesia and that steps must be taken to ensure that the block is working before surgery begins.

In conclusion, the Swedish study provides information about the incidence of major complications occurring following regional anesthesia and the number of problems was greater than generally expected. However, the true incidence of these complications is probably underestimated because of inadequate or lost reports.

The study shows that the judgment of risk must refer to materials of relevant composition.

Is it true that the risk of developing a spinal hematoma after epidural cannulation is 1:190,000[14]?

Yes, it is true if you are referring to obstetric patients.

No, it is false if you are referring to elderly women undergoing total knee joint replacement, a well-defined patient group. Here, the risk was found to be 1:3600, which is 44 times greater compared with the group of young, obstetric females.

Irrespective of age and gender, the risk of severe complications in connection with spinal anesthesia never exceeds 1:20,000. Epidural blockades are about five times more often hampered by severe complications when compared with spinal blockades.

Referring to compressive or toxic trauma to the nervous system, it is recommended to seriously consider the advantages of using central blockades for the following categories:

- Patients with derangements in the coagulation
- Patients with osteoporosis or spinal stenosis
- Patients with ongoing neurologic defects within the region to be blocked
- Patients with deranged spinal anatomy, including surgical scarring
- Patients who reject the treatment

If postoperative surveillance is without the capacity to apprehend signs of an expanding process in the patient's back, epidural blockade should be executed with restriction.

## References

1. Moen V, Dahlgren N, Irestedt L. Severe neurological complications after central neuraxial blockades. Anesthesiology 2004;101:950–959.
2. Holmström B, Rawal N, Arnér S. The use of regional anesthesia techniques in Sweden: results of a nation-wide survey. Acta Anaesthesiol Scand 1997;41:565–572.
3. Caplan RA, Ward RJ, Posner K, Cheney FW. Unexpected cardiac arrest during spinal anesthesia: a closed claims analysis of predisposing factors. Anesthesiology 1988;68: 5–11.
4. Aromaa U, Lahdensuu M, Cozanitis DA. Severe complications associated with epidural and spinal anaesthesias in Finland 1987–1993. A study based on patient insurance claims. Acta Anaesthesiol Scand 1997;41:445–452.
5. Riegler ML, Drasner DH, Krejcie TC, et al. Cauda equina syndrome after continuous spinal anesthesia. Anesth Analg 1991;72:275–281.
6. Schneeberger PM, Janssen M, Voss A. Alpha-hemolytic streptococci: a major pathogen of iatrogenic meningitis following lumbar puncture. Infection 1996;24:29–33.

7. Broadbent CR, Maxwell WB, Ferrie R, Wilson DJ, Gawne-Cain M, Russel R. Ability of anaesthetists to identify a marked lumbar interspace. Anaesthesia 2000;55: 1122–1126.
8. Cottrell JE, Smith DS. Anesthesia and Neurosurgery. 3rd ed. St. Louis: Mosby; 1994. Chapter 4.
9. Schroeder DR. Statistics: detecting a rare adverse drug reaction using spontaneous reports. Reg Anesth Pain Med 1998;23(suppl 2):183–189.
10. Reynolds F. Dural puncture and headache. In: Reynolds F, ed. Regional Analgesia in Obstetrics. A Millennium Update. London: Springer-Verlag; 2000:307–319.
11. Hawkins JL, Koonin LM, Palmer SK, Gibbs CP. Anesthesia related deaths during obstetric delivery in the United States 1979–1990. Anesthesiology 1997;86:277–284.
12. Auroy Y, Narchi P, Messiah A, Litt L, Rouvier B, Samii K. Serious complications related to regional anesthesia. Anesthesiology 1997;87:479–486.
13. Selander D, Sjöstrand J. Longitudinal spread of intraneurally injected local anesthetics. Acta Anaesthesiol Scand 1978;22:622.
14. Wulf H. Epidural anesthesia and spinal hematoma. Can J Anaesth 1996;43:126–171.

# Section 5

## Medicolegal Claims: Summary of an Australian Study

Albert H. Santora

Cass reported on "222 medicolegal claims involving 160 anaesthetist members of Victoria's largest medical indemnity organization during the period 1980–1999."[1] Of this group, claims had been made against 35% of the anesthetists. Claims were classified as closed, withdrawn by the plaintiff, or proceeding at the time of the paper's writing.

Exact settlement amounts were not specified but the claims were assigned to one of five settlement "bands." For example, Band I: Settlements up to A$1000 versus Band V: Settlements exceeding A$100,000. Table 23-5-1 lists the settlement stratification.

Table 23-5-2 lists the complaints with 10 or more claims and Table 23-5-3 lists complaints with fewer than 10 claims. Table 23-5-4 was generated to summarize the regional anesthesia–related data.

The author does not report settlement data for all types of claims.

TABLE 23-5-1. Settlements of Claims by Band

| Band | Range in A$ |
|---|---|
| I | Up to 1,000 |
| II | 1,000–10,000 |
| III | 10,000–50,000 |
| IV | 50,000–100,000 |
| V | Exceeding 100,000 |

*Source:* Cass.[1] Used with permission from the Australian Society of Anaesthetists.

TABLE 23-5-2. Ten or More Complaints

| Claim | Closed | Withdrawn | Open | Total |
|---|---|---|---|---|
| Dental | 70 | 14 | | 84 |
| Awareness | 7 | 4 | | 11 |
| Deaths under anesthesia | 9 | 1 | 2 | 12 |
| Epidural | 12 | 8 | 2 | 22 |
| Inquests | 28 | | | 28 |
| Joined with surgeon | 17 | 4 | 1 | 22 |
| Nerve palsy | 9 | 4 | | 13 |
| Postoperative complications | 7 | 2 | 3 | 12 |
| Totals | 159 | 37 | 8 | 204 |

*Source:* Cass.[1] Used with permission from the Australian Society of Anaesthetists.
*Note:* Several claims fall into more than one category, e.g., Deaths under Anesthesia and Inquests.

TABLE 23-5-3. Less than 10 Claims Filed

| Claim | Closed | Withdrawn | Open | Total |
|---|---|---|---|---|
| Assault | 1 | | | 1 |
| Assistance at resuscitation | 2 | | | 2 |
| Bradycardia | 1 | | | 1 |
| Disconnection | 1 | | | 1 |
| Drug overdose | 2 | | | 2 |
| Electrolyte disturbance | 1 | | | 1 |
| Endoscopy | 5 | | | 5 |
| Extravasation | 1 | | | 1 |
| Eye injury | 6 | | | 6 |
| Fall off table | 3 | 1 | | 4 |
| Gas embolism | 2 | | | 2 |
| Hypotensive event | 1 | | | 1 |
| Immune reaction | 5 | | | 5 |
| Informed consent | 4 | 2 | | 6 |
| Local anesthetic toxicity | 1 | | | 1 |
| Miscellaneous | 3 | | | 3 |
| Operative hemorrhage | 3 | | | 3 |
| Pneumothorax | 4 | | | 4 |
| Postoperative hemorrhage | 1 | | | 1 |
| Preoperative assessment | 2 | | | 2 |
| Respiratory complications | 6 | | | 6 |
| Retained foreign body | 3 | | | 3 |
| Sedation | 7 | 1 | 1 | 9 |
| Spinal anesthesia | 7 | 2 | | 9 |
| Therapeutic treatment | 2 | | | 2 |
| Wrong site | 1 | | 1 | 2 |
| Wrongs claim | 5 | | | 5 |
| Totals | 79 | 10 | 2 | 91 |

*Source:* Cass.[1] Used with permission from the Australian Society of Anaesthetists.

TABLE 23-5-4. Summary of Regional Anesthesia–Related Cases

| Block | Total | Closed | Withdrawn | Open | Lost to follow-up | Settlement |
|---|---|---|---|---|---|---|
| Epidural | 22 | 12 | 8 | 2 | | (Ave.: A$37,620) |
| Dural puncture | | | | | | |
| Cauda equina damage | | 2 | | | | Band V |
| Blood patch | | 1 | | | | |
| Epidural hematoma | | 1 | | | | |
| Obstetric related | | | | | | |
| Inadequate block | | 4 | | | | (Ave.: A$58,121) |
| Headache–muscle weakness | | 1 | | | | Band IV |
| Cauda equina damage | | 1 | | | | |
| Hypotension | | 1 | | | | |
| Multiple attempts | | 1 | | | | Band I |
| Eye | 6 | 6 | | | | |
| Block related | | 3 | | | | |
| 2/3 blindness | | | | | | (Ave.: A$99,581) |
| Peripheral block | 8 | 8 | | | | |
| "Arm" block with local anesthesia | | | | | | |
| Palsy | | 4 | | | | (Ave.: A$18,437) |
| Sensory loss | | 1 | | | | Band II |
| Axillary (seizure) | | 1 | | | | Band III |
| Supraclavicular (pneumothorax) | | 1 | | | | A$4,212 |
| Subclavicular (pneumothorax) | | 1 | | | | A$4,212 |
| Spinal block | 9 | 6 | 2 | | 1 | (Ave.: A$7,869) |
| Inadequate block | | 1 | | | | Band I |
| Cauda equina damage (informed consent problem) | | 1 | | | | Band V |
| Inadequate block (cesarean) | | 2 | | | | Band III |
| Foot drop–sensory loss | | 1 | | | | Band II |
| Fatal brain syndrome | | 1 | | | | (Judged unrelated to block) |

*Source:* Cass.[1] Used with permission from the Australian Society of Anaesthetists.

## Conclusion

The Australian study shared many of the limitations of other closed claims analyses. It is somewhat limited in scope. However, a few conclusions regarding regional anesthesia can be drawn.

1. Neuraxial blocks were the most frequently cited techniques related to malpractice claims.
2. Inadequate analgesia with neuraxial blocks was a repeated source of litigation.
3. Injury related to eye blocks had a relatively high settlement cost.

## Reference

1. Cass NM. Medicolegal claims against anaesthetists: a 20 year study. Anaesth Intensive Care 2004;32(1):47–58.

# Section 6

# Regional Anesthesia Morbidity Study: France

Yves Auroy and Dan Benhamou

Regional anesthesia is both an old and a new technique. It is now a well-established technique of anesthesia and its use has increased very much during the last 20 years.[1] Providing estimates of the incidence of the various complications related to regional anesthesia is not a new concern. In two classic studies, each assessing a large number of spinal blocks, Dripps and Vandam[2] assessed the risk associated with the use of procaine and tetracaine in 10,098 patients, whereas Phillips et al.[3] monitored 10,440 patients after lidocaine spinal anesthesia. The main message of these prospective studies was that complications related to spinal anesthesia are very rare. Such results and the numerous advantages associated with regional anesthesia have contributed to the perception that regional anesthesia is "safe," and this has translated into an increasing number of regional anesthesia procedures performed worldwide. However, one should be very careful before extrapolating these old results to our current practice. The comparison cannot probably be made, not only because of methodologic concerns, but also because of tremendous quantitative and technical changes during this 30-year period. This factor also restricts our ability to conduct metaanalysis studies.[4]

Unfortunately, the number of recent prospective studies assessing the incidence of severe complications related to regional anesthesia is low, and this is particularly true when peripheral nerve blocks are concerned. Severe complications are rare and this is the main factor explaining the low number of studies. Indeed, the number of monitored procedures has to be very large in order to estimate the level of risk with sufficient statistical power.[5] In the case of rare events, other approaches that have been developed in other fields of research need to be used to understand and to control the risk associated with regional anesthesia techniques.[6,7]

## SOS Regional Anesthesia Service

After a first large epidemiologic study had been performed in France in 1996 in order to evaluate the incidence of serious complications related to regional anesthesia and to define their characteristics,[8] an original and new service named SOS Regional Anesthesia (RA) Service was created in 1998.[9] This service first included a hot line and three experts (Pr Samii, Pr Ecoffey, and Pr Benhamou) rotated each week to respond to any question asked by participants on regional anesthesia at any time (even at night if necessary) and 7 days a week (even Sunday if necessary). SOS RA Service had four main goals: 1) to provide an online clinical help for the practitioner facing a severe complication, 2) to obtain immediately relevant clinical information for every complication reported (and obviate the loss of pertinent information related to late collection as this occurred in the first survey), 3) to provide advice on difficult clinical cases before any anesthesia is given (generally at the time of the preanesthetic visit), 4) to estimate incidence of complications from a prospective declaration of all regional techniques performed by practitioners who had subscribed to the service. The SOS RA Service works currently according to the three first initial goals, as the calculation of incident rates was not maintained after the first 10-month period because of the complexity related to exhaustive case collection. Even with this insufficiency, this expert system remains highly demanded by practitioners (one phone call each day as a mean) and is very useful for detecting the emergence of "new" complications.

From the voluntary participation of 487 anesthesiologists who performed 158,083 regional blocks in a 10-month period, 56 major complications (including four deaths) were reported in the SOS RA survey.

### *Cardiac Arrest*

The incidence of cardiac arrest that occurred after spinal anesthesia was 2.7/10,000. Interestingly, the clinical situations associated with cardiac arrests were homogeneous because bradycardia was recorded before each cardiac arrest that occurred during spinal anesthesia, and cardiac arrest causing death occurred in the course of a central block performed during hip surgery in an elderly patient. The factors involved in cardiac arrest occurring during central blocks are several and the risk probably increases from the beginning of the procedure to its ends. Factors causing hemodynamic instability superimpose on those previously present. In cardiac arrests occurring more "lately," an additional factor (cementing or position change) often decompensated an already unstable situation because of sympathetic blockade and hemorrhage. Special attention should therefore be given to correct each factor that might contribute to decompensation.

One case of cardiac arrest and two respiratory complications (not leading to cardiac arrest) occurred during a lumbar plexus block performed via the posterior approach, and and the incidence of 80/10,000 seen after posterior lumbar plexus block is obviously much higher than after spinal anesthesia. Complications were related to cephalad diffusion of the local anesthetic in the epidural or intrathecal space.[10] Although it was difficult to draw any definite conclusion regarding this block, French anesthesiologists were warned against the high rate of complications that was found with the posterior lumbar plexus block and were advised to manage this block with at least the same vigilance as for a central block.[11]

### *Systemic Local Anesthetic Toxicity*

Systemic local anesthetic toxicity consisted of seizures only, without cardiac toxicity. The results suggested a decreased rate of local anesthetic-induced systemic toxicity when compared with the first previous survey, although methodologic differences between the two studies preclude any definitive conclusion. If this result proves to be true, the low incidence of toxic systemic complications may be related to better physician information, improved practice patterns (lower doses, slow injection, test dose, fractionated injection . . .), and the introduction of ropivacaine in clinical practice (at the time the first study was performed, ropivacaine was not available in France). In the face of these reassuring results, two main points were emphasized at that time: i) the most important factor for increased safety is to maintain the high level of vigilance even if the use of ropivacaine is considered a progress to prevent systemic toxicity,[12] ii) the "good" prognosis of these complications (neither cardiac arrest nor death were reported) could become worse if such complications occur outside the operating theater (i.e., in case of postoperative analgesia on the wards). A few years after, however, case reports describing cardiac arrest following high doses of ropivacaine injected in multiple block techniques were published.[13–17] Although the safety of ropivacaine can be questioned after the report of these cardiac arrests, it should be noted that both patients were easily resuscitated, a characteristic that is obviously different from bupivacaine. This also shows that the absence of event in large surveys cannot lead to the conclusion that the incidence is zero. Calculation of the incidence of rare complications thus remains difficult and might be underestimated, again suggesting that epidemiologic surveys are not the only way to study rare events.

### *Neurologic Complications*

Lidocaine spinal anesthesia was associated with more neurologic complications than bupivacaine spinal anesthesia (14.4 versus 2.2/10,000). Most neurologic complications were transient. These results about transient neurologic symptoms and neurologic toxicity of lidocaine contributed to the declining use of intrathecal lidocaine in France.

Among 12 complications that occurred after peripheral nerve blocks, nine were observed in patients in whom a nerve stimulator had been used, demonstrating that nerve stimulation is not a definitive guarantee against neurologic complications. Moreover, the exact incidence of neurologic complications after nerve stimulation (versus other techniques) cannot be calculated from this study because of the low number of cases. In cases reported in our files since 1998, inadequate patient positioning and/or noncooperative patients, insufficient physician experience, insufficient patient information on the procedure, excessive sedation, or a nongentle technique are often critical factors that contribute to increased risk of neurologic complications. Obviously, these factors hold true also when a nerve stimulator is used. The use of nerve stimulation was already accepted in European institutions and a relatively new debate emerged related to the significance of a paresthesia occurring during puncture. This debate is far from being closed. Experts using ultrasound guidance have, for example, added to the discussion by reporting several cases in which the needle had made physical contact with a nerve, but no paresthesia was felt by the patient.[18] Others have also recently shown that intraneural injection can follow a puncture in which nerve stimulation has been used without any warning sign.[19]

## Limitations of Reporting Systems

Reporting systems to study a rare event come up against several difficulties.

To collect enough cases, these studies require covering a large number of institutions and must probably be implemented at a nationwide level (or even at a multinational level as is already done in studies related to aviation safety). At present, voluntary declaration is often the solution used to gather information about complications associated with regional anesthesia. Because there is no "black box" system, an obvious bias of underreporting exists and different sources of information probably have to be merged.[20] However, voluntary declaration has some advantages to improve safety culture and to conduct in-depth causal analysis because results are often debated at the proximity level of the medical unit.

Because of the difficulty in gathering cases, investigators are tempted to pool the reported cases, with the risk of pooling very different patient populations or pooling very different regional anesthesia procedures. It is now clear that the obstetric population should be studied separately. Moen et al.[20] in their retrospective study on central neuraxial blocks demonstrated that major complications were observed in obstetric patients at a much lower incidence than in nonobstetric females cases.

One significant problem is the difficulty in attributing a complication to regional anesthesia. On one hand, it is important to define whether the complication is related or not to regional anesthesia, particularly for insurance judgment. One clinically significant and frequent situation is obstetric nerve injuries. Regional anesthesia is often blamed first, whereas the relative incidences of complications related to procedure or delivery are 5- to 10-fold higher. On the other hand, reducing the analysis of cases to the single question of causal relation limits our view and conclusions that could be drawn to avoid future complications. Compartment syndromes are severe complications occurring after lower limb orthopedic surgery, in particular if a cast is needed.[21,22] In several cases reported to the SOS RA Service, it was clear that an intense postoperative analgesia, often associated with motor blockade, was a factor of bad prognosis, delaying the diagnosis of this complication. In these cases, the main question is not, "Is this complication related or not to regional anesthesia?" but "What happened?" To explore in depth the last question, all staff involved (anesthesiologists, surgeons, nurses) should analyze together facts that contributed to the incident. Another challenge to improve safety is to enlarge our point of view. Looking at published data surprisingly shows that very few cases associated with human errors have been recorded. To explain these findings, it can be hypothesized either that the incidence of such complications is very low or that a classification bias exists (i.e., complications as consequences of human being considered as unrelated to regional anesthesia technique). During the last 3 years, 25 cases with drug injection errors were reported to SOS RA Service. Fortunately, most of these cases had a good prognosis but some of the patients had after-effects. All of the wrongly injected drugs were transparent and usually located on the anesthetic tray near the syringes containing the local anesthetic drugs.

## A Systems Analysis Approach

To explore more widely the causes of complications, we have to keep in mind that behind the outcome is the process of care and that a complication can be considered as a window on the healthcare system. We thus have to move from the "What happened?" question to "Why did it happen?"[5] This requires a change of our investigation tools. The systems analysis used by Vincent[7] is a typical example of innovative methods to investigate in depth a complication, and especially to study system errors. This approach remains useful for extremely rare events, whereas the epidemiologic approach does not work because of the difficulty (or impossibility) of gathering enough similar cases to obtain sufficient statistical power.

Using Vincent's methods for analyzing several cases reported to SOS RA Service, we identified several root causes specific to regional anesthesia. Five of them were often noticed:

1. An important dispersion in "how to do" the block within a single group of anesthesiologists: Many techniques or drugs are often available for a given block procedure. The anesthesia technique changes according to the anesthesiologist's preferences or experience. And this large dispersion could be considered a latent factor leading to human errors.[23]
2. Insufficiently defined aims and protocols: A regional anesthesia technique can be performed for both anesthesia allowing a surgical procedure and/or postoperative analgesia. However, there are some differences (type of drugs, drugs concentration, sites of puncture . . .) according to the chosen aim. This can be a source of confusion and sometimes of mistakes (i.e., a too high concentration of a local anesthetic used for postoperative analgesia leading to side effects that will occur during the patient stay on the ward or at home.
3. Prolonged effects of regional anesthesia: The long duration of postoperative analgesia is often an argument in favor of the use of regional anesthesia. However, after the patient has left the operating theater to go on the ward or at home, the

medical and nursing organization should be prepared to care for these prolonged anesthetic effects. For example, the timing at which neurologic complications become apparent is often delayed. In several cases reported to the SOS RA Service, neurologic complications were discovered long after the block was performed and only after discontinuation of a continuous infusion. This has been seen to occur also in institutions where anesthesiologists are highly trained and where surgeons have a high confidence toward RA but where monitoring and nurses' training are not adequately organized to allow for rapid diagnosis of complications. It is as if physicians do place a greater emphasis on performing the block than on organizing the postoperative surveillance.

4. Regional anesthesia is a technique: As with all techniques, regional anesthesia needs first to be learned (in particular, excellent knowledge of anatomy is critical) and this initial training period should be associated with adequate supervision. The next step is a stabilization period of how to do in order to avoid unnecessary changes without real benefit for the patient. It is still too often that physicians try for the first time in their next patient a new block for which the technique was described (as being easy to do, safe – a conclusion often reached after several hundred performed procedures – and with a high rate of success) by an enthusiastic speaker in a meeting that they had recently attended.

5. Regional anesthesia is a technique that can fail. Whereas it is considered that general anesthesia always works (although awareness is a known adverse event), it is clear that regional anesthesia can fail. In several cases associated with insufficient anesthesia reported to us, the poor outcome was related to the lack of preoperative definition of an alternative anesthesia strategy.

The interest of such approaches is to identify common causes (each of them leading to different types of complications). Controlling the side effects of one cause is a way to manage the risk related to regional anesthesia, often decreasing the risk of several types of complications.

## Conclusion

Large epidemiologic studies are always necessary. Many strategies such as improved training, use of safer devices and drugs, technologic innovation, and use of quality-improvement programs have been implemented to control the risks of RA. This probably explains why severe complications are now very rare in healthy patients (e.g., obstetric patients). In particular for "rare events," other approaches are available to explore complications and increase safety culture.

## References

1. Clergue F, Auroy Y, Pequignot F, Jougla E, Lienhart A, Laxenaire MC. French survey of anesthesia in 1996. Anesthesiology 1999;91:1509–1520.
2. Dripps RD, Vandam LD. Long term follow-up of patients who received 10,098 spinal anesthetics: failure to discover major neurological sequelae. JAMA 1954;156:1486–1491.
3. Phillips OC, Ebner H, Nelson A, Black MH. Neurologic complications following spinal anesthesia with lidocaine: a prospective review of 10,440 cases. Anesthesiology 1969;30:284–289.
4. Rodgers A, Walker N, Schug S, et al. Reduction of postoperative mortality and morbidity with epidural or spinal anaesthesia: results from overview of randomised trials. BMJ 2000;321:1493.
5. Auroy Y, Benhamou D, Amaberti R. Risk assessment and control require analysis of both outcomes and process of care. Anesthesiology 2004;101:815–817.

6. Vincent C, Taylor-Adams S, Chapman EJ, et al. How to investigate and analyse clinical incidents: clinical risk unit and association of litigation and risk management protocol. BMJ 2000;320:777–781.
7. Vincent CA. Analysis of clinical incidents: a window on the system not a search for root causes. Qual Saf Health Care 2004;13:242–243.
8. Auroy Y, Narchi P, Messiah A, Litt L, Rouvier B, Samii K. Serious complications related to regional anesthesia: results of a prospective survey in France. Anesthesiology 1997; 87:479–486.
9. Auroy Y, Benhamou D, Bargues L, et al. Major complications of regional anesthesia in France: The SOS Regional Anesthesia Hotline Service. Anesthesiology 2002;97: 1274–1280.
10. Gentili M, Aveline C, Bonnet F. Total spinal anesthesia after posterior lumbar plexus block [French]. Ann Fr Anesth Reanim 1998;17:740–742.
11. Auroy Y, Bargue L, Benhamou D, et al. Recommendation of the SOS ALR Group on the use of locoregional anesthesia [French]. Ann Fr Anesth Reanim 2000;19:621–623.
12. Mulroy MF. Systemic toxicity and cardiotoxicity from local anesthetics: incidence and preventive measures. Reg Anesth Pain Med 2002;27:556–561.
13. Abouleish EI, Elias M, Nelson C. Ropivacaine-induced seizure after extradural anaesthesia. Br J Anaesth 1998;80:843–844.
14. Ruetsch YA, Fattinger KE, Borgeat A. Ropivacaine-induced convulsions and severe cardiac dysrhythmia after sciatic block. Anesthesiology 1999;90:1784–1786.
15. Reinikainen M, Hedman A, Pelkonen O, Ruokonen E. Cardiac arrest after interscalene brachial plexus block with ropivacaine and lidocaine. Acta Anaesthesiol Scand 2003;47: 904–906.
16. Polley LS, Santos AC. Cardiac arrest following regional anesthesia with ropivacaine: here we go again! Anesthesiology 2003;99:1253–1254.
17. Chazalon P, Tourtier JP, Villevielle T, et al. Ropivacaine-induced cardiac arrest after peripheral nerve block: successful resuscitation. Anesthesiology 2003;99:1449–1451.
18. Schafhalter-Zoppoth I, Zeitz ID, Gray AT. Inadvertent femoral nerve impalement and intraneural injection visualized by ultrasound. Anesth Analg 2004;99:627–628.
19. Shah S, Hadzic A, Vloka JD, Cafferty MS, Moucha CS, Santos AC. Neurologic complication after anterior sciatic nerve block. Anesth Analg 2005;100:1515–1517.
20. Moen V, Dahlgren N, Irestedt L. Severe neurological complications after central neuraxial blockades in Sweden 1990–1999. Anesthesiology 2004;101:950–959.
21. Hyder N, Kessler S, Jennings AG, De Boer PG. Compartment syndrome in tibial shaft fracture missed because of a local nerve block. J Bone Joint Surg Br 1996;78:499–500.
22. Strecker WB, Wood MB, Bieber EJ. Compartment syndrome masked by epidural anesthesia for postoperative pain. Report of a case. J Bone Joint Surg Am 1986;68: 1447–1448.
23. Amalberti R, Auroy Y, Berwick D, Barach P. Five system barriers to achieving ultrasafe health care. Ann Intern Med 2005;142:756–764.

## Chapter Conclusion

This chapter presents morbidity information associated with the practice of regional anesthesia. Study design limitations such as the sources of data (sometimes voluntary), retrospective data analysis, lack of clinical denominators and controls, as well as biases and interrater reliability issues are addressed forthrightly. These studies are important for many reasons. They deal with large patient populations and some analyze data collected in systematic manner for three decades. The largest study, that of the American Society of Anesthesiologists, is ongoing. In some cases, patterns of practice that may lead to morbidity are proposed and examined. The fundamental goal of the studies is to enhance awareness of the morbidity associated with the practice of regional anesthesia and to propose ways to improve patient safety with better vigilance and the proper use of perioperative monitoring.

# 24 Medicolegal Aspects of Regional Anesthesia

Albert H. Santora

The purpose of this chapter is to present basic medicolegal principles, to report published guidelines that establish professional standards, and to summarize recent publications concerning medicolegal issues specific to the practice of regional anesthesia. Those interested in reading a meticulous dissertation concerning the legal aspects of medicine should consult a law text covering that field of jurisprudence. One could peruse a contemporary textbook of anesthesiology; such publications devote at least one exhaustive chapter to the subject.

## The Physician–Patient Relationship

Fundamentally, the physician–patient relationship is ethical in nature. One of the first people to offer his perception of the relationship was Hippocrates (c. 460–370 B.C.). He did so not in his famous "Physicians' Oath," but in another of his works, *Epidemics*, book 1, section 11:

> "As to diseases, make a habit of two things – to help, or at least to do no harm."[1]

To support this teaching, his "Physicians' Oath" contains two references to the "do no harm" doctrine. Taken out of context, these references have been translated as follows:

> I will apply dietetic measures for the benefit of the sick according to my ability and judgement; I will keep them from harm and injustice.

And

> Whatever houses I may visit, I will come for the benefit of the sick, remaining free of all intentional injustice, of all mischief . . .[2]

Hippocrates was Greek. Therefore, the famous Latin phrase "Primum non nocere" cannot be attributed to his original work. Nevertheless, Hippocrates' ancient admonition to do no harm still constitutes the ethical tenet on which the physician–patient relationship is based.

Unfortunately, some patients do experience harm while under the care of a physician. This fact has led to the establishment of the massive and complex medicolegal system that exists today to deal with "malpractice." The medicolegal ramifications of harm resulting from the practice of regional anesthesia will be discussed later in this chapter. First, a few basic legal principles and professional guidelines will be set forth to lay the foundation for further considerations.

### *The Legal Definition of the Physician–Patient Relationship*

A legal relationship is established when a physician accepts the duty to care for a patient. The patient (or his legal surrogate), after fulfilling the requirement of understanding and accepting the terms and information included in an informed consent disclosure, voluntarily agrees to enter into a physician–patient relationship. The duties of the physician to the patient include the following[2]:

1. To adhere to accepted "standards of care"
2. To practice in a "reasonable and prudent" manner
3. To obtain informed consent from the patient before entering into the relationship
4. To maintain medical records
5. To examine the patient
6. To use consultants and referring physicians when appropriate

Many situations will arise when the conditions set forth in this section will be difficult, impossible, or inappropriate to fulfill. For example, in an emergency, when an unconscious patient cannot respond to the physician and no surrogate is present, informed consent cannot be obtained. Another patient may be unable to understand the information contained on the hospital's standard "Informed Consent" statement. Moreover, the patient may not be of legal age and his parent may demand a standard of care that the physician considers immoral or unreasonable. Many other factors may confound the establishment of a normal physician–patient relationship. In general, when the care to be rendered is elective in nature, the physician must fulfill all of the requirements necessary to establish a legal physician–patient relationship. When the care to be given is emergent in nature, the physician must assume the duty to care for the patient and to practice within the "standards of care" at all times.

### *Informed Consent*

Over the past 48 years, the concept of informed consent has evolved to its current definition.[3] Informed consent is rendered by an autonomous, reasonable patient who has been appropriately informed about the procedure or treatment plan he is to undergo. The physician must assure that the patient receives and understands all of the "information that the hypothetical reasonable patient would consider important to make a decision."[3] Included in this information is a description of ". . . those risks which are reasonably likely to occur in any patient under the circumstances, and to those which are reasonably likely to occur in particular patients because of their condition."[2] Benefits to be expected from the procedure must be set forth as well as alternative treatment plans. An anesthesiologist should inform the patient if he or she, or another care team member, is to administer the anesthetic. If a patient does not want to hear all of the "gory details," the physician must document that the patient does not wish to be informed, note such on the chart, and ask the patient to countersign the chart.[2] Verbal, written, and implied informed consent is valid. However, it is obvious that a written consent is easiest to prove should the necessity arise.

Much has been written concerning the ethical considerations of informed consent. The American Society of Anesthesiologists' *Syllabus on Ethics*,[4] 1999, devotes an entire section to the informed consent issue. A pertinent quotation from this publication follows[4]:

> The most common theory of suit relating to informed consent is negligence. Negligence means that the anesthesiologist did not provide sufficient disclosure to permit a patient to make an informed decision.

The anesthesiologist should treat the patient as a reasonable, autonomous person. The quality as well as the quantity of the information presented to the patient must be considered. With respect to regional anesthesia, it may not be enough to tell a patient that one risk of neuraxial anesthesia is "epidural hematoma." The patient may think that a "hematoma" is some sort of vegetable! It is more honest, accurate, and ethical to tell the patient what an "epidural hematoma" is and to describe the complications that it can cause. Speak to the patient in his language.

## Professional Guidelines and Statements

A professional society publishes guidelines and statements that codify principles considered fundamental to defining its purpose and existence. The American Society of Anesthesiologists (ASA) has published many guidelines and statements that address the Society's position on every aspect of anesthesia practice. All of these can be examined on the Society's Web site: www.asahq.org. Guidelines and statements do not carry the weight of law. They do not represent rules of practice expounded by the Society. In fact, ASA specifically states that certain circumstances may be encountered when the guidelines do not apply. However, in general, the guidelines of the ASA do establish standards of care.

All physicians who practice regional anesthesia should read and understand all of the guidelines and statements of the professional societies with which they are affiliated. Particularly pertinent to the practice of regional anesthesia are these published by the ASA:

1. Guidelines for the Ethical Practice of Anesthesiology[4]
2. Guidelines for Regional Anesthesia in Obstetrics[5]
3. Statement on Regional Anesthesia[6]

These Guidelines and Statement are presented in the Appendices of this chapter.

To deviate from the guidelines is permissible. If a practitioner does so, he or she should document *in writing* the reasons for their decision.

## Risk Management and Quality Assurance

The purpose of risk management and quality assurance programs is to decrease the likelihood of causing preventable injury to patients and to assure that the level of care rendered meets or exceeds the expected standards. Excellent chapters covering these topics are published in standard anesthesiology textbooks.[7–9] The ASA has published its Quality Management Template: October 2004[10] that deals comprehensively with the subjects. Physicians who incorporate risk management and quality assurance programs into their practices will at least fulfill institutional, legal, organizational, and professional obligations. The impact of a malpractice lawsuit may very well be moderated to the benefit of the defendant if appropriate risk management and quality assurance programs are in effect before an untoward event happens. Hopefully, these programs will help physicians to adopt new policies, practice habits, and protocols to make anesthesia delivery safer for the patient.

## Malpractice: Basic Legal Considerations

Although physicians may become involved with the criminal legal system, the vast majority of medical malpractice litigation deals with civil concerns dealt with by tort laws. Although grounds for medical malpractice may include battery and abandonment, most of the time negligence on the part of the physician is claimed by the plaintiff. To prove medical malpractice, a plaintiff must establish the following[9] (with modification):

1. Duty: That the physician owed him a duty
2. Breach of duty: That the physician failed to fulfill his duty
3. Proximate cause: That a reasonably close causal relation existed between the physician's acts and the resultant injury
4. Damages: That actual damages resulted because of the acts of the physician

The following legal definitions are presented as these terms turn up in every article on the subject of medical malpractice. All of the definitions are quoted from Black's Law Dictionary, 8th Edition, 2004.[12]

1. Tort: A civil wrong, other than breach of contract, for which a remedy may be obtained, usually in the form of damages; a breach of duty that the law imposes on persons who stand in a particular relation to one another.

2. Duty: A legal obligation that is owed or due to another and that needs to be satisfied; an obligation for which somebody else has a corresponding right.

3. Malpractice: An incidence of negligence or incompetence on the part of a professional. To succeed in a malpractice claim, a plaintiff must also prove proximate cause and damages. Medical malpractice: A doctor's failure to exercise the degree of care and skill that a physician or surgeon of the same medical specialty would use under similar circumstances.

4. Negligence: The failure to exercise the standard of care that a reasonably prudent person would have exercised in a similar situation.

5. Standard of care: In the law of negligence, the degree of care that a reasonable person should exercise.

6. Damages: Money claimed by, or ordered to be paid to, a person as compensation for loss or injury. Damages may be actual, discretionary (for pain and suffering), or exemplary (punitive).

7. Proximate cause: A cause that is legally sufficient to result in liability; an act or omission that is considered in law to result in a consequence so that liability can be imposed on the actor.

The most common allegation of a medical malpractice complaint is that the plaintiff was injured by a physician who acted negligently. The physician's practice deviated from accepted standards of care causing injury to the patient. Compensation for the injury has a monetary value in the form of damages.

Because plaintiff attorneys usually receive a percentage of the damage settlement, the damages are set as high as possible.

### *What to Do if Sued*

One of the most enduring and thoughtful theses on this subject was written by John H. Tinker, MD and William W. Hesson, JD.[13] Their disquisition should be read in its entirety and is referenced for that purpose. In the limited scope of this chapter, a few of their more pertinent quotations, observations, and suggestions are presented.

Quotations from Tinker and Hesson[13]:

1. It is important to understand, at the outset of this chapter, that anyone can sue anyone for anything.[13]

2. In other words, after we [physicians] create expectations of excellence, when something goes awry, it is natural for the patient to assume that something has been done wrong – somebody was negligent, either by omission or commission.[13]

3. It is a basic tenet that it is extremely unlikely, if not impossible, to perform procedures with a zero complication rate.[13]

4. The message here is to expect litigation from poor results or complications, whether expected or unexpected, whether the patient was informed or not.[13]

5. When a physician gets sued, he or she must not allow any recriminations that may occur to affect care of present or future patients.[13]

6. Throughout the whole process, though many physicians have become quite cynical, it must be remembered that underneath the inevitable mountain of paper, the oscillation of emotions, the sometimes misleading testimony, and numerous other problems there is a patient. That patient or family *still deserves our attention and care even if they have brought suit against us.*[13]

Tinker and Hesson address many other topics such as the trial process, the attorney defendant relationship, expert witness testimony, and how to prepare for a deposition and an appearance in the courtroom. They advise the physician-defendant on how to act as well as how to react. Their presentation is prudent and essential reading. To summarize their suggestions, the physician should act professionally, honestly, and cooperatively with his attorney. He should not take the allegations of the suit personally. He should not let it ruin his life and career. He should allow his attorney to do his job. He should do everything possible to discover the facts. Finally, he should not forget that a *patient* feels that he has been wronged. That patient is entitled to learn the truth.

### *The Expert Witness*

Expert witnesses are used by plaintiff and defense attorneys to render opinions as to whether or not standards of care have been breached. If breached, did the physician's act or omission cause an injury to the patient? Qualifications of an expert witness vary. Must the expert be in active practice? Is a retired physician competent to be an expert? Must the expert be board certified? Does he need certification in the same specialty as the defendant? How much money does the physician make from expert testimony? Does the expert have any conflicts of interest with either party in the suit? Each state has its own set of rules and qualifications required of the expert witness.

The ASA has published guidelines concerning expert witness testimony (see Appendices of this chapter).[14] Interestingly, the Society has adopted review procedures for expert witness testimony.[15] An ASA member may file a complaint with the Society if he deems that "sworn expert testimony"[15] rendered in a legal proceeding is in violation of the Society's guidelines. The complaint can be filed only after all judicial proceedings of the suit from which the complaint had arisen have been completed. Eventually, if the Society's Judicial Council determines that an expert witness's testimony is in violation of guidelines, the Council may recommend "an appropriate sanction – censure or suspension or revocation of membership – to the Board of Directors for final action."[14] All of the preliminary proceedings of the Society are confidential. "Only if the board imposes a sanction shall that fact be made public."[14] For an honorable expert witness, a sanction from the Board of the ASA would constitute a significant reprimand. For the less than honorable witness, such a sanction would be inconsequential. The Society has set reasonable and fair standards that its members should observe if they accept the responsibility and the pecuniary rewards of serving as an expert witness.

## Medicolegal Aspects of Regional Anesthesia: Conclusions from Morbidity Studies

Many international studies present morbidity data associated with regional anesthesia. Chapter 23 of this book reports findings from the major studies. Because much of the data is derived from medicolegal sources, pertinent comments concerning each study's implications are presented in this chapter. The reader may refer to the previous chapter to review each study in more detail.

## American Society of Anesthesiologists' Closed Claims Project

Publications authored by investigators of the ASA's Closed Claims Project constitute the most thorough and scholarly body of literature dealing with the medicolegal aspects of American anesthesia practice.

The ASA's Closed Claims Project has been collecting anesthesia malpractice claim data for more than 30 years.[15] The database for the Project consists of a standardized collection of information obtained from the detailed analyses of more than 6000 anesthesia malpractice law suits that had been "closed" by the time each analysis had been conducted.[16] "Closed" is defined as settled. Data are obtained voluntarily from insurance carriers who cover approximately 50% of American anesthesiologists.

The limitations of the study have been published elsewhere.[15–18] These include the lack of a denominator, reliance on voluntary cooperation offered by the insurance carriers, and concerns over biases relating to changing patterns of practice, poor interrater reliability, the study's retrospective design, and outcome severity. Nevertheless, the Project's investigators have uncovered patterns and trends that "... discern how the process of care contributes to the genesis of adverse outcomes."[16] Some of the objectives of the Project have been to define the damaging events and adverse outcomes associated with the delivery of anesthesia care, to hypothesize the mechanism of the events, to ascertain whether current standards of patient monitoring could have prevented some of the events, to report financial settlement patterns, and to evaluate the appropriateness of care rendered. Much other information is presented in the Project's many publications. Suffice it to say that the ASA's Closed Claims Project collects, analyzes, and reports data eventuated by interactions at the anesthesiology practice/medicolegal system interface.

### *Conclusions*

Conclusions drawn from analysis of the ASA's Closed Claims Project regional anesthesia data[19] include the following:

1. "Nearly half of the damaging events for both obstetric and nonobstetric neuraxial anesthesia claims were block related."[19]
2. "The most common damaging event for these high severity injuries in obstetric and nonobstetric groups was neuraxial cardiac arrest."[19]
3. "Ninety percent of claims for neuraxial cardiac arrest resulted in death or permanent brain damage."[19] The authors cautioned that appropriate early treatment with epinephrine "... may not guarantee a good outcome during neuraxial cardiac arrest."[19]
4. "Unintentional intravascular injection was the second most common damaging event in obstetric claims but accounted for only 2% of nonobstetric claims with high-severity outcome."[19]
5. Regional anesthesia techniques associated with neuraxial cardiac arrest included the following:
    a. Spinal: 70%
    b. Lumbar epidural: 25%
    c. Caudal epidural: 2%
    d. Thoracic epidural: 1%
    e. Combined spinal/epidural: 1%
6. With respect to neuraxial cardiac arrest, "Resuscitation was delayed in 91% of obstetrics claims compared with 45% of nonobstetric claims as judged by two or more ASA Closed Claims Project Committee reviewers."[19]
7. Despite the widespread availability of capnography and pulse oximetry in the 1990s, outcome for neuraxial cardiac arrest was not significantly different between the 1980s and 1990s.[19]

8. "Combined analysis of obstetric and nonobstetric neuraxial claims associated with hematoma revealed that almost three fourths of these claims had evidence of either an intrinsic (one obstetric claim with severe preeclampsia) or iatrogenic coagulopathy."[19]

9. Data of the Closed Claims Project demonstrates that "an increased motor block out of proportion to the infused local anesthetic is the most common presenting symptom"[19] of a potentially problematic epidural hematoma although many have suggested that back pain is the cardinal symptom. Early treatment of an epidural hematoma is essential to favorable outcome!

10. Eye "injuries were usually permanent and related to the block technique, and more than half of the claims resulted in blindness."[19]

11. Damaging events might have been prevented by better use of available monitors, the application of safer techniques (such as topical anesthesia for cataract surgery), and a more vigilant practice of anesthesia.

Of the lumbar and thoracic epidural blocks, 52% were associated with unintentional subarachnoid injection. Therefore, 84% of the neuraxial cardiac arrest claims were associated with subarachnoid injections.

### *ASA's Closed Claims Project: Chronic Pain Management*

Fitzgibbon et al.[21] reported a Closed Claims Project analysis of injuries associated with chronic pain management. Many of these claims are associated with regional anesthetic techniques.

Relevant clinical suggestions based on the findings of their study include:

1. A test dose should be used when administering a regional block.
2. The volume of solution injected into the epidural space should not exceed that of a typical intrathecal test dose.
3. The addition of local anesthetics and opioids to epidural steroid injections can lead to more severe outcomes (death and brain damage). Are these adjunctive drugs really necessary?
4. ". . . It is important to establish a monitoring system for pneumothorax and to instruct patients as to the symptoms and signs of a pneumothorax after intercostal nerve blocks, stellate ganglion blocks, trigger point injections, and brachial plexus blocks."[21]

### *ASA's Closed Claims Project: Obstetric Anesthesia*

Davies et al.[22] presented Closed Claims Project data analyzing 792 obstetric-related claims from the 1970s, 1980s, and 1990s.

Although an in-depth analysis of damaging events and specific injury patterns was not presented, the abstract reported significant data related to regional anesthesia.

**Results**

1. The proportion of cesarean delivery claims associated with general anesthesia decreased in the 1980s and 1990s as compared with the 1970s, whereas the proportion of regional anesthesia claims increased.
2. Lumbar epidurals were more common in cesarean delivery claims in the 1980s and 1990s as compared with the 1970s.
3. Spinal anesthesia for cesarean delivery data showed no differences between epochs.
4. The proportion of vaginal delivery claims associated with regional anesthesia increased over the decades.
5. Claims for maternal death decreased over the decades.
6. Claims for maternal nerve injury and back pain increased in the 1990s compared with the 1970s.
7. Newborn brain damage decreased in the 1990s compared with the 1980s.

**Conclusions**

Davies et al.[22] summarized their findings as follows:

1. The change in cesarean delivery–related claims reflected the increased use of regional anesthesia versus the declined use of general anesthesia for cesarean delivery.
2. This change may have been related to the decreased number of claims for maternal death and neonatal brain damage.
3. The increased use of regional anesthesia may have accounted for the increased number of claims of maternal nerve damage and back pain.
4. ". . . Changing medicolegal strategies and other factors may also have contributed to the reduction in severe outcomes in OB claims over the decades."[22]

Hopefully, a more detailed analysis of obstetric-related claims will be forthcoming.

### *Canadian Closed Claims Review: Regional Anesthesia Morbidity*

Smedstad (Chapter 23) suggests that an anesthesiologist can minimize the risk of a lawsuit by obtaining appropriate consent, by good record keeping, by taking note of preexisting conditions, by utilizing appropriate monitoring, and by avoiding the use of the wrong drugs. A few other conclusions are offered in the article by Peng and Smedstad[23]:

1. "Good communication before, during, and after the procedure may prevent a malpractice claim."[23]
2. Before an anesthesiologist performs an eye block, he or she should be fully trained and familiar with the anatomy as well as the potential complications of the various techniques.
3. With respect to neuraxial blocks, should a patient experience pain on needle insertion or injection of local anesthetic or steroid, follow-up contact with the patient should be conducted.
4. Thorough documentation at all steps of anesthetic care must be recorded in the chart. Neat, thorough charting in the operating room can prevent an unfavorable legal outcome.

**Medicolegal Claims: An Australian Study**

A review of the Australian study published by Cass[24] is presented in Chapter 23. Medicolegal conclusions from his study follow.

***Conclusions***

The Australian study shared many of the limitations with the closed claims studies discussed previously. It is also somewhat limited in scope. However, the following observations can be made in summarizing the data:

1. Neuraxial blocks were the most frequently cited techniques related to malpractice claims.
2. Inadequate analgesia with neuraxial blocks was a repeated source of litigation.
3. Injury related to eye blocks had a relatively high settlement cost.

### *Overall Conclusions of the Malpractice Claims Studies*

Closed claims analyses reveal, organize, and evaluate fallout from interactions between anesthesiologists and the legal system. Although the studies cited in this chapter suffer from methodologic limitations, they impart valuable information. They analyze medicolegal data associated with claims resulting from the practice of regional anesthesia. Analysis of the data suggests "trends" on how the practice of anesthesia might be made safer. Studies should be designed to test hypotheses that are formulated after consideration of these suggestions. Future claims reports from localities in which all misadventure, injury, and poor outcome must be reported by law will be extremely useful. These data will be more complete and a known denominator will allow investigators to document the incidences and the true magnitude of the types of problems that lead to lawsuits.

## Additional Considerations Regarding the Practice of Regional Anesthesia: Medicolegal Implications

The practitioner of regional anesthesia should consider the medicolegal implications of three additional controversial subjects.

### *Performing Regional Blocks on Anesthetized Patients*

Regional blocks are routinely performed on anesthetized pediatric patients.[24] In addition, many anesthesiologists perform a multitude of blocks on anesthetized or heavily sedated adult patients. They offer the block under anesthesia with due consideration to the comfort of the patient. Advocates of the practice claim that it should be left up to the individual practitioner to consider the risks and benefits involved. They cite breaches of judgment and technique as the main causative factors of poor outcome with respect to the practice.[25] However, the safety of this practice has been questioned by many authors in the recent literature.[26–31] These authors argue that the general anesthetic or heavy sedation would mask typical patient responses to needle trauma or the deposition of local anesthetic in the wrong place. Philip Bromage[32] has termed this type of injury "... an example of the most florid form of 'masked mischief,'" Rosenquist and Birnbach[31] ask in an editorial, "Will your patient thank you?" should the practice lead to a serious neurologic injury. They further opine, "If and when more safety data [concerning the practice] are available, this point should be revisited."[31] Debate over administering blocks to anesthetized patients is ongoing and is heated at times. Keep in mind that should an anesthesiologist be faced with a lawsuit resulting from this practice, the plaintiff will have absolutely no problem finding an expert witness to condemn him. This knowledge should not dictate the way an anesthesiologist practices. However, one should remember the ancient advice *primum non nocere* before electing to administer a block to an anesthetized patient. Safety of the practice has been questioned by many.

### *Awareness "Under Anesthesia"*

The regional anesthesia practitioner must be aware that there is a movement afoot that is gaining momentum: the phenomenon of awareness under anesthesia. Companies that market various types of electroencephalogram monitors, talk-show hosts, certain hospital regulatory authorities, and especially trial lawyers are aware of this specter and are doing their best to warn the public of its existence. Those who practice regional anesthesia may be particularly vulnerable to lawsuits concerning awareness because their patients are usually not "asleep." The closed claims studies clearly documented that lawsuits claiming "inadequate anesthesia/analgesia" have already been adjudicated. Was there a component of unexpected awareness related to the claim? In the process of obtaining informed consent, due consideration should be given to discussing with the patient the proposed degree of sedation, what the patient will feel when a block is administered, what the patient may "feel," hear, or otherwise sense in the operating room, and what he or she might remember of the perioperative experience. Often a patient will say something like, "I'll agree to a spinal, but I don't want to hear, feel, or remember anything in the operating room." The anesthesiologist must address these concerns. Finally, BEWARE of what the surgeon has told the patient.

He might have said to the patient: "Anesthesia will pop in an epidural. You won't feel a thing. You'll be asleep anyway!" If the physician takes the time to listen, he would be surprised to hear what the patient has to tell him.

### *Can Regional Anesthesia Worsen Medicolegal Risk?*

A provocative article by Wedel[33] asks: "Can Regional Anesthesia Worsen Outcome? Medicolegal Risk." In certain cases, perhaps it might. The ASA's Closed Claims Project has documented that most nerve injury claims involved general anesthesia (general anesthesia 61% versus regional anesthesia 36%).[33] Most of the time, the etiology of the injury could not be specified. This causes "breach of duty" and "causation" problems for the plaintiff. However, when a nerve injury occurs after administration of a regional block, the plaintiff's lawyer may invoke the doctrine of res ipsa loquitur "the thing speaks for itself." If the theory is proven, the burden of proof shifts to the defendant to show that he did not cause the injury. This may prove difficult. After all, "he stuck a needle into the patient!" Wedel writes, "Whether an increased medicolegal risk is associated with regional as compared with general anesthesia is unclear. Analyses of closed claim data are simultaneously reassuring and concerning."[33] Although this warning should be considered, the anesthesiologist cannot allow himself to practice "legal medicine." Clearly, regional anesthesia has certain advantages over general anesthesia in many cases. In the end, how one practices anesthesia is a medical, not a legal issue.

## Recommendations

The following recommendations are made concerning ways to avoid a lawsuit, to practice safer anesthesia, and to better understand the legal system.

1. Act professionally at all times.
2. Keep meticulous records.
3. Know the guidelines and statements of your specialty.
4. Practice only the standards of care.
5. Adopt risk management and quality assurance protocols.
6. Understand your duties to the patient: physician/patient relationship.
7. Consider your informed consent obligations seriously.
8. Never coerce a patient into accepting a given anesthetic plan.
9. Examine the patient. Document preexisting conditions.
10. Know the patient's history and medication regimen.
11. Examine all laboratory data preoperatively (e.g., coagulation status of the patient).
12. Practice only those techniques in which you are fully trained and proficient.
13. Carry adequate malpractice insurance.
14. Make the acquaintance of an excellent malpractice defense lawyer before you need him. If you require his professional expertise, listen to him and do what he tells you to do!
15. If possible, establish a professional relationship with a malpractice defense attorney that will allow you to review legal/medical records generated in a lawsuit. This practice is often helpful to the lawyer and always educational for the physician. Learn how lawyers think, write, and speak.
16. Be honest.
17. As a defendant, do not let the rigors of a lawsuit affect your care of patients.
18. Expect to be sued at some point in your career. Be prepared to deal with it.
19. Often, a lawsuit is just a matter of money (some for the plaintiff, a lot for the lawyers). If you know that you have acted properly, do not take it personally.
20. Remember: If you are sued, there exists a patient who feels that he has been wronged. He is entitled to know the truth.

## Conclusion

This chapter has discussed the medicolegal aspects of regional anesthesia. Basic legal principles have been presented. Standards of care have been addressed. Closed claims data have been analyzed. These data were obtained from examinations of lawsuits that involved claims alleging malpractice related to the administration of regional anesthetics. It is hoped that these analyses demonstrated how practitioners of regional anesthesia have become involved with the medicolegal system. Closed claims studies report historical findings. In the future, controlled, prospective studies may better define the types of practices that could bring an anesthesiologist into contact with that system. Hopefully, future research will define ways not only to avoid legal problems, but to make the practice of regional anesthesia safer for patients.

## References

1. Respectfully Quoted: A Dictionary of Quotations Requested from the Congressional Research Service. Washington DC: Library of Congress; 1989. Bartleby.com, 2003. Available at: www.bartleby.com/73/847.html. Accessed February 9, 2006.
2. Edelstein L. The Hippocratic Oath: Text, Translation, and Interpretation. Baltimore: Johns Hopkins Press; 1943. Available at: www.pbs.org/wgbh/nova/doctors/oath_classical.html. Accessed February 9, 2006.
3. American Society of Anesthesiologists. Professional Liability and the Anesthesiologist. Park Ridge, IL: ASA; 1992:2–3. Available at: www.asahq.org/publicationsAnd Services/professional.html. Accessed February 9, 2006.
4. American Society of Anesthesiologists. Syllabus on Ethics. Park Ridge, IL: ASA; 1999: A-1.
5. American Society of Anesthesiologists. Guidelines for the Ethical Practice of Anesthesiology. Park Ridge, IL: ASA; 2003.
6. American Society of Anesthesiologists. Guidelines for Regional Anesthesia in Obstetrics. Park Ridge, IL: ASA; 2000.
7. American Society of Anesthesiologists. Statement on Regional Anesthesia. Park Ridge, IL: ASA; 2002.
8. Eichhorn JH. Risk management. In: Benumof JL, Saidman LJ, eds. Anesthesia and Perioperative Complications. St. Louis: Mosby Year Book; 1992.
9. Vitez TS. Quality assurance. Risk management. In: Benumof JL, Saidman LJ, eds. Anesthesia and Perioperative Complications. St. Louis: Mosby Year Book; 1992.
10. Kroll DA, Cheney FW. Medicolegal aspects of anesthetic practice. In: Barash PG, Cullen BF, Stoelting RK, eds. Clinical Anesthesia. 2nd ed. Philadelphia: Lippincott-Raven; 1996:115–125.
11. American Society of Anesthesiologists. Quality Management Template. Park Ridge, IL: ASA; 20 as Ref. 15: 115.
12. Garner BA. Black's Law Dictionary. 8th ed. St. Paul: Thompson/West; 2004.
13. Tinker JH, Hesson WW. What to do if sued: an analysis of the allegations of malpractice brought against an anesthesia provider. Risk management. In: Benumof JL, Saidman LJ, eds. Anesthesia and Perioperative Complications. St. Louis: Mosby Year Book; 1992.
14. American Society of Anesthesiologists. Guidelines for Expert Witness Qualifications and Testimony. Park Ridge, IL: ASA; 2003.
15. Scott M. ASA adopts review procedure for expert witness testimony. ASA Newslett 2003;67(12). Available at: www.asahq.org/Newsletter/2003/12-03/scott.html. Accessed February 9, 2006.
16. Posner KL. Data reveals trends in anesthesia malpractice payments. ASA Newslett 2004;68(6). Available at: www.asahq.org/Newsletter/2004/06_04/posner06_04.html. Accessed February 9, 2006.
17. Caplan RA. The ASA closed claims project: lessons learned. ASA Annual Meeting Refresher Course Lectures 2004; Lecture 118:1–7.

18. Cheney FW. The American Society of Anesthesiologists Closed Claims Project: what have we learned, how has it affected practice, and how will it affect practice in the future? Anesthesiology 1999;91:552–556.
19. Lee LA, Domino KB. The closed claims project. Has it influenced anesthetic practice and outcome? Anesthesiol Clin North Am 2002;20(3):485–501.
20. Lee LA, Posner KL, Domino KB, Caplan RA, Cheney FW. Injuries associated with regional anesthesia in the 1980s and 1990s. Anesthesiology 2004;101:143–152.
21. Fitzgibbon DR, Posner KL, Domino KB, Caplan RA, Lee LA, Cheney FW. Chronic pain management. Anesthesiology 2004;100:98–105.
22. Davies JM, et al. Trends in obstetric anesthesia malpractice claims of the last three decades. Anesthesiology 2004;101:A1231.
23. Peng PWH, Smedstad KG. Litigation in Canada against anesthesiologists practicing regional anesthesia. A review of closed claims. Can J Anaesth 2000;47(2):105–112.
24. Cass NM. Medicolegal claims against anaesthetists: a 20 year study. Anaesth Intensive Care 2004;32(1):47–58.
25. Markakis DA. Regional anesthesia in pediatrics. Anesthesiol Clin North Am 2000; 18(2):355–381.
26. Fischer HBJ. Performing epidural insertion under general anaesthesia. Anaesthesia 2000; 55:288–289.
27. Benumof JL. Permanent loss of cervical spinal cord function associated with interscalene block performed under general anesthesia. Anesthesiology 2000;93(6):1541–1544.
28. Bromage PB, Benumof JL. Letter: paraplegia following intracord injection during attempted epidural anesthesia under general anesthesia. Reg Anesth Pain Med 1998; 23(5):520–521.
29. Benumof JL. Comment on "perioperative interscalene blockade: an overview of its history and current clinical use." J Clin Anesth 2003;15:489.
30. Kao MC, Tsai SK, Tsou MY, Lee HK, Guo WY, Hu JS. Paraplegia after delayed detection of inadvertent spinal cord injury during thoracic epidural catheterization in an anesthetized elderly patient. Anesth Analg 2004;99:580–583.
31. Rosenquist RW, Birnbach DJ. Editorial: epidural insertion in anesthetized adults – will your patients thank you? Anesth Analg 2003;96:1545–1546.
32. Bromage PR. Masked mischief. Reg Anesth 1996;21(6S):62–63.
33. Wedel DJ. Can regional anesthesia worsen outcome? Medicolegal risk. Reg Anesth 1996; 21(6S):71–74.
34. Kroll DA, Caplan RA, Posner K, Ward RJ, Cheney FW. Nerve injury associated with anesthesia. Anesthesiology 1990;72:202–207.

## Bibliography

Sanbar SS, ed. Legal Medicine. 6th ed. Philadelphia: Mosby; 2004.

## Appendices

All of the appended documents are publications of the American Society of Anesthesiologists, Park Ridge, IL. Reproduced here with permission.

### *Appendix I: Guidelines for the Ethical Practice of Anesthesiology*

(Approved by House of Delegates on October 3, 1967, and last amended on October 15, 2003.)

#### Preamble

Membership in the ASA is a privilege of physicians who are dedicated to the ethical provision of health care. The Society recognized the Principles of Medical Ethics of the American Medical Association (AMA) as the basic guide to the ethical conduct of its members.

### AMA Principles of Medical Ethics

The medical profession has long subscribed to a body of ethical statements developed primarily for the benefit of the patient. As a member of this profession, a physician must recognize responsibility not only to patients but also to society, to other health professionals and to self. The following principles adopted by the AMA are not laws but standards of conduct that define the essentials of honorable behavior for the physician.

I. A physician shall be dedicated to providing competent medical care with compassion and respect for human dignity.
II. A physician shall uphold the standards of professionalism, be honest in all professional interactions, and strive to report physicians deficient in character or competence, or engaging in fraud or deception to appropriate entities.
III. A physician shall respect the law and also recognize a responsibility to seek changes in those requirements which are contrary to the best interests of the patient.
IV. A physician shall respect the rights of patients, colleagues, and other health professionals and shall safeguard patients' confidence within the constraints of the law.
V. A physician shall continue to study, apply, and advance scientific knowledge, maintain a commitment to medical education, make relevant information available to patients, colleagues, and the public, obtain consultation, and use the talents of other health professionals when indicated.
VI. A physician shall, in the provision of appropriate patient care except in emergencies, be free to choose whom to serve, with whom to associate, and the environment in which to provide medical care.
VII. A physician shall recognize a responsibility to participate in activities contributing to improvement of the community and betterment of public health.
VIII. A physician shall, while caring for a patient, regard responsibility to the patient as paramount.
IX. A physician shall support access to medical care for all people.

### AMA, 2001

The practice of anesthesiology involves special problems relating to the quality and standards of patient care. Therefore, the Society requires its members to adhere to the AMA Principles of Medical Ethics and any other specific ethical guidelines adopted by the Society.

### Medical Direction

Medical Direction is anesthesia direction, management, or instruction provided by an anesthesiologist whose responsibilities include:

a. Preanesthetic evaluation of the patient.
b. Prescription of the anesthesia plan.
c. Personal participation in the most demanding procedures in this plan, especially those of induction and emergence, if applicable.
d. Following the course of anesthesia administration at frequent intervals.
e. Remaining physically available for the immediate diagnosis and the treatment of emergencies.
f. Providing indicated postanesthesia care.

An anesthesiologist engaged in medical direction should not personally be administering another anesthetic and should use sound judgment in initiating other concurrent anesthetic and emergency procedures.

**ASA Ethical Guidelines**

*There may be specific circumstances when elements of the following guidelines may not apply and wherein individualized decisions may be appropriate.*

I. Anesthesiologists have ethical responsibilities to their patients.

1. The patient–physician relationship involves special obligations for the physician that include placing the patient's interests foremost, faithfully caring for the patient, and being truthful.
2. Anesthesiologists respect the right of every patient to self-determination. Anesthesiologists should include patients, including minors, in medical decision making that is appropriate to their developmental capacity and the medical issues involved. Anesthesiologists should not use their medical skills to restrain or coerce patients who have adequate decision-making capacity.
3. Anesthetized patients are particularly vulnerable, and anesthesiologists should strive to care for each patient's physical and psychological safety, comfort, and dignity. Anesthesiologists should monitor themselves and their colleagues to protect the anesthetized patient from any disrespectful or abusive behavior.
4. Anesthesiologists should keep confidential patients' medical and personal information.
5. Anesthesiologists should provide preoperative evaluation and care and should facilitate the process of informed decision making, especially regarding the choice of anesthetic technique.
6. If responsibility for a patient's care is to be shared with other physicians or nonphysician anesthesia providers, this arrangement should be explained to the patient. When directing nonphysician anesthesia providers, anesthesiologists should provide or ensure the same level of preoperative evaluation, care, and counseling as when personally providing these same aspects of anesthesia care.
7. When directing nonphysician anesthesia providers or physicians in training in the actual delivery of anesthetics, anesthesiologists should remain personally and continuously available for direction and supervision during the anesthetic; they should directly participate in the most demanding aspects of the anesthetic care.
8. Anesthesiologists should provide for appropriate postanesthetic care for their patients.
9. Anesthesiologists should not participate in exploitive financial relationships.
10. Anesthesiologists share with all physicians the responsibility to provide care for patients irrespective of their ability to pay for their care. Anesthesiologists should provide such care with the same diligence and skill as for patients who do pay for their care.

II. Anesthesiologists have ethical responsibilities to medical colleagues.

1. Anesthesiologists should promote a cooperative and respectful relationship with their professional colleagues that facilitates quality medical care for patients. This responsibility respects the efforts and duties of other care providers, including physicians, medical students, nurses, technicians, and assistants.
2. Anesthesiologists should provide timely medical consultation when requested and should seek consultation when appropriate.
3. Anesthesiologists should cooperate with colleagues to improve the quality, effectiveness, and efficiency of medical care.
4. Anesthesiologists should advise colleagues whose ability to practice medicine becomes temporarily or permanently impaired to appropriately modify or discontinue their practice. They should assist, to the extent of their own abilities, with the reeducation or rehabilitation of a colleague who is returning to practice.

5. Anesthesiologists should not take financial advantage of other physicians, non-physician anesthesia providers, or staff members. Verbal and written contracts should be honest and understandable, and should be respected.

III. Anesthesiologists have ethical responsibilities to the healthcare facilities in which they practice.

1. Anesthesiologists should serve on healthcare facility or specialty committees. This responsibility includes making good-faith efforts to review the practice of colleagues and to help develop departmental or healthcare facility procedural guidelines for the benefit of the healthcare facility and all of its patients.
2. Anesthesiologists share with all medical staff members the responsibility to observe and report to appropriate authorities any potentially negligent practices or conditions that may present a hazard to patients or healthcare facility personnel.
3. Anesthesiologists personally handle many controlled and potentially dangerous substances and, therefore, have a special responsibility to keep these substances secure from illicit use. Anesthesiologists should work within their healthcare facility to develop and maintain an adequate monitoring system for controlled substances.

IV. Anesthesiologists have ethical responsibilities to themselves.

1. The achievement and maintenance of competence and skill in the specialty is the primary professional duty of all anesthesiologists. This responsibility does not end with completion of residency training or certification by the American Board of Anesthesiology.
2. The practice of quality anesthesia care requires that anesthesiologists maintain their physical and mental health and special sensory capabilities. If in doubt about their health, then anesthesiologists should seek medical evaluation and care. During the period of evaluation or treatment, anesthesiologists should modify or cease their practice.

V. Anesthesiologists have ethical responsibilities to their community and society.

1. An anesthesiologist shall recognize a responsibility to participate in activities contributing to an improved community.
2. An anesthesiologist who serves as an expert witness in a judicial proceeding shall possess the qualifications and offer testimony in conformance with the ASA "Guidelines for Expert Witness Qualifications and Testimony."

## *Appendix II: Guidelines for Regional Anesthesia in Obstetrics*

(Approved by House of Delegates on October 12, 1988, and last amended on October 18, 2000.)

These guidelines apply to the use of regional anesthesia or analgesia in which local anesthetics are administered to the parturient during labor and delivery. They are intended to encourage quality patient care but cannot guarantee any specific patient outcome. Because the availability of anesthesia resources may vary, members are responsible for interpreting and establishing the guidelines for their own institutions and practices. These guidelines are subject to revision from time to time as warranted by the evolution of technology and practice.

### Guideline I

REGIONAL ANESTHESIA SHOULD BE INITIATED AND MAINTAINED ONLY IN LOCATIONS IN WHICH APPROPRIATE RESUSCITATION EQUIPMENT AND DRUGS ARE IMMEDIATELY AVAILABLE TO MANAGE PROCEDURALLY RELATED PROBLEMS.

Resuscitation equipment should include, but is not limited to, sources of oxygen and suction, equipment to maintain an airway and perform endotracheal intubation, a means to provide positive pressure ventilation, and drugs and equipment for cardiopulmonary resuscitation.

**Guideline II**

REGIONAL ANESTHESIA SHOULD BE INITIATED BY A PHYSICIAN WITH APPROPRIATE PRIVILEGES AND MAINTAINED BY OR UNDER THE MEDICAL DIRECTION[a] OF SUCH AN INDIVIDUAL.

Physicians should be approved through the institutional credentialing process to initiate and direct the maintenance of obstetric anesthesia and to manage procedurally related complications.

**Guideline III**

REGIONAL ANESTHESIA SHOULD NOT BE ADMINISTERED UNTIL: 1) THE PATIENT HAS BEEN EXAMINED BY A QUALIFIED INDIVIDUAL[b]; AND 2) A PHYSICIAN WITH OBSTETRIC PRIVILEGES TO PERFORM OPERATIVE VAGINAL OR CESAREAN DELIVERY, WHO HAS KNOWLEDGE OF THE MATERNAL AND FETAL STATUS AND THE PROGRESS OF LABOR AND WHO APPROVES THE INITIATION OF LABOR ANESTHESIA, IS READILY AVAILABLE TO SUPERVISE THE LABOR, AND MANAGE ANY OBSTETRIC COMPLICATIONS THAT MAY ARISE.

Under circumstances defined by departmental protocol, qualified personnel may perform the initial pelvic examination. The physician responsible for the patient's obstetric care should be informed of her status so that a decision can be made regarding present risk and further management.[b]

**Guideline IV**

AN INTRAVENOUS INFUSION SHOULD BE ESTABLISHED BEFORE THE INITIATION OF REGIONAL ANESTHESIA AND MAINTAINED THROUGHOUT THE DURATION OF THE REGIONAL ANESTHETIC.

**Guideline V**

REGIONAL ANESTHESIA FOR LABOR AND/OR VAGINAL DELIVERY REQUIRES THAT THE PARTURIENT'S VITAL SIGNS AND THE FETAL HEART RATE BE MONITORED AND DOCUMENTED BY A QUALIFIED INDIVIDUAL. ADDITIONAL MONITORING APPROPRIATE TO THE CLINICAL CONDITION OF THE PARTURIENT AND THE FETUS SHOULD BE USED WHEN INDICATED. WHEN EXTENSIVE REGIONAL BLOCKADE IS ADMINISTERED FOR COMPLICATED VAGINAL DELIVERY, THE STANDARDS FOR BASIC ANESTHETIC MONITORING[c] SHOULD BE APPLIED.

**Guideline VI**

REGIONAL ANESTHESIA FOR CESAREAN DELIVERY REQUIRES THAT THE STANDARDS FOR BASIC ANESTHETIC MONITORING[c] BE APPLIED AND THAT A PHYSICIAN WITH PRIVILEGES IN OBSTETRICS BE IMMEDIATELY AVAILABLE.

**Guideline VII**

QUALIFIED PERSONNEL, OTHER THAN THE ANESTHESIOLOGIST ATTENDING THE MOTHER, SHOULD BE IMMEDIATELY AVAILABLE TO ASSUME RESPONSIBILITY FOR RESUSCITATION OF THE NEWBORN.[c]

The primary responsibility of the anesthesiologist is to provide care to the mother. If the anesthesiologist is also requested to provide brief assistance in the care of the newborn, the benefit to the child must be compared with the risk to the mother.

**Guideline VIII**

A PHYSICIAN WITH APPROPRIATE PRIVILEGES SHOULD REMAIN READILY AVAILABLE DURING THE REGIONAL ANESTHETIC TO MANAGE ANESTHETIC COMPLICATIONS UNTIL THE PATIENT'S POST-ANESTHESIA CONDITION IS SATISFACTORY AND STABLE.

**Guideline IX**

ALL PATIENTS RECOVERING FROM REGIONAL ANESTHESIA SHOULD RECEIVE APPROPRIATE POSTANESTHESIA CARE. AFTER CESAREAN DELIVERY AND/OR EXTENSIVE REGIONAL BLOCKADE, THE STANDARDS FOR POSTANESTHESIA CARE[d] SHOULD BE APPLIED.

1. A postanesthesia care unit (PACU) should be available to receive patients. The design, equipment, and staffing should meet requirements of the facility's accrediting and licensing bodies.
2. When a site other than the PACU is used, equivalent postanesthesia care should be provided.

**Guideline X**

THERE SHOULD BE A POLICY TO ASSURE THE AVAILABILITY IN THE FACILITY OF A PHYSICIAN TO MANAGE COMPLICATIONS AND TO PROVIDE CARDIOPULMONARY RESUSCITATION FOR PATIENTS RECEIVING POSTANESTHESIA CARE.

[a]The Anesthesia Care Team (approved by ASA House of Delegates 10/26/82 and last amended 10/17/01).
[b]For Perinatal Care (American Academy of Pediatrics and American College of Obstetricians and Gynecologists, 1988).
[c]Standards for Basic Anesthetic Monitoring (approved by ASA House of Delegates 10/21/86 and last amended 10/21/98).
ASA House of Delegates 10/21/86 and last amended 10/21/98.
[d]Standards for Postanesthesia Care (approved by ASA House of Delegates 10/12/88 and last amended 10/19/94).

## *Appendix III: Statement on Regional Anesthesia*

(Approved by ASA House of Delegates on October 12, 1983, and last amended on October 16, 2002.)

Although scope of practice is a matter to be decided by appropriate licensing and credentialing authorities, the ASA, as an organization of physicians dedicated to enhancing the safety and quality of anesthesia care, believes it is appropriate to state its views concerning the provision of regional anesthesia. These views are founded on the premise that patient safety is the most important goal in the provision of anesthesia care.

Anesthesiology, in all of its forms, including regional anesthesia, is the practice of medicine. Regional anesthesia involves diagnostic assessment, the consideration of indications and contraindications, the prescription of drugs, and the institution of corrective measures and treatment in response to complications. Therefore, the successful performance of regional anesthesia requires medical as well as technical expertise. The medical component generally comprises the elements of medical direction and includes:

a. Preanesthetic evaluation of the patient
b. Prescription of the anesthetic plan
c. Personal participation in the technical aspects of the regional anesthetic when appropriate
d. Following the course of the anesthetic
e. Remaining physically available for the immediate diagnosis and treatment of emergencies
f. Providing indicated postanesthesia care

The technical requirements for regional anesthesia will vary with the procedure to be performed.

The decision as to the most appropriate anesthetic technique for a particular patient is a judgment of medical practice that must consider all patient factors, procedure requirement, risks and benefits, consent issues, surgeon preferences, and competencies of the practitioners involved. The decision to perform a specific regional anesthetic technique is best made by a physician trained in the medical specialty of anesthesiology. The decision to interrupt or abort a technically difficult procedure, recognition of complications and changing medical conditions, and provision of appropriate postprocedure care is the duty of a physician. Regional anesthetic techniques are best performed by an anesthesiologist who possesses the competence and skills necessary for safe and effective performance.

## *Appendix IV: Guidelines for Expert Witness Qualifications and Testimony*

(Approved by ASA House of Delegates on October 14, 1987, and last amended on October 15, 2003.)

### **Preamble**

The integrity of the litigation process in the United States depends in part on the honest, unbiased, responsible testimony of expert witnesses. Such testimony serves to clarify and explain technical concepts and to articulate professional standards of care. The ASA supports the concept that such expert testimony by anesthesiologists should be readily available, objective, and unbiased. To limit uninformed and possibly misleading testimony, experts should be qualified for their role and should follow a clear and consistent set of ethical guidelines.

A. Expert Witness Qualifications

1. The physician (expert witness) should have a current, valid, and unrestricted state license to practice medicine.

2. The physician should be board certified in anesthesiology or hold an equivalent specialist qualification.

3. The physician should be familiar with the clinical practice of anesthesiology at the time of the occurrence and should have been actively involved in clinical practice at the time of the event.

B. Guidelines for Expert Testimony

1. The physician's review of the medical facts should be truthful, thorough, and impartial and should not exclude any relevant information to create a view favoring either the plaintiff or the defendant. The ultimate test for accuracy and impartiality is a willingness to prepare testimony that could be presented unchanged for use by either the plaintiff or defendant.

2. The physician's testimony should reflect an evaluation of performance in light of generally accepted standards, reflected in relevant literature, neither condemning

performance that clearly falls within generally accepted practice standards nor endorsing or condoning performance that clearly falls outside accepted medical practice.

3. The physician should make a clear distinction between medical malpractice and adverse outcomes not necessarily related to negligent practice.

4. The physician should make every effort to assess the relationship of the alleged substandard practice to the patient's outcome. Deviation from a practice standard is not always causally related to a poor outcome.

5. Fees for expert testimony should relate to the time spent and in no circumstances should be contingent upon outcome of the claim.

6. The physician should be willing to submit such testimony for peer review.

# Index

## N

Printed in the United States of America.